# ATHEROGENESIS

Edited by **Sampath Parthasarathy**

**Atherogenesis**
Edited by Sampath Parthasarathy

**Published by InTech**
Janeza Trdine 9, 51000 Rijeka, Croatia



**Publishing Process Manager** Marija Radja

**Technical Editor** Teodora Smiljanic

**Cover Designer** InTech Design Team

Additional hard copies can be obtained from orders@intechopen.com

Atherogenesis, Edited by Sampath Parthasarathy
p. cm.
978-953-307-992-9

For EU product safety concerns:
IN TECH d.o.o., Prolaz Marije Krucifikse Kozulić 3, 51000 Rijeka, Croatia,
info@intechopen.com or visit our website at intechopen.com.

# Meet the editor

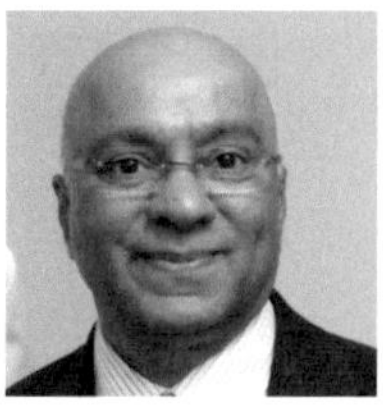

Dr. Parthasarathy is a scientist internationally recognized for his work in the area of atherosclerosis. As one of the originators of the oxidative hypothesis of atherosclerosis, he is credited with the co-discovery of oxidized low-density lipoprotein (ox-LDL) and has published extensively on oxidative stress in chronic diseases including atherosclerosis and endometriosis. He has published over 225 full-length publications and has authored a book on modified lipoproteins. He holds several patent rights and has been continuously funded by NIH for over 20 years. He is one of the highly cited authors and has trained over 200 scientists from around the world. Dr Parthasarathy has held endowed positions in many universities and currently holds the Florida Hospital endowed chair in cardiovascular sciences at the University of Central Florida.

# Contents

# Preface

Cardiovascular disease in general and atherosclerosis in particular have been a topic of great interest for decades. During the later half of the past century, we noted great advances in defining steps involved in the biosynthesis of cholesterol to the discovery of lipoproteins. The latter led to the identification of key cell types which are involved in the uptake of the lipoproteins and specific cell membrane receptors that determine their entry. The lipid clinics played a major role in identifying the risk factors, particularly in identifying high plasma cholesterol and low HDL cholesterol, in the etiology of the disease.

On the one hand, drugs such as statins, life style modulation in the form of reduced fat intake, decreased smoking, and increased physical activity, continue to show marked impact on the incidence of cardiovascular diseases. While on the other hand, the emerging understanding of the roles of chronic inflammation, diet, increases in the incidence of diabetes, and the environment, are factors that we need to be concerned about in the future.

Although prevention is always better than cure, the beneficial roles of HDL are still only partly uncovered. In addition to promoting reverse cholesterol transport, it appears to influence inflammatory and oxidative pathways. The latter poses paradoxical and conflicting implications. While most non-clinical studies seem to stress its importance, the use of antioxidants in human clinical trials has not been encouraging to propose antioxidants as a therapeutic means. Caution should be exercised in making judgments as inflammatory and oxidative stress seem to go hand in hand.

This monograph will bring out the state-of-the-art advances in the dynamics of cholesterol transport and will address several important issues that pertain to oxidative stress and inflammation. The book is divided into three major sections; the first section deals with the pathophysiology of atherosclerosis with emphasis on epigenetics and nutrigenomics. The second section discusses cholesterol influx-efflux pathways and inflammation and immune mechanisms of atherosclerosis. The last section discusses oxidative stress and vascular mechanisms involved in cardiovascular disease development. The book will offer insights into the roles of specific cytokines, inflammation, and oxidative stress in atherosclerosis and is intended for new researchers who are curious about atherosclerosis as well as for established senior researchers and clinicians who would be interested in novel findings that may link various aspects of the disease.

**Dr. Sampath Parthasarathy**
Florida Hospital Endowed Chair in
Cardiovascular Sciences at the University of Central Florida
USA

# Part 1

## Atherosclerosis-Models and Concepts

# 1

# Mouse Models of Experimental Atherosclerosis as a Tool for Checking a Putative Anti-Atherogenic Action of Drugs

Jacek Jawien
*Jagiellonian University School of Medicine, Chair of Pharmacology, Krakow, Poland*

## 1. Introduction

Studies concerning the pathogenesis of atherosclerosis entered a new phase at the turn of the 21st century. The 20$^{th}$ century was the age of cholesterol and lipoproteins, which has been concluded in a number of clinical studies carried out on a large scale, and they demonstrated unequivocally that normalization of hypercholesterolemia significantly decreased the incidence and mortality of coronary artery disease (Prevention of cardiovascular events and death with pravastatin in patients with coronary heart disease and a broad range of initial cholesterol levels. The Long-Term Intervention with Pravastatin in Ischaemic Disease (LIPID) Study Group. 1998; Scandinavian Simvastatin Survival Study Group. Randomised trial of cholesterol lowering in 4444 patients with coronary heart disease: The Scandinavian Simvastatin Survival Study (4S). 1994) Nearly to the end of the nineties, atherosclerosis had been assumed to develop as the so-called chronic response to injury (response-to-injury hypothesis) that resulted in the loss of endothelial cells which line the inner side of the vessels (Ross & Glomset, 1976).
Atherosclerosis had been considered first of all a degenerative disease (Ross et al., 1977; Ross et al. 1984; Ross, 1986). However, approximately 20 years ago, the trials started to focus to a large extent on another pathogenetic mechanism of atherosclerosis, not considered so far – the inflammatory process.

## 2. The first indications

In 1986, with the use of monoclonal antibodies, the small cells with round nucleus present in the atheromatous plaque, known before as "small monocytes", were demonstrated to be T lymphocytes (Jonasson et al., 1986). Several years later it was shown that these lymphocytes "recognize" as antigens the oxidized molecules of low-density lipoproteins (LDL) – oxLDL (Stemme et al., 1995). Moreover, the correlation between atherosclerosis and the presence of at least two types of infectious microorganisms: *Chlamydia pneumoniae* and *Herpes simplex virus* were observed (Thom et al., 1991; Hendrix et al., 1990). It raised the question if the inflammatory process participate in atherosclerosis. Speculations of this kind were initially received with great scepticism because there was no spectacular and unequivocal evidence of a significant role of inflammation in atherosclerosis.

This evidence was delivered by a new technique – gene targeting, for the invention of which Mario R. Capecchi (Italy), Martin J. Evans (United Kingdom) and Oliver Smithies (USA) received the Nobel Prize in Physiology or Medicine in 2007.

## 3. Additional evidence for the presence of inflammation in atherosclerosis

The newest model of atherosclerosis (described precisely at the end of the paper) enabled the investigators to create apoE-knockout mice, an ideal animal model to test the influence of singular proteins participating in the inflammatory response on the development of atherosclerosis. These studies showed, for example, that the absence of only one cytokine – interferon γ (IFN-γ), reduced atherosclerosis even by 60% (Gupta et al., 1997).
The overexpression of adhesive molecules (vascular adhesion molecule 1 and intercellular adhesion molecule 1) at sites with atheromatous changes was also observed in apoE-knockout mice (Nakashima et al., 1998). Monocyte chemotactic protein was shown to play an important part in the progression of atheromatous lesions (Aiello et al., 1999; Ni et al., 2001). Moreover, it was observed that interleukin-18 knockout decreased atherosclerosis by 35% (Elhage et al., 2003; Tenger et al., 2005).
Inhibition of CD40 signaling reduced atherosclerosis (Mach et al., 1998). This was explained by the fact that ligation of CD40 molecule (tumor necrosis factor α [TNF-α] receptor superfamily member) – found in the atheromatous plaque, on endothelial cells, vascular smooth muscle cells, antigen-presenting cells, platelets – with CD40L activates a number of transcription factors: NF-κB, AP-1, STAT-1 or Egr-1. Therefore, it influences, for example, the endothelial cell, which, in consequence, acquires proinflammatory and proatherosclerotic phenotype leading to the expression of adhesive molecules and tissue factor on its surface. It creates new possibilities of therapeutic approach, consisting in inhibition of the CD40–CD40L pathway (Welt et al., 2004; Alber et al., 2006; Tousoulis, et al. 2007). In mice the effect of CD40 is also antagonized by transforming growth factor β (Robertson et al., 2003).
Finally, in apoE-knockout mice with severe combined immunodeficiency (SCID) atherosclerosis was reduced by 70% in comparison to the control group, due to a significantly lower number of lymphocytes in mice with SCID. It was demonstrated that transfer of T cells to these mice aggravated atherosclerosis even by 164% (Zhou et al., 2000).

## 4. Atherosclerosis as an inflammatory process

These and other facts made the investigators realize unequivocally that inflammation was essential for atherogenesis. Therefore, in 1999, just before his death, Russell Ross (the author of the previous theory of atherosclerosis as a chronic response to injury) officially proclaimed that atherosclerosis was an inflammatory disease (Ross, 1999).
Whereas the deposition of atheromatous lipids and the accumulation of foam cells – macrophages filled with such lipids – in intima is the main morphological hallmark of atherosclerosis, the more subtle changes in the environment of the arterial wall, stimulated by the influx of inflammatory cells and local release of cytokines and other inflammatory mediators are currently recognized as the crucial causative factors of atherogenesis (Glass & Witztum, 2001; Binder et al., 2002).

Inflammation occurs in response to a factor that destabilizes the local homeostasis. The factors that cause Toll-like receptor dependent macrophage activation in the arterial wall include oxLDL, heat shock protein 60 (HSP60) and bacterial toxins (Hansson, 2005).

The first stage of atherogenesis consists in endothelial dysfunction (Ross, 1999). It involves first of all the regions of arterial bifurcations where the blood flow is not laminar. Hence, these localizations are prone to develop atherosclerosis. In such places LDL is stored in the subendothelial space. Low-density lipoprotein accumulation is increased if serum LDL level is elevated. Low-density lipoprotein is transported by passive diffusion and its accumulation in the vascular wall seems to depend on the interaction between apolipoprotein B of the LDL molecule and proteoglycans of the matrix (Boren et al., 1998).

There is evidence that unchanged LDL are "collected" by the macrophages too slowly to activate their transformation into foam cells. Therefore, it has been suggested that LDL molecule is "modified" in the vascular wall. The most significant modification is lipid oxidation, resulting in the formation of so-called "minimally oxidized" LDL (Gaut & Heinecke, 2001). The generation of these "aliens" for the body molecules leads to the development of inflammatory response, with participation of monocytes and lymphocytes in the first place (Fredrikson et al., 2003; Pentikäinen et al., 2000). The inflammation is triggered by accumulation of the minimally oxidized LDLs in the subendothelial space, thus stimulating the endothelial cells to produce a number of proinflammatory molecules (Lusis, 2000).

Before the "minimally oxidized" LDL have been phagocytised by the macrophages, they have to be modified into "highly oxidized" LDL. The scavenger receptors are responsible for the rapid uptake of the modified LDL (Suzuki et al., 1997).

During the following phase macrophages "present the antigen" to T lymphocytes. This antigen may be a fragment of oxidized LDL "digested" by the macrophages, HSP60, β2-glycoprotein I or the fragments of bacterial antigens (Hansson, 2001). The interaction between the immunological cells requires the presence of CD40 receptor on the surface of macrophages and its ligand CD40L on the surface of T lymphocytes (Schonbeck et al., 2000; Phipps et al., 2000). It is currently believed that the immunological response of Th1 type and its mediators: IFN-γ, TNF-α, interleukin-1, interleukin-12 as well as interleukin-18 accelerate atherosclerosis, whereas the response of Treg type and its mediators: interleukin-10 and TGF-β inhibit the development of atherosclerosis (Daugherty & Rateri, 2002; Laurat et al., 2001; Pinderski et al., 2002). Therefore, there has arisen an idea of vaccination as a future treatment against atherogenesis (Hansson, 2002).

The next phase of atherogenesis is the development of fibrous atheroma. The deposition of extracellular cholesterol and its esters is then intensified as well as the migration of smooth muscle cells from media to intima, proliferation of these cells and finally production of the extracellular matrix by the smooth muscles cells.

A stable atheromatous plaque is most commonly covered with a fairly thick fibrous layer, protecting the lipid nucleus from contact with the blood. In an unstable plaque there is a big lipid nucleus with a fairly thin fibrous layer. In atheromatous plaque, changed as described above, the proinflammatory factors produced by T lymphocytes (such as IFN-γ) seem to play a crucial role. They decrease production of the extracellular matrix by smooth muscles and at the same time increase production of the metalloproteinases by macrophages (Shishehbor & Bhatt, 2004).

## 5. Is atherosclerosis an autoimmunological disease?

The role of HSP60 as an initiator of atherogenesis is currently intensively investigated. Its "molecular mimicry" with HSP of *Chlamydia* has been observed (Wick et al., 1995).
Moreover, the anti-oxLDL antibodies resemble antiphospholipid antibodies, therefore the concept of atherosclerosis as an autoimmunological disease has been established (Hansson, 2001; Kobayashi K et al., 2007; Wick G et al., 2001). The investigators also emphasize a high pathogenetic similarity of atherosclerosis to rheumatoid arthritis ( Shoenfeld et al., 2001).

## 6. The new experimental model of atherosclerosis

Since 1992 the mouse has become an excellent object for the studies on atherosclerosis, replacing the previous animal models. (Paigen et al., 1994; Moghadasian, 2002; Jawien et al., 2004).
Then, the first line of mice with a switched off gene for apolipoprotein E (apoE-knockout) was developed almost contemporaneously in two laboratories in the United States. (Piedrahita et al., 1992; Plump et al., 1992).
These mice were soon described as "reliable and useful, the best animal model of atherosclerosis in present times" (Meir & Leitersdorf, 2004).
During the generation of apoE-knockout mice (known also as apoE null or apoE deficient mice) the normal gene coding apolipoprotein E is replaced by a mutated gene which does not produce this molecule. Such mice are called apoE knockout because they have a knockout, switched-off, null or inactivated gene coding apolipoprotein E. For clarity, in the following sections of this paper we will use the most popular name: apoE-knockout mice.
The year 1992, in which apoE-knockout mice were invented by a homological exchange of genes, was a real breakthrough year in the studies on the pathogenesis of atherosclerosis (Savla, 2002).
The apoE-knockout mice were formed by homological recombination of embryonic stem cells. The changed cells were implanted into the blastocyst of a mouse of C57BL/6J strain which were subsequently implanted into the uterus. The offspring was a "chimera" that was next crossbred with a mouse of C57BL/6J strain (wild type), which led to the formation of apoE-knockout, homozygous mice in the second generation (Capecchi, 2001).
The inactivation of the gene coding apoE resulted in the formation of mice with a phenotype with a complete suppression of apoE, but with preservation of fertility and vitality (Breslow, 1996).
The apoE-knockout mice, in contrast to all of other animal models, develop atherosclerosis spontaneously, without high-cholesterol diet (Hansson et al., 2002).
The generation of such a model changed the nature of the studies on the pathogenesis of atherosclerosis and enabled the investigators to formulate a new definition of atherosclerosis as a chronic inflammation (Savla, 2002).
In a number of reports on atherogenesis published so far there has been a tendency to consider this process as the effect of dyslipidemia or inflammation alone. It is an erroneous dichotomy. It should be emphasized that atherosclerosis results from both lipid disorders and enhanced inflammation. Therefore, atherosclerosis is a chronic inflammatory disease, in most cases initiated and aggravated by hypercholesterolemia. In the review published in Nature Medicine hypercholesterolemia and inflammation were described as "partners in crime" (Steinberg, 2002).

The inflammatory concept of atherosclerosis has been formulated just in the recent years. However, it is currently an unquestionable achievement of science which also have specific therapeutic implications (Fan & Watanabe, 2003; Libby, 2000; Libby, 2002; Libby P et al., 2002; Jawien et al., 2006; Alpert & Thygesen, 2007).

## 7. Animal models of atherosclerosis

Atherosclerotic cardiovascular disease, the major cause of death in Western society, results from complex interactions among multiple genetic and environmental factors.

Numerous animal species have been used to study the pathogenesis and potential treatment of the lesions of atherosclerosis. The first evidence of experimental atherosclerosis came into view as early as in 1908 when Ignatowski (Ignatowski, 1908) reported thickening of the intima with formation of large clear cells in the aorta of rabbits fed with a diet rich in animal proteins (meat, milk, eggs). The most useful animal models have thus far been restricted to relatively large animals, such as nonhuman primates, swine, and rabbits. Hamsters and pigeons have been used occasionally but present problems peculiar to their species. Rats and dogs are not good models for atherosclerosis because they do not develop spontaneous lesions and require heavy modifications of diet to produce vascular lesion. Despite the fact that rabbits do not develop spontaneous atherosclerosis, they are useful because they are highly responsive to cholesterol manipulation and develop lesions in a fairly short time (Drobnik et al., 2000).

The lesions are much more fatty and macrophage-rich (inflammatory) than the human lesions and plasma cholesterol levels are extraordinarily high (very dissimilar to humans). Pigs and monkeys are better suited to model human atherosclerotic lesions. However, nowadays monkeys are not widely used due to obvious species - specific concerns (risk of extinction) and cost. The pig is a very good model - when fed with cholesterol, they reach plasma levels and atherosclerotic lesions that are quite similar to those seen in humans. Problems with the pig model are costs, the difficulties involved in maintaining the colonies and in their handling.

What has been traditionally lacking was a small, genetically reproducible, murine model of atherosclerosis. Such a model could help to overcome the many problems and deficiencies of larger animals and, in particular, would permit studies of possible therapies that require relatively large numbers of animals.

Until 1992, the majority of atherosclerotic research focused on mechanisms in rabbits, with a lesser number of studies in pigs and nonhuman primates. These large animal models have provided invaluable insight. The use of pig models of the disease initially revealed that monocyte infiltration was one of the primary cellular events in the atherogenic process (Gerrity, 1981).

Studies in monkeys and rabbits have been pivotal in defining the cellular events in the initiation and development of lesions (Faggiotto & Ross, 1984; Rosenfeld et al., 1987). In recent years, there has been an explosion in the number of *in vivo* studies that is largely attributable to the use of mouse models to study atherogenic mechanisms.

## 8. Mouse as a model of atherosclerosis

Mice are highly resistant to atherosclerosis. The only exception in mice is the C57BL/6 strain. When fed a very high cholesterol diet containing cholic acid, however, the vascular lesions in the C57BL/6 differ from the human condition in the histologic nature and location and are possibly attributed to a chronic inflammatory state rather than a genetic predisposition.

The earliest mouse model of atherosclerosis was the diet - induced model that was first characterized during the 1960s in Wissler's laboratory. Special diet contained 30% fat, 5% cholesterol, and 2% cholic acid led to atherosclerosis in C57BL/6 mice. However, this was a very toxic diet on which the mice lost weight and often got sick with morbid respiratory infections. Paigen et al. modified this diet by blending it one part to three parts with a 10% fat diet to yield what is called the "Paigen diet" which consists of 15% fat, 1.25% cholesterol, and 0.5% cholic acid (Paigen et al., 1985).

Although there were many uses of this model, there were also many disadvantages. The lesions are very small in mice at 4 to 5 months of age, in order of 200 to 1 000 square microns in the aortic root. The lesions are largely confined to the aortic root, and they usually do not develop beyond the early foam-cell, fatty-streak stage. The diet is also unphysiological with regard to its extremely high cholesterol content, 1.25%, and the presence of cholic acid. In addition, Lusis et al. have shown that this diet is in itself inflammatory, as leads to the induction of hepatic NF-kB activation and the expression of acute phase reactants, such as serum amyloid A (Liao et al., 1993).

Paigen et al. colleagues also developed assays that are widely used to quantify atherosclerosis in the mouse model. The most standard assay is the measurement of the cross-sectional lesion area in the aortic root (Paigen et al., 1987).

In this assay, freshly perfused and isolated hearts are fixed in formalin, embedded in gelatin, frozen, and cut into thin sections at anatomically defined sites in the aortic sinus and valve region. These sections are stained for lipids, and the lesion area is measured microscopically. Although this model has been widely employed and is of significant use in the study of atherosclerosis, the pathology of the lesions are not ideally suited as a model for human atherosclerosis. This shortcoming led many investigators to downplay the role of the mouse as a good model of atherosclerosis. Lesion formation in the diet - induced model is largely limited to the aortic root after feeding the Paigen - diet for periods of 14 weeks to 9 months. The lesions are quite small, only several hundred to a few thousand square micrometers, and they consist almost entirely of macrophage foam cells with little evidence for smooth muscle cell involvement. Thus, this model is largely limited to the fatty streak stage and does not progress to resemble human intermediate lesions.

For many years the mouse was not used as an experimental model for atherosclerosis research because of the beliefs that mice could not survive on high - fat atherogenic diets, that lesions were not reproducible, that most mice did not get lesions, and that lesion pathology did not resemble atherosclerosis in humans. However, the use of lower - fat diets solved the survival problem; the use of inbred strains rather than random - bred mice solved the reproducibility problem; the use of susceptible strains resulted in most mice getting lesions; and longer experimental times showed that lesions with fibrous caps were produced.

The following is a list of questions that can be used to judge the usefulness of animal models of atherosclerosis: 1) What is the nature of the experimental lesions and their similarity to human lesions; 2) is the plasma lipoprotein profile and metabolism similar to metabolism in humans; 3) what is the time frame necessary for lesions to form, and how long does it take to breed the animals for the studies; 4) what is the cost of acquiring and maintaining the

animals; 5) what is the ability to perform in vivo manipulations and imaging; and 6) what is the ability of the model to take advantage of classical and molecular genetic approaches ?
The mouse as a model meets many of these criteria, but first it is important to acknowledge many important differences between mice and humans. The average lifespan of a mouse is about 2 years, compared to about 75 years in humans. Mice weigh much less, about 30 grams for the adult. The lipid profile in the mouse is very different from that in humans, who carry about 75% of their plasma cholesterol on LDL. Mice carry most of their cholesterol on high-density lipoprotein (HDL), which we know in humans is protective against atherosclerosis. Thus, mice fed their normal low-fat chow diet do not get atherosclerosis, while it is a common disease in humans. One difference, which is an advantage of all animal models, is the ability to control the environment and diet in mouse studies, which is impossible for long-term human studies. Human genetic studies are limited in range to various types of association studies. With mice, on the other hand, many additional kinds of genetic experiments are possible, including breeding and genetic engineering.
There are many advantages of using mice for experimental atherosclerosis research, including their relative ease and thriftiness to acquire and maintain. Their generation time is short, at about 9 weeks, 3 weeks for gestation and about 6 weeks until sexual maturity. It is easy to breed very large cohorts for experimental studies, and mice can develop atherosclerosis in a very short timeframe, as discussed below. Classical genetics in the mouse is very well established and is aided immensely by the availability of hundreds of inbred strains. Moreover, in 2002, The Mouse Genome Sequencing Consortium published the culmination of international efforts - a high quality sequence and analysis of the genome of the C57BL/6J mouse strain (Waterson et al., 2002).
With the coming of age of molecular genetics, it is now possible to add exogenous transgenes into mice, which can also be done in many other species. However, uniquely in mice, it is also possible to knock out or replace endogenous genes; this is one of the main advantages of working in the mouse model. The major disadvantage of the mouse model is their small size, which makes it difficult but not impossible to perform surgical manipulations and *in vivo* imaging. But there have been recent advances in these techniques that have overcome many of the size limitations, such as the ability to perform imaging of abdominal atherosclerotic lesions in living mice, cardiac catheterization to determine cardiovascular function in free-ranging mice, and surgical ligature of coronary arteries giving rise to myocardial ischemia.

## 9. Apolipoprotein E–knockout mice: A breakthrough

It has been a longstanding goal of many investigators around the world to create better mouse models for lipoprotein disorders and atherosclerosis and to identify genes that may modify atherogenesis and lesion progression. In 1992 apoE - deficient mice were generated by inactivating the apoE gene by targeting (Piedrahita et al., 1992).
They inactivated the apoE gene in mouse embryonic stem (ES) cells by homologous recombination. Two targeting plasmids were used, pJPB63 and pNMC109, both containing a neomycin-resistance gene that replaced a part of the apoE gene and disrupted its stucture. ES cell colonies targeted after electroporation with plasmids were identified by the polymerase chain reaction (PCR) followed by genomic Southern analysis. Chimeric mice were generated by blastocyst injection with targeted lines. They gave strong chimeras, which transmitted the

disrupted apoE gene to their progeny. Mice homozygous for the disrupted gene were produced from the heterozygotes. The facts that homozygous animals have been born at the expected frequency and that they appeared to be healthy were important. They demonstrated that lack of apoE was compatible with normal development, and they also provided another tool for studies of the phenotypic consequences of apoE deficiency. At the same time another group created also apoE - deficient mice (Plump et al., 1992).

Mice homozygous or heterozygous for the disrupted apoE gene appeared healthy. No difference in their body weights compared to normal mice was observed. However, significant phenotypic differences between normal animals and the homozygous mutants were observed in their lipid and lipoprotein profiles. The apoE-knockout mice had markedly increased total plasma cholesterol levels, which were five times those of normal litter mates. These levels were unaffected by the age or sex of the animals. Although the total plasma cholesterol levels were greatly elevated in the mutants, the high density lipoprotein (HDL) cholesterol levels were only 45% the normal level. The triglyceride levels were 68% higher than those of normal animals. (These apoE-deficient mice have had a dramatic shift in plasma lipoproteins from HDL, the major lipoprotein in control mice, to cholesterol - enriched remnants of chylomicrons and VLDL.

Mice naturally have high levels of HDL and low levels of LDL, in contrast to humans who are high in LDL and low in HDL. In addition, mice apparently lack the cholesteryl ester transfer protein, en enzyme that transfers cholesterol ester from HDL to VLDL and LDL. Despite these differences, apoE - deficient mice have phenotypes remarkably similar to those of apoE - deficient humans.

A chronological analysis of atherosclerosis in the apoE - deficient mouse has shown that the sequential events involved in lesion formation in this model are strikingly similar to those in well - established larger animal models of atherosclerosis and in humans (Nakashima et al., 1994). Animals as young as 5-6 weeks of age have monocytic adhesions to the endothelial surface of the aorta that can be appreciated readily with electron microscopy (EM). EM also has demonstrated transendothelial migration of blood monocytes in similarly aged mice. By 6-10 weeks of age, most apoE - deficient mice have developed fatty - streak lesions comprised primarily of foam cells with migrating smooth muscle cells. These fatty - streak lesions rapidly progress to advanced lesions, which are heterogeneous but are typically comprised of a necrotic core surrounded by proliferating smooth muscle cells and varying amounts of extracellular matrix, including collagen and elastin.

These lesions have well - formed fibrous caps made up of smooth muscle cells and extracellular matrix that often have groups of foam cells at their shoulders. It is not uncommon for the inflammatory lesion to erode deep into the medial wall of the aorta, and some of these animals develop aortic aneurysms. Many of the lesions found in older mice develop calcified foci (Reddick et al., 1994).

Other characteristics of the lesions in the apoE - deficient mouse, such as indications of oxidative change, merit attention as well (Palinski et al., 1994).

The atherosclerotic lesions in this mouse contain oxidation - specific epitopes. In young lesions these epitopes are predominantly localized in macrophage - rich areas, whereas in advanced lesions they are localized in necrotic regions. In addition, high titers of antibodies against the oxidized epitopes are present in the plasma of the apoE - deficient mice.

The complexity of lesions in the apoE - deficient mouse, together with the benefits of using the mouse as a model of human disease, makes it a desirable system in which to study both environmental and genetic determinants of atherosclerosis. Initial studies examined the effects of grossly different diets on susceptibility to atherosclerosis in this animal. These studies confirmed the validity of this mouse as a model of human atherosclerotic disease and laid the groundwork for future dietary studies.

Hayek et al. developed a more physiological than Paigen diet - "western-type" diet for mouse studies, which is similar in composition to an average American diet of several years ago, consisting of 21% fat by weight, 0.15% cholesterol, and no cholic acid. When fed this diet, wild-type mice have a two-fold elevation in plasma cholesterol, while apoE-deficient mice have over a three-fold elevation, to about 2 000 mg/dl, again, mostly in βVLDL, but there is also an increase in LDL (Plump et al., 1992).

The post-prandial clearance of intestinally derived lipoproteins is dramatically impaired in apoE - deficient mice. The apoE - deficient mouse responds appropriately to a human - like western - type diet (Nakashima et al., 1994). On this diet, lesion formation is greatly accelerated and lesion size is increased. In 10-week old animals fed this diet for only 5 weeks, lesions are 3-4 times the size of those observed in mice fed a low - fat diet. In addition, monocytic adhesions and advanced lesions develop at a significantly earlier age. The results of this dietary challenge demonstrate that the mouse model responds in an appropriate manner, i.e. increased fat leads to increased plasma cholesterol, which in turn leads to increased atherosclerosis. Moreover, the data suggest that in addition to its histological similarity to humans, the mouse model exhibits a response to environmental cues resembling that of humans.

Lesions in the apoE-deficient mouse, as in humans, tend to develop at vascular branch points and progress from foam cell stage to the fibroproliferative stage with well-defined fibrous caps and necrotic lipid cores, although plaque rupture has not been observed in apoE - deficient mice or in any other mouse model. Progression of lesions appears to occur at a faster rate than in humans atherosclerosis; the rapidity of lesion progression can be advantageous in many experimental situations.

The genetic background has a major effect on atherosclerosis susceptibility in strains of apoE - deficient mice. For example, lesions from 16-week chow diet C57BL/6 apoE-KO were relatively larger than from FVB apoE-KO mice and in contrast to FVB mice there was evidence of early development of fibrous caps in these mice. In older mice, fibrous plaques from C57BL/6 apoE-KO mice were larger in size and had larger necrotic cores compared with FVB apoE-KO mice. Comparing humans and apoE - deficient mice, lesion progression and cell types are similar, as is the presence of oxidized lipoproteins. The major difference of this mouse model, as is the presence of oxidized lipoproteins. The major difference of this mouse model, as is the case for most of the other models of experimental atherosclerosis, is that plaque rupture is not observed, whereas plaque rupture is fairly common in humans and can lead to heart attacks. One potential reason for the lack of plaque rupture in mice is that the diameter of the aorta is less than 1 mm, which is even smaller than the diameter of the major coronary arteries in humans. As the vessel diameter decreases, the surface tension increases exponentially; thus, in the mouse there may be so much surface tension that plaque rupture would not be likely to occur.

ApoE-knockout mice are considered to be one of the most relevant models for atherosclerosis since they are hypercholesterolemic and develop spontaneous arterial lesions (Nakashima et al., 1994).

Heterozygous apoE-deficient mice do not exhibit elevated plasma cholesterol levels on the chow or Western-type diet, suggesting that when mice are fed a physiological diet, a 50% decrease in apoE is not sufficient to influence fasting plasma lipids (Van Ree et al., 1994).
The apoE-deficient mouse contained the entire spectrum of lesions observed during atherogenesis and was the first mouse model to develop lesions similar to those of humans. This model provided opportunity to study the pathogenesis and therapy of atherosclerosis in a small, genetically defined animal.
In 1995 Kashyap et al. (Kashyap et al., 1995) described the successful correction of apoE deficiency in apoE-deficient mice by using an alternative approach involving systemic delivery to mouse liver of recombinant adenovirus vectors expressing human apoE. Thus, the single genetic lesion causing apoE absence and severe hypercholesterolemia is sufficient to convert the mouse from a species that is highly resistant to one that is highly susceptible to atherosclerosis (Breslow, 1994).
The method of measure atherosclerosis by using the aortic root atherosclerosis assay was originally developed by Paigen et al. (Paigen et al., 1987). The aortic root cross sectioning assay is widely used in murine studies of atherosclerosis, allows for coincident inspection of lesion histology, and is amenable in studies using large numbers of mice. Alternative measures of atherosclerosis, such as the en face method, correlate with aortic root measurements. However, these methods are less amenable for studies using large numbers of mice and do not allow for inspection of lesion histology.

## 10. LDL receptor deficient mice

Gene targeting in embryonic stem cells has recently been used to create LDL receptor - knockout (LDLR-KO) mice, a model of familial hypercholesterolemia. LDL receptor - deficient mice was made in 1993 by Ishibashi et al. (Ishibashi et al.1993). These mice have a more modest lipoprotein abnormality than the apoE - deficient mice, with increases in LDL and VLDL cholesterol leading to a total plasma cholesterol of about 250 mg/dl on a chow diet. On this diet, and at that level of plasma cholesterol, LDL receptor - deficient mice do not get atherosclerosis. However, this is a very diet-responsive model. After these mice are fed the Paigen diet, their plasma cholesterol levels soar to about 1 500 mg/dl, and large atherosclerotic lesions form (Ishibashi et al., 1994). It has also been shown that feeding the less toxic western-type diet also leads to the development of large lesions, with plasma cholesterol levels of about 400 mg/dl. The lesion pathology in this model is not as well characterized as in the apoE - deficient model, but it does appear similar in that the lesions can progress beyond the foam - cell fatty-streak stage to the fibro-proliferative intermediate stage.

## 11. Other mouse models

Overexpression of human apoA-I in apoE - deficient mice increased HDL cholesterol levels twofold and substantially decreased fatty streak and advanced fibroproliferative lesion formation (Paszty et al. 1994; Plump et al., 1994).
By 4 months of age, all but 3-5% of apoE - deficient mice have had detectable fatty streaks that vary considerably in size; some are barely detectable, whereas others occlude as much as 8% of the aortic lumen. In apoE - deficient mice that overexpress human apoA-I, more than 50% of animals have no lesions by 4 months of age, and the animals that do develop

atherosclerosis have lesions that are barley detectable. By 8 months of age, apoE - deficient mice have lesions that are highly organized and that occlude on average 25% of the aortic lumen. Those apoE - deficient mice that overexpress human apoA-I have mainly immature fatty - streak lesion that occlude on average only 5% of the aortic lumen. Collectively, these data suggest that overexpression of apoA-I can diminish lesion size and slow the initiation of fatty streak formation.

More recently, apoE and LDL-receptor (LDLr) double – knockout (apoE/LDLr-DKO) mice have been created (Ishibashi et al., 1994), representing a new mouse model that develops severe hyperlipidaemia and atherosclerosis (Bonthu et al., 1997).

It has been reported that, even on a regular *chow diet*, the progression of atherosclerosis is usually more marked in apoE/LDLr-DKO mice than in mice deficient for apoE alone (Witting et al., 1999).

Thus, the apoE/LDLr-DKO mouse is a suitable model in which to study the anti-atherosclerotic effect of compounds without having to feed the animals an atherogenic diet.

To study the contribution of endothelial nitric oxide synthase (eNOS) to lesion formation Kuhlencordt et al. (Kuhlencordt et al., 2001). created apoE / eNOS double - knockout mice. It has occured that chronic deficiency of eNOS increases atherosclerosis in apoE-KO mouse model. Furthermore, in the absence of eNOS, peripheral coronary disease, chronic myocardial ischemia, heart failure, and an array of vascular complications develop that have not been observed in apoE-KO animals.

Recently, Veniant et al. (Veniant et al., 2000) managed to even up the cholesterol levels in chow-fed apoE-KO mice and LDLR-KO mice. They did so by making both mouse models homozygous for the apolipoprotein B-100 allele, which ameliorates the hypercholesterolemia in the setting of apoE deficiency but worsens it in the setting of LDLR deficiency. Moreover, the LDLR-KO Apob100/100 mice developed extensive atherosclerosis even on a chow diet. So far this model seems to be the best as concerns the development of atherosclerosis in mice.

Therefore, gene - targeted mouse models has changed the face of atherosclerotic research (Savla U, 2002) and helped in creation of the new theory of atherosclerosis - as an inflammatory disease (Ross, 1999)

## 12. The experimental use of gene targeted mice

The apoE - deficient mouse model of atherosclerosis can then be used to: 1) identify atherosclerosis susceptibility modifying genes, by the candidate-gene and gene-mapping methods; 2) identify the role of various cell types in atherogenesis; 3) identify environmental factors affecting atherogenesis; and 4) assess therapies that might block atherogenesis or lesion progression.

ApoE-deficient mice have also been used to look for environmental and drug effects on atherosclerosis and to test novel therapies. One of the first observations was paradoxical effects of probucol on atherogenesis in both apoE-KO (Moghadasian et al., 1999) and LDL receptor deficient (Bird et al., 1998) mice. Probucol with strong antioxidant and cholesterol - lowering effects increased atherogenesis in apoE-KO mice by 3 folds (Moghadasian et al., 1999). Several other compounds reduced the extent and severity of atherosclerotic lesions without affecting plasma cholesterol levels in apoE–KO mice. For example, administration of antioxidant N,N'-diphenyl 1,4 - phenylenediamine (DPPD) to apoE-KO mice resulted in a significant decrease in atherosclerosis without reducing plasma cholesterol levels (Tangirala et al., 1995).

A marked reduction in atherosclerosis by dietary vitamin E was accompanied by no change in plasma cholesterol levels in apoE-KO mice (Pratico et al., 1998).

Likewise, antiatherogenic effects of the angiotensin - converting enzyme inhibitors (Hayek et al. 1998; Keidar et al. 2000; Hayek et al. 1999) or the angiotensin II receptor antagonist (Keidar et al. 1997) in apoE-KO mice were independent of plasma cholesterol lowering effects.

Since inflammation plays an important role in atherogenesis, during recent years it has become apparent that the 5-lipoxygenase (5-LO) pathway may take significant part in modifying the pathogenesis of atherosclerosis. Enzymes associated with the 5-LO pathway are abundantly expressed in arterial walls of patients afflicted with various lesion stages of atherosclerosis of the aorta and of coronary arteries. These data raised the possibility that antileukotriene drugs may be an effective treatment regimen in atherosclerosis (Mehrabian et al., 2002).

Of special interest for atherosclerosis is the arachidonate 5-LO which was originally identified in polymorphonuclear leukocytes, but which over-expression was recently demonstrated in macrophages, dendritic cells, foam cells, mast cells and neutrophils within atherosclerotic vessels. This enzyme generates an unstable epoxide intermediate compound leukotriene A4 (LTA4), which is an important precursor of LTB4, LTC4 and other cysteinyl leukotrienes. Initial observations and the use of drugs affecting the 5-LO metabolism were mainly connected with asthma and other inflammatory diseases (De Caterina & Zampolli, 2004).

However, a growing understanding of the role of inflammation in atherosclerosis has brought attention to the potential role of leukotrienes and their metabolism. In 2002 Mehrabian et al. identified the 5-LO as a crucial enzyme, contributing to atherosclerosis susceptibility in mice (Mehrabian et al., 2002; Spanbroek et al., 2003).

This observation, after a long pause (De Caterina R et al., 1988) has again focused the attention of researchers on the role of leukotrienes in the pathogenesis of atherosclerotic plaque (Radmark, 2003; Zhao & Funk, 2004; Zhao et al., 2004; Kuhn et al., 2005; Kuhn H, 2005; Lotzer et al., 2005; Back & Hansson, 2006; Radmark & Samuelsson, 2007). Therefore, the speculations have been risen that anti-asthmatic drugs could have beneficial effects on atherogenesis (Spanbroek & Habenicht, 2003; Wickelgren, 2004; Funk, 2005; Back, 2006).

Indeed, it has been recently demonstrated that the 5-LO substantially contribute to atherosclerosis in both mouse models and humans (Mehrabian & Allayee, 2003; Dwyer et al., 2004). Later Aiello et al. showed that LTB4 receptor antagonism reduced monocytic foam cells in mice (Aiello et al., 2002). Lotzer et al. pointed that macrophage-derived LTs differentially activate cysLT2-Rs via paracrine stimulation and cysLT1-Rs via autocrine and paracrine stimulation, during inflammation and atherogenesis (Lotzer et al., 2003).

Therefore, a hypothesis has been formulated that leukotriene-inhibiting drugs developed to treat asthma might protect the heart. There are numerous potential targets that could be useful in the intervention in leukotriene metabolism in atherosclerosis. Interestingly, the 18 kDa microsomal protein - five lipoxygenase activating protein (FLAP) was found to be critical for the regulation of 5-LO activity and biosynthesis of leukotrienes. The role of FLAP in atherosclerosis was additionally confirmed in humans by Helgadottir et al. (Helgadottir et al., 2004) who showed that genetic polymorphisms of FLAP are associated with myocardial infarction and stroke by increasing leukotriene production and inflammation in the arterial wall.

The 5-LO is abundantly expressed in atherosclerotic lesions of apoE and LDLR deficient mice, appearing to co-localize with a subset of macrophages but not with all macrophage-staining regions. Indeed, the results of our studies showed that the inhibition of FLAP by MK-886 or BAYx1005 can significantly prevent the development of atherosclerosis in gene-targeted apoE/LDLR-DKO mice ( Jawien et al., 2006; Jawien et al., 2007).
Moreover, this study showed that cysteinyl leukotriene receptor blocker montelukast decreases atherosclerosis in apoE/LDLR-double knockout mice (Jawien et al., 2008). These results derived also from our numerous studies, concerned with atherosclerotic mice (Elhage et al., 2004; Elhage et al., 2005; Guzik et al., 2005; Jawien et al., 2005; Jawien et al., 2007).
The findings of the study concerning MK-886 were confirmed by Back et al. on their model of transgenic apoE-/- mice with the dominant negative transforming growth factor β type II receptor, which displays aggravated atherosclerosis (Back et al, 2007).
Colin D. Funk's research team questioned the hypothesis concerning leukotrienes, 5-LO and their role in atherogenesis in gene-targeted mice, stating that in mouse plaques there is no 5-LO overexpression detectable (Cao et al., 2008).
Finally, Poeckel & Funk in 2010, they tried to explain the whole complicated phenomenon.

## 13. Limitations of animal models

Animal models potentially bear the risk of compensatory mechanisms due to genetic modification of the target gene that render the results difficult to interpret. Another caveat is species differences between mice and humans. For instance, 5-LO expression in intimal atherosclerotic lesions varies between mice and humans; also, 5-LO and 12/15-LO appear to be differentially regulated in inflammatory cells of mice and humans with the murine 12/15-LO producing mainly 12-HPETE, while its human counterpart primarily synthesizes 15-HPETE. Notably, both products may have opposing effects in inflammation (Conrad DJ, 1999).
Moreover, atherogenesis in mice differs in several facets from the human pathology. Thus, T cells, whose presence in all stages of atherosclerotic lesions is acknowledged, are underrepresented in murine models of atherosclerosis (Daugherty & Hansson, as cited in Dean & Kelly, 2000; Roselaar et al., 1996).
Despite these shortcomings, animal models afford an invaluable means to study the effects of directed genetic overexpression, deletion or pharmacological inhibition of key enzymes of the LT cascade in a physiological setting that cannot be achieved in humans.
5-LO/LT pathway shows important disparities between murine and human atherosclerosis. Advanced human plaques show differences in 5-LO expression compared with mouse lesions. In human lesions, 5-LO (+) cells were identified in macrophages, DCs, mast cells, and neutrophils (Spanbroek et al, 2003) and notably, these 5-LO (+) cells are present in the neointimal region, whereas in mice, they are restricted to the adventitial layer (Zhao et al., 2004). With increasing age, these adventitial macrophages form clusters with T cells, independent of the severity of atherosclerosis. Intimal inflammatory reactions are connected to distinct adventitial inflammation responses, whereby B lymphocytes, plasma cells, and T cells conglomerate with macrophages. 5-LO (+) cells accumulate around new blood vessels, a common feature between mice and humans.
In human atherosclerotic plaque specimens, the quantity of 5-LO (+) cells even increased during progression from early to late phase coronary heart disease (Spanbroek et al., 2003).

Moreover, the elevated 5-LO activity was found to be associated with BLT1-mediated matrix metalloproteinase release from T cells, promoting plaque instability (Cipollone et al., 2005). Human lesions demonstrate detectable expression levels for all major components of the LT cascade, i.e., FLAP, $LTA_4$ hydrolase, and $LTC_4$ synthase, as well as $BLT_1$/$BLT_2$ and $CysLT_1$/$CysLT_2$ receptors.

Taken together, in advanced human atherosclerosis, a role for 5-LO is likely, which is distinct from its role in early atherogenesis. This presence of the 5-LO/LT pathway in advanced lesions is not found in mouse models, which might be due to: (i) rapid progression of atheroma growth in mice vs. slower, often interrupted progression in humans (i.e., initial fatty streaks might remain dormant for many years in humans, until certain factors promote the progression of some lesions into an advanced state) (Libby, 2006; Libby & Sasiela, 2006) (ii) advanced human plaques display a higher degree of instability and risk to rupture than murine plaques; (iii) temporal dissociation in the Th1/Th2 'balance' at distinct lesion stages between mice and humans (Kus et al., 2009; Toton-Zuranska et al., 2010; Smith et al. 2010).

## 14. Future directions

During the last few years there has been a resurgent focus on the 5-LO/LT pathway as a potential target in coronary vascular disease (CVD). The complexity of the 5-LO/LT pathway participation in mechanisms contributing to CVD is evident based on the many studies (Poeckel & Funk, 2010). Limitations of these studies often result from the 'snapshot' punctual nature of analysing a single time point in CVD pathogenesis that makes it difficult to gain systematic insight into 5-LO-driven or -independent processes.

Murine and human CVD etiology differ with respect to the 5-LO/LT pathway, and even within murine studies, the nature of the applied model (for atherosclerosis, abdominal aortic aneurysm (AAA), or ischemia/reperfusion injury) influences the conclusions. Whereas a role for 5-LO-derived LTs in early stages of murine and human atherosclerosis, AAA, and reperfusion injury is cogent based on their effects in chemotaxis and induction of pro-inflammatory responses, the 5-LO pathway appears to play a distinct role in advanced human atherosclerosis, but not in advanced murine disease. Targeting specific leukotriene G protein-coupled receptors rather than upstream targets involved in LT synthesis may be a superior strategy for future CVD therapeutic interventions, based on extensive past experience with other pathways (e.g., via angiotensin II and adrenergic receptors), although this remains to be determined. Conditional knockouts and comprehensive translational studies should serve better than the traditional, simplistic 'one model' approach to understand the complex effects exerted by 5-LO products. Understanding the cytokine milieu during distinct stages of CVD progression will be crucial to elucidate how the expression of members of the 5-LO/LT pathway is regulated. There is little doubt that 5-LO plays important roles in many facets of CVD, but the challenge for future studies will be to clearly dissect these activities in a temporal and cell- and tissue- specific context in order to provide a solid basis for potential therapeutic interventions.

## 15. Acknowledgments

This article was supported by the grant form Polish Ministry of Science and Higher Education nr: N N401548340 for the years 2011-2012.

## 16. References


Aiello R.J., Bourassa P.A., Lindsey S., et al. (1999). Monocyte chemoattractant protein-1 accelerates atherosclerosis in apolipoprotein E-deficient mice. *Arterioscler Thromb Vasc Biol*, 19, 1518-1525.

Aiello R.J., Bourassa P.A., Lindsey S., Weng W., Freeman A. & Showell HJ. (2002) Leukotriene B4 receptor antagonism reduces monocytic foam cells in mice. *Arterioscler Thromb Vasc Biol*, 22, 443-449.

Alber H.F., Frick M., Suessenbacher A., et al. (2006) Effect of atorvastatin on circulating proinflammatory T-lymphocyte subsets and soluble CD40 ligand in patients with stable coronary artery disease - a randomized, placebo-controlled study. *Am Heart J*, 151, 139.

Back M. (2006) Leukotrienes: potential therapeutic targets in cardiovascular diseases. *Bull Acad Natl Med*, 190, 1511-1518.

Back M. & Hansson G.K. (2006) Leukotriene receptors in atherosclerosis. *Ann Med*, 38, 493-502.

Back M., Sultan A., Ovchinnikova O. & Hansson GK. (2007) 5-lipoxygenase-activating protein. A potential link between innate and adaptive immunity in atherosclerosis and adipose tissue inflammation. *Circ Res*, 100, 946-949.

Binder CJ, Chang MK, Shaw PX, et al. (2002) Innate and acquired immunity in atherogenesis. *Nat Med*, 8, 1218-1226.

Bird D.A., Tangirala R.K., Fruebis J., Steinberg D., Witztum J.L., & Palinski W. (1998) Effect of probucol on LDL oxidation and atherosclerosis in LDL receptor - deficient mice. *J Lipid Res*, 39: 1079-1090.

Bonthu S., Heistad D.D., Chappell D.A., Lamping K.G., & Faraci F.M. (1997) Atherosclerosis, vascular remodeling, and impairment of endothelium - dependent relaxation in genetically altered hyperlipidemic mice. *Arterioscler Thromb Vasc Biol*, 17, 2333-2340

Boren J., Olin K., Lee I., et al. (1998) Identification of the principal proteoglycan-binding site in LDL. A single-point mutation in apo-B100 severly affects proteoglycan interaction without affecting LDL receptor binding. *J Clin Invest*, 101, 2658-2664.

Breslow J.L. (1994) Lipoprotein metabolism and atherosclerosis susceptibility in transgenic mice. *Curr Opin Lipidol*, 5: 175-184.

Breslow J.L. (1996) Mouse models of atherosclerosis. *Science*, 272, 685-688.

Cao R.Y., St Amand T., Grabner R., Habenicht A.J., & Funk C.D. (2008) Genetic and pharmacological inhibition of the 5-lipoxygenase/leukotriene pathway in atherosclerotic lesion development in apoE deficient mice. *Atherosclerosis*, 203, 395-400.

Capecchi M.R. (2001) Generating mice with targeted mutations. *Nature Med*, 7, 1086-1090.

Cipollone F., Mezzetti A., Fazia M.L., et al. (2005) Association between 5-lipoxygenase expression and plaque instability in humans. *Arterioscler Thromb Vasc Biol*, 25, 1665-1670.

Conrad D.J. (1999) The arachidonate 12/15 lipoxygenases. A review of tissue expression and biologic function. *Clin Rev Allergy Immunol*, 17, 71-89.

Daugherty A. & Hansson G.K. (2000) Lymphocytes in atherogenesis, In: *Atherosclerosis*, RT Dean R.T & Kelly D., pp. 230-249, New York, Oxford Press.

Daugherty A., & Rateri D.L. (2002) T lymphocytes in atherosclerosis. The Yin-Yang of Th1 and Th2 influence on lesion formation. *Circ Res*, 90, 1039-1040.

De Caterina R., Mazzone A., Giannessi D., Sicari R., Pelosi W., Lazzerini G., Azzara A., Forder R., Carey F. & Caruso D. (1988) Leukotriene B4 production in human atherosclerotic plaques. *Biomed Biochim Acta*, 47, S182-S185.

De Caterina R. & Zampolli A. (2004) From asthma to atherosclerosis - 5-lipoxygenase, leukotrienes, and inflammation. *N Engl J Med*, 350, 4-7.

Dwyer J.H., Allayee H., Dwyer K.M., et al. (2004) Arachidonate 5-lipoxygenase promoter genotype, dietary arachidonic acid, and atherosclerosis. *N Engl J Med*, 350, 29-37.

Elhage R., Jawien J., Rudling M., et al. (2003) Reduced atherosclerosis in interleukin-18 deficient apolipoprotein E-knockout mice. *Cardiovasc Res*, 59, 234-240.

Elhage R., Gourdy P., Brouchet L., et al. (2004) Deleting TCR alpha beta+ or CD+ T lymphocytes leads to opposite effects on site-specific atherosclerosis in female apolipoprotein E - deficient mice. *Am J Pathol*, 165, 2013-2018.

Elhage R., Gourdy P., Jawien J., et al. (2005) The atheroprotective effect of 17-estradiol depends on complex interactions in adaptive immunity. *Am J Pathol*, 167, 267-274.

Faggiotto A. & Ross R. (1984) Studies of hypercholesterolemia in the nonhuman primate. II. Fatty streak conversion to fibrous plaque. *Arteriosclerosis*, 4, 341-356.

Fan J. & Watanabe T. (2003) Inflammatory reaction in the pathogenesis of atherosclerosis. *J Atheroscler Thromb*, 10, 63-71.

Fredrikson G.N., Soderberg I., Lindholm M., et al. (2003) Inhibition of atherosclerosis in apoE null mice by immunization with apoB-100 peptide sequences. *Arterioscler Thromb Vasc Biol*, 23, 879-884.

Funk C.D. (2005) Leukotriene modifiers as potential therapeutics for cardiovascular disease. *Nature*, 4, 664-672.

Gaut J.P. & Heinecke J.W. (2001) Mechanisms for oxidizing low-density lipoprotein. Insights from patterns of oxidation products in the artery wall and from mouse models of atherosclerosis. *Trends Cardiovasc Med*, 11, 103-112.

Glass C.K. & Witztum J.L. (2001) Atherosclerosis: the road ahead. *Cell*, 104, 503-516.

Gupta S., Pablo A.M., Jiang X., et al. (1997) IFN-gamma potentiates atherosclerosis in ApoE knock-out mice. *J Clin Invest*, 99, 2752-2761.

Hansson G.K. (2001) Immune mechanisms in atherosclerosis. *Arterioscler Thromb Vasc Biol*, 21, 1876-1890.

Hansson G.K. (2002) Vaccination against atherosclerosis: science or fiction? *Circulation*, 106, 1599-1601.

Hansson G.K. (2005) Inflammation, atherosclerosis, and coronary artery disease. *N Engl J Med*, 352, 1685-1695.

Hansson G.K., Libby P., Schonbeck U., & Yan ZQ. (2002) Innate and adaptive immunity in the pathogenesis of atherosclerosis. *Circ Res*, 91, 281-291.

Hayek T., Attias J., Coleman R. et al. (1999) The angiotensin - converting enzyme inhibitor, fosinopril, and the angiotensin II receptor antagonist, losartan, inhibit LDL oxidation and attenuate atherosclerosis independent of lowering blood pressure in apolipoprotein E deficient mice. *Cardiovasc Res*, 44, 579-587.

Helgadottir A., Manolescu A., Thorleifsson G., et al. (2004) The gene encoding 5-lipoxygenase activating protein confers risk of myocardial infarction and stroke. *Nat Genet*, 36, 233-239.

Hendrix M.G., Salimans M.M., van Boven C.P., & Bruggeman CA. (1990) High prevalence of latently present cytomegalovirus in arterial walls of patients suffering from grade III atherosclerosis. *Am J Pathol*, 136, 23-28.

Ignatowski A.C. (1908) Influence of animal food on the organism of rabbits. *S Peterb Izviest Imp Voyenno-Med. Akad*, 16, 154-173.

Ishibashi S., Brown M.S., Goldstein J.L., Gerard R.D., Hammer R.E., & Herz J. (1993) Hypercholesterolemia in low density lipoprotein receptor knockout mice and its reversal by adenovirus - mediated gene delivery. *J Clin Invest*, 92, 883-893.

Ishibashi S., Herz J., Maeda N., Goldstein J.L., & Brown MS. (1994) The two-receptor model of lipoprotein clearance: tests of the hypothesis in "knockout" mice lacking the low density lipoprotein receptor, apolipoprotein E, or both proteins. *Proc Natl Acad Sci USA*, 91, 4431-4435.

Jawien J., Nastalek P. & Korbut R. (2004) Mouse models of experimental atherosclerosis. *J Physiol Pharmacol*, 55, 503-517.

Jawień J., Gajda M., Mateuszuk L., et al. (2005) Inhibition of nuclear factor-kappaB attenuates artherosclerosis in apoE/LDLR - double knockout mice. *J Physiol Pharmacol*, 56, 483-489.

Jawien J., Gajda M., Rudling M., et al. (2006) Inhibition of five lipoxygenase activating protein (FLAP) by MK-886 decreases atherosclerosis in apoE/LDLR double knockout mice. *Eur J Clin Invest*, 36, 141-146.

Jawien J., Gajda M., Olszanecki R. & Korbut R. (2007) BAYx1005 attenuates atherosclerosis in apoE/LDLR - double knockout mice. *J Physiol Pharmacol* 58: 583-538.

Jawien J., Csanyi G., Gajda M., et al. (2007) Ticlopidine attenuates progression of atherosclerosis in apolipoprotein E and low density lipoprotein receptor double knockout mice. *Eur J Pharmacol*, 556, 129-135.

Jawien J., Gajda M., Wolkow P.P., Zuranska J., Olszanecki R. & Korbut R. (2008) The effect of montelukast on atherogenesis in apoE/LDLR - double knockout mice. *J Physiol Pharmacol*, 59, 633-639.

Jawień J. (2008) New insights into immunological aspects of atherosclerosis. *Pol Arch Med Wewn*, 118, 127-131.

Jawień J. (2009) The putative role of leukotrienes in experimental atherogenesis. *Pol Arch Med Wewn*, 119, 90-93.

Jawień J. & Korbut R. (2010) The current view on the role of leukotrienes in atherogenesis. *J Physiol Pharmacol*, 61: 647-650.

Jonasson L., Holm J., Skalli O., et al. (1986) Regional accumulations of T cells, macrophages, and smooth muscle cells in the human atherosclerotic plaque. *Arteriosclerosis*, 6, 131-138.

Kashyap V.S., Samantarina-Fojo S., Brown D.R. et al. (1995) Apolipoprotein E deficiency in mice: gene replacement and prevention of atherosclerosis using adenovirus vectors. *J Clin Invest*, 96, 1612-1620.

Keidar S., Attias J., Smith J., Breslow J.L, & Hayek T. (1997) The angiotensin-II receptor antagonist, losartan, inhibits LDL lipid peroxidation and atherosclerosis in apolipoprotein E – deficient mice. *Biochem Biophys Res Comm*, 236, 622-625.

Keidar S., Attias J., Coleman R., Wirth K., Scholkens B., & Hayek T. (2000) Attenuation of atherosclerosis in apolipoprotein E - deficient mice by ramipril is dissociated from

its antihypertensive effect and from potentiation of bradykinin. *J Cardiovasc Pharmacol* 35, 64-72.
Kobayashi K., Tada K., Itabe H., et al. (2007) Distinguished effects of antiphospholipid antibodies and anti-oxidized LDL antibodies on oxidized LDL uptake by macrophages. *Lupus*, 16: 929-938.
Kuhlencordt P.J., Gyurko R., Han F. et al. (2001) Accelerated atherosclerosis, aortic aneurysm formation, and ischemic heart disease in apolipoprotein E/endothelial nitric oxide synthase double knockout mice. *Circulation* 104: 448-454.
Kuhn H. (2005) Biologic relevance of lipoxygenase isoforms in atherogenesis. *Expert Rev Cardiovasc Ther*, 3, 1099-1110.
Kuhn H., Romisch I. & Belkner J. (2005) The role of lipoxygenase isoforms in atherogenesis. *Mol Nutr Food Res*, 49, 1014-1029.
Kus K., Gajda M., Pyka-Fosciak G., et al. (2009) The effect of nebivolol on atherogenesis in apoE - knockout mice. *J Physiol Pharmacol*, 60, 163-165.
Laurat E., Poirier B., Tupin E., et al. (2001) In vivo downregulation of T helper cell 1 immune responses reduces atherogenesis in apolipoprotein E-knockout mice. *Circulation*, 104, 197-202.
Liao F., Andalibi A., deBeer F.C. et al. (1993) Genetic control of inflammatory gene induction and NF kappa B-like transcription factor activation in response to an atherogenic diet in mice. *J Clin Invest*, 91, 2572-2579.
Libby P. (2000) Changing concepts of atherogenesis. *J Intern Med*, 247, 349-358.
Libby P. (2002) Inflammation in atherosclerosis. *Nature*, 420, 868-874.
Libby P., Ridker P.M., & Maseri A. (2002) Inflammation and atherosclerosis. *Circulation*, 105, 1135-1143.
Libby P. (2006) Atherosclerosis: disease biology affecting the coronary vasculature. *Am J Cardiol*, 98, 3Q-9Q.
Libby P. & Sasiela W. (2006) Plaque stabilization: can we turn theory into evidence? *Am J Cardiol*, 98, 26P-33P.
Lotzer K., Spanbroek R., Hildner M., et al. (2003) Differential leukotriene receptor expression and calcium responses in endothelial cells and macrophages indicate 5-lipoxygenase dependent circuits of inflammation and atherogenesis. *Arterioscler Thromb Vasc Biol*, 23, e32-e36.
Lotzer K., Funk C.D. & Habenicht A.J. (2005) The 5-lipoxygenase pathway in arterial wall biology and atherosclerosis. *Biochim Biophys Acta*, 1736, 30-37.
Lusis A.J. (2000) Atherosclerosis. *Nature*, 407, 233-241.
Mach F., Schönbeck U., Sukhova G.K., et al. (1998) Reduction of atherosclerosis in mice by inhibition of CD40 signalling. *Nature*, 394, 200-203.
Mehrabian M., Allayee H., Wong J., Shi W., Wang X.P., Shaposhnik Z., Funk C.D. & Lusis A.J. (2002) Identification of 5-lipoxygenase as a major gene contributing to atherosclerosis susceptibility in mice. *Circ Res*, 91, 120-126.
Mehrabian M. & Allayee H. (2003) 5-lipoxygenase and atherosclerosis. *Curr Opin Lipidol*, 14, 447-457.
Meir K.S., Leitersdorf E. (2004) Atherosclerosis in the apolipoprotein E - deficient mouse. A decade of progress. *Arterioscler Thromb Vasc Biol*, 24, 1006-1014.
Moghadasian M.H., McManus B.M., Godin D.V., Rodrigues B., & Frohlich J.J. (1999) Proatherogenic and antiatherogenic effects of probucol and phytosterols in

apolipoprotein E - deficient mice. Possible mechanisms of action. *Circulation*, 99, 1733-1739.

Moghadasian M.H. (2002) Experimental atherosclerosis: a historical overview. *Life Sci*, 70, 855-865.

Nakashima Y., Plump A.S., Raines E.W., Breslow J.L., & Ross R. (1994) ApoE - deficient mice develop lesions of all phases of atherosclerosis throughout the arterial tree. *Arterioscler Thromb*, 14: 133-140.

Nakashima Y., Raines E.W., Plump A.S., et al. (1998) Upregulation of VCAM-1 and ICAM-1 at atherosclerosis-prone sites on the endothelium in the ApoE-deficient mouse. *Arterioscler Thromb Vasc Biol*, 18, 842-851.

Ni W., Egashira K., Kitamoto S., et al. (2001) New anti-monocyte chemoattractant protein-1 gene therapy attenuates atherosclerosis in apolipoprotein E-knockout mice. *Circulation*, 103, 2096-2101.

Olszanecki R., Jawień J., Gajda M., et al. (2005) Effect of curcumin on atherosclerosis in apoE/LDLR – double knockout mice. *J Physiol Pharmacol*, 56, 627-635.

Paigen B., Morrow C., Brandon C., et al. (1985) Variation in susceptibility to atherosclerosis among inbtred strains of mice. *Atherosclerosis* 57: 65-73.

Paigen B., Morrow A., Holmes P.A., Mitchell D., & Williams R.A. (1987) Quantitative assessment of atherosclerotic lesions in mice. *Atherosclerosis*, 68, 231-240.

Paigen B., Plump A.S. & Rubin E.M. (1994) The mouse as a model for human cardiovascular disease and hyperlipidemia. *Curr Opin Lipidol*, 5, 258-264.

Palinski W., Ord V.A., Plump A.S., Breslow J.L., Steinberg D., & Witztum J.L. (1994) ApoE - deficient mice are a model of lipoprotein oxidation in atherogenesis. Demonstration of oxidation – specific epitopes in lesions and high titers of autoantibodies to malondialdehyde - lysine in serum. *Arterioscler Thromb*, 14, 605-616.

Paszty C., Maeda N., Verstuyft J., & Rubin E.M. (1994) Apolipoprotein AI transgene corrects apolipoprotein E deficiency - induced atherosclerosis in mice. *J Clin Invest*, 94, 899-903.

Pentikäinen M.O., Öörni K., Ala-Korpela M., & Kovanen P.T. (2000) Modified LDL-trigger of atherosclerosis and inflammation in the arterial intima. *J Intern Med*, 247, 359-370.

Piedrahita J.A., Zhang S.H., Hagaman J.R., Oliver P.M. & Maeda N. (1992) Generation of mice carrying a mutant apolipoprotein E gene inactivated by gene targeting in embryonic stem cells. *Proc Natl Acad Sci USA*, 89, 4471-4475.

Phipps R.P. (2000) Atherosclerosis: the emerging role of inflammation and the CD40-CD40L system. *Proc Natl Acad Sci*, 97, 6930-6932.

Pinderski L.J., Fischbein M.P., Subbanagounder G., et al. (2002) Overexpression of interleukin-10 by activated T lymphocytes inhibits atherosclerosis in LDL receptor-deficient mice by altering lymphocyte and macrophage phenotypes. *Circ Res*, 90, 1064-1071.

Plump A.S., Smith J.D., Hayek T., et al. (1992) Severe hypercholesterolemia and atherosclerosis in apolipoprotein E – deficient mice created by homologous recombination in ES cells. *Cell*, 71, 343-353.

Plump A.S., Scott C.J., & Breslow J.L. (1994) Human apolipoprotein A-I gene expression increases high density lipoprotein and suppresses atherosclerosis in the apolipoprotein E - deficient mouse. *Proc Natl Acad Sci USA*, 91, 9607-9611.

Poeckel D. & Funk CD. (2010) The 5-lipoxygenase/leukotriene pathway in preclinical models of cardiovascular disease. *Cardiovasc Res*, 86, 243-253.

Pratico D., Tangirala R.K., Rader D.J., Rokach J., & Fitzgerald G.A. (1998) Vitamin E suppresses isoprostane generation in vivo and reduces atherosclerosis in apoE - deficient mice. *Nature Med*, 4, 1189-1192.

Prevention of cardiovascular events and death with pravastatin in patients with coronary heart disease and a broad range of initial cholesterol levels. The Long-Term Intervention with Pravastatin in Ischaemic Disease (LIPID) Study Group. (1998) *N Engl J Med*, 339, 1349-1357.

Radmark O. (2003) 5-lipoxygenase-derived leukotrienes. Mediators also of atherosclerotic inflammation. *Arterioscler Thromb Vasc Biol*, 23, 1140-1142.

Radmark O. & Samuelsson B. (2007) 5-lipoxygenase: regulation and possible involvement in atherosclerosis. *Prostaglandins Other Lipid Mediat*, 83, 162-174.

Reddick R.L., Zhang S.H., & Maeda N. (1994) Atherosclerosis in mice lacking apoE. Evaluation of lesional development and progression. *Arterioscler Thromb*, 14, 141-147.

Robertson A.K., Rudling M., Zhou X., et al. (2003) Disruption of TGF-beta signaling in T cells accelerates atherosclerosis. *J Clin Invest*, 112, 1342-1350.

Roselaar S.E., Kakkanathu P.X. & Daugherty A. (1996) Lymphocyte populations in atherosclerotic lesions of apoE -/- and LDL receptor -/- mice. Decreasing density with disease progression. *Arterioscler Thromb Vasc Biol*, 16, 1013-1018.

Rosenfeld M.E., Tsukada T., Chait A. et al. (1987) Fatty streak expansion and maturation in Watanabe heritable hyperlipidemic and comparably hypercholesterolemic fat-fed rabbits. *Arteriosclerosis* 1987, 7, 24-34.

Ross R. & Glomset J.A. (1976) The pathogenesis of atherosclerosis. *N Engl J Med*, 295, 369-377.

Ross R., Glomset J., & Harker L. (1977) Response to injury and atherogenesis. Am J Pathol, 86, 675-684.

Ross R., Faggiotto A., Bowen-Pope D., & Raines E. (1984) The role of endothelial injury and platelet and macrophage interactions in atherosclerosis. *Circulation*, 70, 77-82.

Ross R. (1986) The pathogenesis of atherosclerosis – an update. *N Engl J Med*, 314, 488-500.

Ross R. (1999) Atherosclerosis – an inflammatory disease. *N Eng J Med*, 340, 115-126.

Savla U. (2002) At the heart of atherosclerosis. *Nat Med*, 8, 1209.

Scandinavian Simvastatin Survival Study Group. Randomised trial of cholesterol lowering in 4444 patients with coronary heart disease: The Scandinavian Simvastatin Survival Study (4S). 1994. *Lancet* 344: 1383-1389.

Schonbeck U., Sukhova G.K., Shimizu K., et al. (2000) Inhibition of CD40 signaling limits evolution of established atherosclerosis in mice. *Proc Natl Acad Sci USA*, 97, 7458-7463.

Shishehbor M.H. & Bhatt D.L. (2004) Inflammation and atherosclerosis. *Curr Atheroscler Rep*, 6: 131-139.

Shoenfeld Y., Sherer Y., & Harats D. (2001) Atherosclerosis as an infectious, inflammatory and autoimmune disease. *TRENDS Immunol*, 22, 293-295.

Smith D.D., Tan X., Tawfik O., Milne G., Stechschulte D.J. & Dileepan K.N. (2010) Increased aortic atherosclerotic plaque development in female apolipoprotein E-null mice is associated with elevated thromboxane A2 and decreased prostacyclin production. *J Physiol Pharmacol*, 61, 309-316.

Spanbroek R., Grabner R., Lotzer K., et al. (2003) Expanding expression of the 5-lipoxygenase pathway within the arterial wall during human atherogenesis. *Proc Natl Acad Sci USA*, 100, 1238-1243.

Spanbroek R. & Habenicht A.J. (2003) The potential role of antileukotriene drugs in atherosclerosis. *Drug News Perspect*, 16, 485-489.

Steinberg D. (2002) Atherogenesis in perspective: hypercholesterolemia and inflammation as partners in crime. *Nat Med*, 8, 1211-1217.

Stemme S., Faber B., Holm J., et al. (1995) T lymphocytes from human atherosclerotic plaques recognize oxidized low density lipoprotein. *Proc Natl Acad Sci USA*, 92, 3893-3897.

Suski M., Olszanecki R., Madej J., et al. (2011) Proteomic analysis of changes in protein expression in liver mitochondria in apoE knockout mice. *J Proteomics*, 74, 887-893.

Suzuki H., Kurihara Y., Takeya M., et al. (1997) A role for macrophage scavenger receptors in atherosclerosis and susceptibility to infection. *Nature*, 386, 292-296.

Tangirala R.K., Casanada F., Miller E., Witztum J.L., Steinberg D., & Palinski W. (1995) Effect of the antioxidant N,N' - diphenyl 1,4-phenylenediamine (DPPD) on atherosclerosis in apoE - deficient mice. *Arterioscler Thromb Vasc Biol*, 15, 1625-1630.

Tenger C., Sundborger A., Jawien J., & Zhou X. (2005) IL-18 accelerates atherosclerosis accompanied by elevation of IFN-gamma and CXCL16 expression independently of T cells. *Arterioscler Thromb Vasc Biol*, 25, 791-796.

Thom D.H., Wang S.P., Grayston J.T., et al. (1991) Chlamydia pneumoniae strain TWAR antibody and angiographically demonstrated coronary artery disease. *Arterioscler Thromb*, 11, 547-551.

Toton-Zuranska J., Gajda M., Pyka-Fosciak G., et al. (2010) AVE 0991 - angiotensin-(1-7) receptor agonist, inhibits atherogenesis in apoE-knockout mice. *J Physiol Pharmacol*, 61, 181-183.

Tousoulis D., Antoniades C., Nikolopoulou A., et al. (2007) Interaction between cytokines and sCD40L in patients with stable and unstable coronary syndromes. *Eur J Clin Invest*, 37, 623-628.

Van Ree J.H., van der Broek W., Dahlmans V. et al. (1994) Diet-induced hypercholesterolemia and atherosclerosis in heterozygous apolipoprotein E - deficient mice. *Atherosclerosis*, 111, 25-37.

Veniant M.M., Withycombe S., & Young SG. (2000) Lipoprotein size and atherosclerosis susceptibility in Apoe-/- and Ldlr-/- mice. *J Clin Invest*, 106, 1501-1510.

Waterson R.H., Lindblad-Toh K., Birney E., et al. (2002) Initial sequencing and comparative analysis of the mouse genome. *Nature*, 420, 520-562.

Welt F.G., Rogers S.D., Zhang X., et al. (2004) GP IIb/IIIa inhibition with eptifibatide lowers levels of soluble CD40L and RANTES after percutaneous coronary intervention. *Catheter Cardiovasc Interv*, 61, 185-189.

Wick G., Schett G., Amberger A., et al. (1995) Is atherosclerosis an immunologically mediated disease? *Immunol Today*, 16: 27-33.

Wick G., Perschinka H., & Millonig G. (2001) Atherosclerosis as an autoimmune disease: an update. *TRENDS Immunol*, 22, 665-669.

Wickelgren I. (2004) Gene suggests asthma drugs may ease cardiovascular inflammation. *Science*, 303: 941.

Witting P.K., Pettersson K., Ostlund-Lindqvist A.M., Westerlund C., Eriksson A.W., & Stocker R. (1999) Inhibition by a coantioxidant of aortic lipoprotein lipid peroxydation and atherosclerosis in apolipoprotein E and low density lipoprotein receptor gene double knockout mice. *FASEB J*, 13, 667-675.

Zhang S.H., Reddick R.L., Piedrahita J.A., & Maeda N. (1992) Spontaneous hypercholesterolemia and arterial lesions in mice lacking apolipoprotein E. *Science*, 258, 468-471.

Zhao L. & Funk C.D. (2004) Lipoxygenase pathways in atherogenesis. Trends Cardiovasc Med, 14, 191-195.

Zhao L., Moos M.P., Gräbner R., Pédrono F., Fan J., Kaiser B., John N., Schmidt S., Spanbroek R., Lötzer K., Huang L., Cui J., Rader D.J., Evans J.F., Habenicht A.J. & Funk C.D. (2004) The 5-lipoxygenase pathway promotes pathogenesis of hyperlipidemia dependent aortic aneurysm. Nat Med, 10, 966-973.

Zhou X., Nicoletti A., Elhage R., Hansson G.K. (2000) Transfer of CD4(+) T cells aggravates atherosclerosis in immunodeficient apolipoprotein E knockout mice. *Circulation*, 102, 2919-2922.

# 2

# Spontaneous Atherosclerosis in Pigeons: A Good Model of Human Disease

J. L. Anderson, S. C. Smith and R. L. Taylor, Jr.
*University of New Hampshire, Durham*
*U.S.A.*

## 1. Introduction

Avian models of human atherosclerosis such as the chicken, turkey, quail, and pigeon are not currently in widespread use, but have a longer and richer history than most mammalian models of cardiovascular disease. In 1874, the first angioplasty surgery of the aortic wall was performed in birds (Roberts & Strauss, 1965). Spontaneous (non-induced) atherosclerosis in the chicken was first described in 1914 (Roberts & Strauss, 1965), and it has been repeatedly observed that avian lesions bear close resemblance to their human counterparts (Clarkson et al., 1959; Herndon et al., 1962; Cornhill et al., 1980b; Qin & Nishimura, 1998). The pigeon (*Columba livia*) is especially suited for genetic studies of atherosclerosis because susceptible and resistant strains exist in the natural population (Herndon et al., 1962; St. Clair, 1983) eliminating the need to construct an artificial phenotype through genetic or dietary manipulation. In fact, it has been suggested that the White Carneau (WC) pigeon may be one of the most appropriate models of early human lesions (Cornhill et al., 1980b; St. Clair, 1998; Moghadasian et al., 2001). This review is comprised of background information on human atherosclerosis, a description of other animal models and details of the pigeon model.

Atherosclerosis is the most common form of heart disease, a general term encompassing a variety of pathologies affecting the heart and circulatory system. More specifically, atherosclerosis is a disease of the blood vessel itself, and is most likely to develop at branch points and other regions of low shear stress along the arterial tree, such as the celiac bifurcation of the aorta, and in coronary and carotid arteries (Bassiouny et al., 1994; Kjaernes et al., 1981). The disease is a chronic and multifactorial result of both environmental and genetic factors, as well as their interactions (Breslow, 2000; Moghadasian et al., 2001). It remains the number one cause of morbidity and mortality in the United States and other developed countries (Gurr, 1992; Wagner, 1978).

Arterial lesions begin to develop during childhood as lipid-filled foam cells making up "fatty streaks" (Napoli et al., 2002; Stary, 1989), and slowly progress into complex plaques consisting of multiple cell types, intra- and extracellular cholesterol esters, calcium deposits, proteoglycans, and extensive connective tissue. The final and terminating atherosclerotic event is blood vessel occlusion, often caused by plaque rupture, which can lead to a heart attack, stroke, or embolism, depending on the location of the affected artery. However, not all fatty streaks progress to advanced lesions (Getz, 2000), and their progression/regression rate, although well correlated with classical risk factors, is unique to each individual.

Clinical symptoms do not usually appear until later in life (Munro & Cotran, 1988; Stary, 1989). Therefore, research and intervention strategies have focused on delaying the progression of plaque formation rather than preventing the appearance of foam cells or fatty streaks. There is a strong familial component to all forms of heart disease, and many genetic disorders have been identified that contribute to lesion progression and the probability of plaque rupture in the general population. However, little is known about the specific genes that determine predisposition to the disease, nor how these genes interact with each other and the environment to initiate atherosclerotic foam cell formation in any one individual.

## 2. Human atherogenesis

### 2.1 The observed beginning: Foam cells and lesion development

In human lesions, early foam cells originate primarily from vascular smooth muscle cells (VSMC) [Wissler et al., 1996]. They are the first cell type to appear in susceptible regions of the aorta (Balis et al., 1964; Ross & Glomset, 1973), and the most abundant cell type in developing fatty streaks (Gabbiani et al., 1984; Katsuda & Okada, 1994; Mosse et al., 1985, 1986; Wissler et al., 1996;). Early electron microscopy studies noted that VSMC were often filled with lipid when there was no lipid in either existing macrophages or in the extracellular space, but the reverse was never observed.

Since those observations, multiple investigators have reported that abnormal VSMC accumulation in susceptible aortic regions precedes the actual lipid accumulation (Mosse et al., 1985; Ross & Glomset, 1973). Atherosclerotic foam cells can be derived from both VSMC and macrophages (Adelman & St. Clair, 1988; Wissler et al., 1996), depending on their physical location (Strong et al., 1999) and the cause of initiation. For example, plaques that develop along the descending thoracic aorta have more macrophages than VSMC, whereas plaques along the abdominal aorta and coronary arteries are comprised mostly of VSMC, with very few macrophages. Human thoracic plaques are very rare, and those that do progress are usually secondary to other chronic conditions such as hypertension and hyperlipidemia (Wissler et al., 1996).

Although VSMC are the first cell type to accumulate lipid and initiate the fatty streak (Doran et al., 2008), much emphasis is placed on macrophage foam cells rather than myogenic foam cells. Macrophage-derived foam cells are quick to develop into lesions and are easy to induce with a high-fat and/or high-cholesterol diet (Knowles & Maeda, 2000; Xu, 2004; Zhang et al., 1992), in common animal models of human atherosclerosis, especially transgenic mice. Unlike VSMC, which can alternate between contractile and synthetic phenotypes, macrophage cells do not change during the disease progression, and so are easier to identify in the laboratory under controlled conditions.

Greater emphasis on macrophage-derived foam cells is problematic because the pathogenic lipid accumulation mechanism appears to be dissimilar for the two cell types. Also, rather than being a primary initiative event in humans, the arrival of macrophages appears to be a secondary response, as they are far more common in advanced plaques than in early lesions (Balis et al., 1964; Nakashima et al., 2007; Stary, 1989; Wissler et al., 1996; Zhang et al., 1992;).

### 2.2 Atherogenesis risk factors

Major physiological conditions such as high blood cholesterol, high blood pressure, diabetes, a skewed lipoprotein profile, heredity, advanced age, and maleness can increase an individual's chance of developing atherosclerosis. Collectively, these risk factors, along with lifestyle patterns such as physical inactivity, smoking, obesity, and stress have been statistically correlated with specific stages of lesion development, plaque stability, and overall disease outcome in the general population. Although genotype clearly influences many quantitative traits such as LDL/HDL levels, blood pressure, and adiposity (Gibbons et al., 2004), progress has been made on minimizing the effects of the controllable risk factors in order to disrupt, delay, reverse, or otherwise deter plaque rupture and aortic occlusion in high risk individuals.

Despite moderate success, especially in the realm of cholesterol-lowering drugs, unknown genetic factors continue to influence both the age of onset as well as the frequency/severity of clinical symptoms (Funke & Assmann, 1999). Unfortunately, by the time most people manifest clinical symptoms, it is too late to implement preventative measures because the disease is well into the progressive stage. Early identification of susceptible individuals allows timely therapeutic treatment. Less than 50% of the mortality risk from coronary heart disease can be explained by currently recognized risk factors (Ridker, 2000), even with early diagnosis.

In order to understand events in the at-risk population that remain unidentified under current screening methods, the specific contributions of heredity, diet, and lifestyle influences on atherogenesis and progression must be determined. Towards this end, research emphasis has recently shifted towards identifying cardiovascular disease markers that may be detectable prior to the manifestation of clinical symptoms. Markers are simply variations in alleles that are known to associate with a specific disease phenotype. Markers do not necessarily cause the disease, but can be used to improve diagnosis and risk assessment (Gibbons et al., 2004). Inflammatory markers such as C-reactive protein (CRP) factors [Tsimikas et al., 2006; Ridker, 2000] plus markers of oxidative damage such as myeloperoxidase (Shao et al., 2006) and paraoxanase (Visvikis-Siest & Marteau, 2006) have already increased clinicians' predictive power. As more markers of atherosclerosis are correlated with disease progression and outcome, the genetic variation contributing to predisposition and initial manifestation will become clear.

Until the genetic basis for susceptibility to atherosclerosis is understood, correlation of various risk factors with specific metabolic or pathological features will be difficult to assess, and efforts for prevention will remain equivocal. Understanding the inheritance mechanisms for atherosclerosis is an important step towards reducing the morbidity and mortality from the disease by customizing intervention strategies for individuals based upon unique genotypes and environmental risk exposures.

## 3. Genetic defects in human atherogenesis

The relative risk for atherosclerosis is clearly higher in individuals with a familial history compared with those having a susceptible lipid profile (Funk & Assmann, 1999; Ordovas & Shen, 2002; Palinski & Napoli, 2002). Many studies have explored the relationship, or concordance, between heredity and atherosclerosis. Heritability for early-onset coronary heart disease has been estimated at 0.63 (Galton & Ferns, 1989). The relationship becomes even clearer after analyzing concordance in twin studies. Twins fertilized from one egg (monozygotic) have a concordance rate of 0.83, whereas twins that arose from two separate fertilizations (dizygotic) demonstrate a concordance rate of 0.22 (Galton & Ferns, 1989).

These concordance values suggest an intimate relationship between the genotype of an individual and the incidence of heart disease. The fact that the concordance rate in monozygotic twins is less than 1.0 (indicating 100% correlation) most likely reflects the attenuating environmental effects on atherosclerosis initiation and progression. This gap in causality underscores the importance of understanding the genetic profile of a client before attempting intervention, because even among those sharing the same set of alleles, the atherosclerosis phenotype will vary depending on individual exposures.

Genetic research on human atherosclerosis has focused primarily on the role of cholesterol metabolism. It is estimated that several hundred genes (Ordovas & Shen, 2002) are involved in the absorption, conversion, transport, deposition, excretion, and biosynthesis, of cholesterol and other lipid substrates in the body (Knowles & Maeda, 2000; Stein et al., 2002). Very few of these genes have been characterized. A defect in any of these pathways may contribute to atherosclerotic susceptibility, because the net result can be a significant increase in plasma lipoprotein concentration, especially LDL, and/or the inappropriate deposition of cholesterol in peripheral tissues such as skin, tendons, and arteries (Garcia et al., 2001).

Blood lipid homeostasis and cellular cholesterol metabolism are highly regulated (Attie, 2001). Genetic defects have been found to impact overall cholesterol metabolism at many steps. In humans, most plasma cholesterol is in the form of LDL, having a half-life of about 2.5 days (Goldstein & Brown, 2001). Some of the cholesterol component of LDL is transferred to HDL via the action of cholesterol ester transfer protein (CETP). However, as much as 70% of LDL is removed from the blood by LDL receptors (LDLR) in the liver (Garcia et al., 2001). A variety of single gene defects have been identified that increase the incidence of atherosclerosis by influencing the LDLR activity (Funke & Assmann, 1999).

Probably the most studied of these LDLR defects is familial hypercholesterolemia (FH), an autosomal dominant Mendelian disorder (Brown et al., 1981; Funke & Assmann, 1999; Goldstein & Brown, 2001). This mutation renders the hepatic receptors nonfunctional, so that they are unable to clear circulating LDL from the blood. A second type of hypercholesterolemia, autosomal recessive hypercholesterolemia (ARH), also impacts the LDLR (Garcia et al., 2001; Goldstein & Brown, 2001). ARH is similar to FH, in that both of these hereditary defects result in chronically elevated blood cholesterol. This imbalance has the potential to change the physiology of the arterial wall, making it exceptionally vulnerable to atherogenesis. However, unlike FH, the LDLR in ARH, are believed to be functional, but their altered location in the liver makes them inaccessible to circulating LDL.

Brown and Goldstein also identified a single gene defect known as familial ligand defective apoB-100, the primary human LDL (Fielding et al., 2000) apoprotein. This inherited defect lies in the composition and binding capacity of the apoB-100 to the LDLR, decreasing the ability of the LDL to be picked up by the LDLR (Goldstein & Brown, 2001; Gurr, 1992). In the healthy human aorta, LDL particles are thought to be incorporated into SMC by receptor mediator endocytosis. Chemically modified or oxidized LDL enters via scavenger receptors. Once inside the cell, the LDL cholesterol esters (CE) are transported to the lysosomes where they are hydrolyzed by lysosomal acid lipase (LAL), also known as acid cholesterol ester hydrolase (ACEH). This enzyme breaks each CE into its free fatty acid (usually linoleate), and free cholesterol. There are several known LAL gene mutations that result in the abnormal accumulation of cholesterol esters in the lysosome.

Two of the more common lysosomal storage disease phenotypes of a LAL mutation are Wolman's Disease (Kuriyama et al., 1990; Lohse et al., 1999) and cholesterol ester storage disease (CESD). Both are inherited as an autosomal recessive trait, although Wolman's disease is usually fatal within the first year of life, and so not directly related to atherogenesis in the general population. However, individuals with CESD do demonstrate premature atherosclerosis, in addition to accumulating CE and triglycerides (TG) in the liver, adrenal glands and intestines (Pagani et al., 1996). Niemann-Pick Type C is a third form of lysosomal storage disease that directly impacts cholesterol metabolism at the cellular level (Blanchette-Mackie et al., 1988). In this condition, the CE is successfully hydrolyzed by ACEH, but the released cholesterol component is unable to leave the lysosome to travel to the endoplasmic reticulum, causing the accumulation of free cholesterol in the lysosome.

Lysosomes are also responsible for the degradation of glycosaminoglycan (GAG) chains after the core proteoglycan has been broken down by extracellular proteases such as matrix metallopeptidases (MMP) and disintigrins (ADAMs) [Arndt et al, 2002; Seals & Courtneidge, 2003). There is an extensive repertoire of catalytic lysosomal enzymes, and their functions have been revealed mostly by observing the consequences of their absence (Santamarina-Fojo et al., 2001). Defective enzymes lead to a wide variety of diseased phenotypes known as mucopolysaccharidoses (MP) ranging from the mild Schie Disease to the severe Hurler Disease, which results in childhood mortality. In these two examples, GAGs are not properly degraded, and so will accumulate in the lysosomes and in the extracellular space. GAGs in the ECM will attract LDL that has entered the intima by binding to apoB-100 as previously described, where the cholesterol is most likely endocytosed by macrophages and SMC within the developing plaque.

Once in the cytoplasm, cholesterol that is not needed for routine cellular functions is esterified by acyl CoA: cholesterol acyltransferase (ACAT) and stored in vacuoles. Intracellular CE remains trapped in the cytoplasm until hydrolyzed by neutral cholesterol ester hydrolase (NCEH). This enzyme releases the free cholesterol so it can be removed by HDL and transported to the liver. A pair of ATP binding cassette proteins has been identified that are believed to control this efflux of cellular cholesterol. One of these, ABCP–1 is defective in Tangier Disease (Faber et al., 2002), an inherited condition where cholesterol is unable to exit the cell via reverse cholesterol transport. There is a moderate risk of atherogenesis associated with Tangier Disease, which is increased in the presence of additional risk factors (Tall et al., 2001)

Research is directed towards a range of HDL-associated apoproteins. Genetic factors account for approximately 50% of the variance of HDL composition and plasma concentration in the general population (Tall et al., 2001). The primary apoprotein in HDL is apoA1, followed by apoA2, apoC, and apoE (Fielding, 2000). ApoE is an important ligand for receptor-mediated clearance of HDL from arterial cells (Moghadasian et al., 2001; Stein et al., 2002), whose role is of great interest to investigators of atherosclerotic resistance because most patients with familial dysbetalipoproteinemia (FD) are homozygous for the E2 isoform of apoE (Johns Hopkins University, 2011). Although this defect has been shown to be relevant in some animal models, especially apoE null mice (Smith et al., 2006; Zhang et al., 1992), only 1-4% of humans with the E2/E2 apoE phenotype actually develop FD (Johns Hopkins University, 2011). The pathological influence of apoE dysfunction is important in these genetically susceptible individuals, but may not be relevant to the more common forms of atherosclerosis in the overall population.

Any of the currently identified monogneic defects that directly or indirectly influence cholesterol metabolism and/or the inflammatory response will increase the likelihood of atherosclerotic events. However, individual genes do not work in a vacuum, and additional genetic and/or environmental factors are often required to determine the overall susceptibility or resistance to disease. Nuclear hormone receptors and other types of transcription factors are under investigation to determine how they exert their regulatory effects (Cohen & Zannis, 2001; Desvergne al., 2006). For example, although the binding capacity of apoB-100 is genetically determined (Goldstein & Brown, 2001), the specific number of hepatic LDLR being expressed at any given time is dependent on dietary and hormonal factors (Gurr, 1992). In a hypothetical situation, the apoB domain of LDL may be functional (non-mutated), but without the adequate expression of the LDLR to bind circulating LDL, the end result could still be high blood cholesterol.

Clinical studies have demonstrated that not all individuals afflicted with FH will develop early onset atherosclerosis. Of those manifesting the heterozygous form of the disease, where circulating LDL levels tend to range between 300-400 mg/dL, only 50% will actually develop cardiovascular disease (Stein et al, 2002). Even though there are both hyper- and hypo- responders to the effects of dietary cholesterol on serum levels, some individuals demonstrate relative resistance to atherogenesis, even in the face of hypercholesterolemia. Equal emphasis should be placed on the search for genes that contribute to individual susceptibility and those that confer resistance.

The ultimate sequence of atherosclerotic events is a result of the combined effects of many genes, regulatory factors, and environmental exposures (Hartman et al., 2001). This synergistic influence on phenotype may give the appearance of a polygenic or multifactorial effect (Funke & Assmann, 1999; Goldstein & Brown, 2001), even when a monogenic abnormality has been clearly implicated. These interactions have made it difficult to establish a universally accepted mechanism of atherogenesis (Peltonen & McKusick, 2001), because the sample sizes needed to test these gene-gene and gene-environment interactions are much larger than those needed for simpler genotype-phenotype associations (Ordovas & Shen, 2002).

Pathways that trigger atherosclerosis in the general population have yet to be elucidated (Visvikis-Siest & Marteau, 2006). Most genomic scale experiments have compared either full-blown plaques against non-affected aortic segments (Archacki et al., 2003; Forcheron et al., 2005; Hiltunen et al., 2002; Shanahan et al., 1997), or they have analyzed differences between ruptured and unruptured plaques (Adams et al., 2006; Faber et al., 2001; Papaspyridonos et al., 2006). In both types of comparisons, differentially expressed genes have been identified that illuminate plaque development and mortality risk. However, genes responsible for initiating foam cell formation could not be discriminated from those involved in later events. This gap is not an oversight by the investigators, but rather reflects the limited availability of human tissue samples at early stages of atherosclerosis for relevant comparative studies. One of the major limitations of elucidating the sequence of events that occur during atherogenesis is that an investigator can "observe and study a single site in the arterial vasculature" only once (Ross & Glomset, 1973). For this and other reasons, most atherogenic research requires animal and in-vitro models of the human disease.

## 4. Animal models of atherogenesis

### 4.1 Mammals

No animal model of human disease can fully encompass the unique complexity of molecular machinery and the wide range of expressed clinical phenotypes. However, many important metabolic pathways have been explained by the judicious use of animal models (Hartman et al., 2001). Therefore, the most appropriate choice of a disease model for genetic inquiry will ultimately depend on the specific hypothesis or research question being investigated.

There are some general guidelines to follow when choosing an animal model of human disease. The phenotype should resemble the human physiological condition as closely as possible in both the normal and diseased state (Moghadasian et al., 2001). There are additional practical issues to consider such as the size of the animal and housing requirements, generation times, and the specific cost of overall maintenance, including food, daily care, and experimental treatment (Moghadasian et al., 2001; Suckling, & Jackson, 1993). These concerns become especially important with the development of transgenic models, in that the associated investment costs are much higher than with traditional animal studies.

Several animal models are used currently to investigate various clinical manifestations and genetic mechanisms of human atherosclerosis. Mice (regular laboratory and transgenic), rabbits, and hamsters, are the most common models but miniature swine, primates, rats, dogs, and pigeons are also employed. These models have been used to elucidate the role of specific molecules in atherogenesis, lesion progression, thrombosis, and plaque rupture by direct hypothesis testing. Selected disease characteristics in animal models with their relationship to the human atherosclerosis are presented in **Table 1**.

Animal lipid metabolism studies become complicated because the majority of circulating cholesterol is in HDL (Suckling & Jackson, 1993) for most species except humans who utilize LDL (Garcia et al., 2001). For example, a decrease in plasma HDL has been associated with a reduced risk of atherosclerosis in mice (Breslow, 2000). It does make sense that relatively low levels of HDL decreased the clinical atherosclerosis incidence because HDL (Moghadasian et al., 2001) is 70% of mouse total cholesterol.

However, in humans, decreased HDL levels are associated with an increased risk of atherosclerosis. Despite this marked inconsistency, the successful extrapolation of animal studies to human atherosclerosis is exemplified by the fact that it was impossible to raise circulating LDL levels, and thus increase atherosclerosis risk in experimental models, without LDLR that were compromised, either genetically or in response to dietary overload (Brown et al., 1981; Goldstein & Brown, 2001). Subsequently, over 600 human LDLR gene mutations similar to FH that trigger varying degrees of hypercholesterolemia have been identified (Goldstein & Brown, 2001). In addition, hamsters, rabbits and primates have repeatedly shown reduced functional capacity of hepatic receptors in response to a high fat (Suckling & Jackson, 1993) diet. Individual LDLR activity varied in response to dietary fat and cholesterol because primates, like humans, dogs, and rabbits can be hypo- or hyper-responsive to diet (Goldstein & Brown, 2001; Moghadasian et al., 2001; Overturf et al., 1990; Stein et al., 2002), with some individuals demonstrating unique resistance.

In newborn humans and many animal species, hepatic LDLR have a maximum operative capacity when circulating LDL levels are approximately 0.25 mg/dL (Khosla & Sundram, 1996). Approximately 60% of plasma LDL in hamsters is removed by hepatic receptors. The clearance rate in hamsters is much faster than that of humans, with the hamster LDLR taking up 3.1 mg/hr whereas the companion human LDLR only removes 0.6 mg/hour

(Suckling & Jackson, 1993). However, the fact that hamsters and humans share a common LDL clearance mechanism makes the hamster a suitable model for this aspect of cholesterol metabolism.
Hamsters and humans also share CETP molecules (Suckling & Jackson, 1993) that transfer the cholesterol component of LDL to HDL, a key step in reverse cholesterol transport. These homologous features are in direct contrast to the mouse, which, despite being fed a high-fat high-cholesterol diet (Pitman et al., 1998) and its evolutionary relationship to hamsters, does not develop advanced atherosclerotic plaques resembling those in humans unless animals with sensitized genetic backgrounds (Xu, 2004) are used.

| | Hamster | Mouse | | Pig | Rabbit | | Pigeon | Human |
|---|---|---|---|---|---|---|---|---|
| | | Normal | Transgenic | | Normal | WHHL/ MI | | |
| **Lipoprotein Profiles** | | | | | | | | |
| Predominant | LDL | HDL | HDL | LDL | HDL | HDL | HDL | LDL |
| CETP | + | - | - | - | + | + | + | + |
| LDLR | + | + | - | + | + | - | - | + |
| ApoE | + | + | - | + | + | + | - | + |
| ApoB100 | + | + | + | + | + | + | + | + |
| ApoB-48 | + | + | + | + | + | + | - | + |
| **Lesions/Foam Cells** | | | | | | | | |
| Primary Location | Arch | Root | Root | Arch | Arch, Thoracic | Arch, Thoracic | Celiac branch | Coronary, Celiac branch |
| **Primary Cell** | | | | | | | | |
| Macrophage | + | + | + | - | + | + | - | - |
| SMC | - | - | - | + | + | + | + | + |
| **Characteristics** | | | | | | | | |
| Spontaneous | - | - | - | + | - | - | + | + |
| Diet-induced | + | + | + | + | + | + | + | + |
| Thrombosis | - | - | + | + | - | + | + | + |
| Myocardial infarction | - | - | + | - | - | +/- | + | + |
| **Genome size (Gbp)** | 3.55 | 3.45 | 3.45 | 3.10 | 3.47 | 3.47 | 1.47 | 3.40 |
| **Wild-type diet** | | | | | | | | |
| Omnivore | + | + | + | + | - | - | + | + |
| Herbivore | - | - | - | - | + | + | - | - |

Table 1. Comparison of selected characteristics of atherosclerosis between animal models and humans.

The mouse is technically advantageous because of its small size, short generation time, large litters, and the availability of many inbred strains (Breslow, 2000). However, laboratory mice fed on a chow diet do not develop spontaneous atherosclerotic lesions. Atherosclerosis must be experimentally induced by feeding a diet containing 15% fat, 1.25% cholesterol, and 0.5% cholic acid. These non-physiological conditions create serious limitations for comparison with human studies. The most important factor may be the presence of cholate in the diet. Cholate is enough, in and of itself, to induce a chronic inflammatory state in mice (Breslow, 2000; Shi et al., 2003) confounding the true atherogenic role of inflammation. This is further exacerbated by the fact that some mice are more sensitive to inflammatory cues (Rader & Pure, 2000) so that some genetic differences between susceptible and resistant mouse strains pertain to the diet used, rather than the atherogenic process as it is observed on Western diets (Breslow, 2000).

These and other genetic differences that exist between mouse strains can cause significant problems when interpreting and comparing the results of gene expression studies (Sigmund, 2000). For example, just because a specific inflammatory marker was identified in an atherosclerotic plaque and not in a healthy aorta does not mean that inflammation is causing the disease. Indeed, the molecule could be there to accelerate the cascade; but it could also be there in an attempt to reverse the pathology, or may even be responding to a cellular signal not specific to plaque progression (Knowles & Maeda, 2000) such as cholate. This is true even with transgenic mice because the foundation stock may be different. Also, because gene insertion is random, knock-in models do not by definition contain the gene of interest at the same locus. Therefore, simple transgenics may not be sufficient to prove the role of any given trait because of positional insertion effects on both absolute gene expression and copy number variation (Warden & Fisler, 1997). Delineating the specific function of a candidate gene is difficult, if not impossible, without being able to precisely correlate the phenotype to the initiating mechanism of foam cell formation. The heterogenic background of the mice combined with the variable responses to the atherogenic diet confound the interpretation.

Despite these often overlooked limitations of extrapolating mouse studies to the human disease, research using transgenic mice has enhanced the concept that atherosclerosis is not a simple lipid disorder. New atherogenic theories must be explored to explain the occurrence of atherosclerotic heart disease in individuals displaying no dyslipidemia. Most of the more than twenty unique quantitative trait loci (QTL) identified in mice (Smith et al., 2006) do not influence plasma lipid levels or blood pressure (Allayee et al., 2003; Colinayo et al., 2003). This finding has been especially interesting because these QTL were identified in hypothesis-driven experiments exploring cholesterol metabolism in LDLR and/or apoE knockout mice. Many of these studies have demonstrated the strong genetic influence in the arterial wall on the susceptible and resistant phenotypic differences between mouse strains (Lusis et al., 2004). For example the major mouse QTL, Ath29 on chromosome 9, in the BXH ApoE(-/-) cross fed a chow diet was associated with early lesion development but not with risk factors including circulating lipids (Wang et al., 2007).

Knockout models theoretically mirror homozygous recessive forms of inherited disease because of the loss of gene function (Knowles & Maeda, 2000). As in familial hypercholesterolemia (FH), LDLR null mice experience a 2X increase in plasma cholesterol levels, even on a regular diet, that is further exacerbated on the high-fat, high-cholesterol atherogenic diet (Knowles & Maeda, 2000). The same is true for apoE null mice, although the mutation's impact on plasma cholesterol is greater than in the LDLR negative mice, with 4-5 times the normal amount of circulating lipoproteins (Knowles & Maeda, 2000; Zhang et al., 1992;). However, preliminary studies revealed no relationship between these elevated lipid levels and lesion size in apoE null mice (Zhang et al., 1994). Only 2% of the homozygous apoE2 null mice developed aortic lesions at all, and the contribution of this mutation to the overall human disease burden has been questioned (Visvikis-Siest & Marteau, 2006). Subsequent studies have shown contradictory results, as the nature of the lesion appears to be dependent on the parental strain used in the experiment rather than the particular knockout gene (Allayee et al., 2003; Getz, 2000; Sigmund, 2000; Smith et al., 2006).

The largest effect in these hyper-cholesterolemic models resulted from the macrophage colony stimulation factor (MCSF) impact on lesion progression (Knowles & Maeda, 2000). MCSF has been reported in advanced human atheromas, and this finding in mice lends experimental support to the role of the inflammatory response in atherosclerosis. However, the role of this molecule in atherogenesis per se is difficult to elucidate in the mouse, because of its chronically inflamed state.

Although not yet yielding consistent results applicable to human therapeutics (Yutzey & Robbins, 2007), transgenic mouse research has reinforced the importance of genetic background in determining atherosclerotic susceptibility or resistance in an individual. These studies have also suggested that the mechanism of foam cell formation varied among individuals under discrete experimental and/or environmental stimuli. The importance of the specific initiating mechanisms on the developing phenotype has been further demonstrated in rabbit models of atherosclerosis.

Rabbits, like hamsters, have CETP and do develop atherosclerotic foam cells when induced by an unnatural diet (Suckling & Jackson, 1993). Unlike the other animal models described in Table 1, rabbits are vegetarian, and so cholesterol is not a normal component of their wild-type diet. The Watanabe Heritable Hyperlipidemic (WHHL) rabbit was developed through selective breeding, and does not have LDLR (Watanabe et al., 1985;). WHHL rabbits get lesions along the aortic arch within six months, but do not experience thrombosis or myocardial infarction. However, these advanced atherosclerotic phenomena are observed in a sub-strain, the WHHLMI rabbit. This rabbit does get a heart attack similar to one of the human atherosclerotic (Shiomi et al., 2003) endpoints.

One of the important contributions of the rabbit model to understanding human disease was the observation that rabbit foam cells can be derived from smooth muscle cells (SMC) or macrophages, depending on the specific dietary perturbation (Weigensberg et al, 1985). This is in direct contrast to the mouse, where the predominant cell type in early lesions is always the macrophage, regardless of diet and genetic strain (Lusis, 2000). Rabbit myogenic foam cells are biochemically and morphologically distinct from macrophage derived foam cells, and both types of early lesions are structurally different from those produced by catheter injury (Weigensberg et al, 1985). Recognizing that different types of foam cells develop in response to different initiating mechanisms should help unravel the controversy of foam cell origin. In all probability, the predominant cell type in early atherogenesis is dependent on the pathological stimulus, and the specific model under study.

A second revelation from rabbit research has been that both macrophages and SMC express receptors for the MCSF protein (Inaba et al., 1992). The proto oncogene c-fms3 induces SMC migration and proliferation, as well as macrophage recruitment to the atherosclerosis-prone regions of the aorta (Mozes et al., 1998). This is important for atherogenesis investigations because the ratio of SMC to macrophages, both found in human lesions, changes as the disease progresses. The fact that both cell types share an activation mechanism means that the presence of MCSF in an experimental sample does not by definition mean that only macrophages will be recruited. This simple fact is not evident from the plethora of mouse studies, and is further evidence that multiple models are needed to grasp the complexity of human atherosclerosis, especially at the initiation stage.

Swine are unique among the other mammals depicted in Table 1 because, although they are LDL carriers like the hamster (Julien et al., 1981), and most lesions develop in the aortic arch, they also develop spontaneous lesions in the abdominal aorta. The initial foam cells are derived from intimal SMC (Scott et al., 1985), and appear similar to those found in early stages of the human disease. Unfortunately, these lesions do not progress to advanced atheromas without being induced by a 4% (w/w) cholesterol diet (Moghadasian et al., 2001). Even after 90 days on a hyperlipidemic diet, less than 5% of the cells are monocytes (Scott et al., 1985). Swine could adequately model the gradual transition from a myogenic fatty streak to an advanced lesion with activated macrophage cells, reflecting the inflammatory response in humans over time.

### 4.2 Pigeons

The WC pigeon is unique among non-primate models in that it develops naturally occurring (spontaneous) atherosclerosis at both the celiac bifurcation of the aorta and in the coronary arteries (Clarkson et al., 1959; Prichard et al., 1964). Foam cells develop into fatty streaks which progress into mature plaques in the absence of elevated plasma cholesterol and other traditional risk factors (Wagner, 1978; Wagner et al., 1979). These non-induced atherosclerotic lesions are morphologically and ultrastructurally similar to those seen in humans and occur at parallel anatomical sites along the arterial tree (Cornhill et al., 1980a, 1980b; Hadjiisky, et al., 1991; Kjaernes et al., 1981). Multiple studies have clearly demonstrated that susceptibility in the WC resides at the level of the arterial wall (St. Clair et al., 1986; Wagner et al., 1973, 1979;). Lesion site specificity, severity, and disease progression as a function of age are also highly predictable (Cooke & Smith, 1968; Santerre et al., 1972).

Show Racer pigeons (SR) are resistant to atherosclerosis, while consuming the same cholesterol-free diet. This susceptibility difference occurs despite similar plasma cholesterol and lipoprotein concentrations in both WC and SR (Barakat & St. Clair, 1985). WC pigeons are one of the few animal models to develop severe atherosclerosis while consuming a cholesterol free diet, and comparing results with the resistant SR enables pathological changes associated with the disease to be distinguished from changes due to the natural pigeon aging process. Virtually all WC and SR differences occur at the arterial tissue level as there are few system level differences (Fronek & Alexander, 1981).

Both pigeon breeds are hypercholesterolemic compared to humans, and, like mice and rabbits, they are primarily HDL carriers. However, pigeons are unique in that for the first three days of life, cholesterol is circulated in the form of LDL, after which time the lipoprotein profile switches to HDL (unpublished data) for the remainder of the pigeon's life. Neither breed has apoE (Randolph et al., 1984) or LDLR (Randolph & St. Clair, 1984; St. Clair et al., 1986), so the effect of these variables in other models of the human disease is not a factor in the pigeon pathology. Combined unpublished data gathered from several hundred birds aged 6 months to 3 years over a twenty-year period shows that the average plasma cholesterol concentration in pigeons ranges from 201 mg/dL in the SR to 242 mg/dL in the WC (+/- 16 mg/dL in both groups). Although these values are borderline significant, they do not change during disease progression, nor does it appear that blood cholesterol induces WC foam cell development. This fact is further supported in wild mourning doves, a close relative of the pigeon, that have 258 mg/dL average plasma cholesterol but do not get atherosclerosis (Schulz et al., 2000). Sterol balance studies have revealed that the WC excretes less neutral sterols than the SR breed (Siekert et al., 1975; Subbiah & Connelly, 1976), but this difference had much greater impact in diet-induced atherosclerosis than in the susceptible phenotype of the WC to the naturally occurring form of the disease (Hulcher & Margolis, 1982).

The most widely studied spontaneous atherosclerotic lesion in susceptible pigeons occurs at the celiac bifurcation of the aorta, and by three years of age reaches a size to be easily visible on gross examination (Nicolosi et al., 1972; Santerre et al., 1972). Early pathological and metabolic changes are apparent microscopically in this site by six months of age (Cooke & Smith, 1968). In contrast, diet-induced lesions in the WC aorta occur at various and unpredictable sites along the descending (Gosselin, 1979; Jerome & Lewis, 1985; Wagner, 1978) and abdominal aortas, and are pathologically very different from non-induced lesions. Foam cells in spontaneous lesions consist primarily of modified SMC (Cooke & Smith, 1968; St. Clair, 1983) while cholesterol-induced foam cells are mostly composed of macrophages (Denholm & Lewis, 1987; Gosselin, 1979; Jerome & Lewis, 1984; St. Clair, 1983).

As with mice, diet-induced lesions develop more rapidly in the pigeon than their spontaneous counterparts (Jerome & Lewis, 1984; Xu, 2004), but different atherogenic mechanisms appear to be involved (Santerre et al., 1972; St. Clair, 1983). One of the primary diet induction effects is to shift the physiological lipoprotein profile from HDL to LDL (Jones et al., 1991; Langelier et al., 1976). In fact, 1% diet supplementation with cholesterol causes such a rapid onset of atherosclerotic foam cells in both breeds that it becomes unfeasible to detect the influence of intrinsic factors (Lofland, 1966) contributing to either WC susceptibility or SR resistance. Therefore, the spontaneous lesion model is best suited for genetic studies to identify candidate genes for susceptibility or resistance as the introduction of an artificial diet confounds the interpretation of the earliest events occurring in atherogenesis.

Since 1959, many studies have been performed to systematically characterize the initiating factor in lesion development in the susceptible WC pigeon. However, the mechanism(s) leading to WC foam cell development is not known, and few studies have been conducted in the spontaneous model to identify the gene(s) or gene product(s) that are specific to initiation. Clarkson and associates (1959) observed that age and heredity were the biggest factors in atherosclerotic susceptibility. Diet, exercise, and gender were not primary factors in the WC pathology.

Further studies of age and heredity effects demonstrated that genetics play a larger role in lesion development than the normal aging process (Goodman & Herndon; 1963). The authors hypothesized that inheritance was a polygenic trait. Wagner and co-workers (1973) compared susceptibility to lesion development between the WC and SR celiac bifurcation of the aorta. The authors found a greater number of advanced lesions in the WC than in the SR, and concluded that the genetic control conferring susceptibility or resistance in the pigeon appeared to be at the level of the artery. Supplementary experiments by that group showed that blood cholesterol, triacylglycerol, and glucose levels were not different between the two breeds (Wagner, 1978), and that elevated blood pressure is actually a consequence of pigeon atherosclerosis, rather than being an initiating factor (Wagner et al., 1979). The latter study provided initial indications that although diet is not the primary factor contributing to atherosclerotic susceptibility in the pigeon, it can impact the severity of a lesion once formed; thus indicating a role in progression.

A range of metabolic differences between the arterial wall of WC and SR pigeons have been identified. In vivo, differences in the WC susceptible foci include increased glycosaminoglycans, especially chondroitin-6-sulfate (Curwen & Smith, 1977), greater lipid content, predominantly in the form of cholesterol esters (Hajjar et al., 1980b; Nicolosi et al., 1972), lower oxidative metabolism(Hajjar et al., 1980a; Santerre et al., 1974), relative hypoxia (Hajjar et al., 1988), decreased acid cholesterol hydrolase (Sweetland et al., 1999), and neutral cholesterol ester hydrolase (Fastnacht, 1993) activities, increased glycolysis (Zemplenyi & Rosenstein, 1975), decreased tricarboxylic acid cycle activity (Zemplenyi & Rosenstein, 1975), and the increased synthesis of prostaglandin E2, which also decreased cholesterol ester hydrolase activity (Subbiah et al., 1980). Although these studies did not distinguish the primary or underlying problem from secondary effects, increases in non-esterified fatty acids (NEFA) and in chondroitin-6-sulfate (C6S) seem to precede many of the other observed differences. The role of excess NEFA and C6S in pigeon atherogenesis is not yet clear, although the presence of C6S in the susceptible pigeon by six weeks of age does support the response to retention theory. Both human and pigeon smooth muscle cells synthesize C6S as part of the ECM (Edwards et al., 1995; Wight, 1985), where it has been observed to complex with plasma LDL entering the vascular wall (Nakashima et al., 2007; Tovar et al., 1998; Wagner et al., 1989; Wight, 1980).

Human atherosclerosis is considered to be a multifactorial disease, with many genes and environmental factors contributing to the specific phenotype and ultimate endpoint. In pigeons, where individual lifestyle choices are not a factor, the numbers and types of genes contributing to baseline susceptibility and resistance may be easier to elucidate. Preliminary crossbreeding studies indicated a polygenic mechanism of inheritance (Goodman & Herndon, 1963) with resistance being the dominant trait. However, the authors noted that each breed responded differently to dietary manipulation (Herndon et al., 1962), so it is possible that the genetic differences observed may have reflected the confounding influence of diet, rather than the spontaneous expression profile.

Pigeons are not as well suited for traditional inheritance studies as mammalian species because the birds mate for life, and do not reach sexual maturity until seven months of age (Brannigan, 1973). Although excess cholesterol esters can be detected biochemically at 12 weeks, three years are required in order to definitively characterize the complete atherosclerotic phenotype. However, the pigeon genome is approximately half the size of its counterpart mammalian models, and comparative genomic studies are facilitated by the published chicken (Gallus gallus) genome, which is similar in size (Hillier et al., 2004) to the pigeon.

A 15-year cross breeding study at the University of New Hampshire examined grossly visible lesions (or lack thereof) at three years of age in the celiac foci of susceptible WC, resistant SR, and in F1, F2, and backcross progeny. The results supported autosomal recessive inheritance of susceptibility to spontaneous atherosclerosis in the pigeon (Smith et al., 2001). This finding contrasted earlier results (Herndon et al., 1962) that indicated a polygenic mechanism based only on the F1 progeny, but the latter researchers carried the experiments through the backcross generations and did not use a cholesterol-supplemented diet (Smith et al., 2001). In addition, and probably of greater importance to the experimental results, all pigeons consumed the same cholesterol-free diet. Parallel investigation of the smooth muscle cells cultured from several tissues of the WC, SR, and F1 pigeons demonstrated that lipid accumulation observed at the celiac bifurcation is a constitutive property of WC (Smith et al., 2001).

The finding that spontaneous atherosclerosis in the susceptible WC appears to be the result of a single gene, and not the net result of many interacting genes, as is thought to be the case in humans, makes the pigeon model a simplest case system. Identification of the gene responsible for predisposition, and an understanding of how this gene influences the described metabolic and morphological changes could reveal an initiating mechanistic pathway that remains undetected in more confounded models of atherogenesis.

Experiments have demonstrated that the SMC monolayers grown in vitro accumulate lipid and synthesize proteoglycans in the same manner as aortic cells in vivo (Cooke & Smith, 1968; Smith et al., 1965; Wight, 1980; Wight et al., 1977) but at an accelerated rate. A comparison of the maturation and degeneration of pigeon aortic cells in vivo and in vitro is presented in **Table 2**. In culture, foam cell development is evident in WC SMC by 8-10 days, where several weeks are needed in order to observe the same phenomena in vivo. Other differences in the WC SMC include more esterified cholesterol present in lipid vacuoles, less arachidonate, and decreased mitochondrial metabolism. Although it has been demonstrated that the act of culturing aortic cells can change the SMC phenotype from contractile to synthetic (Worth et al., 2001), this has not been observed in primary cultures, where the lack of sub-culture minimizes potential genetic alterations. WC aortic cells obtained in vitro demonstrate a similar degenerative progression as those cells observed in the celiac bifurcation (Cooke & Smith, 1968; Wight et al., 1977), offering further evidence that the gene expression profile is comparable between the two model systems.

In vitro, there is no signal communication between SMC and endothelial cells, monocytes, hormones, neurotransmitters, other humoral factors, and whole body feedback systems (Shanahan & Weissberg, 1998; Thyberg et al., 1990). The only source of interaction is between the SMC and the media components, resulting in cell growth and ECM synthesis. This makes it possible to observe the intrinsic characteristics of WC and SR aortic cell development in a controlled, time-compressed setting, while limiting the number of genes under investigation to those specific to aortic SMC. Interestingly, although only the SMC of the WC celiac and coronary bifurcations are susceptible to atherogenesis in vivo, SMC taken from other WC tissue such as the gizzard or small intestine exhibit features in vitro similar to atherogenesis in aortic cells. This is not the case in the SR, where neither SMC from the celiac foci, nor SMC from any other tissue undergo phenotype modification when cultured under identical conditions.

The aforementioned experiments provide additional evidence that the genetic defect predisposing the WC to atherosclerosis is conditionally expressed in SMC. Factors that stimulate the expression of atherogenic genes at the celiac bifurcation in vivo appear to be present in vitro, as the cultured WC cells undergo degeneration parallel to their counterparts in aortic tissue (Cooke & Smith, 1968; Wight et al., 1977). Genetic factors denoting resistance in the SR remain expressed in both experimental environments.

| Approximate Age *(in vivo)* variable starting at 6 weeks | Salient Morphological Features | | Approximate Age *(in vitro)* |
|---|---|---|---|
| 1-10 days | Myoblasts<br>↓ | | 1-2 days |
| 10-18 days | Myofilaments increase<br>Organelles increase<br>Myofilaments align<br>↓<br>Formation of myofibrils<br>Dilation of ER<br>↓ ↓ | | 2-4 days |
| | Show Racer | White Carneau | |
| 1 day–6 months | Myofibrils enlarge<br>↓ | Extension & dilation of ER<br>Modified smooth muscle cell<br>↓ | 4-6 days |
| 2 weeks–2 years | Myofibrils increase<br>Organelles decrease<br>↓ | Pinched off cisternae of ER<br>Loss of ribosomes<br>Mitochondrial abnormalities<br>Lipid inclusions, vacuoles<br>Cell rounding<br>↓ | 6-8 days |
| | Mature smooth muscle cell | Foam cell | 8-10 days |

Table 2. Maturation and degeneration of pigeon aortic cells.

Anderson (2008) analyzed differential gene expression in vitro at day seven of cellular growth. Ninety-one genes were uniquely expressed in the susceptible WC cells compared to 101 genes exclusive to the resistant SR. There was a marked difference in energy metabolism between the two breeds. The SR VSMC expressed genes related to oxidative phosphorylation such as cytochrome B, cyctochrome C oxidase subunit I, NADH dehydrogenase subunit 4, ubiquinone, and ATP synthase subunit 4B. This was in direct contrast to the glycolytic genes expressed by the WC which included enolase, glucose phosphate isomerase, and lactate dehydrogenase subunit B.

In addition, genes expressed by the SR were indicative of a contractile VSMC phenotype whereas susceptible WC pigeons expressed genes that reflected a synthetic phenotype. Spondin, decorin, vimentin and beta actin were upregulated in the WC. Myosin heavy chain, myosin light chain kinase, tropomyosin, and alpha actin were expressed in the SR. The resistant SR appeared to develop and maintain an extracellular matrix with structural integrity, whereas the susceptible WC was already expressing proteases and immune signals.

Although many genes were different between the two breeds, the compressed time frame made it difficult to determine what happens first: changes in energy metabolism or changes in cellular phenoptye. Future in vivo studies are necessary to elucidate the chronological sequence of events and determine the single gene responsible for atherogenesis in the WC pigeon.

Analysis of SMC soluble proteins from WC and SR pigeons revealed differential expression between the two breeds. Eight discrete zones of molecular weight versus pI were identified, five which included only proteins unique to susceptible cells and three which included proteins unique to resistant cells. Eighty-eight differentially-expressed proteins were found in susceptible cells with 41 located in unique zones. Resistant cells had 29 of 82 differentially-expressed proteins in unique zones. Some annotated proteins, including smooth muscle myosin phosphatase, myosin heavy chain, fatty acid binding protein, ribophorin, heat shock protein, TNF alpha-inducing factor, and lumican, corresponded to genes identified previously or to current hypotheses to explain atherogenesis (Smith et al., 2008).

Additional research to identify the causative gene for spontaneous atherosclerosis will be facilitated by pigeon genome sequencing. Comparative studies between the resistant versus susceptible breeds may reveal sequence variation contributing to the disease. The pigeon remains an important model to study the genetic role at the site of lesion development that is associated with human atherosclerosis.

## 5. Acknowledgements

This is Scientific Contribution Number 2455 from the New Hampshire Agricultural Experiment Station.

## 6. References

Adams, L.D., Geary, R.L., Li, J., Rossini, A., & Schwartz, S.M. (2006). Expression profiling identifies smooth muscle cell diversity within human intima and plaque fibrous cap: loss of RGS5 distinguishes the cap. *Arteriosclerosis Thrombosis and Vascular Biology*, Vol. 26, 319-325

Adelman, S., & St. Clair, R. (1988). Lipoprotein metabolism by macrophages from atherosclerosis-susceptible White Carneau and resistant Show Racer pigeons. *Journal of Lipid Research*, Vol. 29, 643-656

Allayee, H., Ghazalpour, A., & Lusis, A.J. (2003). Using mice to dissect genetic factors in atherosclerosis. *Arteriosclerosis Thrombosis and Vascular Biology*, Vol. 23, 1501-1509

Anderson, J. L. (2008). Differentially expressed genes in aortic cells from atherosclerosis-resistant and atherosclerosis-susceptible pigeons. *Ph. D. Dissertation*, University of New Hampshire, Durham

Archacki, S.R., Angheloiu, G., Tian, X.L., Tan, F.L., DiPaola, N., Shen, G.Q., Moravec, C., Ellis, S., Topol, E.J., & Wang, Q. (2003). Identification of new genes differentially expressed in coronary artery disease by expression profiling. *Physiological Genomics*, Vol. 15, 65-74

Arndt, M., Lendeckel, U., Röcken, C., Nepple, K., Wolke, C., Spiess, A., Huth, C., Ansorge, S., Klein, H.U. & Goette, A. (2002). Altered Expression of ADAMs (a disintegrin and metalloproteinase) in fibrillating human atria. *Circulation*, Vol. 105, 720-725

Attie, A.D. (2001). *Atherosclerosis modified*. Circulation Research, Vol. 89, 102-104

Balis, J.U., Haust, M.D., & More, R.H. (1964). Electron-microscopic studies in human atherosclerosis: cellular elements on aortic fatty streaks. *Experimental and Molecular Pathology*, Vol. 3, 511-525

Barakat, H., & St. Clair, R. (1985). Characterization of plasma lipoproteins of grain- and cholesterol-fed White Carneau and Show Racer pigeons. *Journal of Lipid Research*, Vol. 26, 1252-1268

Bassiouny, H., Zarins, C., Kadowaki, M., & Glagov, S. (1994). Hemodynamic stress and experimental aortoiliac atherosclerosis. *Journal of Vascular Surgery*, Vol. 19, 426-434

Blanchette-Mackie, E.J., Dwyer, N.K., Amende, L.M., Kruth, H.S., Butler, J.D., Sokol, J., Comly, M.E., Vanier, M.T., August, J.T., Brady, R.O., & Pentchev, P.G. (1988). Type-C Niemann-Pick disease: low density lipoprotein uptake is associated with premature cholesterol accumulation in the golgi complex and excessive cholesterol storage in lysosomes. *Proccedings of the National Academy of Sciences USA*, Vol. 85, 8022-8026

Brannigan, D. (1973). Reproductive behavior and squab development in atherosclerosis-susceptible White Carneau and atherosclerosis-resistant show racer pigeons. *Ph. D. Dissertation*, University of New Hampshire, Durham

Breslow, J.L. (2000). Genetic differences in endothelial cells may determine atherosclerosis susceptibility. *Circulation*, Vol. 102, 5-6

Brown, M., Kovanen, P., & Goldstein, J. (1981). Regulation of plasma cholesterol by lipoprotein receptors. Science, Vol. 212, 628-635

Clarkson, T.B., Prichard, R.W., Netsky, M.G., & Lofland, H.B. (1959). Atherosclerosis in pigeons: its spontaneous occurrence and resemblance to human atherosclerosis. *American Medical Association Archives of Pathology*, Vol. 68, 143-147

Cohen, J.C., & Zannis, V.I. (2001). Genes affecting atherosclerosis. *Current Opinion in Lipidology*, Vol. 12, 93-95

Colinayo, V., Qiao, J.H., Wang, X., Krass, K.L., Schadt, E., Lusis, A.J., & Drake, T.A. (2003). Genetic loci for diet-induced atherosclerotic lesions and plasma lipids in mice. *Mammalian Genome*, Vol. 14, 464-471

Cooke, P., & Smith, S. C. (1968). Smooth muscle cells: source of foam cells in atherosclerotic White Carneau pigeons. *Experimental and Molecular of Pathology*, Vol. 8, 171-189

Cornhill, J., Akins, D., Hutson, M., & Chandler, A. (1980a). Localization of atherosclerotic lesions in the human basilar artery. *Atherosclerosis*, Vol. 35, 77-86

Cornhill, J., Levesque, M., & Nerem, R. (1980b). Quantitative study of the localization of sudanophilic coeliac lesions in the White Carneau pigeon. *Atherosclerosis*, Vol. 35, 103-10

Curwen, K., & Smith, S. (1977). Aortic glycosaminoglycans in atherosclerosis-susceptible and -resistant pigeons. *Experimental and Molecular Pathology*, Vol. 27, 121-133

Denholm, E., & Lewis, J. (1987). Monocyte chemoattractants in pigeon aortic atherosclerosis. *American Journal of Pathology*, Vol. 126, 464-475

Desvergne, B., Michalik, L., & Wahli, W. (2006). Transcriptional regulation of metabolism. *Physiological Reviews*, Vol. 86, 465-514

Edwards, I. J., Xu, H., Obunike, J. C., Goldberg, I. J., & Wagner, W. D. (1995). Differentiated macrophages synthesize a heparan sulfate proteoglycan and an oversulfated chondroitin sulfate proteoglycan that bind lipoprotein lipase. *Arteriosclerosis Thrombosis and Vascular Biology*, Vol. 15, 400-409

Faber, B., Heeneman, S., Daemen, M., & Cleutjens, K. (2002). Genes potentially involved in plaque rupture. *Current Opinion in Lipidology*, Vol. 13, 545-552

Faber, B.C., Cleutjens, K., Niessen, R.L., Aarts, P., Boon, W., Greenberg, A.S., Kitslaar, P., Tordoir, J. & Daemen, M. (2001). Identification of genes potentially involved in rupture of human atherosclerotic plaques. *Circulation Research*, Vol. 89, 547-554

Fastnacht, C. (1993). Egasyn-esterase activity in atherosclerosis-susceptible White Carneau and atherosclerosis-resistant Show Racer pigeon aortas. *M.S. Thesis*, University of New Hampshire, Durham

Fielding, C. (2000). Lipoprotein synthesis, transport, and metabolism, In: *Genetic Biochemical and Physiological Aspects of Human Nutrition,* M. Stipanuk, (Ed). pp 351-364, W.B. Saunders, ISBN 072164452X, Philadelphia

Forcheron, F., Legedz, L., Chinetti, G., Feugier, P., Letexier, D., Bricca, G., & Beylot, M. (2005). Genes of cholesterol metabolism in human atheroma: overexpression of perilipin and genes promoting cholesterol storage and repression of ABCA1 expression. *Arteriosclerosis Thrombosis and Vascular Biology,* Vol. 25, 1711-1717

Fronek, K. & Alexander, N. (1981). Genetic difference in the sympathetic nervous activity and susceptibility to atherosclerosis in pigeon. *Atherosclerosis*, Vol. 39, 25-33

Funke, H. & Assmann, G. (1999). Strategies for the assessment of genetic coronary artery disease risk. *Current Opinion in Lipidology*, Vol. 10, 286-291

Galton, D.J., & Ferns, G.A. (1989). Candidate genes for atherosclerosis, In: *Genetic Factors in Atherosclerosis: Approaches and Model Systems,* R.S. Sparkes & A.J. Lusis, (Eds). pp 95-109, Karger, ISBN 3805548907, Basel

Garcia, C.K., Wilund, K., Arca, M., Zuliani, G., Fellin, R., Maioli, M., Calandra, S., Bertolini, S., Cossu, F., Grishin, N., Barnes, R., Cohen, J.C., & Hobbs, H.H. (2001). Autosomal recessive hypercholesterolemia caused by mutations in a putative LDL receptor adaptor protein. *Science*, Vol. 292, 1394-1398

Getz, G.S. (2000). When is atherosclerosis not atherosclerosis? *Arteriosclerosis Thrombosis and Vascular Biology*, Vol. 20, 1694

Gibbons, G.H., Liew, C.C., Goodarzi, M.O., Rotter, J.I., Hsueh, W.A., Siragy, H.M., Pratt, R., & Dzau, V.J. (2004). Genetic markers: progress and potential for cardiovascular disease. *Circulation*, Vol. 109, 47-58

Goldstein, J.L., & Brown, M.S. (2001). The cholesterol quartet. Science, Vol. 292, 1310-1312

Goodman, H. O. & Herndon, C. N. (1963). Genetic aspects of atherosclerosis in pigeons. Federation Proceedings Vol. 22, Abstract 1336, Atlantic City, April 1963

Gosselin, E. J. (1979). A morphological and ultrastructural study of spontaneous and cholesterol-aggravated atherosclerosis in susceptible and resistant pigeons. *M.S. Thesis*, University of New Hampshire, Durham

Gurr, M.I. (1992). Dietary lipids and coronary heart disease: old evidence, new perspective. *Progress in Lipid Research*, Vol. 31, 195-243

Hadjiisky, P., Bourdillon, M., & Grosgogeat, Y. (1991). Experimental models of atherosclerosis. Contribution, limits and trends. *Archive Mal Coeur Vaiss*, Vol. 84, 1593-1603

Hajjar, D., & Smith, S. (1980a). Focal differences in bioenergetic metabolism of atherosclerosis-susceptible and -resistant pigeon aortas. *Atherosclerosis*, Vol. 36, 209-22

Hajjar, D., Farber, I., & Smith, S. (1988). Oxygen tension within the arterial wall: relationship to altered bioenergetic metabolism and lipid accumulation. *Archives of Biochemistry and Biophysics*, Vol. 262, 375-380

Hajjar, D., Wight, T., & Smith, S. (1980b). Lipid accumulation and ultrastructural change within the aortic wall during early spontaneous atherogenesis. *American Journal of Pathology*, Vol. 100, 683-706

Hartman, J.L., IV, Garvik, B., & Hartwell, L. (2001). Principles for the buffering of genetic variation. *Science*, Vol. 291, 1001-1004

Herndon, C. N., Goodman, H. O., Clarkson, T. B., Lofland, H. B., & Prichard, R. W. (1962). Atherosclerosis resistance and susceptibility in two breeds of pigeons. Genetics, Vol. 47, 958

Hillier, L. W. 171 co-authors., (2004). International Chicken Genome Sequencing Consortium. Sequence and comparative analysis of the chicken genome provide unique perspectives on vertebrate evolution. Nature, Vol. 432, 695-716

Hiltunen, M., Tuomisto, T.T., Niemi, M., Brasen, J.H., Rissanen, T.T., P Toronen, P., Vajanto, I., & Yla-Herttuala, S. Changes in gene expression in atherosclerotic plaques analyzed using DNA array. *Atherosclerosis*, Vol. 165, 23-32 (2002).

Hulcher, F., & Margolis, R. (1982). Rate-limiting, diurnal activity of hepatic microsomal cholesterol-7 alpha-hydroxylase in pigeons with high serum cholesterol. *Biochimica et Biophysica Acta*, Vol. 712, 242-249

Inaba, T., Yamada, N., Gotoda, T., Shimano, H., Shimada, M., Momomura, K., Kadowaki, T., Motoyoshi, K., Tsukada, T., & Morisaki, N. (1992). Expression of M-CSF receptor encoded by c-fms on smooth muscle cells derived from arteriosclerotic lesion. *Journal of Biological Chemistry*, Vol. 267, 5693-5699

Jerome, W., & Lewis, J. (1984). Early atherogenesis in White Carneau pigeons. I. leukocyte margination and endothelial alterations at the celiac bifurcation. *American Journal of Pathology*, Vol. 116, 56-68

Jerome, W., & Lewis, J. (1985). Early atherogenesis in White Carneau pigeons. II. ultrastructural and cytochemical observations. *American Journal of Pathology* 119, 210-222

Johns Hopkins University, (2011). Apolipoprotein E, MIM ID +107741, In: Online Mendelian Inheritance in Man (OMIM), 5/23/2011, Available from: http://www.ncbi.nlm.nih.gov/omim

Jones, N., Jerome, W., & Lewis, J. (1991). Pigeon monocyte/macrophage lysosomes during beta VLDL uptake. induction of acid phosphatase activity. a model for complex arterial lysosomes. *American Journal of Pathology*, Vol. 139, 383-392

Julien P, Downar E, & Angel A. (1981). Lipoprotein composition and transport in the pig and dog cardiac lymphatic system. Circulation Research, Vol. 49, 248-54

Katsuda, S., & Okada, Y. (1994). Vascular smooth muscle cell migration and extracellular matrix. *Journal of Atherosclerosis and Thrombosis*, Vol. 1 Suppl 1, S34-38

Khosla, P., & Sundram, K. (1996). Effects of dietary fatty acid composition on plasma cholesterol. *Progress in Lipid Research*, Vol. 35, 93-132

Kjaernes, M., Svindland, A., Walloe, L., & Wille, S. (1981). Localization of early atherosclerotic lesions in an arterial bifurcation in humans. *Acta Pathologica Microbiologica Scandanavia [A]*, Vol. 89, 35-40

Knowles, J.W., & Maeda, N. (2000). Genetic modifiers of atherosclerosis in mice. *Arteriosclerosis, Thrombosis and Vascular Biology,* Vol. 20, 2336-2345

Kuriyama, M., Yoshida, H., Suzuki, M., Fujiyama, J., & Igata, A. (1990). Lysosomal acid lipase deficiency in rats: lipid analyses and lipase activities in liver and spleen. *Journal of Lipid Research,* Vol. 31, 1605-1642

Langelier, M., Connelly, P., & Subbiah, M. (1976). Plasma lipoprotein profile and composition in White Carneau and Show Racer breeds of pigeons. *Canadian Journal of Biochemistry,* Vol. 54, 27-31

Lofland, H. B., Jr. (1966). Irradiation and atherosclerosis in pigeons. Nutrition Reviews, Vol. 24, 178-179

Lohse, P., Maas, S., Lohse, P., Sewell, A.C., van Diggelen, O.P., & Seidel, D. (1999). Molecular defects underlying Wolman disease appear to be more heterogeneous than those resulting in cholesteryl ester storage disease. *Journal of Lipid Research,* Vol. Res 40, 221-228

Lusis, A.J. (2000). Atherosclerosis. *Nature,* Vol. 407, 233-241

Lusis, A.J., Fogelman, A.M., & Fonarow, G.C. (2004). Genetic basis of atherosclerosis: part I: new genes and pathways. *Circulation,* Vol. 110, 1868-1873

Moghadasian, M.H., Frohlich, J.J., & McManus, B. M. (2001). Advances in experimental dyslipidemia and atherosclerosis. *Laboratory Investigation,* Vol. 81, 1173-1183

Mosse, P., Campbell, G., & Campbell, J. (1986). Smooth muscle phenotypic expression in human carotid arteries. II. Atherosclerosis-free diffuse intimal thickenings compared with the media. *Arteriosclerosis, Thrombosis and Vascular Biology,* Vol. 6, 664-669

Mosse, P., Campbell, G., Wang, Z., & Campbell, J. (1985). Smooth muscle phenotypic expression in human carotid arteries. I. Comparison of cells from diffuse intimal thickenings adjacent to atheromatous plaques with those of the media. *Laboratory Investigation,* Vol. 53, 556-562

Mozes, G., Mohacsi, T., Gloviczki, P., Menawat, S., Kullo, I., Spector, D., Taylor, J., Crotty, T.B., & O'Brien, T. (1998). Adenovirus-mediated gene transfer of macrophage colony stimulating factor to the arterial wall in vivo. *Arteriosclerosis Thrombosis and Vascular Biology,* Vol. 18, 1157-1163

Munro, J., & Cotran, R. (1988). The pathogenesis of atherosclerosis: atherogenesis and inflammation. *Laboratory Investigation,* Vol. 58, 249-261

Nakashima, Y., Fujii, H., Sumiyoshi, S., Wight, T.N., & Sueishi, K. (2007). Early human atherosclerosis: accumulation of lipid and proteoglycans in intimal thickenings followed by macrophage infiltration. *Arteriosclerosis Thrombosis and Vascular Biology,* Vol. 27, 1159-1165

Napoli, C., deNigris, F., Welch, J.S., Calaria, F.B., Stuart, R.O., Glass C.K., & Palinski, W. (2002). Maternal hypercholesterolemia during pregnancy promotes early atherogenesis in LDL receptor-deficient mice and alters aortic gene expression determined by microarray. *Circulation,* Vol. 105, 1360-1367

Nicolosi, R. J., Santerre, R. F., & Smith, S. C. (1972). Lipid accumulation in muscular foci in White Carneau and Show Racer pigeon aortas. Experimental and Molecular of Pathology, Vol. 17, 29-37

Ordovas, J., & Shen, A. (2002). Genetics, the environment, and lipid abnormalities. *Current Cardiology Reports,* Vol. 4, 508-513

Overturf, M., Smith, S.A., Gotto, A.M., Jr., Morrisett, J.D., Tewson, T., Poorman, J., & Loose-Mitchell, D.S. (1990). Dietary cholesterol absorption, and sterol and bile acid excretion in hypercholesterolemia-resistant white rabbits. *Journal of Lipid Research,* Vol. 31, 2019-2027

Pagani, F., Garcia, R., Pariyarath, R., Stuani, C., Gridelli, B., Paone, G., & Baralle, F.E. (1996). Expression of lysosomal acid lipase mutants detected in three patients with cholesteryl ester storage disease. *Human Molecular Genetics,* Vol. 5, 1611-1617

Palinski, W., & Napoli, C. (2002). The fetal origins of atherosclerosis: maternal hypercholesterolemia and cholesterol-lowering or antioxidant treatment during pregnancy influence in utero programming and postnatal susceptibility to atherogenesis. *FASEB Journal,* Vol. 16, 1348-1360

Papaspyridonos, M., Smith, A., Burnand, K.G., Taylor, P., Padayachee, S., Suckling, K.E., James, C.H., Greaves, D.R., & Patel, L. (2006). Novel candidate genes in unstable areas of human atherosclerotic plaques. *Arteriosclerosis Thrombosis and Vascular Biology,* Vol. 26, 1837-1844

Peltonen, L., & McKusick, V.A. (2001). Genomics and medicine: dissecting human disease in the postgenomic era. *Science,* Vol. 291, 1224-1229

Pitman, W.A., Hunt, M.H., McFarland, C., & Paigen, B. (1998). Genetic analysis of the difference in diet-induced atherosclerosis between the inbred mouse strains SM/J and NZB/BlNJ. *Arteriosclerosis Thrombosis and Vascular Biology,* Vol. 18, 615-620

Prichard, R., Clarkson, T., Goodman, H., & Lofland, H. (1964). Aortic atherosclerosis in pigeons and its complications. *Archives of Pathology,* Vol. 77, 244-257

Qin, Z., & Nishimura, H. (1998). Ca2+ signaling in fowl aortic smooth muscle increases during maturation but is impaired in neointimal plaques. *Journal of Experimental Biology,* Vol. 201, 1695-1705

Rader, D.J., & Pure, E. (2000). Genetic susceptibility to atherosclerosis: insights from mice. Circulation Research, Vol. 86, 1013-1015

Randolph, R. & St. Clair, R. (1984). Pigeon aortic smooth muscle cells lack a functional low density lipoprotein receptor pathway. *Journal of Lipid Research,* Vol. 25, 888-902

Randolph, R., Smith, B., & St. Clair, R. (1984). Cholesterol metabolism in pigeon aortic smooth muscle cells lacking a functional low density lipoprotein receptor pathway. *Journal of Lipid Research,* Vol. 25, 903-912

Ridker, P. (2000). New clue to an old killer: inflammation and heart disease. *Nutrition Action* Vol. 27, 3-5

Roberts, J.C., Jr., & Straus, R., (Eds). (1965). *Comparative Atherosclerosis; the Morphology of Spontaneous and Induced Atherosclerotic Lesions in Animals and its Relation to Human Disease,* Harper & Row, New York

Ross, R., & Glomset, J.A. (1973). Atherosclerosis and the arterial smooth muscle cell. *Science,* Vol. 180, 1332-1339

Santamarina-Fojo, S., Remaley, A. T., Neufeld, E. B. & Brewer, H. B., Jr. (2001). Regulation and intracellular trafficking of the ABCA1 transporter. *Journal of Lipid Research,* Vol. 42, 1339-1345

Santerre, R., Nicolosi, R., & Smith, S. (1974). Respiratory control in preatherosclerotic susceptible and resistant pigeon aortas. *Experimental and Molecular of Pathology,* Vol. 20, 397-406

Santerre, R., Wight, T., Smith, S., & Brannigan, D. (1972). Spontaneous atherosclerosis in pigeons. A model system for studying metabolic parameters associated with atherogenesis. *American Journal of Pathology*, Vol. 67, 1-22

Schulz, J., Bermudez, A., Tomlinson, J., Firman, J., & He, Z. (2000). Blood plasma chemistries from wild mourning doves held in captivity. *Journal of Wildlife Diseases,* Vol. 36, 541-545

Scott, R., Kim, D., & Schmee, J. (1985). Endothelial and lesion cell growth patterns of early smooth-muscle cell atherosclerotic lesions in swine. *Archives of Pathology and Laboratory Medicine,* Vol. 109, 450-453

Seals, D.F., & Courtneidge, S.A. (2003). The ADAMs family of metalloproteases: multidomain proteins with multiple functions. *Genes and Development*, Vol., 17, 7-30

Shanahan, C.M., & Weissberg, P.L. (1998). Smooth muscle cell heterogeneity: patterns of gene expression in vascular smooth muscle cells in vitro and in vivo. *Arteriosclerosis, Thrombosis and Vascular Biology,* Vol. 18, 333-338

Shanahan, C.M., Carey, N.R., Osbourn, J.K., & Weissberg, P.L. (1997). Identification of osteoglycan as a component of the vascular matrix. *Arteriosclerosis Thrombosis and Vascular Biology,* Vol. 17, 2437-2447

Shao, B., Oda, M., Oram, J., & Heinecke, J. (2006). Myeloperoxidase: an inflammatory enzyme for generating dysfunctional high density lipoprotein. *Current Opinion in Cardiology*, Vol. 21, 322-328

Shi, W., Brown, M.D., Wang, X., Wong, J., Kallmes, D.F, Matsumoto, A.H., Helm, G.A., Drake, T.A., & Lusis, A.J. (2003). Genetic backgrounds but not sizes of atherosclerotic lesions determine medial destruction in the aortic root of apolipoprotein E-deficient mice. *Arteriosclerosis Thrombosis and Vascular Biology,* Vol. 23, 1901-1906

Shiomi, M., Ito, T., Yamada, S., Kawashima, S., & Fan, J. (2003). Development of an animal model for spontaneous myocardial infarction (WHHLMI Rabbit). *Arteriosclerosis Thrombosis and Vascular Biology,* Vol. 23, 1239-1244

Siekert, R., Dicke, B., Subbiah, M., & Kottke, B. (1975). Cholesterol balance in atherosclerosis-susceptible and atherosclerosis-resistant pigeons. *Research Communications in Chemical Pathology and Pharmacology,* Vol. 10, 181-184

Sigmund, C.D. (2000). Viewpoint: are studies in genetically altered mice out of control? *Arteriosclerosis Thrombosis and Vascular Biology,* Vol. 20, 1425-1429

Smith, J.D., Bhasin, J.M., Baglione, J., Settle, M., Xu, Y., & Barnard, J. (2006). Atherosclerosis susceptibility loci identified from a strain intercross of apolipoprotein E-deficient mice via a high-density genome scan. *Arteriosclerosis Thrombosis and Vascular Biology,* Vol. 26, 597-603

Smith, S. C., Smith, E. C. Gilman, M. L. Anderson, J. L., and Taylor, R. L., Jr. (2008). Differentially expressed soluble proteins in aortic cells from atherosclerosis-susceptible and resistant pigeons. *Poultry Science*, Vol. 87, 1328-1334

Smith, S.C., Smith, E.C., & Taylor, R.L., Jr. (2001). Susceptibility to spontaneous atherosclerosis in pigeons: an autosomal recessive trait. *Journal of Heredity*, Vol. 92, 439-442

Smith, S.C., Strout, R.G., Dunlop, W.R., & Smith, E.C. (1965). Fatty acid composition of cultured aortic smooth muscle cells from White Carneau and Show Racer pigeons. *Journal of Atherosclerosis Research*, Vol. 5, 379-387

St Clair, R. (1983). Metabolic changes in the arterial wall associated with atherosclerosis in the pigeon. *Federation Proceedings*, Vol. 42, 2480-2485

St Clair, R. (1998). The contribution of avian models to our understanding of atherosclerosis and their promise for the future. *Lab Animal Science*, Vol. 48, 565-568

St. Clair, R., Leight, M., & Barakat, H. (1986). Metabolism of low density lipoproteins by pigeon skin fibroblasts and aortic smooth muscle cells. comparison of cells from atherosclerosis- susceptible and atherosclerosis-resistant pigeons. *Arteriosclerosis Thrombosis and Vascular Biology*, Vol. 6, 170-177

Stary, H. (1989). Evolution and progression of atherosclerotic lesions in coronary arteries of children and young adults. *Arteriosclerosis, Thrombosis and Vascular Biology* Vol. 9, 19-32

Stein, O., Thiery, J., & Stein, Y. (2002). Is there a genetic basis for resistance to atherosclerosis? *Atherosclerosis*, Vol. 160, 1-10

Strong, J.P., Malcom, G.T., McMahon, C.A., Tracy, R.E., Newman, W.P., Herderick, E.E., & Cornhill, J.F. (1999). Prevalence and extent of atherosclerosis in adolescents and young adults: implications for prevention from the pathobiological determinants of atherosclerosis in youth study. *Journal of the American Medical Association*, Vol. 281, 727-735

Subbiah, M., & Connelly, P. (1976). Effect of dietary restriction on plasma cholesterol and cholesterol excretion in the White Carneau pigeon. *Atherosclerosis*, Vol. 24, 509-13

Subbiah, M., Schweiger, E., Deitmeyer, D., Gallon, L. & Sinzinger, H. (1980). Prostaglandin synthesis in aorta of atherosclerosis susceptible and atherosclerosis resistant pigeons. *Artery*, Vol. 8, 50-55

Suckling, K.E., & Jackson, B. (1993). Animal models of human lipid metabolism. *Progress in Lipid Research*, Vol. 32, 1-24

Sweetland, R. (1999). Lysosomal acid lipase activity in atherosclerosis susceptible and resistant pigeon aortas. *M.S. Thesis*, University of New Hampshire, Durham

Tall, A., Breslow, J.L., & Rubin, E.M. (2001). Genetic disorders affecting plasma high-density lipoproteins, In: *The Metabolic and Molecular Bases of Inherited Disease*, C.R. Scriver, A.L. Beaudet, W.S. Sly, & D. Valle, (Eds). pp 2915-2936, McGraw-Hill, ISBN 0079130356, New York

Thyberg, J., Hedin, U., Sjolund, M., Palmberg, L., & Bottger, B. (1990). Regulation of differentiated properties and proliferation of arterial smooth muscle cells. *Arteriosclerosis, Thrombosis and Vascular Biology*, Vol. 10, 966-990

Tovar, A. M. F., Cesar, D. C. F., Leta, G. C., & Mourao, P. A. S. (1998). Age-related changes in populations of aortic glycosaminoglycans : species with low affinity for plasma low-density lipoproteins, and not species with high affinity, are preferentially affected. *Arteriosclerosis Thrombosis and Vascular Biology*, Vol. 18, 604-614

Tsimikas, S., Willerson, J.T., & Ridker, P. M. (2006). C-Reactive protein and other emerging blood biomarkers to optimize risk stratification of vulnerable patients. *Journal of the American College of Cardiology*, Vol. 47, 19-31

Visvikis-Siest, S. & Marteau, J. (2006). Genetic variants predisposing to cardiovascular disease. *Current Opinion in Lipidology*, Vol. 17, 139-151

Wagner, W. D., Clarkson, T. B., Feldner, H. B., Lofland, H. B., & Prichard, R. W. (1973). The development of pigeon strains with selected atherosclerosis characteristics. *Experimental and Molecular Pathology*, Vol. 19, 304-319

Wagner, W. D., Conner, J., & Labutta, T. (1979). Blood pressure in atherosclerosis-susceptible and -resistant pigeons. *Proceedings of the Society for Experimental Biology & Medicine*, Vol. 162, 101-104

Wagner, W.D. (1978). Risk factors in pigeons genetically selected for increased atherosclerosis susceptibility. *Atherosclerosis*, Vol. 31, 453-463

Wang, S.S., Shi, W., Wang, X., Velky, L., Greenlee, S., Wang, M.T., Drake. T.A., & Lusis, A.J. (2007). Mapping, genetic isolation, and characterization of genetic loci that determine resistance to atherosclerosis in C3H mice. *Arteriosclerosis Thrombosis and Vascular Biology*, Vol. 27, 2671-2676

Warden, C.H., & Fisler, J.S. (1997). Integrated methods to solve the biological basis of common disease. *Methods in Enzymology*, Vol. 13, 347-357

Watanabe, Y., Ito, T., & Shiomi, M. (1985). The effect of selective breeding on the development of coronary atherosclerosis in WHHL rabbits. An animal model for familial hypercholesterolemia. *Atherosclerosis*, Vol. 56, 71-9

Weigensberg, B., Lough, J., & More, R. (1985). Modification of two types of cholesterol atherosclerosis in rabbits by blocking lipoprotein lysine epsilon-amino groups. *Atherosclerosis*, Vol. 57, 87-98

Wight, T. (1980). Differences in the synthesis and secretion of sulfated glycosaminoglycans by aorta explant monolayers cultured from atherosclerosis-susceptible and -resistant pigeons. *American Journal of Pathology*, Vol. 101, 127-142

Wight, T. (1985). Proteoglycans in pathological conditions: atherosclerosis. *Federation Proceedings*, Vol. 44, 381-385

Wight, T., Cooke, P., & Smith, S. (1977). An electron microscopic study of pigeon aorta cell cultures: cytodifferentiation and intracellular lipid accumulation. *Experimental and Molecular Pathology*, Vol. 27, 1-18

Wissler, R.W., Hiltscher, L., Oinuma, T., and the PDAY Research Group. (1996). The lesions of atherosclerosis in the young: from fatty streaks to intermediate lesions, In: *Atherosclerosis and Coronary Artery Disease,* V. Fuster, R. Ross, & E.J. Topol, (Eds). pp 475–489, Lippincott-Raven Press, ISBN 978-078-1702-66-9, New York

Worth, N., Rolfe, B., Song, J.& Campbell, G. (2001). Vascular smooth muscle cell phenotypic modulation in culture is associated with reorganisation of contractile and cytoskeletal proteins. *Cell Motility and Cytoskeleton*, Vol. 49, 130-145

Xu, Q. (2004). Mouse models of arteriosclerosis: from arterial injuries to vascular grafts. *American Journal of Pathology,* Vol. 165, 1-10

Yutzey, K.E., & Robbins, J. (2007). Principles of genetic murine models for cardiac disease. *Circulation*, Vol. 115, 792-799

Zemplenyi, T., & Rosenstein, A. (1975). Arterial enzymes and their relation to atherosclerosis in pigeons. *Experimental and Molecular of Pathology*, Vol. 22, 225-41

Zhang, S., Reddick, R., Burkey, B., & Maeda, N. (1994). Diet-induced atherosclerosis in mice heterozygous and homozygous for apolipoprotein E gene disruption. *Journal of Clinical Investigation*, Vol. 94, 937-945

Zhang, S., Reddick, R., Piedrahita, J., & Maeda, N. (1992). Spontaneous hypercholesterolemia and arterial lesions in mice lacking apolipoprotein E. *Science,* Vol. 258, 468-471

# 3

# Illuminating Atherogenesis Through Mathematical Modeling

L. R. Ritter[1], Akif Ibragimov[2], Jay R. Walton[3]
and Catherine J. McNeal[4]
[1]*Department of Mathematics, Southern Polytechnic State University*
[2]*Department of Mathematics & Statistics, Texas Tech University*
[3]*Department of Mathematics, Texas A & M University*
[4]*Department of Internal Medicine, Division of Cardiology and Department of Pediatrics, Division of Endocrinology, Scott & White Hospital*
*USA*

## 1. Introduction

Mathematical Medicine is a relatively new and expanding area of Applied Mathematics research with a growing number of mathematicians, experimentalist, biomedical engineers, and research physicians involved in collaborative efforts on a global scale. Mathematical models are playing an increasing role in our understanding of such complex biological processes as the onset, progression, and mitigation of various diseases. The cardiovascular system is particularly intricate, and the formulation and analysis of mathematical models presents a myriad of challenges to the investigator. (See (Quarteroni, 2001) for a survey on the subject.) Mathematical studies of the cardiovascular system have included continuum mechanical models of vascular soft tissue (Holzapfel et al., 2000; Humphery & Rajagopal, 2002; Taylor & Humphrey, 2009), fluid dynamical models of the interaction between blood flow and vessel walls (Baek et al., 2007; Quarteroni, 2001; Veneziani, 1998), and mathematical models, such as that of the present work, of biochemical characteristics of the vasculature (Ibragimov et al., 2005; Neumann et al., 1990; Saidel et al., 1987). The disease of atherosclerosis, and its initiation atherogenesis, involves a complex interplay between mechanical, genetic, pathogenic, and biochemical processes. A comprehensive view of atherosclerosis will ultimately require integration of these various modeling perspectives. Herein, we focus on the inflammatory component of atherogenesis, in particular the role of immune cells–primarily macrophages–in the presence of oxidatively modified low density lipoproteins (LDL cholesterol) within the intimal layer of large muscular arteries. We present a mathematical model of the key inflammatory spiral that characterizes the initiation of atherosclerosis, and perform some analyses of this model.

It is well accepted that atherosclerosis is marked by chronic inflammation (Creager & Braunwald , eds.; Fan & Watanabe, 2003; Ross, 1995; 1999; Wilson , ed.). Changes in the permeability of the endothelial layer and subsequent deposition of lipids in the intima cause an up-regulation of chemoattractants such as monocyte chemotactic protein 1, interleukin-8 and macrophage colony-stimulating factor that are secreted by the endothelial and other cells. In addition, LDL molecules become trapped in the subendothelial intima where they are subject to oxidative modification by reactive oxygen species. Macrophages begin to accumulate in the region where they assume a pro-inflammatory phenotype. The stimulation of macrophages may be due to the presence of inflammatory extra-cellular matrix fragments. In addition, oxidized LDL is recognized by a macrophage scavenger receptor with some degree of interindividual variation (Boullier et al., 2001; Martín-Fuentes et al., 2007; Mosser & Edwards, 2008; Podrez et al., 2002). Macrophages attempting to internalize these particles may become engorged with cholesterol and transform into foam cells. In this state, these immune cells are incapable of performing the customary immune function and become part of a developing atherosclerotic lesion. The immune response is mediated by those chemical signals emitted by endothelial cell, immune cells, and immune cell derived foam cells. The *corruption* [1] of the immune process caused by ingestion of oxidized LDL can trigger an inflammatory response which results in increased immune cell migration to the site, possible further corruption, and ultimately accumulation of debris (necrotic, apoptotic, and lipid laden cells) characterizing plaque onset. This inflammatory spiral facilitated by chemotaxis, the process modeled herein, is a hallmark of atherogenesis.

It will become evident that our model incorporates many parameters characterizing such things as the rate at which macrophages move within the intimal tissue (independent of and in response to chemokines), rates of phenotype changes for macrophages, rates of phagocytosis and uptake of lipids by immune cells, degratation rates of various chemicals, chemical reaction rates and so forth. Some of these have value ranges that are known *in vitro* or *in vivo*, but many are unknown. The analytical techniques employed at present are linear stability studies. This allows us to obtain criteria based on the *relative* values of parameters and to interpret these criteria in terms of the propensity for a lesion to initiate—or not. These criteria will take the form of various inequalities in section 4.

In the next section, we lay out the disease paradigm and the assumptions upon which the mathematical model is constructed. This is followed by a presentation of the general model in the form of a system of nonlinear, primarily parabolic partial differential equations with mixed third type boundary conditions. In section 4, we perform stability analyses of the model under two different assumptions regarding the source of inflammatory components. Two stability theorems are given along with a bio-medical interpretation of the criteria derived. Also included is a discussion of the existence of unstable equilibria with a focus on the role of an antioxidant presence and the competing processes of macrophage motility (unrelated to chemotaxis) and chemotaxis. The chapter closes with a brief conclusion.

## 2. The disease paradigm and model basis

The large muscular arteries most vulnerable to atherosclerotic lesions can be considered as thick walled tubes consisting of three distinct layers. The outermost layer, called the adventitia, provides structural integrity through a strong collagen network. The middle layer, the media, provides flexibility and adaptability through layers of smooth muscle cells enmeshed in an elastin and collagen network. And the thin, innermost layer, called the intima, is where the atherosclerotic lesions begin to develop. A monolayer of endothelial cells forms an interface between the intima and the lumen through which blood flows. These endothelial cells are highly active in the circulatory process providing a smooth surface for fluid flow,

[1] The term "corruption" refers to the formation of foam cells due to the failure of the scavenger receptor to down regulate in response to excess cellular cholesterol content (Steinberg, 2002), and to the ability of C-reactive protein and oxLDL to increase the inflammatory properties of monocytes (Zhang & Wahl, 2006).

secreting anticoagulant, procoagulant, and inflammatory factors and regulating the exchange of cells and molecules between the blood and arterial wall. Insult to the endothelium and so called endothelial dysfunction is a precursor to atherosclerosis. A number of pathological conditions, genetic factors, and behavioral practices may result in endothelial dysfunction (Davignon & Ganz, 2004). This process appears to be characterized by a change in the permeability of the endothelial layer that allows lipids to migrate into the subendothelial layer followed by an influx of the cells that comprise the immune response. Following endothelial dysfunction and migration of lipoproteins and immune cells, we identify two significant steps to atherogenesis. These are oxidative modification of LDL, and the initiation of an inflammatory spiral.

### 2.1 Lipoprotein oxidation

Lipoproteins are micellar particles which contain regulatory proteins that direct the blood trafficking of cholesterol and other lipids to various cells in the body.. There are four major classes of lipoprotein–chylomicrons, very low-density lipoproteins (VLDL), low-density lipoproteins, and high-density lipoproteins (HDL)—but the bulk of cholesterol is contained in the latter two. Low density lipoproteins consist of a lipid core, a surface protein and a number of antioxidant defenses. LDLs deposit cholesterol in the tissues for cell metabolism. High density lipoproteins contain most of the remaining cholesterol in the body. These particles take excess lipids from tissues and return them to the liver for processing—the process referred to as reverse transport. Elevated plasma levels of LDL indicate a high risk of disease primarily because of their susceptibility to becoming trapped within the intima and subsequently attacked by radical oxygen species. The inflammation of atherosclerotic lesions occurs in areas of intimal thickening enriched by deposits of oxidized LDL.

The modification of LDL is a complicated process that has been the subject of several studies, and the reader is directed to the articles (Parthasarathy et al., 1992; Steinberg, 1997) and the review (Young & McEneny, 2001) and the references therein for a more complete and detailed description. Cobbold, Sherratt and Maxwell provided a mathematical model of the *in vitro* cascade of oxidation of LDL cholesterol in 2002 formulated according to a linear chemical reaction process (Cobbold et al., 2002). This model is adapted and included in the present model of atherogenesis. In brief, the mechanics of the process can be described as follows: In the tissue, where the concentration of reactive oxygen species (ROS) may be relatively high and external antioxidant defenses low, each interaction of an ROS and an LDL molecule will result in oxidizing one of the vitamin E molecules on the lipid surface. It is also possible that an oxidized vitamin E molecule ($\alpha$-tocopherol radical) may be reduced back to a vitamin E molecule by an antioxidant present (Niki et al., 1984; Watanabe et al., 1999). If, through a finite sequence of oxidation of vitamin E molecules, an LDL molecule losses all of its innate defense against free radical attack, it is susceptible to peroxidation of its lipid core. Once fully modified, the oxidized LDL is both attractive to macrophages and unable to leave the intima (unlike oxidized HDL particles (Tall, 1998)).

### 2.2 The inflammatory response

Accompanying the permeability changes to the endothelium and the influx of lipids is the immune response. Various white blood cells (monocytes, T-lymphocytes, neutrophils) migrate into tissues in response to chemical signals. Once in the subendothelial intima, monocytes differentiate into macrophages. Under normal healthy conditions, these immune cells aid in the degradation of apoptotic cells as well as the removal of foreign agents such as bacteria or viruses through phagocytosis. As stated, macrophages have a high affinity for oxidized LDL. However, attempts to take up the modified lipids by the process of phagocytosis are unsuccessful, and the lipid laden macrophages transform into foam cells (Goldstein et al., 1977; Podrez et al., 2002; Steinberg, 1997). Unable to perform their normal immune function, these lipid-laden cells signal other immune cells to the site precipitating accumulation of fatty tissue and the progression toward plaque growth. Additional chemical signals secreted by the foam cells and endothelial cells summon more immune cells to the site. Additional macrophages migrate to the localized site of inflammation. The chemical mediators of inflammation can increase binding of oxidized LDL to cells in the arterial wall (Hajjar & Haberland, 1997). Hence, the new macrophages become engorged with oxidized LDL and the cycle of chemical signaling continues.

The role of macrophages in initiation of an atherosclerotic lesion is complicated and far from singular. [2] In addition to foam cells, apoptotic macrophages are regularly found in lesions. Apoptosis of cells (macrophage and others) within a plaque is found to have both stabilizing as well as destabilizing affects (Cui et al., 2007; Tabas, 2004). Phagocytosis of apoptotic cells (not necessarily macrophages) may induce resistance to foam cell formation among macrophages. This occurs when during phagocytosis, the macrophage takes in high levels of membrane-derived cholesterol as opposed to lipoprotein-derived cholesterol. In Cui *et al.* , the authors report that ingestion of apoptotic cells induced a survival response in the macrophages in their experiments (Cui et al., 2007). It is also known that macrophages appear in different phenotypes that are non-static in the sense that they may change types—a process that is reversible (Kadl et al., 2010; Mosser & Edwards, 2008; Stout et al., 2005), and that the different types serve opposing functions (e.g. inflammatory versus anti-inflammatory). Moreover, the sources of additional immune cells include transport across the endothelium as well as migration via the vasa vasorum that provides blood to the artery wall. The mathematical model is constructed to allow for the diverse functions of the immune cells. (For a mathematical study similar to that presented here that focuses primarily on the competing role of inflammatory and anti-inflammatory macrophages, we direct you to the article (Ibragimov et al., 2008).)

## 3. The mathematical model

We begin by identifying the key chemical and cellular species involved in atherogenesis. For each species, an evolution equation is derived through the classical approach of imposing a mass balance in an arbitrary control volume and subsequent reduction to a pointwise statement. We do not consider here the volume of a lesion but rather the concentration of each species at any point.

Our model consists of five classes of generalized species–two cellular and three chemical–that have critical roles in the initiation of an atherosclerotic lesion. These classes are labeled and denoted as follows:

$\mathcal{I}$ Immune cells: These are primarily monocyte derived macrophages but may include other white blood cells (T-cells and perhaps neutrophils).

$\mathcal{D}$ Debris: This is the bulk of a forming lesion consisting of apoptotic cells, macrophage derived foam cells, and potentially necrotic tissue . Our use of the term *debris* is unconventional in the sense that we do not intend to suggest that these are inert cells

[2] The reader is directed to the article Mosser & Edwards (2008) for an excellent review of the array of macrophage phenotypes and functions.

or simply a byproduct of some process and merely occupy space. As will be seen in the mathematics to follow, this species type plays a pivotal role in the inflammatory feedback.

$\mathcal{C}$ Chemoattractant: This chemical species represents any of a number of cytokines and chemotactic molecules including macrophage colony stimulating factor, monocyte chemotactic protein-1, and various interleukin proteins. Any chemical that is used in the regulation of the immune response primarily through inducing chemotaxis is included in this species type.

$\mathcal{L}$ & $\mathcal{L}_{ox}$ Low density lipoproteins: The LDL species consists of two major sub-types, those in a native (un-oxidized) state, and those molecules that have undergone full peroxidation of the lipid core.

$\mathcal{R}$ Reactive oxygen species: These are free radical molecules that induce oxidative damage to the lipoproteins present. This species is a byproduct of various metabolic processes within the arterial wall.

Also included in the model are several input parameters. Of particular interest are the parameters $A_{ox}$, that is a level of antioxidants such as vitamins C, E, and beta-carotene, and $\mathcal{L}_B$ representing the serum concentration of LDL.

Each of the representative variables here is a vector with each component representing a specific member of the class. For example,

$$\mathcal{I} = (\mathcal{I}_1, \mathcal{I}_2, \ldots, \mathcal{I}_{N_I})^T$$

where each component $\mathcal{I}_i$, $i = 1, \ldots, N_I$ may be a different specific white blood cell, a different phenotype, or may represent cells in different roles. We allow for $\mathcal{I}$ to have $N_I$ components, $\mathcal{D}$ to have $N_D$, $\mathcal{C}$ to have $N_C$, $\mathcal{L}$ to have $N_L + 1$[3], and each of $\mathcal{L}_{ox}$ and $\mathcal{R}$ are scalar valued.

If we isolate any representative variable $u$ from this list, we construct an equation of the form

$$\frac{\partial u}{\partial t} = -\nabla \cdot \mathbf{J}_u + Q_u$$

that equates the evolution of the concentration of species $u$ to a spatial flux field $\mathbf{J}_u$ and any net source $Q_u$ due to cellular interactions, chemical secretion or uptake, chemical reactions, and the like. The flux fields and source terms are outline below for each variable.

### 3.1 Governing equations

The equations governing these species and based upon the disease paradigm outlined in section 2 are

$$\frac{\partial}{\partial t}\mathcal{I}_i = \mu_{I_i}\nabla^2\mathcal{I}_i - \nabla \cdot \left( \sum_{k=1}^{N_c} \chi_{ik}(\mathcal{C}_k, \mathcal{I}_i)\nabla\mathcal{C}_k \right) - \\ - \sum_{k=1}^{N_D} a_{ik}\mathcal{D}_k\mathcal{I}_i - \sum_{k=1, k\neq i}^{N_I} b_{ik}\mathcal{I}_k\mathcal{I}_i - c_i\mathcal{I}_i\mathcal{L}_{ox} - d_{1i}\mathcal{I}_i, \qquad (3.1)$$

[3] The model of LDL oxidation presented by Cobbold, Sherratt and Maxwell includes LDL molecules in a fully native state containing $N_L$ vitamin E molecules. Studies show the number of such antioxidant defenses is on average 6 per LDL molecule but may vary from 3 to 15 (Esterbauer et al., 1992; Stocker, 1999). We then consider $\mathcal{L}_i$ to contain $i$ vitamin E molecules where $\mathcal{L}_0$ represents LDL molecules completely depleted of native vitamin E that has yet to undergo full oxidation of its core.

$$\frac{\partial}{\partial t}\mathcal{D}_i = \mu_{D_i}\nabla^2\mathcal{D}_i + \tau_i\sum_{k=1}^{N_I}(c_k + f_k)\mathcal{I}_k\mathcal{L}_{ox} - \sum_{k=1}^{N_I}\hat{a}_{ik}\mathcal{I}_k\mathcal{D}_i - d_{2i}\mathcal{D}_i, \tag{3.2}$$

$$\frac{\partial}{\partial t}\mathcal{C}_i = \mu_{C_i}\nabla^2\mathcal{C}_i + \sum_{k=1}^{N_D}p_{ik}\mathcal{D}_k\mathcal{C}_i - \sum_{k=1}^{N_I}e_{ik}\mathcal{I}_k\mathcal{C}_i - d_{3i}\mathcal{C}_i, \tag{3.3}$$

$$\frac{\partial}{\partial t}\mathcal{L}_{N_L} = \mu_{L_{N_L}}\nabla^2\mathcal{L}_{N_L} - k_R\mathcal{R}\mathcal{L}_{N_L} + k_A A_{ox}\mathcal{L}_{N_L-1} - d_{4N_L}\mathcal{L}_{N_L}, \tag{3.4}$$

$$\frac{\partial}{\partial t}\mathcal{L}_i = \mu_{L_i}\nabla^2\mathcal{L}_i + k_R\mathcal{R}(\mathcal{L}_{i+1} - \mathcal{L}_i) - k_A A_{ox}(\mathcal{L}_i - \mathcal{L}_{i-1}) - - d_{4i}\mathcal{L}_i, \quad 1 \leq i \leq N_L - 1 \tag{3.5}$$

$$\frac{\partial}{\partial t}\mathcal{L}_0 = \mu_{L_0}\nabla^2\mathcal{L}_0 + k_R\mathcal{R}\mathcal{L}_1 - k_A A_{ox}\mathcal{L}_0 - k_{Ro}\mathcal{R}\mathcal{L}_0 - d_{40}\mathcal{L}_0, \tag{3.6}$$

$$\frac{\partial}{\partial t}\mathcal{L}_{ox} = \mu_{L_{ox}}\nabla^2\mathcal{L}_{ox} + k_{Ro}\mathcal{R}\mathcal{L}_0 - \sum_{k=1}^{N_I}f_k\mathcal{I}_k\mathcal{L}_{ox}, \tag{3.7}$$

$$\frac{\partial}{\partial t}\mathcal{R} = \mu_R\nabla^2\mathcal{R} - \sum_{k=1}^{N_L}k_R\mathcal{R}\mathcal{L}_k - k_{Ro}\mathcal{R}\mathcal{L}_0 - hA_{ox}\mathcal{R} + \mathbf{p}_R. \tag{3.8}$$

The various parameters appearing in (3.1)–(3.8) require explanation; a succint description of each is given in table 1. Each species is subject to diffusion, or diffusive motility in the case of immune cells, and this is reflected in the flux terms $\mu_u\nabla^2 u$ ($u$ represents any of the various state variables $\mathcal{I}$–$\mathcal{R}$) with the coefficient $\mu$ with a subscript a measure of the motility or diffusive capability of the respective species.

| | |
|---|---|
| $\chi_{ik}$ | chemotactic sensitivity of immune species $i$ to chemical stimulant $k$ |
| $a_{ik}, \hat{a}_{ik}$ | binding of immune cells to the lesion for removal |
| $b_{ik}$ | measure of subspecies interaction for immune cells |
| $c_i, f_i$ | rates of foam cell formation |
| $d_{ni}$ | cell turn over or chemical degradation rate |
| $p_{ik}$ | rate of chemical attractant production due to the lesion presence |
| $e_{ik}$ | uptake of chemoattractant during chemotaxis |
| $k_R, k_{R_0}, k_A$ | rate of oxidation, peroxidation, and reverse (anti-oxidation), respectively |
| $d_{ni}$ | cell turn over or chemical degradation rate |
| $p_{ik}$ | rate of chemical attractant production due to the lesion presence |
| $e_{ik}$ | uptake of chemoattractant during chemotaxis |
| $\tau_i, h$ | efficiency factors |
| $p_R$ | production of free-radicals due to normal metabolism |

Table 1. Bio-physiological Interpretation of Parameters

The terms $\chi_{ik}(\mathcal{C}_k, \mathcal{I}_i)\nabla\mathcal{C}_k$ are the contribution to the flux field for macrophages due to chemotaxis. The coefficient $\chi_{ik}(\mathcal{C}_k, \mathcal{I}_i)$ is the chemo-tactic sensitivity of immune cell $i$ to chemoattractant $k$. This is the classic Keller-Segal model of chemotaxis (Keller & Segel, 1971). The dependence of $\chi_{ik}$ on the immune cells is generally taken to be linear, however there is no present need to specify a particular form for these functions. Each of the immune cells, debris, chemoattractants, and native LDL species may undergo natural turnover or chemical degradation represented by the last terms in equations (3.1)–(3.6).

The immune cell equations contain three significant cross interaction terms. The terms $a_{ik}\mathcal{D}_k\mathcal{I}_i$ capture binding of macrophages with debris—in particular, these and the analogous terms $\hat{a}_{ik}\mathcal{I}_k\mathcal{D}_i$ in (3.2), account for phagocytosis of debris by healthy macrophages and removal for future processing in the liver. We also allow for inter-species interactions via the terms $b_{ik}\mathcal{I}_k\mathcal{I}_i$

in (3.1). This accounts, for example, for potential change of phenotype of macrophages during the inflammatory process. Recent studies have demonstrated that such changes may occur (reversibly) in vitro and in animal models (Kadl et al., 2010; Stout et al., 2005). Finally, the formation of foam cells through binding with oxidized LDL appears in equations (3.1) and (3.7) in the removal terms $c_i\mathcal{I}_i\mathcal{L}_{ox}$ and $f_k\mathcal{I}_k\mathcal{L}_{ox}$. This foam cell formation appears as a source term in equation (3.2) as $\tau_i \sum_{k=1}^{N_I}(c_k + f_k)\mathcal{I}_k\mathcal{L}_{ox}$, where $0 \leq \tau_i \leq 1$, $\sum_{i=1}^{N_D} \tau_i = 1$. The parameter $\tau_i$ allows us to catagorize different contributions to the lesion—different types of *debris*.
The equation for the chemoattractants includes (in addition to those terms already mentioned) a source term reflecting production of these chemicals in response to the presence of debris $p_{ik}\mathcal{D}_k\mathcal{C}_i$. The removal terms $e_{ik}\mathcal{I}_k\mathcal{C}_i$ represent the reduction of the chemoattractant concentration by binding with macrophages during chemotaxis.
As stated, the equations governing the lipid oxidation reactions (3.4)–(3.8) are a modification of the model of lipoprotein oxidation presented by Cobbold, Sherratt and Maxwell in 2002 (Cobbold et al., 2002). The chemical kinetics are assumed to be a linear reaction model in which an LDL molecule containing $i$ vitamin E particles reacts with a reactive oxygen species, with reaction rate $k_R$ to produce an LDL molecule with $i-1$ vitamin E molecules. This model also allows for the reverse oxidation reaction in that an LDL molecule with $i < N_L$ vitamin E molecules may react with the antioxidant species $A_{ox}$, with reaction rate $k_A$, to produce an LDL molecule with $i+1$ vitamin E defenses. Any LDL molecule that has been completely depleted of its native antioxidant defenses contributes to the concentration $\mathcal{L}_0$. A subsequent reaction of an $\mathcal{L}_0$ molecule with an ROS (with reaction rate $k_{R_0}$) results in peroxidation of the lipid core and a fully modified LDL particle. The ROS is depleted through these reactions and through direct reaction with the anti-oxidant species–the latter occurring with the rate of reaction $h$ appearing in equation (3.8). The primary source of ROS is as a byproduct of metabolic processes within the intima. The term $\mathbf{p}_R$ represents this source. The reader is encouraged to see (Cobbold et al., 2002) for a detailed construction of the model.
The modifications of Cobbold-Sherratt-Maxwell model presented here are two fold. First, we allow for spatial variation through a standard Fickian diffusion. More significant to the study of atherogenesis, we include the uptake of modified LDL by macrophages leading to foam cell formation and subsequent inflammation. The terms $f_k\mathcal{I}_k\mathcal{L}_{ox}$ represent removal of oxidized LDL through macrophage binding and the contribution to the forming lesion as seen in (3.2), (3.7) and (3.8).

### 3.2 Domain and boundary conditions

The system (3.1)–(3.8) can be considered in two or three spatial dimensions. In (Ibragimov et al., 2005), the current authors performed numerical simulations of a simplified model accounting only for immune cells, debris, chemoattractant, and later smooth muscle cells (a species not considered here as we are interested only with the earliest onset of cellular aggregation). Such simulations were performed in a two dimensional annular domain, and demonstrated the ability of the model to produce such features as localization of immune cells during inflammation and localized aggregation. The subsequent focus has been on illuminating the interplay of the various parameters by considering the initiation of inflammation as due to an instability in an equilibrium state. The general spatial regime considered is a deformed annulus (in two dimensions) or a deformed annular tube (in three spatial dimensions). In either case, the mathematical domain $\Omega$ is intended to represent the tunica intima, the innermost subendothelial layer of an arterial wall. The annulus, or annular tube, has an inner and outer boundary denoted by $\Gamma_I$ and $\Gamma_O$, respectively. The inner boundary $\Gamma_I$ corresponds to the monolayer of endothelial cells that form the interface between the arterial wall and the lumen, while the boundary $\Gamma_O$ represents the inner elastic lamina that separates the intima from the media. In the following analyses, we will assume that there is no transport of any species across the boundary $\Gamma_O$. While there may well be some transport across this elastic lamina—in particular of free radicals due to metabolic processes within the media—we will assume here that any such contribution is negligible relative to production, consumption, and inter-species reactions within the intima.

Influx through the inner boundary $\Gamma_I$ is for some species a significant source in the model. In particular, the chemoattractant and native LDL are subject to a third type boundary condition on $\Gamma_I$ modeling transport in response to a chemical potential across the endothelial cells. This corresponds mathematically to the conditions

$$-\mu_{C_i}\frac{\partial \mathcal{C}_i}{\partial \mathbf{n}} = \alpha_{C,i}(\mathcal{C}_i - \mathcal{C}_*), \quad \text{and} \tag{3.9}$$

$$-\mu_{L_{N_L}}\frac{\partial \mathcal{L}_{N_L}}{\partial \mathbf{n}} = \alpha_L(\mathcal{L}_{N_L} - \mathcal{L}_B). \tag{3.10}$$

Here, $\mathbf{n}$ is the outward unit normal to $\Gamma_I$, $\mathcal{C}_*$ is a baseline level of chemoattractant present at the endothelium, and $\mathcal{L}_B$ is the serum level of LDL. The parameters $\alpha_{C,i}$ are assumed to be non-negative. However, the sign of $\alpha_L$ is not specified so that (3.10) may correspond with either forward transport of native LDL into the subendothelial intima or reverse transport of native LDL into the blood. We assume here that LDL in the blood stream is fully native (has undergone no free radical attack) so that only native LDL is capable of either forward or reverse transport.

The immune cells are also subject to transport across the endothelium. The mechanism here is a chemo-tactic sensitivity regulated by the level of chemoattractant at the endothelium. The boundary condition is therefore a mixed third type condition with the flux of immune cells dependent on the chemoattractant species.

$$-\mu_{I_i}\frac{\partial \mathcal{I}_i}{\partial \mathbf{n}} = -\alpha_{I,i}(\mathcal{C}). \tag{3.11}$$

Each function $\alpha_{I,i}(\mathcal{C})$, $i = 1, \ldots, N_I$ is a nonnegative monotone function of the vector $\mathcal{C}$ of chemoattractants [4].

The remaining boundary conditions are

$$\frac{\partial Y}{\partial \mathbf{n}} = 0, \quad Y = \mathcal{D}, \mathcal{L}_i, \mathcal{L}_{ox}, \mathcal{R} \quad i = 0, \ldots, N_L - 1, \quad \text{on} \quad \Gamma_I$$

$$\frac{\partial Y}{\partial \mathbf{n}} = 0, \quad Y = \mathcal{I}, \mathcal{C}, \mathcal{D}, \mathcal{L}, \mathcal{L}_{ox}, \mathcal{R} \quad \text{on} \quad \Gamma_O. \tag{3.12}$$

This is the mathematical representation of the previous statement that no transport of any species across the inner elastic lamina separating the intima and the media is considered significant relative to the interactions within the intima, and that only fully native LDL,

[4] We can state the boundary condition for the immune cells in the more general form

$$\mathbf{J}_{I_i} \cdot \mathbf{n} = -\bar{\alpha}_{I,i}(\mathcal{C})$$

where $\mathbf{J}_{I_i} = -\left(\mu_{I_i}\nabla\mathcal{I}_i - \sum_{k=1}^{N_c}\chi_{ik}(\mathcal{C}_k, \mathcal{I}_i)\nabla\mathcal{C}_k\right)$ is the flux field for the $i^{th}$ immune cell species, and $\bar{\alpha}_{I,i}$ is a corresponding reformulation of the right hand side of (3.11).

immune cells and chemoattractant enter into the system via the endothelial layer. We may further consider the completely homogeneous Neumann conditions under the conditions that $\alpha_{C,i} = \alpha_L = \alpha_{I,i} = 0$. This closed system requires a modification of (3.1) to include a source term. This may be interpreted as modeling the vasa vasorum as the sole source of immune cells contributing to the inflammatory process. In reality, supply both via the vasa vasorum and via transport across the endothelium occur simultaneously. Study of the two extreme cases considered here is done to illuminate both the biological and mathematical differences these two delivery mechanisms make in the modeling and analysis.

## 4. Mathematical analysis of the model

There are several approaches to analyzing a particular mathematical model including numerical simulations, asymptotic and perturbation methods, and stability analyses. As suggested, the last of these, stability analyses, is particularly applicable under the present circumstances since we do not have experimental data from which to glean relevant ranges for many of the parameters. A classical approach to mathematical models of biological phenomena—especially those characterized by pattern formation, morphogenesis, and aggregation (Keller & Segel, 1971; Murray, 2002; Turing, 1952), is to consider significant state changes as resulting from a mathematical instability. This will result in the criteria based on relative parameter ranges. The inequalities will depend not only on the relationships between parameter ranges, but also on the source of inflammatory factors, and on the size of the domain (intimal thickness).

We present stability analyses of the system (3.1)–(3.8) under some specified conditions. The system considered throughout this section will be simplified to account for one of each of the species types $\mathcal{I}, \mathcal{D}, \mathcal{C}$, one native LDL species (which may be considered an averaging over each of $\mathcal{L}_i$), an oxidized LDL species, and free-radicals. The system of equations is

$$\frac{\partial \mathcal{I}}{\partial t} = \mu_I \nabla^2 \mathcal{I} - \nabla \cdot (\chi(\mathcal{I}, \mathcal{C}) \nabla \mathcal{C}) - d_1 \mathcal{I} - c\mathcal{I}\mathcal{L}_{ox} - a\mathcal{I}\mathcal{D} + M\phi_0 \tag{4.1}$$

$$\frac{\partial \mathcal{D}}{\partial t} = \mu_D \nabla^2 \mathcal{D} + \hat{c}\mathcal{I}\mathcal{L}_{ox} - \hat{a}\mathcal{I}\mathcal{D} - d_2 \mathcal{D} \tag{4.2}$$

$$\frac{\partial \mathcal{C}}{\partial t} = \mu_C \nabla^2 \mathcal{C} + p\mathcal{D} - e\mathcal{C}\mathcal{I} - d_3 \mathcal{C} \tag{4.3}$$

$$\frac{\partial \mathcal{L}}{\partial t} = \mu_L \nabla^2 \mathcal{L} - k_R \mathcal{L}\mathcal{R} + k_A A_{ox} r \mathcal{L}_{ox} - d_4 \mathcal{L} \tag{4.4}$$

$$\frac{\partial \mathcal{L}_{ox}}{\partial t} = \mu_{L_{ox}} \nabla^2 \mathcal{L}_{ox} + k_{R_0} \mathcal{L}\mathcal{R} - A_{ox} r \mathcal{L}_{ox} - f\mathcal{I}\mathcal{L}_{ox} \tag{4.5}$$

$$\frac{\partial \mathcal{R}}{\partial t} = \mu_R \nabla^2 \mathcal{R} - k_R \mathcal{L}\mathcal{R} - h A_{ox} \mathcal{R} + p_{\mathcal{R}}. \tag{4.6}$$

The modification to (3.1) appearing in (4.1) includes the source term of macrophages via the vasa vasorum as previously indicated (which may be set to zero if appropriate.) Since we are considering only one native LDL species, we also modify the equations to allow for reverse oxidation of oxidized LDL and allow for an efficiency factor $r$ for such reactions. Subscripts have been eliminated where they are no longer needed. For ease of notation $\hat{c} = c + f$.

Our analysis of (4.1)–(4.6) consists of a linear stability analysis using an energy estimate—i.e. Lyapunov functional—approach. That is, we consider certain equilibrium solutions of this system as characterizing a *healthy* state free from certain inflammatory markers. We then ask whether such equilibria are linearly, asymptotically stable.

#### 4.1 Stability with zero transport across the endothelium

We consider a uniform, *healthy* equilibrium solution of (4.1)–(4.6) subject to the boundary conditions (3.9), (3.10), (3.11), and (3.12) in the special case that $\alpha_C = \alpha_L = \alpha_I = 0$. We label this equilibrium solution $(\mathcal{I}_e, \mathcal{D}_e, \mathcal{C}_e, \mathcal{L}_e, \mathcal{L}_{oxe}, \mathcal{R}_e)$, and introduce the perturbation variables $u, v, w, z, y, s$ which are defined by

$$\mathcal{I} = \mathcal{I}_e + u, \quad \mathcal{D} = \mathcal{D}_e + v, \quad \mathcal{C} = \mathcal{C}_e + w,$$

$$\mathcal{L} = \mathcal{L}_e + z, \quad \mathcal{L}_{ox} = \mathcal{L}_{oxe} + y, \quad \text{and} \quad \mathcal{R} = \mathcal{R}_e + s.$$

Substituting the assumed form for $\mathcal{I}$–$\mathcal{R}$ into (4.1)–(4.6) and keeping only terms that are linear in the perturbation variables results in the system of equations

$$\frac{\partial u}{\partial t} = \mu_I \nabla^2 u - \nabla \cdot (\chi \nabla w) - Au - Bu - Cu - Dv - Ey \tag{4.7}$$

$$\frac{\partial v}{\partial t} = \mu_D \nabla^2 v + Fu - Gu - Hv - Iv + Jy \tag{4.8}$$

$$\frac{\partial w}{\partial t} = \mu_C \nabla^2 w - Ku + Lv - Mw - Nw \tag{4.9}$$

$$\frac{\partial z}{\partial t} = \mu_L \nabla^2 z - P_1 z + P_2 y - P_3 s \tag{4.10}$$

$$\frac{\partial y}{\partial t} = \mu_{L_{ox}} \nabla^2 y - Q_1 u + Q_2 z - Q_3 y - Q_4 y + Q_5 s \tag{4.11}$$

$$\frac{\partial s}{\partial t} = \mu_R \nabla^2 s - R_1 z - R_2 s - R_3 s \tag{4.12}$$

with the boundary conditions

$$\frac{\partial u}{\partial \mathbf{n}} = \frac{\partial v}{\partial \mathbf{n}} = \frac{\partial w}{\partial \mathbf{n}} = \frac{\partial z}{\partial \mathbf{n}} = \frac{\partial y}{\partial \mathbf{n}} = \frac{\partial s}{\partial \mathbf{n}} = 0 \quad \text{on} \quad \Gamma_I \cup \Gamma_O. \tag{4.13}$$

The various parameters appearing here are the rates at equilibrium given by

$$A = d_1, \quad B = c\mathcal{L}_{oxe}, \quad C = a\mathcal{D}_e, \quad D = a\mathcal{I}_e, \quad E = c\mathcal{I}_e,$$

$$F = c_{15}\mathcal{L}_{oxe}, \quad G = \hat{a}\mathcal{D}_e, \quad H = \hat{a}\mathcal{I}_e, \quad I = d_2, \quad J = \hat{c}\mathcal{I}_e,$$

$$K = e\mathcal{C}_e, \quad L = p, \quad M = e\mathcal{I}_e, \quad N = d_3, \quad P_1 = k_R\mathcal{R}_e + d_4, \quad P_2 = k_A A_{ox} r,$$

$$P_3 = k_R\mathcal{L}_e, \quad Q_1 = f\mathcal{L}_{oxe}, \quad Q_2 = k_{R_0}\mathcal{R}_e, \quad Q_3 = A_{ox} r, \quad Q_4 = f\mathcal{I}_e,$$

$$Q_5 = k_{R_0}\mathcal{L}_e, \quad R_1 = k_R\mathcal{R}_e, \quad R_2 = k_R\mathcal{L}_e, \quad R_3 = hA_{ox},$$

and $\chi = \chi(\mathcal{I}_e, \mathcal{C}_e)$. Each of these constants is assumed to be nonnegative, and due to balance of mass $F = B + Q_1$, $J = E + Q_4$, $Q_2 = (P_1 - d_4) + R_1$, and $Q_5 = P_3 + R_2$.
Let $\mathbf{U} = (u, v, w, z, y, s)$. Before proceeding, we define stability in the following way:

**Definition 4.1.** *The equilibrium state is called asymptotically stable if every solution of the linearized initial boundary value problem (4.7)–(4.13) for the perturbation variables vanishes at infinity in the sense that there exists a positive functional*

$$\mathcal{F}(\mathbf{U}) = \Phi(t) \quad \textit{such that} \quad \lim_{t \to \infty} \Phi(t) = 0.$$

Our study of (4.7)–(4.13) requires the construction of an appropriate functional $\mathcal{F}$, and this construction gives rise to the inequalities involving the parameters including intimal thickness. In the interest of brevity, much of the computational details are omitted here. The main results are stated with a discussion.

We begin by assuming that the product terms $uv$ and $uw$ are nonnegative within $\Omega$. Physically, this can be interpreted as saying that an increase in debris ($v > 0$) and an increase in chemoattractant ($w > 0$) results in an increase in immune cells ($u > 0$). Likewise a decrease in debris and chemoattractant ($v < 0$, $w < 0$) is met with a decrease in immune cells ($u < 0$). This is a rather minor and biologically reasonable condition. However it can be dropped, and a weaker stability theorem obtained (Ibragimov et al., 2010a).

The transition matrix characterizing the species interactions associated with the system (4.7)–(4.12) is

$$\Lambda = \begin{bmatrix} -(A+B+C) & -D & 0 & 0 & -E & 0 \\ F-G & -(H+I) & 0 & 0 & J & 0 \\ -K & L & -(M+N) & 0 & 0 & 0 \\ 0 & 0 & 0 & -P_1 & P_2 & -P_3 \\ Q_1 & 0 & 0 & Q_2 & -(Q_3+Q_4) & Q_5 \\ 0 & 0 & 0 & -R_1 & 0 & -(R_2+R_3) \end{bmatrix}$$

We will assume that the eigenvalues of $\Lambda$ have negative real part. (The implication of this and other imposed conditions will be discussed later.) In the following construction, this ensures that integrals of the form $\int_\Omega U_i \to 0$ as $t \to \infty$ for $U_i = u, v, w, z, y$, or $s$. This follows from Green's theorem and the homogeneous Neumann boundary conditions. This constraint does not guarantee stability of the system or even point-wise boundedness of each $U_i$. We will also assume here that $\mu_D = 0$ which is consistent with the immobile nature of the lesion core.

A sequence of inequalities is obtained by multiplying (4.7) by $u$ (4.8) by $v$, and so forth and integrating over the domain $\Omega$ to secure bounds on the rate of change of the total energy of the perturbations. In so doing, we introduce consideration of the geometry and size of the domain through use of the Poincaré inequality

$$\text{(Poincaré)} \quad \int_\Omega u^2 \leq \frac{1}{|\Omega|}\left(\int_\Omega u\right)^2 + C_p \int_\Omega |\nabla u|^2.$$

Here, $|\Omega|$ is the volume of the domain, and the parameter $C_p$ is dependent on the geometry of the domain [5].

For ease of notation, we set

$$A_1 = A+B+C, \quad G_1 = G-F, \quad H_1 = H+I, \quad \text{and} \quad M_1 = M+N.$$

And in addition to the condition imposed upon the matrix $\Lambda$, suppose that

$$\text{[Condition 4.1.1]} \;\; E < 1, \quad \text{[Condition 4.1.2]} \;\; \frac{\chi L}{2\mu_C} < \frac{1}{4}, \quad \text{[Condition 4.1.3]} \;\; \frac{\chi K}{2M_1\mu_C} < \frac{1}{8},$$

$$\text{[Condition 4.1.4]} \;\; L < 1, \quad \text{[Condition 4.1.5]} \;\; G_1 > 0, \quad \text{and} \quad \text{[Condition 4.1.6]} \;\; J < 1.$$

[5] When an $L^2$ norm is considered, $C_p$ is related to the inverse of the first positive eigenfrequency of a free membrane (Acosta & Durán, 2003).

Following a systematic construction of integral inequalities from the equations (4.7)–(4.12) we arrive at the principal inequality essential to the present analysis.

$$\frac{d}{dt}\int_\Omega \left[\left(\frac{1}{2}+\frac{\chi K}{2\mu_C D}+\frac{A_1}{2C}\right)u^2+\left(\frac{1}{2}+\frac{H_1}{2G_1}\right)v^2+\left(\frac{1}{2}+\frac{\chi M_1^2}{2K\mu_C D}\right)w^2\right.$$

$$\left.+\frac{1}{2}z^2+\frac{1}{2}y^2+\frac{1}{2}s^2+(uv)+\frac{\chi M_1}{\mu_C D}(uw)+\frac{\mu_I}{2D}|\nabla u|^2+\frac{\chi M_1}{2KD}|\nabla w|^2\right]\leq$$

$$-\int_\Omega \Big[C_u u^2+C_v v^2+C_w w^2+C_z z^2+C_y y^2+C_s s^2+$$

$$C_{uv}(uv)+C_{uw}(uw)+C_{\nabla u}|\nabla u|^2+C_{\nabla w}|\nabla w|^2\Big]. \tag{4.14}$$

The coefficients on the right hand side of the inequality (4.14) are

$$\begin{array}{llll}
C_u = A_1+\frac{C_p}{2}\left(\mu_I-\frac{\chi}{2}\right)-\frac{D+E+Q_1}{2}, & & C_s = R_2+R_3+\mu_R C_p-\frac{P_3+Q_5+R_1}{2}, \\
C_v = H_1-\frac{D+J+L}{2}-\frac{\chi L}{2\mu_C D}-\frac{\chi M_1 L}{2K\mu_C D}, & & C_{uv} = G_1, \\
C_w = M_1+\frac{C_p}{2}\left(\mu_C-\frac{\chi}{2}\right)-\frac{L}{2}, & & C_{uw} = K, \\
C_z = P_1+\mu_L C_p-\frac{P_2+P_3+Q_2+R_1}{2}, & & C_{\nabla u} = \frac{1}{2}\left(\mu_I-\frac{\chi}{2}\right), \\
C_y = Q_3+Q_4+\mu_{L_{ox}} C_p-\frac{P_2+Q_1+Q_2+Q_5+E+J}{2}-\frac{E}{2D}-\frac{J}{2G_1}, & & C_{\nabla w} = \frac{1}{2}\left(\mu_C-\frac{\chi}{2}\right).
\end{array} \tag{4.15}$$

We are now able to state our first major result.

**Theorem 4.1.** *The equilibrium solution* $(\mathcal{I}_e, \mathcal{D}_e, \mathcal{C}_e, \mathcal{L}_e, \mathcal{L}_{oxe}, \mathcal{R}_e)$ *of (4.1)–(4.6) subject to the homogeneous Neumann boundary conditions is asymptotically stable provided*

*(i)* $\int_\Omega uv > 0$ *and* $\int_\Omega uw > 0$

*(ii) all eigenvalues of* $\Lambda$ *have negative real part,*

*(iii)Conditions 4.1.1–4.1.6 hold, and*

*(iv)*$M = min\{C_u, C_v, C_w, C_z, C_y, C_s, C_{uv}, C_{uw}, C_{\nabla u}, C_{\nabla w}\} > 0$

The proof requires a definition of the functional as the obvious modification of the left hand side of (4.14). Of interest are the physical interpretations of the sufficiency conditions stated here. The meaning of the conditions on the products $uv$ and $uw$ has already been given. It can also be noted that each of the coefficients appearing in the array (4.15) is written as a positive term minus a non-negative term to highlight the relationships necessary between the parameters to guarantee stability.

The condition on the matrix $\Lambda$—that its eigenvalues have negative real part—has distinct bio-medical interpretation. Parameters $E$, $J$, and $Q_1$ are the rates of foam cell production by binding of macrophages to oxidized LDL. If these are large, then they are a source to the lesion. If each of these is small (conditions 4.1.1 and 4.1.6), then to leading order $\Lambda$ is block diagonal. The parameters $Q_2$ and $R_1$ are the oxidation rates of LDL. If $Q_2 << 1$ and $R_1 << 1$–so that $C_z, C_s > 0$, then the eigenvalues of the lower $3 \times 3$ block has negative eigenvalues $-P_1$, $-(Q_3 + Q_4)$, and $-(R_2 + R_3)$. A healthy system would be dominated by the antioxidant reactions which correspond to large values of $P_1, Q_3, Q_4, R_2$, and $R_3$. If in addition $L << 1$ (condition 4.1.4), then the production of chemoattractant due to the presence of the lesion is small, and the eigenvalues of the upper $3 \times 3$ block are to leading order

$$-M_1, \quad -\frac{1}{2}(H_1 + A_1) \pm \sqrt{(H_1 + A_1)^2 - 4(A_1 H_1 - DG_1)}.$$

Large $M_1$ indicates a fast degradation of chemoattractant and sufficient uptake of chemokines by macrophages to minimize immune cell migration (reduce inflammation.) The parameters $D$ and $G_1$ are large (condition 4.1.5) when the uncorrupted, healthy immune function dominates through normal phagocytosis of lesion debris. Similarly, large values for $A_1$ (due to dependence on $A$ and $C$) and large $H_1$ correspond to degradation of the lesion and clearing by macrophages. The sufficient condition for stability is the inequality

$$\sqrt{(H_1 - A_1)^2 + 4DG_1} < H_1 + A_1.$$

Several of the requirements for stability rest on the interplay between chemotactic effects and diffusion/motility. This is typical of systems characterized by chemotaxis. Conditions 4.1.2 and 4.1.3 as well as the positivity of each parameter in the array (4.15) provide a minimal requirement of the diffusivity of the intimal layer and the motility of macrophages—motility unrelated to chemotaxis—to guarantee that a perturbation off of the healthy equilibrium state decays.

#### 4.2 Stability with transport of macrophages and LDL across the endothelium

We again consider the simplified system (4.1)–(4.6) and perturb off of a healthy equilibrium solutions $(\mathcal{I}_e, \ldots, \mathcal{R}_e)$. However, we consider the boundary conditions (3.9), (3.10), (3.11), and (3.12) with $\alpha_C > 0$, $\alpha_L \neq 0$, and the form of $\alpha_I$ appearing in (3.11) as

$$\alpha_I(\mathcal{C}) = \alpha_I^0(\mathcal{C} - \mathcal{C}_*) \tag{4.16}$$

where $\mathcal{C}_*$ is a base line serum level of chemoattractant and $\alpha_I^0$ is a positive constant. If the level of chemotaxis inducing agents at the endothelial interface is greater than an average level in the blood stream, then macrophages (or monocytes which differentiate) will enter into the subendothelial intima.

The perturbation variables, $u, \ldots, s$ are defined in the same manner as in 4.1, and the linearized system (4.7)–(4.12) is again studied. However, the boundary conditions on $\Gamma_I$ for the variables $u$, $w$, and $z$ (corresponding to immune cells, chemoattractant, and native LDL, respectively) in the present analysis are nonhomogeneous and must be derived from (3.9), (3.10), and (3.11). It should be noted that the existence of a spatially uniform equilibrium requires

$$\mathcal{C}_e = \mathcal{C}_* \quad \text{and} \quad \mathcal{L}_e = \mathcal{L}_B$$

with $\mathcal{C}_*$ and $\mathcal{L}_B$ the serum levels of chemoattractant and native LDL introduced in section 3.2. From (3.11)

$$\mu_I \frac{\partial(\mathcal{I}_e + u)}{\partial \mathbf{n}} = \alpha_I^0(\mathcal{C}_e + w - \mathcal{C}_*) \quad \text{so that} \quad \mu_I \frac{\partial u}{\partial \mathbf{n}} = \alpha_I^0 w. \tag{4.17}$$

Similarly

$$\mu_C \frac{\partial w}{\partial \mathbf{n}} = -\alpha_C w, \quad \text{and} \quad \mu_L \frac{dz}{d\mathbf{n}} = -\alpha_L z \quad \text{on } \Gamma_I. \tag{4.18}$$

The additional boundary conditions on both $\Gamma_I$ and on $\Gamma_O$ remain as in section 4.1.

The approach applied previously must be modified here to account for the effect of the boundary terms on the total energy of each perturbation variable. In addition to the Poincaré inequality, we require the well known Sobolev trace and generalized Friedrich's inequalities

$$\text{(Sobolev Trace)} \quad \int_{\partial\Omega} u^2\, ds \leq C_1 \left( \int_\Omega u^2 + |\nabla u|^2 \right) dx, \quad \text{and}$$

$$\text{(Generalized Friedrich)} \quad C_2 \int_\Omega u^2\, dx \leq \int_\Omega |\nabla u|^2\, dx + C_3 \int_{\partial\Omega} u^2\, ds.$$

We note that these inequalities also depend on the geometry of the domain through the constants $C_1$, $C_2$, and $C_3$. The consideration of best estimates for these constants has received much attention (Acosta & Durán, 2003; Mazya, 1985). For the tubular domain considered herein, the present authors provide estimates of the constants appearing in each of these inequalities (including the Poincaré inequality) in (Ibragimov et al., 2010b).

The procedure is similar to that used in 4.1, and we obtain a set of inequalities relating the parameters of the system that provide sufficient conditions under which the perturbations will decay. Again, much of the computational details are omitted (the interested reader is referred to (Ibragimov et al., 2010a) and to (Ibragimov et al., 2008; 2010b) for similar results). Instead, we highlight a number of inequalities in light of the bio-medical significance and state the primary result.

To facilitate the analysis, we assume that the decrease of oxidized LDL due to attempted phagocytosis by macrophages is negligible compared the increase and decreases resulting from the chemical reactions with free-radical and antioxidant species. (This is to say that uptake by macrophages is a minor effect on the oxidized LDL concentration, not that foam cell formation is negligible especially as it relates to debris growth or decay.) This is equivalent to the previous case where $Q_1$ is small and corresponds to $f = 0$ so that $c = \hat{c}$, $Q_1 = Q_4 = 0$. Here, we no longer consider the transition matrix because we cannot impose any physically reasonable constraints to guarantee that the integrals $\left(\int_\Omega y\right)^2$ and $\left(\int_\Omega s\right)^2$ can be ignored throughout the construction. (The terms $\frac{1}{|\Omega|}\int_\Omega y$ and $\frac{1}{|\Omega|}\int_\Omega s$ are the average values of the total perturbations of oxidized LDL and free radicals, respectively, over the entire domain.) Instead, these are treated in the same manner as each of the perturbation variables.

The competing effects of diffusion (cellular motility) and chemotaxis are prominent in the result in section 4.1, and the same is true when considering boundary transport. In the present case, however, the sufficient conditions require the diffusion to overcome both chemotaxis within the intima as well as that across the endothelial layer. In particular, stability will rest on the conditions

$$\text{[Condition 4.2.1]} \quad \mu_I - C_1\left(\alpha_I^0 + \frac{\chi\alpha_C}{\mu_C}\right) - \frac{\chi}{2} \equiv \bar{\mu}_I \geq 0$$

and

$$\text{[Condition 4.2.2]} \quad \mu_C - \frac{\chi}{2} \equiv \bar{\mu}_C > 0.$$

The latter condition arose in the previous result, however the former relates the impact of chemotaxis at the boundary through the parameters $\alpha_I^0$ and $\alpha_C$ on the net motility of macrophages within the intima. A direct comparison with $C_{\nabla u}$ appearing in (4.15) reveals the additional requirement on this motility to overcome chemotactic effects when boundary transport is accounted for.

The diffusion and degradation of chemoattractant are also required to be significantly increased in this case. Set $C(\bar{\alpha}, \bar{\mu}_C) = \min(\frac{\bar{\alpha}}{C_3}, \bar{\mu}_C)$ where

$$\bar{\alpha} = \alpha_C\left[1 - \frac{1}{2}\left(\frac{\alpha_I^0}{\alpha_C} + \frac{\chi}{\mu_C}\right)\right].$$

($C_3$ is the constant from the Friedrich inequality.) The function $C(\bar{\alpha}, \bar{\mu}_C)$ is nondecreasing in $\bar{\alpha}$ and $\bar{\mu}_C$ independently, and will increase if both of these increase. The condition $C_w > 0$ in theorem 1 will be replaced by

$$M_1 + C(\bar{\alpha}, \bar{\mu}_C)C_2 - \frac{L}{2} > 0.$$

Recall that $M_1$ is the rate at which the chemoattractant is reduced within the intima due to natural degradation and through uptake by macrophages during chemotaxis. The added source of chemoattractant from the endothelial boundary is reflected in the new requirement on the size of this parameter.

Of particular interest are the two cases of LDL transport—forward and reverse—that can be admitted by allowing $\alpha_L$ to be either positive or negative. When $\alpha_L < 0$, LDL enters into the intima through the endothelial layer. Stability in this case will require

$$\text{[Condition 4.2.3(-)]} \quad \mu_L > |\alpha_L| \quad \text{and} \quad P_1 - |\alpha_L|C_1 - \frac{P_2 + P_3 + R_1 + Q_2}{2} - \frac{(R_1 + Q_2)|\Omega|}{2} > 0.$$

The second in condition 4.2.3(-) gives a specific requirement on the removal rate of LDL ($P_1$), especially due to chemical degradation, relative to influx across the endothelial layer ($\alpha_L$), the oxidation kinetics within the intima ($\frac{P_2+P_3+R_1+Q_2}{2}$), and the size of the intima ($|\Omega|$). This particular inequality indicates that intimal thickening is destabilizing mathematically. The role of diffuse intimal thickening (DIT) as a precursor to, and in the early stages of, atherosclerosis has been the subject of a number of studies (Nakashima et al., 2008). Those arteries that are prone to atherosclerotic lesions such as the abdominal aorta, carotid, and coronary arteries are observed to express DIT whereas arteries known to be resistant to atherosclerosis do not (Nakashima et al., 2002). Accumulation of oxidized LDL relative to native LDL in the deep region of DIT in human coronary arteries has been observed (Fukuchi et al., 2002).

The stability requirement on the degradation of LDL in the case of reverse transport is significantly weaker provided the rate of diffusion of LDL and the rate at which LDL leaves the intima through the endothelial boundary are sufficiently high. Let

$$\phi_0 = \frac{P_2 + P_3 + R_1 + Q_2 + (R_1 + Q_2)|\Omega|}{2}.$$

Then $\phi_0$ is a measure of the total oxidation rate of LDL and depends on the thickness of the intima. If LDL is transported from the intima back to the blood stream, then stability will require

$$\text{[Condition 4.2.3(+)]} \quad \mu_L > \phi_0/C_2, \quad \alpha_L > \phi_0 C_3/C_2, \quad \text{and} \quad P_1 > 0, \quad \text{if} \quad \alpha_L > 0.$$

If conditions 4.2.1, 4.2.2, and the appropriate version of 4.2.3 (- or +) hold, and we follow the techniques used in section 4.1, we obtain our primary inequality

$$\begin{aligned} &\frac{1}{2}\frac{d}{dt}\int_\Omega \left[u^2 + v^2 + w^2 + z^2 + y^2 + s^2\right] + \frac{1}{2}\frac{d}{dt}\left[\left(\int_\Omega y\right)^2 + \left(\int_\Omega s\right)^2\right] \leq \\ &- \left[C_u \int_\Omega u^2 + C_v \int_\Omega v^2 + C_w \int_\Omega w^2 + C_z \int_\Omega z^2 + C_y \int_\Omega y^2 + C_s \int_\Omega s^2 \right. \\ &\left. + (D + G_1)\int_\Omega uv + E\int_\Omega uy + K\int_\Omega uw + C_{\int y}\left(\int_\Omega y\right)^2 + C_{\int s}\left(\int_\Omega s\right)^2\right]. \end{aligned} \tag{4.19}$$

The coefficients appearing on the right hand side are defined by

$$\begin{aligned}
C_u &= A_1 - \tfrac{C_1}{2}\left(\alpha_I^0 + \tfrac{\chi\alpha_C}{\mu_C}\right), & C_s &= \tfrac{\mu_R}{C_p} + R_2 + R_3 - \tfrac{P_3+R_1+Q_5}{2}, \\
C_v &= H_1 - \tfrac{J+L}{2}, & C_{\int y} &= Q_3 - \tfrac{Q_2+Q_5}{2}, \\
C_w &= M_1 + C(\bar{\alpha},\bar{\mu}_C)C - \tfrac{L}{2}, & C_{\int s} &= R_2 + R_3 - \tfrac{R_1+Q_5}{2}, \\
C_y &= \tfrac{\mu_{Lox}}{C_p} + Q_3 - \tfrac{J+P_2+Q_2+Q_5}{2},
\end{aligned} \tag{4.20}$$

and

$$C_z = \begin{cases} P_1, & \alpha_L > 0 \\ P_1 - |\alpha_L| C_1 - \frac{P_2+P_3+R_1+Q_2}{2} - \frac{(R_1+Q_2)|\Omega|}{2}, & \alpha_L < 0. \end{cases}$$

Provided

$$\text{[Condition 4.2.4]} \quad \min\{C_u, C_v, C_w, C_z, C_y, C_s, C_{\int y}, C_{\int s}\} > 0,$$

we define the parameters

$$\beta_u = \sqrt{\frac{1}{3}C_u}, \quad \beta_v = \sqrt{C_v}, \quad \beta_w = \sqrt{C_w}, \quad \text{and} \quad \beta_y = \sqrt{C_y}.$$

The primary result of the current anaylsis is

**Theorem 4.2.** *The equilibrium solution $(\mathcal{I}_e, \mathcal{D}_e, \mathcal{C}_e, \mathcal{L}_e, \mathcal{L}_{oxe}, \mathcal{R}_e)$ of (4.1)–(4.6) subject to the nonhomogeneous Neumann boundary conditions (3.9), (3.10), (3.11) and (4.16) is asymptotically stable provided conditions 4.2.1–4.2.4 hold and*

$$\beta_u\beta_v \geq D + G_1, \quad \beta_u\beta_w \geq K, \quad \text{and} \quad \beta_u\beta_y \geq E.$$

The proof involves the pair of functionals

$$\mathcal{F}_1(\mathbf{V}) = \left(\sum_{i=1}^{6} \int_\Omega V_i^2\right) + V_7^2 + V_8^2,$$

and

$$\mathcal{F}_2(\mathbf{V}) = \int_\Omega \frac{1}{2}(\beta_u u + \beta_v v)^2 + \frac{1}{2}(\beta_u u + \beta_w w)^2 + \frac{1}{2}(\beta_u u + \beta_y y)^2 +$$

$$+M\left[\int_\Omega (z^2 + s^2) + \left(\int_\Omega y\right)^2 + \left(\int_\Omega s\right)^2\right]$$

where $\mathbf{V} = (u, v, w, z, y, s, \int_\Omega y, \int_\Omega s)$ and $M = \min\{C_z, C_s, C_{\int y}, C_{\int s}\}$. The hypotheses of theorem 4.2 ensure

$$\frac{d}{dt}\mathcal{F}_1(\mathbf{V}) \leq -\mathcal{F}_2(\mathbf{V})$$

establishing asymptotic stability for this case.

### 4.3 Instability of the equilibrium solution

The theorems obtained in sections 4.1 and 4.2 establish sufficient conditions under which the uniform healthy state is guaranteed to be stable to small perturbations. It is not readily clear whether the inequalities derived are tight—in the sense that they are *nearly* necessary conditions. One can ask the degree to which these conditions must be violated to result in the existence of a perturbation that will blow up.

The existence of perturbations that blow up, in particular spatially nonhomogeneous perturbations, is typically addressed through construction of an explicit example. The classical approach is adopt the ansatz for the perturbation variables

$$u(\mathbf{x},t) = e^{\sigma t}\bar{u}(\mathbf{x}), \quad v(\mathbf{x},t) = e^{\sigma t}\bar{v}(\mathbf{x}), \quad \ldots, \quad s(\mathbf{x},t) = e^{\sigma t}\bar{s}(\mathbf{x}). \tag{4.21}$$

Expressing the perturbation as $\mathbf{U}$ as in definition 4.1, this gives $\mathbf{U}(\mathbf{x},t) = e^{\sigma t}\bar{\mathbf{U}}(\mathbf{x})$, and the system (4.7)–(4.12) can be written in the vector/matrix formulation as

$$\sigma\bar{\mathbf{U}} = \nabla\cdot(\mathbf{M}_e\nabla\bar{\mathbf{U}}) + \Lambda\bar{\mathbf{U}}. \tag{4.22}$$

The diffusion-chemotaxis coefficient matrix $\mathbf{M}_e$ has the diffusion coefficients on the main diagonal, $\chi(\mathcal{I}_e,\mathcal{C}_e)$ in the first row and third column, and zeroes everywhere else. When considering the case without boundary transport, using the fact that $\mathbf{M}_e$ and $\Lambda$ are constant matrices, the ansatz can be further refined to seek solutions of the form

$$\bar{\mathbf{U}} = \phi_\lambda(\mathbf{x})\vec{\xi}.$$

Here $\vec{\xi}$ is a constant vector and $\phi_\lambda$ an eigenfunction of the Laplacian on $\Omega$,

$$-\nabla^2\phi_\lambda = \lambda\phi_\lambda,$$

subject to the completely homogeneous Neumann boundary conditions (4.13). The system (4.7)–(4.12) reduces to the algebraic equation in $\sigma$, $\lambda$, and $\vec{\xi}$

$$\sigma\vec{\xi} = (\Lambda - \lambda\mathbf{M}_e)\vec{\xi}. \tag{4.23}$$

Solutions to (4.23) for which the real part of $\sigma$ is positive will grow; this is the classic Turing instability problem (Turing, 1952). For the Turing stability problem, one considers the case for which $\Lambda$ has only negative eigenvalues and $\mathbf{M}_e^s$, the symmetric part of $\mathbf{M}_e$, has only positive eigenvalues. (This latter condition will hold if and only if $\chi(\mathcal{I}_e,\mathcal{C}_e) < 2\sqrt{\mu_I\mu_C}$, and this inequality follows from the conditions $C_{\nabla u} > 0$ and $C_{\nabla w} > 0$ appearing in theorem 4.1.)

For any domain $\Omega$, the first eigenpair is $\lambda_0 = 0$ and $\phi_0 = \mathit{constant}$, and it is well known that there is an enumerable set of positive eigenvalues $0 < \lambda_1 < \lambda_2 < \cdots$ and corresponding eigenfunctions $\{\phi_{\lambda_n}\}$ that form an orthonormal basis for $L^2(\Omega)$. In the case that $\Lambda$ has only negative eigenvalues, an instability must come from one of the larger eigenvalues. Unfortunately, finding these eigenvalues explicitly for a general domain is not possible. For an annulus ($\mathbb{R}^2$), or an annular cylinder ($\mathbb{R}^3$), they can be found by separation of variables. The corresponding eigenmodes in these cases are nonaxisymmetric suggesting that lesion initiation should also be nonaxisymmetric—this is consistent with clinical observations.

For the present case with no transport of any species across the endothelial layer, we can study the effect of the antioxidant level on the stability of the healthy state. If $M\phi_0$ in equation (4.1) is replaced with $M\phi_0\mathcal{C}$ (to make the source explicitly dependent on the chemoattractant), or if $M\phi_0 = 0$, then the equilibrium solution is $(\mathcal{I}_e,\mathcal{D}_e,\mathcal{C}_e,\mathcal{L}_e,\mathcal{L}_{oxe},\mathcal{R}_e) = (0,0,0,\mathcal{L}_e,\mathcal{L}_{oxe},\mathcal{R}_e)$.

We can, after some lengthy calculations, show that in the limiting cases as $A_{ox} \to 0^+$ and $A_{ox} \to \infty$ (Ibragimov et al., 2010b)

$$\mathcal{L}_{oxe} \propto A_{ox}^{-1}, \quad \text{and} \quad \mathcal{R}_e \propto p_R, \quad \text{as} \quad A_{ox} \to 0^+$$

and

$$\mathcal{L}_{oxe} \propto A_{ox}^{-2}, \quad \text{and} \quad \mathcal{R}_e \propto A_{ox}^{-1}, \quad \text{as} \quad A_{ox} \to \infty.$$

The latter result demonstrates that the antioxidants strongly control free radical production and LDL oxidation. When studying the spectrum of $\Lambda - \lambda \mathbf{M}_e$, this asymptotic result shows that for $A_{ox}$ sufficiently large, the lower $3 \times 3$ block corresponding to the lipid chemistry produces no eigenvalues with positive real part. The question of most interest is what conditions are required for stability (or produce an instability) for the full system in the case that the lipid chemistry alone is stable. If $(\mathcal{L}_e, \mathcal{L}_{oxe}, \mathcal{R}_e)$ is a stable equilibrium for the lipid equations in isolation, what effect does the antioxidant level have on the stability of the equilibrium $(0, 0, 0, \mathcal{L}_e, \mathcal{L}_{oxe}, \mathcal{R}_e)$? In the limit as the antioxidant level vanishes, the equilibrium will be unstable whenever

$$(\lambda \mu_D + d_2)(\lambda \mu_C + d_3) < (\lambda \chi(0,0) - M\phi_0) \left( \frac{\hat{c}p}{c} \right). \tag{4.24}$$

The critical and competing roles of diffusion and chemotaxis are prominent in this criterion providing an unstable equilibrium. For any positive eigenvalue $\lambda$ and diffusive capacity of the chemoattractant $\mu_C$, if the chemotactic sensitivity $\chi(0,0)$ is large enough, the perturbation will grow away from the healthy equilibrium to some other state.

An analysis like the above can be employed with any variation of the system (3.1)–(3.8) provided the boundary conditions considered are completely homogeneous of Neumann type. For example, in (Ibragimov et al., 2008) the present authors consider a system characterized by two distinct macrophage phenotypes each subject to diffusion, chemotaxis, the potential to change phenotypes, but for which only one subspecies was subject to foam cell formation. We showed that the stability result provided therein—that analogous to theorem 4.1 here—was strongly dependent on the dominance of diffusion over chemotaxis. As is seen here, for any set of other parameter values, the chemotactic sensitivity coefficient can always be taken sufficiently large to produce an unstable equilibrium.

The question of unstable equilibria for the case with boundary transport can likewise be considered. Not surprisingly this presents a far more complicated situation mathematically. Even if we only consider constant equilibria, the special approach based on the ansatz (4.21) and the spectral analysis above does not yield any instability examples. Moreover, the coupled boundary conditions provide a Laplacian that is not self-adjoint and does not allow us the option to expand all of the perturbation variables using any single family of eigenfunctions. Nevertheless, a careful construction within the appropriate mathematical framework will provide conditions for which an unstable equilibrium exists. The effect of antioxidant concentration on stability can be analyzed. The reader is encouraged to see (Ibragimov et al., 2010b) for a construction in this case.

## 5. Conclusion

The purpose of this work is twofold. We have formulated a mathematical model of the inflammatory process that characterizes atherogenesis. This model given in equations (3.1)–(3.8) is presented in general terms to provide a framework for the ongoing modeling process. With this in mind, adaptations are easily included as our understanding of this complex medical process increases. We believe that mathematical modeling provides a useful tool to meet the goals of medical research on atherogenesis—identifying vulnerability to disease, development of treatments, and promotion of preventative interventions. Computer simulation (*in silico* analysis) requires a model consistent with and able to capture the characteristics of disease as observed *in vivo*.

Here, we have also studied the model by performing stability analyses under two different assumptions regarding the supply of inflammatory components—macrophages, chemotactic chemokines, and LDL. Taking the vasa vasorum as the sole source of these species, we arrive at a distinct set of inequality conditions on the system parameters that will guarantee that perturbations off of the healthy equilibrium state will decay. Bio-medically, the perturbations are interpreted as the start of inflammation, and the starting equilibrium as a disease-free state. A stable equilibrium is then seen as representing a cellular configuration that is robust—where a lesion is unlikely to develop in the short term. An unstable one suggests that (bio-chemically) the location is vulnerable to atherogenesis and the potential for development of a fibrofatty lesion or latter fibrous plaque. In addition to the positive stability criteria obtained using the energy estimate, we offer a negative result in the form of construction of an instability example. This latter condition highlights the inflammation mitigating effects of antioxidant presence and the significant interplay between chemotaxis and diffusion when the antioxidant level becomes negligible.

We also raise this same stability question under the assumption that the supply of inflammatory components is from influx from the blood flow via the endothelial interface. We again produce several inequalities that when satisfied by the system parameters ensure that the equilibrium solution is linearly asymptotically stable to small perturbations. Of particular interest in this latter case is the stabilizing effect of reverse transport of native LDL from the intima back to the blood stream. That reverse transport of LDL is stabilizing is not surprising given the corruptive nature of oxidized LDL on macrophage function. Our finding further supports the development of treatment modalities aimed at not only reducing serum LDL levels but at facilitating reverse transport of cholesterol (Superko, 2006). Although the conditions are numerous, clinical values of the various parameters can be easily compared in light of the various inequalities derived and presented in theorems 4.1 and 4.2.

The availability of clinical values for several parameters is lacking. Moreover, the parameters appearing in table 1 need not be constant, and determination of appropriate functional forms is an important and difficult task. This will require a process of "fine tuning" through collaboration with clinicians and experimental scientists.

## 6. References

Acosta G. & Durán, R. G. (2003). An optimal Poincaré inequality in $L^1$ for convex domains, *Proc. Am. Math. Soc.* 132(1): 195–202.

Baek, S., Gleason, R. L., Rajagopal, K. R., & Humphrey, J. D. (2007). Theory of small on large: Potential utility in computations of fluidâĂŞsolid interactions in arteries *Comput. Methods Appl. Mech. Engrg.* 196(31-32): 3070–3078

Boullier, A., Bird, D. A., Chang, M., Dennis, E. A., Friedman, P., Gillotte-Taylor, K., Hörkkö, S., Palinski, W., Quehenberger, O., Shaw, P., Steinberg, D., Terpstra, V., & Witztum, J. L. (2001). Scavenger receptors, oxidized LDL, and atherosclerosis, *Ann. N. Y. Acad. Sci.* 947: 214–223

Cobbold, C. A., Sherratt, J. A., & Maxwell, S. J. R. (2002). Lipoprotein oxidation and its significance for atherosclerosis: a mathematical approach, *Bull. Math. Biol.* 64: 65–95.

M. A. Creager, M. A. & Braunwald, E. eds. (2003). *Atlas of Vascular Disease*, Current Medicine, Inc. 2nd edition

Cui, D., Thorp, E., Li, Y., Wang, N., Yvan-Charvet, L., Tall, A. R., & Tabas, I. (2007). Pivital advance: Macrophages become resistant to cholesterol-induced death after phagocytosis of apoptotic cells, *J. Leuk.Bio.* 82: 1040–1050

Davignon, J. & Ganz, P. (2004). Role of endothelial dysfunction in atherosclerosis, *Circulation* 109(3 supplement 1): 27–32

Esterbauer, H., Gebicki, J., Puhl, H. & Jurgens, G. (1992). Review Article: The role of lipid peroxidation and antioxidants in oxidative modification of LDL, *Free Radic. Biol. Med.* 13: 341–390

Fan, J., & Watanabe, T. (2003). Inflammatory reactions in the pathogenesis of atherosclerosis, *JAT* 10(2): 63–71.

Fukuchi, M., Watanabe, J., Kumagai, K., Baba, S., Shinozaki, T., Miura, M., Kagaya, Y. & Shirato, K. (2002). Normal and oxidized low density lipoproteins accumulate deep in physiologically thickened intima of human coronary arteries, *Lab Invest* 82(10): 1437–1447

Goldstein, J. L., Ho, Y. K., Basu, S. K. & Brown, M. S. (1977). Binding site on macrophages that mediates uptake and degradation of acetylated low density lipoproteins, producing massive cholesterol deposition, *Proc. Natl. Acad. Sci. USA* 76: 333–337

Hajjar, D. P. & Haberland, M. E. (1997). Lipoprotein trafficking in vascular cells; Molecular trojan horses and cellular saboteurs, *J. Bio. Chem.* 272: 22975–22978.

Holzapfel, G. A., Gasser, T. C. & R. W. Ogden, R. W. (2000). A new constitutive framework for arterial wall mechanics and a comparative study of material models, *J. Elast.* 61: 1–48

Humphery, J. D. & Rajagopal, K. R. (2002). A constrained mixture model for growth and remodeling of soft tissues, *Math. Models Methods Appl. Sci.* 12: 407–430.

Ibragimov, A. I., McNeal, C. J., Ritter, L. R. & Walton, J. R. (2005). A mathematical model of atherogenesis as an inflammatory response, *Math. Med. and Biol.* 22: 305–333

Ibragimov, A. I., McNeal, C. J., Ritter, L. R. & Walton, J. R. (2008). Stability analysis of a model of atherogenesis: An energy estimate approach, *J. of Comp. and Math. Meth. in Med.* 9(2): 121–142

Ibragimov, A. I., McNeal, C. J., Ritter, L. R. & Walton, J. R. (2010). Stability analysis of a model of atherogenesis: An energy estimate approach ii, *J. of Comp. and Math. Meth. in Med.* 11(1): 67–88

Ibragimov, A. I., Ritter, L. R. & Walton, J. R. (2010). Stability analysis of a reaction-diffusion system modeling atherogenesis, *SIAM J. Appl. Math.* 70(7): 2150–2185

Kadl, A., Meher, A. K., Sharma, P. R., Lee, M. Y., Doran, A. C., Johnstone, S. R., Elliott, M. R., Gruber, F., Han, J., Chen, W., Kensler, T., Ravichandran, K. S., Isakson, B. E., Wamhoff, B. R. & Leitinger, N. (2010). Identification of a novel macrophage phenotype that develops in response to atherogenic phospholipids via Nrf2, *Circ. Res.* 107(6): 737–746

Keller, E. F. & Segel, L. A. (1971). Model for chemotaxis, *J. Theor. Biol.* 30: 235–248

Martín-Fuentes, P., Civeire, F., Recalde, D., García-Otín, A. L., Jarauta, E., Marzo, I. & Cenarro, A. (2007). Individual Variation of Scavenger Receptor Expression in

Human Macrophages with Oxidized Low-Density Lipoprotein Is Associated with a Differential Inflammatory Response *J. Immunol.* 179: 3242–3248

Mazya, V. G. (1985). *Sobolev Spaces*, Springer-Verlag, Berlin (Russian version: Leningrad Univ., Leningrad)

Mosser, D. M., & Edwards, J. P. (2008). Exploring the full spectrum of macrophage activation, *Nature Rev. Immunol.* 8: 958–969

Murray, J. D. (2002). *Mathematical Biology II: Spatial models and biomedical applications* 3rd ed., Springer-Verlag, New York, Berlin

Nakashima, Y., Chen, X. Y., Kinukawa, N., & Sueishi, K. (2002). Distribution of diffuse intimal thickening in human arteries: preferential expression in atherosclerosis-prone arteries from an early age, *Virchows Arch* 441: 279–288

Nakashima, Y., Wight, T. N., & Sueishi, K. (2008). Early atherosclerosis in humans: role of diffuse intimal thickening and extracellular matrix proteoglycans, *Cardiovasc Res.* 79(1): 14–23

Neumann, S. J., Berceli, S. A., Sevick, E. M., Lincoff, A. M., Warty, V. S., Brant, A. M., Herman, I. M. & Borovetz, H. S. (1990). Experimental determination and mathematical model of the transient incorporation of cholesterol in the arterial wall, *Bull. Math. Biol.* 52: 711–732.

Niki, E., Saito, T., Kawakami, A. & Kamiya, Y. (1984). Inhibition of oxidation of methyl linoleate in solution by vitamin E, *J. Biol. Chem.* 259: 4177–4182

Parthasarathy, S., Steinberg, D., & Witztum, J. L. (1992). The role of oxidized low-density lipoproteins in the pathogenesis of atherosclerosis, *Annu. Rev. Med.* 43: 219–225

Podrez, E. A., Poliakov, E., Shen, Z., Zhang, R., Deng, Y., Sun, M., Finton, P. J., Shan, L., Gugiu, B., Fox, P. L., Hoff, H. F., Salomon, R. G. & Hazen, S. L. (2002). Identification of a novel family of oxidized phospholipids that serve as ligands for the macrophage scavenger receptor CD36, *J. Biol. Chem.* 277: 38503–38516

Quarteroni, A. (2001). Modeling the cardiovascular system: a mathematical challenge, *in* Engquist, B. & Schmid, W. (eds.) *Mathematics Unlimited- 2001 And Beyond: 2001 And Beyond*, Springer-Verlag, Berlin, New York, pp. 961–972

Ross, Russell (1995). Cell biology of atherosclerosis, *Annu. Rev. Physiol.* 57: 791–804.

Ross, Russell (1999). Atherosclerosis–An inflammatory disease, *N. Engl. J. Med.* 340(2): 115–126

Saidel, G. M., Morris, E. D. & Chisolm, G. M. (1987). Transport of macromolecules in arterial wall in vivo: a mathematical model and analytic solutions, *Bull. Math. Biol.* 49: 153–169.

Steinberg, D. (1997). Low density lipoprotein oxidation and its pathobiological significance, *J. Biol. Chem.* 272: 20963–20966

Steinberg, D. (2002). Atherogenesis in perspective: hypercholesterolemia and inflammation as partners in crime, *Nat. Med.* 8: 1211–1217

Stocker, R. (1999). The ambivalence of vitamin E in atherogenesis, *Trends Biochem. Sci.* 24: 219–223

Stout, R. D., Jiang, C., Matta, B., Tietzel, I., Watkins, S. K. & Suttle, J. (2005). Macrophages sequentially change their functional phenotype in response to changes in microenvironmental influences, *J. Immunol.* 175(1): 342–349

Superko, H. R. (2006). The Failure of LDL Cholesterol Reduction and the Importance of Reverse Cholesterol Transport. The Role of Nicotinic Acid, *Br. J. Cardiol.* 13(2): 131–136

Tabas, I. (2004). Apoptosis and plaque destabilization in atherosclerosis: the role of macrophage apoptosis induced by cholesterol, *Cell Death and Differentiation* 11: S12–S16

Tall, A. R. (1998). An overview of reverse cholesterol transport, *Euro. Heart J.* 19(A): A31–A35

Taylor, C. A. & Humphrey, J. D. (2009). Open problems in computational vascular biomechanics: Hemodynamics and arterial wall mechanics, *Comput. Methods Appl. Mech. Engrg.* 198(45-46): 3514–3523

Turing, A. (1952). The chemical basis of morphogenesis, *Phil. Trans. Royal Soc. Lond.* B237: 37–72

Veneziani, A. (1998). Mathematical and numerical modeling of blood flow problems, Ph.D. Thesis, Politecnico di Milano, Italy

Watanabe, A., Noguchi, N., Takahashi, M. & Niki, E. (1999). Rate constants for hydrogen atom abstraction by $\alpha$-tocopherol radical from lipid, hydroperoxide and ascorbic acid, *Chem. Lett.* 7: 613–614

Wilson, P. W. F. (ed.) (2000). *Atlas of Atherosclerosis: Risk Factors and Treatments*, Current Medicine, Inc. 2 edition

Young, I. S., & McEneny J. (2001). Lipoprotein oxidation and atherosclerosis, *Biochem. Soc. Trans.* 29: 358–362

Zhang, Y. & Wahl, L. M. (2006). Synergistic enhancement of cytokine-induced human monocyte matrix metalloproteinase-1 by C-reactive protein and oxidized LDL through differential regulation of monocyte chemotactic protein-1 and prostaglandin E2, *J. Leukoc. Bio.* 79: 105–113

# 4

# Parametric Determination of Hypoxic Ischemia in Evolution of Atherogenesis

Lawrence M. Agius
*Department of Pathology, Mater Dei Hospital, Tal-Qroqq, University Of Malta Medical School, Msida, Malta*

## 1. Introduction

Atherosclerosis constitutes a primarily destructive phenomenon inherently arising from dynamics of pathobiologic effect within the intima of elastic and muscular arteries. It is significant to view the development of elevated intimal lesions within dimensions of ongoing further injury to the endothelium.

Considerable interactivity evolves within plaques in consequence to neovascularization in particular. The outline evolution of individual atherosclerotic plaques would considerably modulate the dynamics of migration of smooth muscle cells to the intima and as a consequence of various agonists such as hypoxia, growth factors and coagulation-anticoagulation-fibrinolysis systems. Also, insulin appears to exert toxicity on the vascular wall and possibly promote atherogenesis (Nandish et al., 2011).

## 2. System pathways of injury

System pathways constitute a representative sequence of events that depend on dysfunctional activation of endothelial cells. It is within scope of parameters of permeability and loss of endothelial cells that a full plethora of forms of injury converge as intimal cell proliferation and as deposition of protein matrix proteoglycans. Oxidative stress and chronic inflammation promote diabetes, hypertension and atherosclerosis (Sewon et al., 2011).

The individual roles played by various agonist actions in the definition of the atherosclerotic plaque would evolve within the specificity of focal injury to the intima in particular. The convergence of such injuries appears a constitutive attribute of the variable expression of sequence prototypes in lesion demarcation.

Developmental parameters of modelling include the delineation of individual pathogenic events in terms that integrally reconstitute the modified anatomy of the individual atherosclerotic plaque. In this regard, Ghrelin improves endothelial function, lowers blood pressure and regulates atherosclerosis (Zhang et al., 2011).

Significance in terms of complicated plaques as constitutive pathways in modelling of plaques includes the essential interactivity of endothelium with smooth muscle cell trophic effect. Macrophages in particular implicate a series of converging events that sequentially re-define in repetitive form the dynamics of atherogenesis. Dyslipidemmia increases lipid content in foam cells found in atherosclerotic plaques (Wong et al., 2011).

Growth factors are instrumental in terms of the emerging morphologic features of the early atherosclerotic plaque and as derivative phenomena of endothelial injury and permeability. The constitutive parameters of re-distribution of trophic effect particularly interact with neovascularization within the plaque core.
Developmental sequences of multifactorial type in atherogenesis are particularly prone to a staged outline evolution that permeates the intima and sustains injury to the endothelium. Such significant interactivity contributes to outline emergence of new sequences in trophic effect and as proliferation and migration of smooth muscle cells.
The macrophage is central to such interactivity and operates primarily in chemotaxis and trophism, and also in terms that dominantly influence in significant fashion the attributes of lipid foam cells. Plant-derived alpha-linolenic acid, for example, restricts plaque T-cell proliferation, differentiation and inflammatory activity (Winnik et al., 2011).

## 3. Focality of inflammation

The inflammatory infiltrates include a representative response to injury as atherogenesis further compounds injury to the vascular intima. The role of endothelium is implicated as dysfunctional response with increased permeability to monocytes in particular. Proteoglycans retain lipoproteins subendothelially (Anggraeni et al., (2011).
Such recruitment of novel forms of injury includes the transforming ability of protein matrix proteoglycans as integral constitution of the injurious agents. It is within the dimensional redistribution of such injury that the endothelium plays a prominent role in sequence selectivity and in modulation of parameters of redefinition of activated dysfunctional states of inflammatory cells within the plaque.
The focality of injury is particularly significant within the neovascularized core of the individual plaque and as parameters in the growth and maturation of smooth muscle cells. Reparative processes allow for a sequential remodelling within such system pathways as coagulation and cellular migration within the vascular intima.
The variability of delineation of injurious agents indicates an activation of new parameters as the plaque evolves. The overall confines further extend parameters in plaque modelling that permits responsive elements in the creation of multiple sequence pathways that evolve in their own right; for example, deletion of microsomal prostaglandin E2 synthase-1 retards atherogenesis (Wang et al., 2011).

## 4. The individual smooth muscle cell/macrophage

The secretory dynamics of smooth muscle cells and of macrophages attribute a central pathogenic role to foam cells within the intima. Both smooth muscle cells and macrophages are recognized source for foam cells that, in turn, predominate in the mature atheromatous plaque. On the other hand, the matrix proteoglycans are also central players in re-defining attributes of the injured endothelium.
The reactivity of macrophages within the protein matrix that accumulate within the intima allows for the emergence of multiple converging agonists that characterize endothelial cell activation. The development of subsequent new forms of injury transforms such endothelial dysfunctionality as parameters of maturation of the plaque. Interleukin 18 is involved in plaque destabilization and regulates the innate immune response (Yamaoka-Tojo et al., 2011).

The central core of the plaque is one dominated by influences exerted by transformations in terms of neovascularization and as compounded maturation leading to lipid core formation within the plaque. Insulin resistance and cardiovascular pathology may share a common genetic background (Bacci et al., 2011).

It is highly significant to view the trophic attributes of injury to the endothelium as source of the evolutionary traits of emerging atherosclerotic plaques; indeed, Insulin-like growth factor-1 stabilizes the atherosclerotic plaque by altering smooth muscle phenotype (von der Thusen et al., 2011). Stages in sequence pathway maturation are central to the outline demarcation of individual plaques in a manner that depends integrally on dynamics of neovascularization of the plaque core.

Hemodynamic shear stress contributes to a redistribution of actin microfilaments within endothelial cells in a manner that modulates dysfunctional issues of activated endothelium.

## 5. Cellular proliferative kinetics

A proliferative smooth muscle cellular response is further significant in the maturation of the atherosclerotic plaque within such sequence steps as redefined injury to the endothelium.

Stages in preparation for subsequent events in the outline of the atherogenesis process would include the delivery of injurious agents to the intima. The sequence pathways are significant parametric factors in defining the dimensions of the endothelial participation in atherogenesis. Endoplasmic reticulum stress and the unfolded protein response characterize endothelial susceptibility to atherogenesis (Civelek et al., 2011).

It is further to the evolving forms of agonist action that atherogenesis modifies in repeatedly staged sequence the pathways of dysfunctional activation of the endothelium.

## 6. Low-density lipoproteins

Neovascularization proves to be a centrally operative agonist in the modified development of atheroma formation and deposition. The added parameters of consequence appear to implicate a primarily evolutionary role for hypoxia and ischemia as plaque re-definition, both morphologically and in dysfunctional forms of endothelial activation.

The inflammatory nature of the intimal deposits elicits a responsive panorama that implicates derivative attributes of low density lipoproteins and cholesterol and as extended participation of the neovascularization of the plaque. MicroRNA-29a targets lipoprotein lipase in oxidized low density lipoprotein and modulates cytokines and scavenger receptors (Chen et al., 2011)

Hypoxia is itself essential for the formation of new vessels within the plaque with the production of growth factors and would additionally contribute to the intimal thickening as further evidence for staged representation of injury to the intima.

Directional re-orientation of active dysfunctional states of endothelial cells compounds hypoxia and ischemia within the vascular intima. By-products of matrix proteoglycans and of lipid metabolism indicate the essential staging events in plaque maturation and as derivative phenomenon to further atherogenesis. Chemokines produced by endothelial cells are associated with leukocyte recruitment and angiogenesis in atherosclerosis (Speyer & Ward, 2011).

## 7. Intimal remodeling

It is as remodelling of the injury to the intima that hypoxia and ischemia further modulate the migration of smooth muscle cells within the intima. The increased permeability of the endothelium is significant as a redefined series of further injuries to the underlying intima.

The orientational redistribution of the agonists in atherogenesis redefine a central plaque contribution to increasing profiles of further hypoxia/ischemia and as evidential remounting of parameters of sequence effect. The multi-factorial injurious events are converging agonists in hypoxic/ischemic core regions of the individual atherosclerotic plaque. In such manner, the multi-staged evolution of plaques correlates with interactive dynamics of further injury within the intima.

Dynamics of action of oxidized lipids correlate closely with emerging new roles for agonist action in developing plaques. The interaction of variably participating agonists contrast with the intimal emergence of incremental hypoxia/ischemia in terms of increasing matrix proteoglycan deposition and cellular proliferation of smooth muscle cells in particular. Atherosclerosis affecting different topographic sites correlate with the type of hyperlipidemia (Van Craeyveld et al., 2011).

The platelet/coagulation systems are incremental sequence events as trophic influence in staged convergence of multiple agonists in intimal injury.

Distributional parameters are particularly significant in the dimensional targeting of the intima in terms of the vasa vasorum supplying the arterial wall.

Component systems of sequential impact would contribute to the emergence of positive feedback effect in agonist action. The endothelial cells participate by the production of various agents such as growth factors, in particular Platelet-Derived Growth Factor. The semblance of such influence dominantly re-characterizes the atherosclerotic plaque that trophically redefines the form of hypoxic/ischemic injury to the intima. miRNA –mediated epigenetic regulation may be implicated in atherogenesis, involving oxidized low-density lipoproteins (Chen et al., 2011).

## 8. Hemodynamics

Hemodynamics within the neovascularized core of the plaque allows for a developmental evolution in terms of so-called complications such as hemorrhage and rupture of the plaque and as staged representation of the endothelial cell injury. Consequential pathways of significance would confirm the agonist nature of hypoxia/ischemia in terms of further emergence of intimal deposition and of cellular proliferation and migration.

A response to injury permits role redefinition as emerging parameters in pathogenesis of the deposition of proteoglycans within the vascular intima. Matrix metalloproteinases participate in plaque destabilization and rupture. Their overexpression is an independent factor in the pathogenesis of acute coronary syndromes (Kulach et al., 2010). A proliferative response in particular illustrates the nature of the vascular wall injury that incrementally progresses as gradients of hypoxia and ischemia within the vessel wall.

## 9. Gradient parameters

Consequential involvement of the lipid deposition phenomenon integrally permits the establishment of gradient parameters of hypoxia/ischemia within the operative fields of emerging neovascularization in the plaque core.

Procedural and technical specificity of individual plaques illustrate dynamic turnover within plaques in terms particularly of agonists and cellular parameters in redefinition of atherogenesis. In this regard, Interferon-alpha upregulates expression of scavenger-A in monocytes/macrophages with foam cell formation (Li et al., 2011).

The specificity of the inflammatory response is sequentially consequent to the interchangeability of agonist-induced parameters in creating a microenvironment of hypoxia and ischemia centered on the intima.

## 10. Cellular endothelial injury

The contributing roles of endothelium especially in cases of trauma to the vessel wall would indicate the prototypical attributes in lesion emergence and of subsequent maturation of the atherogenesis phenomenon. Atherogenesis is contributory phenomenon to an ongoing migratory involvement of the intima. This is well-testified by smooth muscle cells that synthesize and secrete matrix proteoglycans, and oxidative stress also induces production of superoxide by endothelial cells with nitric oxide synthase uncoupling (Zweier et al., 2011).

Significant participation in atherogenesis involves mirror-imaged targeting of multiple component systems within the vessel wall that developmentally integrate as regions of hypoxia and ischemia, including the thioredoxin system that correlates with cellular apoptosis in endothelial cell lines in hypoxic stress (Park et al., 2011). Neovascularization proves a permissive phenomenon in development of gradients of ischemia that redefine the individual plaque as compounding parameters of progression to further injury to the vascular wall.

Permissive dynamics are characteristic of oxidation of lipids and particularly of low-density lipoproteins and as evolution of deposition within the intima. Targeting of subsets of cells indicates a selectivity process of progression within sequential pathways of incremental further injury to the vessel wall. Disrupted endoplasmic reticulum equilibrium engages the unfolded protein response in such cells as monocytes (Carroll et al., 2011).

## 11. Vulnerability issues

System reproduction indicates vulnerability selectivity in the evolution of atheromatous plaques in terms ranging from cell kinetics to proliferative migration of smooth muscle cells directed to the intima and a sensitivity of endothelial cells to responsive pathway generation and trophic factor production. The macrophage system is especially representative of novel pathway events that induce a sequential series of models in manipulative further compromise of viability of the endothelial cells.

Within such scopes of pathogenic representation, there would emerge a parametric remodelling based on aberrant reconstitution of injury as further projected by responses to injury to the intima and endothelium. Within such context, the unfolded protein response is implicated in all stages of atherogenesis and plaque progression (Lhotak et al., 2011).

## 12. Pathway activation

The operative essentiality of the intimal involvement in atheroma formation calls into operation the developmental dimensions of both endothelium and also of medial smooth muscle cells. The sequence attributes of multiple different pathways contribute to the subsequent emergence of activation phenomena as well represented by the macrophage and foam cell systems. Mast cells, macrophages and neutrophils release TNF-alpha, IFN-gamma and IL-6 with expression of adhesion molecules and leukocyte recruitment (Zhang et al., 2011). Synthetic and contractile phenotypes of the individual smooth muscle cell indicate specialized forms of series determination in reconstitution of the damaged or injured subintima and also modelled parametric fashioning of the overlying endothelium. Hemodynamics of blood flow localizes such injured endothelium as representative and constitutive foci of persistent pathway activation that delivers dysfunctional attributes to the multi-components of the early atheromatous plaque.

## 13. Eventual sequence emergence

Contrasting sequentiality is triggered by an aberrant selectivity for trophic effect reproduction in terms of ongoing creation of hypoxia/ischemic gradients across both the endothelium lining the vascular lumen and also within critical regions of operative effect in the involved vascular intima. Such representation calls into evidence gradient pathways of projected reproduction that specifically induce focality of involvement of the plaque within systems of cascade effect. A complex interaction of genetic and environmental factors operates (Chyu & Shah, 2011)

The platelet and coagulation systems conclusively demonstrate a participating series of roles culminating in organization of adherent thrombus within the plaque as incorporated dynamics of trophic potential.

Incremental attributes of further compromise of the viability of the intima are demonstrable as evidential pathways of increasing impact in terms of enhanced intimal thickness. In this regard, cells proliferate in atherosclerotic lesions and also in vascular tissue bordering the plaque (Zettler et al., 2010).

Scope of representative projection is conclusively constituted by the end-stage plaque with a central atheromatous core that consists of cholesterol lipid, lipoprotein and oxidized molecular entities of variable derivation. Increasing representation of inflammatory dynamics is largely dependent on initiating events within the foci of intima underlying dysfunctionally activated endothelium. The dynamics of spread and of replication of individual endothelial cells constitutes a further pathway model for gradient creation between flowing blood and vascular wall intima. Pancoronary arterial instability implicates multifocal disease in acute coronary syndromes (Puri et al., 2011).

## 14. Concluding remarks

Re-distribution and retargeting events are primary modelling systems in sequence pathways and as multi-staged involvement of the intima of arterial vessel walls. The intimal thickness and remodelling of pathways allow for incremental redistribution of agonists that target differential systems such as endothelium and smooth muscle cells. Macrophages are constitutive systemic parameters that focally re-orientate the targeting dynamics of hypoxia and ischemia in intimal lesion creation. Oxidation-specific epitopes present on apoptotic cells induce the selection of Pattern Recognition Receptors and damage-associated molecular patterns that may be targeted by innate immunity (Miller et al., 2011).

Only in terms of ensuing neovascularization of the individual atherosclerotic plaque can system specificity in atherogenesis permit the emergence of converging pathways of injury and attempted reconstitution of the vessel wall and endothelium.

Macrophages induce transformational events within micro-environmental conditions of propagated susceptibility patterns that relate in particular to selective sites of vascular involvement such as near-arterial branch points of exit. It is such representation that illustrates the evolving vulnerability of focal sites of intima and endothelium in the generation of multiple atheromatous plaques; these subsequently promote self-involvement in dynamic transformation to the so-called complicated plaque.

Regional pathways of spread and further expansion contrast with the maturation of plaque morphology within such systems as macrophage and endothelial cell activation, with the creation of the synthetic/secretory phenotype of the individual smooth muscle cell within the intima.

Distributional dynamics in generation of the atheromatous plaque are developmental issues as indicated by activation of the proto-oncogenes c-fos and c-myc. The considerable heterogeneity of component cell subpopulations within any atheromatous plaque also permits the emergence of monoclonal groups of smooth muscle cells that trophically sustain growth of the plaque within dimensional confines of the involved intima and of injured overlying endothelium.

Hypoxia-ischemia is a powerful component series of systems in evolution of the susceptibility pattern determination of plaque localization and remodelling, as well-typified by the marked eventual thickening of the involved intima.

Gradient generation is a key mechanistic system in generation of projected effects of hypoxia-ischemia that coordinate the convergence of injurious agonists in terms of trophic and destructive elements within the intima of the arterial wall.

## 15. References


Anggraemi VY, Emoto N, Yagi K, Mayasari DS, Nakayama K, Izumikawa T et al. "Correlation of C4ST-1 and ChGn-2 expression with chondroitin sulphate chain elongation in atherosclerosis" Biochem Biophys Res Commun 2011 Jan 29.

Bacci S, Rizza S, Prudente S, Spoto B, Powers C, Facciorusso A et al. "The ENPPI Q121 variant predicts major cardiovascular events in high-risk individuals: evidence for interaction with obesity in diabetic patients" Diabetes 2011 Jan31.

Carroll TP, Greene CM, McEloaney NG "Measurement of the unfolded protein response (UPR) in monocytes" Methods Enzymol 2011;489:83-95.

Chen KC, Wang YS, Hu CY, Chang WC, Liao YC, Dai CY et al. "OxLDL up-regulates microRNA-29b, leading to epigenetic modifications of MMP-2/MMP-9 genes: a novel mechanism for cardiovascular diseases" FASEB J 2011 Jan25.

Chen T, Li Z, Tu J, Zhu W, Ge J, Zheng X et al. "MicroRNA-29a regulates pro-inflammatory cytokine secretion and scavenger receptor expression by targeting LPL in oxLDL-stimulated dendritic cells" FEBS Lett 2011 Jan27.

Chyu KY, Shah PK "Emerging therapies for atherosclerosis prevention and management" Cardiol Clin 2011 Feb;29(1):123-35.

Civelek M, Manduchi E, Grant GR, Stoeckert CJ Jr, Davies PF "Discovery approaches to UPR in athero-susceptible endothelium in vivo" Methods Enzymol 204;489:109-26.

Kulach A, Dabek J, Glogowska-Ligus J, Garczorz W, Gasior Z "Effects of standard treatment on the dynamics of matrix metalloproteinases gene expression in patients with acute coronary syndromes" Pharmacol Rep 2010 Nov-Dec;62(6):1108-16.

Lee S, Park Y, Zuidema MY, Hannink M, Zhang C "Effects of interventions on oxidative stress and inflammation of cardiovascular diseases" World J Cardiol 2011 Jan 26;3(1):18-24.

Lhotak S, Zhou J, Austin RC "Immunohistochemical detection of the unfolded protein response in atherosclerotic plaques" Methods Enzymol 2011;489:23-46.

Li J, Fu Q, Cui H, Qu B, Pan W, Shen N et al. "Interferon-alpha priming promotes lipid uptake and macrophage-derived foam cell formation: A novel link between interferon-alpha and atherosclerosis in lupus" Arthritis Rheum 2011 Feb;63(2):492-502.

Miller YI, Choi SH, Wiesner P, Fang L, Harkewicz R, Hartvigsen K et al. "Oxidation-specific epitopes are danger-associated molecular patterns recognized by pattern recognition receptors of innate immunity" Circ Res 2011 Jan21; 108(2):235-48.

Nandish S, Barlon O, Wyatt J, Smith J, Stevens A, Lujan M et al. "Vasculotoxic effects of insulin and its role in atherosclerosis: what is the evidence?" Curr Atheroscler Rep 2011 Feb2.

Park KJ, Kim YJ, Choi EJ, Park NK, Kim GH, Kim SM et al. "Expression pattern of the thioredoxin system in human endothelial progenitor cells and endothelial cells under hypoxic injury" Korean Circ J 2010 Dec;40(12):651-8.

Puri R, Worthley MI, Nicholls SJ "Intravascular imaging of vulnerable coronary plaque: current and future concepts" Nat Rev Cardiol 2011 Jan25.

Speyer CL, Ward PA "Role of endothelial chemokines and their receptors during inflammation" J Invest Surg 2011;24(1):18-27.

Van Craeyveld E, Gordts SC, Jacobs F, DeGeest B "Correlation of atherosclerosis between different topographic sites is highly dependent on the type of hyperlipidemia" Heart Vessels 2011 Jan26.

Von der Thusen JH, Borensztajn KS, Mormas S, van Heiningen S, Teeling P, van Berkel TJ et al. "IGF-1 has plaque stabilizing effects in atherosclerosis by altering vascular smooth muscle cell phenotype" Am J Pathol 2011 Feb;178 | (2):924-34.

Wang M, Ihida-Stansbury K, Kothapalli D, Tamby MC, Yn Z, Chen L et al. "Microsomal prostaglandin E2 synthase-1 modulates the response to vascular injury" Circulation 2011 Jan31.

Winnik S, Lohmann C, Richter EK, Schafer N, Song WL, Leiber F etal., „Dietary {alpha}-linolenic acid diminishes experimental atherogenesis and restricts T-cell-driven inflammation" Eur Heart J 2011 Jan31.

Wong BX, Kyle RA, Croft KD, Quinn CM, Jessup W, Yeap BB "Modulation of macrophage fatty acid content and composition by exposure to dyslipidemia serum in vitro" Lipids 2011 Feb1.

Yamaoka-Tojo M, Tojo T, Wakaume K, Kameda R, Nemoto S et al. "circulating interleukin-18: A specific biomarker for atherosclerosis-prone patients with metabolic syndrome" Nutr Metab (Lond) 2011 Jan20;8(1):3.

Zettler ME, Merchant MA, Pierce GN « Augmented cell cycle protein expression and kinase activity in atherosclerotic rabbit vessels » Exp Clin Cardiol 2010 Winter ;15(4) :e139-44.

Zhang G, Yin X, Qi Y, Pendyale L, Chen J, Hou D et al. «Ghrelin and cardiovascular diseases «

Zhang J, Alcaide P, Liu L, Sun J, He A, Luscinskas FV et al. « Regulation of endothelial cell adhesion molecule expression by mast cells, macrophages, and neutrophils » PLoS One 2011 Jan14 ;6(1) :e14525.

Zweier J, Chen CA, Druhan LJ "S-Glutathionylation reshapes our understanding of eNOS uncoupling and NO/ROS mediated signaling" Antioxid Redox Signal 2011 Jan24.

5

# Emerging Epigenetic Therapy for Vascular Proliferative Diseases

Kasturi Ranganna[1], Frank M. Yatsu[2] and Omana P. Mathew[1]
[1]*Texas Southern University, Department of Pharmaceutical Sciences,*
[2]*University of Texas Health Science Center at Houston, Texas, Department of Neurology*
*USA*

## 1. Introduction

Atherosclerosis and restenosis, complex pathologies of blood vessels, are multifactorial diseases triggered by the inflammatory response to injury of endothelium. Remodeling of the injured vessel, proliferation and migration of vascular smooth muscle cells (VSMC) and elaboration and accumulation of extracellular matrix proteins are main traits of these diseases (Dzau et al., 2002; Libby, 2002; Pons et al., 2009; Ranganna et al., 2006; Ross, 1995;). Despite the substantial progress in understanding the etiology and the clinical management of atherosclerosis and restenosis, they are still life threatening diseases. Precise reasons are not still fully transparent. Different cell types; distinct cellular pathways and processes; and multiple genes within each participating cell types that are vulnerable to both genetic and environmental risk factors participate in the pathogenesis of atherosclerosis and restenosis.
Recently, it is recognized that besides the genetic control epigenetic mechanisms regulate development and maintenance of organisms or their interaction with surrounding environment through the coordination of a set of reversible modifications that turn parts of the genome 'off' and 'on' at strategic times and at specific sites causing changes in gene expression with no changes in DNA sequences (Ekstrom, 2009; Pons et al., 2009; Ranganna et al., 2006; Turunen, 2009). The two well-known epigenetic mechanisms, DNA methylation and histone modifications change the chromatin structure and dynamics that alter gene functions by influencing gene expressions. Dysregulation of epigenetic processes has been linked to human diseases, which influences many aspects of cell biology including cell growth, cell cycle control, proliferation, differentiation, and cell death. Reversing the dysregulation of epigenetic mechanisms may offer effective treatment strategy for many diseases including cardiovascular disease due to atherosclerosis and restenosis. This review presents the current advancement in the epigenetics of VSMC proliferation and potential use of histone epigenetic modifiers in the intervention of atherosclerosis and restenosis.

## 2. Overview of pathogenesis of atherosclerosis

Atherosclerosis, a disease of medium to large arterial vessels, accounts for over 55% of all deaths in western countries. It is typically asymptomatic for decades but ultimately result in life-threatening pathological outcomes like myocardial infarction and stroke, both with tissue infarction because of intra-arterial thrombosis provoked by atherosclerosis.

Atherosclerosis is a complex progressive disease in which intimal thickening of the arterial wall promotes luminal stenosis by vascular remodeling, accumulation of cellular and extracellular substances and VSMC proliferation and migration. Integrity of arterial wall is crucial for the regulation of vascular tone, control inflammation, thrombosis, and angiogenesis, enhance regional blood flow, and inhibit cancer metastasis. Arterial wall is composed of three tunics that surround a central lumen through which blood flows. The innermost layer is the tunica intima composed of endothelial cells that form a smooth lining that minimizes interaction with circulating cellular and non-cellular components as blood moves through the vessel. The middle layer, tunic media, is composed of vascular smooth muscle cells (VSMC) and layers of flexible proteins, which enables the lumen to contract and dilate to regulate blood flow in the body. The outer layer, tunica adventitia is a protective layer of connective tissue that anchors the blood vessel to surrounding structures.

Under normal conditions, a delicate balance between proliferation and apoptosis of local vascular cell types maintains the thickness of arterial vessel wall. A number of regulatory factors produced by the endothelial cells are responsible for the homeostatic balance by controlling vessel tone, coagulation state, leukocyte trafficking, and cellular proliferative response. Any damage to the vessel wall by mechanical, biochemical, or immunological insults triggers endothelial dysfunction or denudation of endothelial layer overwhelming the normal homeostatic balance, thus, upsets the normal vascular tone setting the stage for the activation of proinflammatory and immune response. Escalating evidence indicates that inflammatory or atherogenic stimuli promote ROS generation in endothelial milieu causing oxidative stress (Freeman & Crapo, 1982; Kehrer, 1993; Kunsch & Medford, 1999; Madamanchi et al., 2005). Inflammatory response fueled by the oxidative stress is also linked to oxidation of lipoproteins. LDL molecules that enter the subendothelial space are oxidized to form oxidized LDL (OxLDL) by different mechanisms including enzymatic and nonenzymatic pathways, which are taken up by macrophages via scavenger receptors to become foam cells. Besides stimulating proinflammatory and proatherogenic effects, OxLDL also appears to elicit highly immunogenic response resulting in the generation of autoantibodies that appears to be of pathogenic significance (Hansson, 2009; Klingenberg, R., & Hansson, G.K. 2009; Steinberg & Witztum, 2010; Witztum, 1997). Moreover, elevated levels of ROS appear to function as second-messenger molecules transmitting the extracellular signals to nucleus via redox-sensitive signaling pathways to turn on the expression of atherogenic gene products such as adhesion molecules and inflammatory cytokines. Expression of these gene products elicit changes in the vessel wall promoting inflammation, infiltration of monocytes and T cells, proliferation, migration and activation of VSMC and matrix alteration (Freeman & Crapo, 1982; Hansson, 2007; Kehrer, 1993; Klingenberg & Hansson, 2009; Kunsch & Medford, 1999; Madamanchi et al., 2005; Steinberg & Witztum, 2010; Witztum, 1997). These processes involve synthesis and release of a host of regulatory molecules, both by cellular components in the blood and vascular cells of the arterial wall triggering autocrine, paracrine, and endocrine type of interactions between cells and the molecules they produce. Outcome of these complex interactions leads to migration of VSMCs from their normal residence in the arterial media to the intima where they change their phenotype from a contractile to a proliferative type (Libby, 2002; March et al., 1999; Ross, 1995). This phenotypic change, in conjunction with excessive production and accumulation of extracellular matrix proteins, is the main contributor to vascular remodeling.

### 2.1 Vascular remodeling in atherosclerosis and restenosis

Atherosclerosis and restenosis both are multifactorial vascular occlusive processes but exhibit certain similarities and differences in the origin and progression of their development (Dzau et al., 2002; Pons et al., 2009). Inflammatory response of activated endothelial cells to injury or insults elicits both these processes. Activation of endothelial cells leads to a cascade of events, which promotes vascular remodeling by changing the size, structure and composition of vessel wall. Moreover, both processes involve proliferation, migration and activation of VSMC and modulation of extracellular matrix by elaborating and accumulating extracellular matrix proteins. Although they share some of the risk factors such as hypertension and diabetes, there is a consensus that atherosclerosis develops in response to elevated low-density lipoproteins (LDL) and cigarette smoke. On the other hand, VSMC proliferation is the primary pathophysiological mechanism in restenosis, which is largely due to transcending wound healing response to clinical procedures such as balloon angioplasty, stent placement and vein graft surgery [Dzau et al., 2002; Pons et al., 2009]. While restenosis appears to be insensitive to circulating lipids, accumulation of oxidized LDL is the characteristic feature of atherosclerosis. Additionally, while development and progression of atherosclerosis is a gradual process, the restenotic process is a relatively a rapid process caused by surgical revascularization procedures such as angioplasty and stent placement. Despite substantial progress in understanding the etiology and the clinical management of atherosclerosis and restenosis, they are still life-threatening diseases. Possible reasons are multiple factors, different cellular pathways and processes, and multiple genes are contributory to these complex vascular disease processes.

### 2.2 VSMC proliferation

VSMC are highly specialized cells, which play vital roles in the regulation of blood pressure, blood flow and in many pathological states. In mature individuals, the typical function of arterial VSMC is contraction and maintenance of vascular tone. As such, VSMC in adult artery exhibit contractile or differentiated phenotype displaying quiescent proliferation state, decreased synthetic activity and expression of proteins unique to contractile phenotype like contractile proteins, ion channels and signaling proteins. However, VSMC retain their remarkable plasticity to undergo reversible phenotypic change in response to alterations in the local environment like during development, physiological conditions like pregnancy or in response to vascular injury. This remarkable flexible persona of VSMC makes them vulnerable to phenotypic modification from contractile to proliferative, synthetic, or de-differentiated phenotype in conjunction with vessel remodeling by altering cell number and composition of vessel wall (Pons et al., 2009; Ross, 1993).

VSMC proliferation is also the primary pathophysiological mechanism in different clinical pathologies such as postangioplasty restenosis, in-stent restenosis, vein bypass graft failure and transplant vasculopathy (Dzau et al., 2002; Holmes, 2003). The clinical procedures performed to clear the occluded vessel fortuitously become precursors for restenosis in 30-40% of the patients, mainly due to proliferation and activation of VSMC. While entry into cell cycle followed by proliferation of VSMC contributes to the formation of neointima, activation of VSMC induces expression of proinflammatory cytokines, adhesion molecules, chemoattractants, proteolytic enzymes and other molecules not usually present in normal, quiescent, contractile VSMC of the medial layer (Kleemann et al., 2008; Li et al., 1993; O'Brien et al., 1996; Zeffer et al., 2004). Expression of these molecules amplifies the inflammatory response, and in turn, increases further proliferation of VSMC and elaboration of vessel remodeling.

### 2.3 Antiproliferative therapeutics to target VSMC proliferation

The current therapies used for atherosclerosis aim to minimize the risk factors that promote atherosclerosis, such as reducing elevated levels of cholesterol or enhancing the blood flow by surgical intervention of an already occluded vessel. Ironically, the surgical procedures performed to clear the occluded vessel become a precursor for restenosis, mainly due to VSMC proliferation, in significant number of patients (Dzau et al., 2002; Ferns et al., 1991). Because proliferation of VSMC is the hallmark of atherosclerosis and clinical conditions such as arterial stenosis, transplant vasculopathy, and bypass graft failure, the suitable therapeutic approach is to develop strategies that inhibit or block VSMC proliferation. Based on the current understanding of the molecular basis of vascular proliferative diseases, there is an abundance of potential therapeutic possibilities. Accordingly, a number of agents are tested for antiproliferative activity including heparins, cytostatic agents, inhibitors of angiotensin converting enzyme, and antagonists to growth factors (Dzau et al., 2002; Ferns et al., 1991; Gershlick, 2002; Stephen et al., 2005; Toshiro et al., 2005). Although some of these agents have shown promise in animal models, they failed to elicit any protection in human clinical studies (Gershlick, 2002). Species differences, potential toxicity, and lack of potency are possible culprits. Furthermore, the probability of successfully treating a multifactorial disease by targeting a single factor is unlikely. Additionally, all vascular cell types secrete growth factors and cytokines that activate signaling pathways that are redundant and thus prevent the success of targeting one or two factors.

### 2.4 Cell cycle as the therapeutic target

Based on the current knowledge of cell cycle mechanisms, it appears that targeting specific parts of the cell cycle is a better strategy to inhibit or block the development of vascular proliferative diseases such as arterial restenosis; in-stent-stenosis and vein bypass graft failure. Moreover, cell cycle is the final common pathway where all the growth regulatory signals converge, and thus, makes a rational target of antiproliferative therapeutics to inhibit vascular proliferative diseases. Some of the experimental studies indeed reveal that inhibition of cell cycle progression emerges as an important therapeutic target for prevention of vascular proliferative diseases (Dzau et al., 2002; Ranganna et al., 2006; Von der Leyen & Dzau, 2001). Different approaches such as pharmacological agents, irradiation, and gene therapy have been used for arresting VSMC proliferation. These approaches inhibit proliferation by cytostatic or cytotoxic mechanism. However, cytostatic mechanism of cell cycle arrest is desired over cytotoxic mechanism to avoid unintended damage to the vessel wall due to cytotoxic treatment. Three different approaches have been tried for arresting VSMC proliferation by targeting cell cycle, which include: 1) brachytherapy, 2) gene therapy, and 3) pharmacotherapy.

#### 2.4.1. Brachytherapy

Endovascular radiotherapy is a promising method for effective antiproliferative treatment of restenosis (Teirstein & King, 2003; Waksman, 2000). Radiotherapy directed at restenosis has two objectives, one to treat restenosis by killing the cells that re-occluded and to prevent further restenosis by inhibiting tissue growth. Brachytherapy with either beta or gamma radiation sources are used to diminish restenosis in patients with post-angioplasty restenosis or with in-stent restenosis. The rationale for using radiation for treating restenosis is that uncontrolled proliferation of VSMC is similar to neoplastic cells that can be targeted for radiation therapy just as transformed cells in cancer tissue. Brachytherapy-induced DNA damage of VSMC can result in arrest of VSMC at the G1 checkpoint or induction of apoptosis through p53 induced p21Cip1 upregulation. A key feature of brachytherapy is that the irradiation only affects a precise localized area around the radiation sources. Exposure to radiation of healthy tissues further away from the sources is therefore, reduced. In addition, brachytherapy is associated with a low risk of serious adverse side effects. More than a dozen randomized trials established its safety and efficacy. However, it exhibits two radiotherapy-related problems, arterial narrowing adjacent to the edge of the target site and unexpected late coronary thrombo-occlusive events (Raizner, 2000).

### 2.4.2 Gene therapy

Gene therapy techniques provide a unique opportunity to genetically engineer vessels and grafts to become impervious to atherosclerosis and neointimal formation that contributes to arterial restenosis, in-stent restenosis and vein graft failure (Dzau et al., 2002; Khanna, 2008; Kishore & Losordo, 2007; Gaffney et al., 2007; Melo et al., 2005; Von der Leyen & Dzau, 2001). Gene therapy approach has potential not only against monogenic diseases, but also against complex diseases where multiple genes are involved in the disease pathogenesis like in cardiovascular diseases and cancer. One of the key challenges of the gene therapy is appropriate vector for the delivery of functional gene or a concoction of genes in multigenic diseases as in cardiovascular diseases. Besides the choice of vector, other parameters such as, appropriate gene targets and efficient methods of vector delivery for a specific target have to be optimized. Vectors can be either viral or non-viral. The ideal vector is the one, which is nonpathogenic, less immunogenic, more efficient, and enhanced tissue specificity.

Delivery of therapeutic genes to the cardiovascular tissues is challenging. To facilitate local gene delivery to lesions in the vasculature catheter-based vector delivery has been tried using a variety of balloon catheters in animal models and human trials (Khanna, 2008; Kishore & Losordo, 2007; Gaffney et al., 2007; Melo et al., 2005). Stents are ideal gear for localized gene delivery to the vascular wall because of their widespread use, safety and permanent scaffold structure. Stents can be coated with genetically engineered cells or plasmid or adenoviral vectors carrying therapeutic genes (Khanna, 2008; Kishore & Losordo, 2007; Gaffney et al., 2007; Melo et al., 2005). Experimental studies have demonstrated usefulness of gene therapy in treating atherosclerosis and restenosis in various animal models and in some clinical trials. It can be used to transfer exogenous genes to express functional gene products to overcome defective or downregulated endogenous gene expressions through vector-based delivery system. It also can be used to knockdown or suppress the expression of gene products that contribute to pathogenesis of disease by one of the several methods of gene silencing. These include antisense oligonucleotides (ODNs), short segments of RNA with enzymatic activity (ribozymes) and small interfering RNAs [siRNA] (Dzau et al., 2002; J.M. Li et al., 2010; Banno, et al., 2006).

A number of studies have shown that gene therapies can be targeted for reducing cholesterol levels, inflammation and thrombosis (Feldman & Isner, 1995); for upregulating apo-A1 and downregulating chemoattractant protein-1 (MCP1)receptor expression (Tangirala, 1999); transferring pleiotropic atheroprotective nitric oxide synthase [NOS]

(Qian, 1999); targeting vascular redox biology through heme oxygenase-1, superoxide dismutase, catalase and glutathione peroxidase antioxidant gene therapy to attenuate oxidative stress (Van Assche, 2011); and lipid-lowering gene therapy to reduce plasma LDL levels (Grossman et al., 1995). Furthermore, neointimal hyperplasia that contributes to pathogenesis of arterial stenosis, in-stent stenosis and vein graft failure is also a good target for gene therapy. A number of potential therapeutic genes, which are key to the development of neointimal hyperplasia, have been identified. The ones that are promising for gene therapy include tissue inhibitors of matrix metalloproteinases (Akowuah et al., 2005; Gaffney et al., 2007; Khanna, 2008); NOS (Cooney, 2006; Dzau et al., 2002; Khanna, 2008; Kishore & Losordo, 2007; Gaffney et al., 2007; Melo et al., 2005; Von der Leyen & Dzau, 2001) and p53 (Gaffney et al., 2007). Importantly, delivery of antiproliferative genes such as those coding for p21Cip1, p27Kip1, and iNOS are used to inhibit stenosis and neointimal hyperplasia (Dzau et al., 2002; Von der Leyen & Dzau, 2001]. Conversely, silencing the genes that contribute to proliferation via antisense ODNs (Dzau et al., 2002; Khanna, 2008; Kishore & Losordo, 2007; Gaffney et al., 2007; Melo et al., 2005) or siRNA approach is also effective in preventing in-stent and graft neointimal hyperplasia (Banno, et al., 2006; F. Li et al., 2005; J.M. Li et al., 2010; Matsumae et al., 2008). Antisense ODNs–based inhibition of cell proliferation-related genes such as PCNA, c-myc, c-myb or different cyclin-dependent kinases (cdks) have been successfully carried out in experimental models of vascular lesion formation (Braun-Dullaeus et al., 1998; Dzau et al., 2002; Morishita et al., 1993; Simons et al., 1994).

RNA interference (RNAi) technology is becoming popular approach to alter gene expressions to interrogate their role in pathogenesis of disease, which has utility in the inhibition of VSMC proliferation and neointimal hyperplasia (Banno, et al., 2006; F. Li et al., 2005; J.M. Li et al., 2010; Matsumae et al., 2008). To determine whether Angiotensin II (ANG II)-induced neointimal thickening is mediated via cytoplasmic phospholipase A2 (cPLA2) - and phospholipase D2 (PLD2)-activated Akt, injured carotid arteries were exposed to a retrovirus containing $cPLA_2$ siRNA or PLD2 siRNA to test whether their knockdown will result in the reduction of ANG II-induced neointimal thickening (F. Li et al., 2005). SiRNA-mediated downregulation of cPLA2 and PLD2 resulted in the reduction of ANG II-induced neointimal thickening. The involvement of CCN1, an extracellular matrix-associated protein, in the development of neointimal hyperplasia is confirmed by siRNA-mediated knockdown approach (Matsumae et al., 2008). The atheroprotective role of midkine (MK), a heparin-binding growth factor, is corroborated by the use of MK-siRNA (Banno, et al., 2006). NADPH oxidase has a critical role in the development of neointimal hyperplasia and restenosis due to its contribution to oxidative stress, which is blocked by siRNA specific to NOX2 gene *Cybb*, an important component of NADPH oxidase (J.M. Li, et al., 2010).

Several experimental gene transfer and gene silencing strategies are evaluated as potential treatments for cardiovascular disease, which resulted in Phase I, and Phase I to Phase III clinical studies for inducible iNOS (Tzeng, 1996; Von der Leyen & Dzau, 2001) and transcription factor E2F, respectively (Dzau et al., 2002; McCarthy, 2001; Mann et al., 1999). E2F, a transcription factor that leads to upregulation of up to 12 cell-cycle genes is an ideal target for cell-cycle blockade. A double-stranded E2F decoy ODN that bears the consensus E2F-binding site (*cis*-elements) was designed as an agent for prevention of vein graft disease. In rabbits, treatment of vein grafts with E2F decoy ODN resulted in inhibition of neointimal hyperplasia and graft atherosclerosis for up to 6 months. This led to phase I

PREVENT trial for human vascular bypass grafts, which resulted in about 75% reduction in VSMC proliferation and fewer graft occlusions. Similar gene manipulation approach was used for coronary bypass grafts in PREVENT II trial. Although the phase 1 trial (PREVENT Trial) showed promising results, later studies were less positive including the phase III, multicentre, randomized double-blinded, placebo-controlled trial of 3014 patients undergoing primary coronary artery bypass graft surgery with at least two planned saphenous grafts (Alexander et al., 2005; Conte et al., 2005, 2006). Although appears to be promising, the use of gene therapy in the treatment of vascular proliferative diseases is still in infancy. Various feasibility and efficacy issues as well as design and delivery of the genes have to be addressed taking into account the complexity of the pathological processes leading to atherosclerosis and restenosis.

### 2.4.3 Pharmacotherapy

A number of pharmacological agents have been used to target injury-induced VSMC proliferation that contributes to neointimal growth in balloon-injured arteries. Among these rapamycin or sirolimus, a cytostatic agent, arrests VSMC proliferation and migration *in vitro* and reduces neointimal growth in animal models of balloon-injury (Dzau et al., 2002; Guerin et al., 2005). Its action appears to be mediated through the inhibition of mammalian target of rapamycin (mTOR). One of the downstream events induced by the inhibition of mTOR is induction of p27Kip1, an inhibitor of cyclin-dependent kinases (cdk), causes cells to arrest in G1 phase of the cell cycle. In doing so, it inhibits cell proliferation. Paclitaxel, a derivative of Taxol, is another promising agent for proliferation arrest, which by collapsing the mitotic spindle formation causes mitotic arrest (Jordan et al., 1993). It prevents neointima formation in animal models, and its clinical effect in the blockade of restenosis is investigated in several human trials (the ELUTES, TAXUS and ASPECT trials) via local delivery through stents coated with paclitaxel (Finn et al., 2007; Wilson et al., 2007).

### 2.4.4 Immunotherapy

Over the past several years, accumulating data have identified involvement of several antigens in the initiation of immune response during atherosclerosis. These include exogenous infectious microbial pathogens like, cytomegalovirus and chlamydia pneumonia and endogenous proteins such as oxLDL, heat shock proteins (HSPs) and $\beta_2$-glycoprotein-1b (Habets et al., 2010). Among these, the epitopes recognized on oxLDL are important because of the role of oxLDL in the pathogenesis of atherosclerosis ((Hansson, 1997; 2007; Steinberg & Witztum, 2010; Witztum, 1997). In addition to its proinflammatory and proatherogenic effects, and participation in the formation of foam cells, oxLDL is also immunogenic due to the presence of several neoepitopes. A number of neoepitopes generated during the oxidation of LDL are highly immunogenic and cause the generation of autoantibodies, which are detected in atherosclerotic lesions. Since the different epitopes of oxLDL induce atherogenic immune response, it may be possible to inhibit proatherogenic effects of oxLDL by modulating the immune response towards oxLDL through the immunization against oxLDL. Several antigens have been identified and investigated for immunization against atherosclerosis in animal models. Immunization against oxLDL show reduction in atherosclerosis in several animal models (Habets et al., 2010). This discovery of atheroprotective immunity has resulted in the emergence of immunotherapy approach against atherosclerosis. Indeed, several animal studies indicate that immunization against oxLDL offers protection against atherosclerosis, which appears to operate both through cellular and humoral immunity (Zhou, 2001). The increased titers of T cell-dependent IgG antibodies to oxLDL (Habets et al., 2010; Zhou, 2001) and natural IgM antibodies to phosphocholine (Binder et al., 2004) are also in agreement with the atheroprotection. Furthermore, two recent studies report promising immunotherapeutic approach for the prevention of atherosclerosis. In one study, LDL-receptor deficient mice were vaccinated with oxLDL-pulsed mature dendritic cells to determine the effect on atherosclerosis (Habets et al., 2010). In the second immunotherapy study, tolerogenic apo-B100-loaded dendritic cells in combination with immunosuppressive cytokine interleukin-10 were injected intravenously to hypercholesterolemic mice. This immunotherapy significantly prevented atherosclerosis by reducing autoimmune response against LDL ( Hermansson et al., 2011) Although, these studies are encouraging and promising from a clinical perspective to translate these promising outcomes to the clinics, antigens that can be easily manufactured under good manufacturing practice conditions and that have a reproducible quality are necessary. However, several clinical studies are currently underway to evaluate the therapeutic implications of immunotherapy.

## 3. Epigenetics and vascular proliferative diseases

Advancement in technological innovations during the past 25 years has resulted in far-reaching in-depth comprehension of the biology and the etiology of vascular diseases, and thus influencing the perception of the pathophysiology of vascular proliferative diseases like atherosclerosis and restenosis. In spite of the substantial understanding of the etiology and the clinical management of these vascular proliferative diseases, they are still life threatening diseases and reasons are not fully evident. Based on the recent finding of the role of epigenetics in human diseases, it is proper to expect that epigenetic mechanisms enforces an additional layer of gene regulation that alters chromatin structure, and dynamics in the pathogenesis of vascular proliferative diseases (Ekstrom, 2009; Pons et al., 2009; Ranganna et al., 2006; Turunen, 2009). Epigenetic mechanisms are essential for the functioning of genomes to regulate normal development and maintenance of organisms, and to facilitate their interaction with surrounding environment. Compilation of the past 10 to 20 years of studies has resulted in the identification of three highly interrelated epigenetic mechanisms that alter the chromatin structure and accessibility. These include, DNA methylation, histone posttranslational modifications and non-coding RNA (ncRNA) expression based mechanisms, each of these mechanisms is essential for regulation of gene expression. Therefore, it is anticipated that the genetic and environmental factors that are relevant to the development of vascular proliferative diseases by their effect on inflammation, VSMC proliferation and vessel remodeling, is regulated by epigenetic mechanisms through the modification of chromatin structure, dynamics and accessibility (Ekstrom, 2009; Pons et al., 2009; Ranganna et al., 2006; Turunen, 2009). Although there is an outbreak of interest and enthusiasm in linking altered epigenetic mechanisms to human pathologies particularly cancers, it is relatively unexplored area regarding cardiovascular diseases. Moreover, deregulation of epigenetic processes are linked to changes in many aspects of cell biology including cell growth, cell cycle control, and cell death by altering the expression and in turn functions of target genes without changing their primary gene structure. Because VSMC proliferation is the hallmark of vascular proliferative diseases, understanding the epigenetics of VSMC proliferation and in particular their susceptibility to perturbation by the epigenetic modifiers may offer novel insights into disease pathogenesis and epigenetic therapeutic approaches. Therefore, it is appropriate to review the current knowledge of epigenetics in the regulation of VSMC proliferation.

### 3.1 VSMC epigenetics

Curiosity in epigenetics has surged during past decade even though the principle question it aims to address has been there for decades. That is, how a multicellular organism maintain drastically different gene expression profile in different cell types of the organism, while all the different cell types of the organism have exactly the same DNA. This is where epigenetics come into picture. Epigenetics refers to the inheritance of gene function/activity/expression that may be stable over long periods, last through several cell divisions or inherit through several generations, all without any change in their primary DNA (Ng & Gurdon, 2008; Probst, 2009). The three interrelated epigenetic mechanisms, which involve: methylation of DNA at CpG dinucleotides at specific position in the DNA molecule suppress expression of nearby genes (Esteller, 2008); posttranslational modifications of histones alters chromatin structure and changes promoter accessibility (Kouzarides, 2007); and small RNA molecules generated from non-coding RNAs (ncRNAs) inhibit gene expression (Mattick et al., 2009). All these mechanisms involved in epigenetic regulation contribute to epigenome. This review focuses on the role of posttranslational modifications of histones in the regulation of VSMC proliferation, and on the epigenetic regulators of histone modifications as potential candidates for drug targeting in the treatment and management of vascular proliferative disease.

### 3.2 Chromatin structure

Chromatin is a nucleoprotein complex consisting of repeating units of nucleosomal core particles. It offers a dynamic platform for all DNA-mediated processes within the nucleus. The nucleosomal core particles are the basic units of chromatin consisting of 147 base pair (bp) of DNA that wraps almost twice around two copies of each of the four core histone proteins, H3, H4, H2A and H2B. Each nucleosome is separated by 10-16 bp long linkers DNA, which gives an appearance of a bead on a string structure that constitutes the chromatin fiber of ~10 nm in diameter. The linker DNA assists further compaction of chromatin structure into higher-order chromatin structure, which is essential for packaging of remarkable lengths of DNA into the cell nucleus. Furthermore, this compact chromatin structure limits accessibility of DNA to DNA-mediated processes like transcription, DNA replication, and DNA repair (Kouzarides, 2007). Evidence accumulated during the past 15 years reveals that three interrelated epigenetic mechanisms alter the highly compacted chromatin structure and facilitate accessibility of DNA for gene transcription. The interrelated epigenetic mechanisms that include DNA methylation, histone modification and ncRNA expression contribute to the epigenome making the epigenome dynamic rather than static like genome and thus, being predisposed to and influenced by environmental factors and extracellular stimuli. Deregulation of epigenetic mechanisms is observed in many different cancers and other human diseases. Thus, understanding of how epigenetic mechanisms contribute to gene regulation will provide insight into the disease process.

### 3.3 Histone modifications

Histones are highly conserved basic proteins that undergo an amazing number and types of posttranslational modifications, which contributes to the active or inactive chromatin (Ekstrom, 2009; Kouzarides, 2007; Pons et al., 2009; Ranganna et al., 2006; Turunen, 2009). Each of the four core histones are composed of a conserved globular domain that forms the nucleosome core, and a highly dynamic amino-terminal tail of 20-35 residues rich in basic amino acids. Additionally, H2A histone has an extended tail of about 35 residues at the carboxy-terminal end. Both amino- and carboxy-terminal tails protrude from nucleosome into the nucleoplasm. Histones tails are the targets of an array of site-specific posttranslational modifications including lysine acetylation/deacetylation, lysine and arginine methylation, serine and threonine phosphorylation, lysine ubiquitylation and sumoylation, and glutamic acid ADPribosylation (Fischle et al., 2003; Ito, 2007; Jenuwein & Allis, 2001; Turner, 2003).

Histone modifications are dynamic and reversible, and their 'off' and 'on" modification states are influenced by different physiological and environmental factors like developmental state, stress condition and environmental cues. Many of histone modifications are associated with transcriptionally active euchromatin regions, while other histone modifications are localized to transcriptionally inactive heterochromatin regions. Even though issues such as how the process of modification is regulated, and how many modifications are required for their biological effect are still elusive, recognition of specific histone modifications by various effector proteins is suggested to mediate specific biological processes like gene activation or gene suppression by altering the chromatin structure and gene accessibility. Generally, conformationally relaxed and decondensed chromatin structure that is associated with histone acetylation and DNA hypomethylation is the feature of transcriptionally active chromatin. On the other hand, compact and condensed chromatin structure that is associated with deacetylation of histones and hypermethylation of DNA is transcriptionally silent. Condensed chromatin structure is essential during cell cycle, mitosis and meiosis, whereas decondensed chromatin structure is required for gene expression, replication, repair and recombination. The combinatorial pattern of the histone modifications indicates the state of the chromatin structure, and thus, regulates the accessibility of the DNA to the transcription-regulatory complexes, through it controls gene expression. The collection of various covalent histone modifications serve as epigenetic marks for the recruitment of different proteins or protein complexes to regulate disparate chromatin functions such as gene expression, gene suppression, mitosis, repair, replication and chromosome segregation (Taverna et al., 2007). Furthermore, there is also crosstalk between different histone modifications like acetylation, methylation and phosphorylation at independent sites forming a "histone code" that is translated to a specific biological event through the mediation of various effector proteins. For example, phosphorylation of serine 10 of histone H3 facilitates acetylation of lysine 14 and methylation of lysine 4, which create an open or relaxed chromatin conformation associated with an active gene. Serine 10-phosphorylation also facilitates the acetylation of lysine 9, thus preventing the repressive lysine 9-methylation associated with an inactive gene (Jenuwein & Allis., 2001; Lund & van Lohuizen, 2004; Mathew et al., 2010; Schreiber & Bernstein, 2002; Turner, 2003).

### 3.4 Chromatin modifying enzymes

Consistent with the variety of posttranslational modifications of histones, a disparate family of enzymes, which are referred as histone modification writers, catalyzes addition of specific functional groups to histones. These modifications of histones alter the chromatin structure and function by two distinct manner: First, by directly altering the charges of histone proteins, certain posttranslational modifications cause localized relaxation of chromatin structure and second, by serving as recognition and binding sites for various classes of effector proteins that participate in chromatin remodeling, certain histone modifications indirectly alter the chromatin structure. However, most histone modification are reversible and diverse families of proteins, which include histone acetyltransferases (HATs) /histone deacetylases (HDACs), histone methyltransferases (HMTs)/demethylases, histone kinases/phosphatases, and ubiquitin ligases, catalyze addition and removal of the modifications from histones. One of the highlights of epigenetics is that it offers new therapeutic targets for diseases including cardiovascular diseases. The epigenetic regulators, HATs/HDACs and HMTs/demethylases, which exhibit counterbalancing activities are essential for the regulation of gene expression, which are required for the basic cellular processes such as cell proliferation and differentiation. This essential role of epigenetic regulators in basic cellular processes identifies potential therapeutic targets for diseases including cardiovascular diseases. Moreover, identification of those HATs and HDACs that plays a role in the transcriptional regulation of genes, products of which contributes to the processes of neointima formation like inflammation, VSMC proliferation, and matrix formation is also important in designing potential epigenetic therapy to target vascular proliferative diseases. Thus, pharmacological inhibition of enzyme activities involved in epigenetic DNA and histone modifications designed to induce or silence the transcription of disease-relevant genes offers an amenable therapeutic intervention for atherosclerosis and restenosis. In addition to modifying the effects of diseased genes, it is possible to change the effects of environmental risk factors by targeting epigenetic mechanisms. Here we will focus on HATs/HDACs, the principal epigenetic regulators that control histone acetylation, a major epigenetic modification for transcriptional control of gene expression. Because HATs/HDACs are essential for the regulation of gene expression, in all probability, they play crucial role in the development of multigene and multifactorial diseases such as atherosclerosis and restenosis.

## 4. Histone acetyltransferases (HATs) and histone deacetylases (HDACs)

One of the best- and most-studied posttranslational histone modifications is lysine acetylation catalyzed by HATs, the modification that is generally associated with gene activation (Ekstrom, 2009; Kouzarides, 2007; Pons et al., 2009; Ranganna et al., 2006; Turunen, 2009). Hyperacetylation of histones causes decondensation of chromatin allowing a more relaxed or open and active chromatin structure, which allows accessibility of DNA to basal transcription initiation machinery (Kouzarides, 2007; Roth, 2001). In contrast, gene repression is mediated by HDACs, and other co-repressors, which cause deacetylation of hyperacetylated histones and offset the activity of HATs resulting in a closed conformation of chromatin structure. Thus, the acetylation status of the chromatin associated with particular genes is dictated by the balance between the activities of HATs and HDACs. These enzymes are shown to regulate expression of genes associated with various cellular processes like inflammation, proliferation and matrix modulation (Cao et al., 2005; Pons et al., 2009; Sahar et al., 2007; Vinh et al., 2008; Waltregny et al., 2005; Xu et al., 2007; Yan et al., 2009). HATs and HDACs are also recruited to gene promoters by multiprotein transcriptional complexes, where they regulate transcription through chromatin modification without directly binding the DNA.

A number of different HATs are identified and organized as families based on the presence of highly conserved structural motifs, which include PCAF/Gcn5, p300/CBP, MYST, SRC, and $TAF_{II}250$ families. While they all differ in their HAT domains and substrate specificity, they all require the assembly of multiprotein complexes for acetylation of nucleosomes (Marmorstein, 2001). Likewise a number of HDACs are identified and are classified into three different classes based on cellular localization, substrates and binding site features (Lindemann et al., 2004; Santini et al., 2007). Class I and class II include zinc-dependent HDACs, and class III includes NAD-dependent HDACs, which are also called as sirtuins. Class I HDACs are widely expressed and include HDACs 1-3 and 8 that are exclusively localized to nucleus. They are known to modulate cell proliferation and survival. Class II HDACs are HDACs 4-7, 9, and 10, which shuttle between the nucleus and cytoplasm in response to certain cellular signals. They may be involved in cell differentiation (Pons et al., 2009; Santini et al., 2007). Class II HDACs are further divided into Class IIa and Class IIb , which include HDACs 4, 5 ,7, and 9, and, HDACs 6 and 10, respectively. While Class IIa members have an extended N-terminal regulatory domain, Class IIb exhibit an extra catalytic domain (Lindemann et al., 2004; Pons et al., 2009; Santini et al., 2007). Class III HDACs are sirtuins (SIRT), which include $NAD^+$-dependent enzymes (SIRT 1-7) potentially involved in apoptosis (Pons et al., 2009).

HATs and HDACs are also recruited to gene promoters by multiprotein transcriptional complexes. There they regulate transcription through chromatin modification without directly binding the DNA (Johnstone & Licht, 2003; Pons et al., 2009). Moreover, HATs and HDACs are also involved in the acetylation status of lysine residues of transcription factors such as p53, E2F1, GATA1, RelA, YY1 and hormone receptors. Acetylation status of these transcription factors affects their DNA binding and transcriptional activity (Glozak et al., 2005; Johnstone & Licht., 2003; Marks, 2001; Pons et al., 2009). Besides histones and transcription factors, several other non-histone proteins like α-tubulin, nuclear import protein importin-α7, and signal transduction protein β-catenin are also modified by HATs and HDACs, but their effects on gene expression is not dependent on chromatin remodeling (Johnstone & Licht., 2003; Marks, 2001).

### 4.1 Epigenetic therapy targeting VSMC proliferation

Because HATs/HDACs are involved in dynamic reversible epigenetic processes that contribute to modulation of gene expression profiles specific to cellular processes like cell proliferation, they probably play important role in cardiovascular pathologies such as atherosclerosis and restenosis. Moreover, epigenetic deregulation affects several aspects of cell biology, including cell growth, cell cycle control, differentiation, DNA repair, and cell death. This elevates the strong possibility that reversing deregulated epigenetic mechanisms may be an effective treatment strategy for proliferative diseases. Incidentally, the property of HDACs, suppression of gene expression by epigenetic mechanism, has been exploited in the field of cancer to reactivate transcriptionally silent tumor suppressor gene to arrest proliferation of cancer cells and growth (Pons et al., 2009; Ranganna, et al., 2005, 2007; Sharma et al., 2010). Moreover, HDAC inhibitors (HDACi) are emerging as a new class of anticancer agents that are under clinical trials for different cancer treatment. Some of the early clinical studies have demonstrated that certain HDACi exhibit promising activity against several neoplasms (Bhalla, 2005). Naturally, it has stimulated great interest to determine how HATs/HDACs regulate transcriptome of different processes that are linked to the development of atherosclerosis and restenosis like inflammation, VSMC proliferation and matrix modification and to assess therapeutic potential of HDACi in these vascular proliferative diseases (Ekstrom, 2009; Pons et al., 2009; Ranganna et al., 2006; Turunen, 2009). The following sections will focus on the role of HATs and HDACs in the transcriptional regulation of genes in the context of their contribution to VSMC proliferation and its disorders as well as on the potential applicability of HDACi in vascular disease management.

#### 4.1.1 Histone deacetylase inhibitors (HDACi)

In the past few years, great effort has been focused on seeking and designing most effective HDACi because of their potential roles in reversing the silenced genes in tumor cells by modulating transcriptional processes. The balance between the acetylated/deacetylated states of histones, which is mediated by the counterbalancing activities of HATs and HDACs, contributes to the transcriptional states of chromatin structure. The structural modification of histones by acetylation/deacetylation of their N-terminal tails is crucial in modulating gene expression, because it affects the accessibility of DNA for the transcription-regulatory protein complexes. HATs preferentially acetylate specific lysine residues of histones, which relaxes the DNA conformation, thus allowing its access to transcription machinery to turn on gene expression. On the contrary, HDACs restore the positive charge on lysine residues by removing acetyl groups, which promotes condensed chromatin structure. This promotes silencing of gene expression by blocking the access of transcription machinery to DNA. Inappropriate silencing of critical genes such as tumor suppressor genes can result in cancer based on the recent understanding of the cancer cell cycle (Kristeleit et al., 2004). This provides a rationale for using inhibition of HDAC activity to release transcriptional repression. As result, a flurry of HDACi has been recognized for their ability to inhibit HDACs activity.

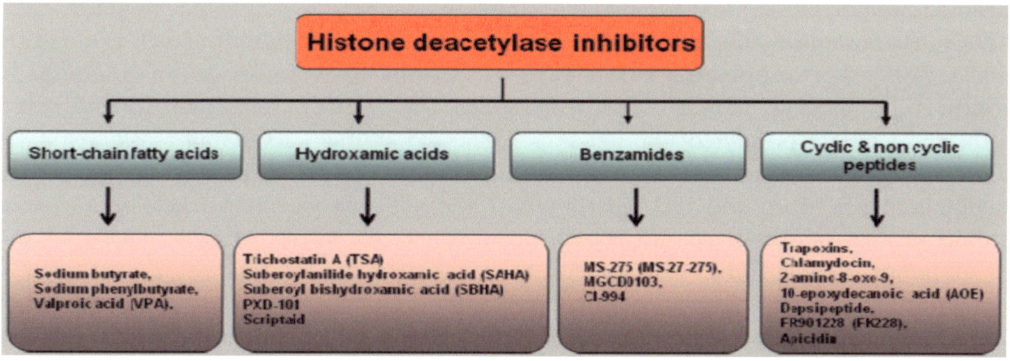


Fig. 1. Structural class of histone deacetylase inhibitors

Structurally diverse classes of naturally occurring and synthetic compounds have been recognized for their ability to bind to the catalytic pocket of HDACs and chelate the zinc ion at its base, thereby inhibiting HDAC activity (Marks et al., 2000). A wide range of structures inhibits activity of class I/II HDAC enzymes with a few exceptions [Figure 1]. The HDACi are classified into structural classes including 1) short-chain fatty acids (carboxylates), 2) hydroxamic acids, 3) benzamides, and 4) cyclic and non-cyclic peptides. The various HDACi studied so far have been shown to inhibit class I (HDACs 1, 2, 3, and 8) and II (HDACs 4, 5, 6, 9, and 10) HDACs. Their activities have been tested in cell lines and preclinical murine models, and appropriate drugs that are selected for clinical trials, demonstrated good tolerance and clinical activity against different human neoplasms (Santini et al., 2007). However, Class III HDACs (SIRT 1, 2, 3, 4, 5, 6, and 7), also known as sirtuins, require NAD rather than zinc as a co-factor for their activity, and are not inhibited by the HDACi. Instead, they are inhibited by Nicotinamide (Luo et al., 2001).

#### 4.1.2 HDACi effects on cellular processes

HDACi exhibit multiple cellular effects, which are linked to chromatin-mediated altered transcriptional activity. In general, most HDACi exhibit inhibition of cell proliferation, stimulation of cell differentiation and/or induction of cell death by selectively modulating gene expression (Bhalla, 2005; Mathew et al., 2010; Ranganna, 2005). HDACi arrest cells at the G1 or G2/M, and promote cell differentiation mainly by stimulating cyclin-dependent kinase inhibitor (cdkI) p21Cip1 expression (Bhalla, 2005; Mathew et al., 2010; Ranganna et al., 2005). HDACi also cause cell cycle blockade through the modulation of mechanisms that involve repression of cyclin D and cyclin A and upregulation of other cdkI like p27Kip1, p16INK4A and p15INK4B, which blocks pRb/E2F pathway, thus preventing the cell cycle progression (Mathew et al., 2010; Bhalla, 2005) [Figure 2]. Now with the array technologies, it is recognized that HDACi selectively modulate about 2% to 10% of all genes, with as many genes upregulated as are downregulated genes in different cell types (Bhalla, 2005; Ranganna et al., 2003). One of the genes that are universally upregulated is the cdkI p21Cip1, in a p53-independent manner, which is necessary for HDACi-induced G1 arrest. Induction of GADD45α and β and upregulation of transforming growth factor beta, which inhibits c-*myc* expression may also contribute to the cell cycle arrest in G1 or G2 (Bhalla, 2005.). HDACi treatment is also shown to transcriptionally downregulate the expression of CTP synthetase and thymidylate synthetase, which are required for DNA synthesis, thus, causing inhibition of S phase progression [Figure 3].

HDACi also stimulate differentiation of several cancer cells by inhibiting cell proliferation (Bhalla, 2005). Again, upregulation of p21Cip1 appears to be essential for differentiation because cells lacking p21Cip1 fail to respond to HDACi treatment (Bhalla, 2005). Furthermore, acute promyelocytic leukemic cells and primary leukemia blasts, expressed differentiated phenotype in response to a combination of ATRA, a retinoid-based chemotherapeutic drug and HDACi (Bhalla, 2005). HDACi stimulated gelsolin, an actin-binding protein required for morphological and cytostructural changes associated with differentiation (Bhalla, 2005).

It is interesting that HDACi induce growth arrest and cell differentiation in some cell, and in others, they cause apoptosis (Bhalla, 2005; Johnstone & Licht, 2003). HDACi-induced apoptosis triggers both the intrinsic and extrinsic pathways of apoptosis. Several types of HDACi, particularly hydroxamic acid analogs are shown to induce mitochondrial permeability transition, which releases prodeath molecules such as cytochrome c, Smac and Omi into cytosol (Bhalla, 2005). This triggers activation of Apaf-1, which leads to the processing and activation of caspases-9 and-3 (Bhalla, 2005). HDACi appear to promote apoptotic cell death not only by upregulating several proteins that participate in apoptotic cell death including Bak, Bax, Bim, DR4, DR5, and TRAIL, but also by attenuating the levels of a number of antiapoptotic proteins such as Bcl-xL, Bcl-2, XIAP, and survivin (Bhalla, 2005).

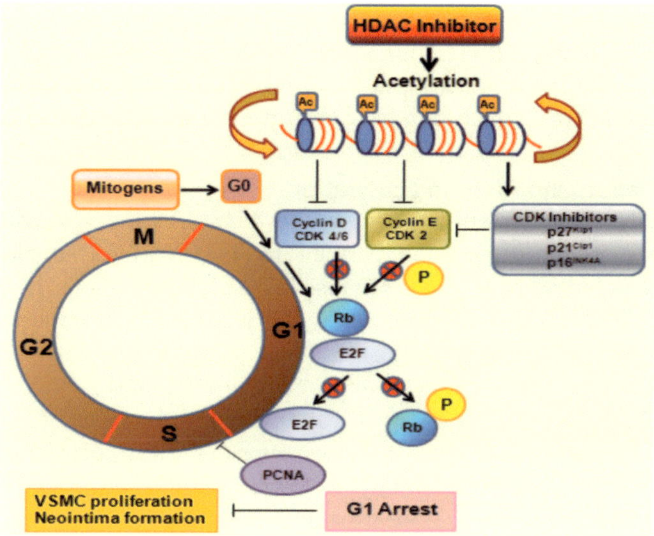


Fig. 2. Display of cell cycle targets of HDAC inhibition.

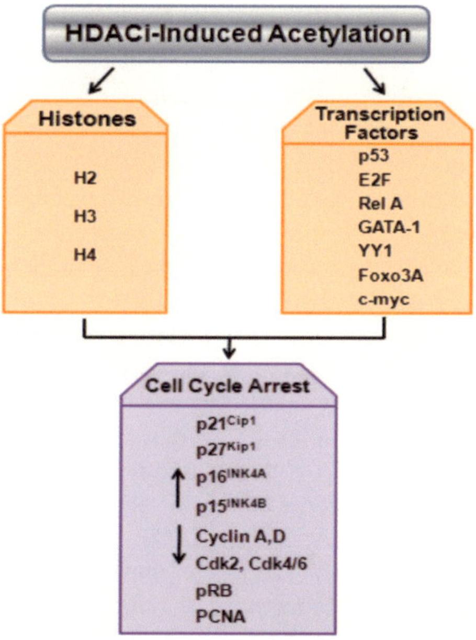


Fig. 3. Cell cycle regulatory proteins that are altered by the HDACi-induced acetylation of histones and transcription factors.

Besides affecting cell proliferation, differentiation and apoptosis, HDACi also alter the function of some of the non-histone transcription factors like p53, RelA, GATA1 and FoxO3A because HDACi enhance their acetylation, which may affect their DNA binding and transcriptional activity (Marks et al, 2001; Lindemann et al., 2004). Similarly, stimulating acetylation status of other non-histone protein such as nuclear import protein importin-α7, signaling protein β-catenin, DNA repair enzyme Ku70, and the cytoskeletal protein β-tubulin, HDACi alter their activity (Bhalla, 2005). Taken together, by inducing acetylation of histones and non-histones, HDACi alter the levels of proteins that control cell cycle progression, differentiation and apoptosis appropriately by transcriptional and post-transcriptional mechanisms, which implicate their potential use in disease treatment.

### 4.2 VSMC proliferation and histone acetylation

Although the common mechanism of pathogenesis shared by the atherosclerosis and cancer are linked to abnormal cell proliferation, very limited information is available with reference to anti-atherogenic potential of HDACi. Because HDACi not only alter gene expressions, but also cause inhibition of cell proliferation and induction of differentiation and/or apoptosis, a number of studies are initiated in the past few years to test the effects of HDACi as potential antiatherogenic agents. Even though both in vitro and in vivo studies have been done with the intention of targeting VSMC proliferation for the intervention and management of vascular proliferative diseases, most of the information that is available currently is from in vitro cell culture studies. There is limited in vivo data supporting the protective role of HDACi but needs further evaluation in models of VSMC injury.

#### 4.2.1 VSMC proliferation

In general, HDACi exhibit almost same effects in VSMC as they do in cancer cells. They arrest cell proliferation, induce differentiation and/or apoptosis, and modulate expression of cell cycle regulators. Several studies have shown that trichostatin A (TSA), a well-known HDACi, arrests VSMC proliferation via upregulation of p21Cip1 and subsequent reduction of the phosphorylation of Rb protein at the G1-S phase (Okamoto et al., 2006; Pons et al., 2009), the effects consistently observed in cancer cell (Bhalla, 2005). In contrast, in one of the studies TSA unexpectedly exhibited paradoxical pro-atherogenic effect on VSMCs via the reduction of thioredoxin 1 instead of antiatherogenic properties (Song et al., 2010).
Besides TSA, butyrate, a well-known dietary HDACi, which has been used in different human cancer and other disease treatments, appears to exhibit potential antiatherogenic effect by arresting VSMC proliferation and appropriately altering both negative and positive cell cycle regulators (Davie, 2003; Mathew et al., 2010; Ranganna et al, 2005). Butyrate belongs to the class of short-chain fatty acids and is a derived from the intestinal microbial fermentation of dietary fiber. A number of epidemiological, animal and interventional studies suggest an inverse relationship between dietary fiber and chronic diseases such as bowel disorders and colorectal cancer, cancer of other tissues, cardiovascular disease, diabetes, obesity and hypertension (Anderson, 2003; Dashwood et al., 2006; Kim, 2000; Ranganna et al., 2005, 2006). Some of the studies suggest that the protective effect of dietary fibers in chronic diseases is linked to bioactivity of butyrate (Anderson, 2003; Dashwood et al., 2006; Kim, 2000; Ranganna et al., 2005, 2006). Butyrate elicits many cytoprotective, chemopreventive and chemotherapeutic activities mainly through inhibition of cell proliferation, stimulation of cell differentiation and/or induction of cell death by selectively

modulating certain gene expressions, but the mechanistic basis for these actions are far from clear. Butyrate has been known to alter chromatin structure and organization via hyperacetylation of histone amino-terminal tails, modulate gene expression and play a protective role in the prevention of cancer and inflammatory diseases of colon for a long time (Ranganna et al., 2005, 2006). However, its importance in the prevention of cancer of other tissues and different diseases has been recognized during the past ten years (Anderson, 2003; Dashwood et al., 2006; Kim, 2000; Ranganna et al., 2005, 2006). On the other hand, no similar studies are performed to indicate the protective role of butyrate in cardiovascular diseases due to atherosclerosis and restenosis.

During last few years, significant interest is focused on potential utility of butyrate and its stable derivatives in the intervention of vascular proliferative diseases, besides their therapeutic applications in other diseases including cancers. Butyrate and its more stable in vivo analogue tributyrin, arrested proliferation and inhibited DNA synthesis of smooth muscle cells in a cAMP-independent manner. Butyrate also abolished serum-induced c-fos, c-myc, and Ki-Ras expression that are important for early G1 events initiated by serum growth factors, but stimulated the expression of PS4 and thromospondin (Feng et al., 1996). Moreover, studies performed in our own lab further supports the efficacy of butyrate and its stable derivatives in vascular proliferative diseases. Treatment of VSMC with butyrate inhibited serum and PDGF-induced proliferation and abolished expression of proliferation markers such as c-myc and proliferating cell nuclear antigen [PCNA] (Ranganna et al., 1995, 2000). Furthermore, our analysis of profiles of VSMC transcriptome by array technology disclosed that butyrate-arrested VSMC proliferation is a multigene and multipathway-mediated process. Our array data identified differential expression of several genes in butyrate arrested VSMC proliferation, which are mainly belonging to four different functional classes: cell proliferation and differentiation; stress response; vascular function; and genes normally present in neuronal cells (Ranganna, et al., 2003). Extension of this study reveals that an upper level regulatory mechanism mediated through epigenetic modification of chromatin structure controls the expression of both positive and negative cell cycle regulatory genes linked to VSMC proliferation arrest by butyrate (Mathew et al., 2010). To establish the mechanistic link between chromatin remodeling and antiproliferation action of butyrate, influence of butyrate on posttranslational modifications of histone H3 and its consequence on G1-specific cell cycle regulators were investigated [Figure 2]. Outcomes of the study indicate interplay between different site-specific posttranslational modifications of histone H3 in butyrate treated VSMCs that seem to alter chromatin structure and organization that supports downregulation of cdk2, cdk4/6, and PCNA, and upregulation of cdkI, p21Cip1 and p15INK4B. This causes inhibition of Rb phosphorylation resulting in arrest of VSMC proliferation [Figure 2 and Figure 3]. The effects of HDACi on cell cycle-related gene expressions appear to be highly selective, leading to transcriptional activation of certain genes such as the cdkIs but repression of others like cdks to efficiently block cell proliferation.

### 4.2.2 Histone acetylation

Hypernuclear acetylation (HNA) also plays a role in proliferation (Kawahara et al., 2003). Presence of increased histone acetylation is observed in VSMC of atherosclerotic lesions unlike in normal arteries. Thrombin, a humoral factor that is known to activate and stimulate VSMC proliferation, strongly induced HNA in cultures of VSMC. MAP kinase pathway and CBP are implicated in thrombin-induced HNA suggesting that coactivators cooperating with signaling-dependent transcription activators play a role in atherosclerosis through HNA (Kawahara et al., 1999).

## 5. Conclusions and perspectives

Over the past few years, it has become abundantly evident that several interdependent epigenetic changes collaborate with genetic changes in the development of human diseases including cardiovascular diseases such as atherosclerosis and restenosis. Since the genetic foundations of diseases are generally immutable, but their epigenetic and chromatin changes are reversible, they are suitable for epigenetic therapy with epigenetic and chromatin modifiers. Therefore, thorough understanding on the roles of epigenetic processes in the etiology of atherosclerosis and restenosis is essential to launch an epigenetic therapy designed to target the epigenetic processes. Although a number of different therapeutic approaches have been investigated in the treatment of atherosclerosis and restenosis such as brachytherapy, pharmacotherapy, gene therapy, and immunotherapy, the therapeutic efficacy of these treatment modalities for atherosclerosis and restenosis is not adequate for a number of patients. Possible reasons are multiple factors, genes, pathways are involved in the disease pathogenesis, and targeting one or two genes or pathways are not sufficient to treat complex vascular pathologies. In these scenarios, epigenetic therapy, which is reversible, appears to be appropriate because HDACi exhibit multiple cellular effects that play major roles in vascular pathogenesis. HDACi exhibit antiproliferative, antioxidant and antiinflammatory effects and cause inhibition of cell proliferation and stimulation of differentiation or apoptosis by modulating expression of multiple genes (Natarajan, 2011; Ranganna, et al.,2005; 2006; 2007). For example, HDACi inhibit cell proliferation by appropriately altering both positive and negative regulators of cell cycle. While cell cycle inhibitors such as p21Cip1, p27kip1, p16INK4a and p15INK4b are upregulated, expressions of cyclin D, cyclin A, cdk2, cdk4/6, PCNA and pRb that promote cell cycle progression are downregulated (Figure 2 and Figure 3). With one single HDACi, multiple genes are altered that control cell cycle progression unlike gene therapy, where a cocktail of genes is required to bring about inhibition of cell proliferation. Furthermore, stents are ideal platform for the localized delivery of HDACi to the vascular wall because of their widespread use and safety in the treatment of restenosis. It is recognized that many of the processes that play critical role in atherosclerosis and restenosis such as VSMC proliferation, migration, inflammation, cellular redox state and matrix protein synthesis (Natarajan, 2011) are regulated by epigenetic mechanisms. As such, they present an exciting opportunity for therapeutic intervention, particularly to refractory or recurrent vascular pathologies such as restenosis and in-stent restenosis and vein graft failure. A number of natural and synthetic HDACi are already in the pipeline for the treatment of cancer either stand alone, or in combination with other anticancer drugs and several clinical trials are in progress. Exploring these particulars will speed the necessary epigenetic treatment strategies for the management of atherosclerosis and restenosis.

## 6. Acknowledgements

The work from our laboratory described in this review is supported by G12RR0345 and C06RR012537-01 grants from National Institutes of Health/National Center for Research Resources.

## 7. References

Akowuah, E.F., Gray, C., Lawrie, A., Sheridan, P.J., Su, C.H., Bettinger, T., et al. (2005). Ultrasound-mediated delivery of TIMP-3 plasmid DNA into saphenous vein leads to increased lumen size in a porcine inteposition graft model. *Gene Therapy* 12, No. 14, (July 2005), pp. 1154–1157, ISSN 0969-7128

Anderson, J.W. (2003). Whole grains protect against atherosclerotic cardiovascular disease. *Proceedings of Nutrition Society*, Vol. 62, No. 1, (February 2003), pp. 135-142, ISSN 0029-6651

Banno, H., Takei, Y., Muramatsu, T., Komori, K., & Kadomatsu, K. (2006). Controlled release of small interfering RNA targeting midkine attenuates intimal hyperplasia in vein grafts. *Journal of Vascular Surgery*, Vol. 44, No. 3 (September 2006), pp. 633-641, ISSN 0741-5214

Bhalla, K.N. (2005). Epigenetic and chromatin modifiers as targeted therapy of hematologic malignancies. *Journal of Clinical Oncology*, Vol. 23, No. 17, (June 2005), pp. 3971-3993, ISSN 0732-183X

Binder, C.J., Hartvigsen, K., Chang, M. K., Miller, M., Broide, D., Palinski, W. et al. (2004). IL-5 links adaptive and natural immunity specific for epitopes of oxidized LDL and protects from atherosclerosis. *Journal of Clinical Investigsation*, Vol.114, No. 3, (August 2004), pp. 427–37 ISSN 0021-9738

Braun-Dullaeus, R.C., Mann, M.J., & Dzau, V.J. (1998). Cell cycle progression: New therapeutic target for vascular proliferative disease. *Circulation*, Vol. 98, No. 1, (July 1998), pp. 82-89, ISSN 0009-7322

Cao, D., Wang, Z., Zhang, C.L., Oh, J., Xing, W., Li, S., et al. (2005). Modulation of smooth muscle gene expression by association of histone acetyltransferases and deacetylases with myocardin. *Molecular and Cellular Biology*, Vol. 25, No. 1, (January 2005), pp. 364 –376, ISSN 0270-7306

Cooney, R., Hynes, S.O., Sharif, F., Howard, L., & O'Brien, T. (2006). Effect of gene delivery of NOS isoforms on intimal hyperplasia and endothelial regeneration after balloon injury. *Gene Therapy*, Vol. 14, No 5, (March 2007), pp. 396–404, ISSN 0969-7128

Dashwood, R.H., Myzak, M.C., & Ho, E. (2006). Dietary HDAC inhibitors: time to rethink weak ligands in cancer chemoprevention? *Carcinogenesis*, Vol. 27, No. 2, (February 2006), pp. 344-349, ISSN 0143-3334

Davie, J.R. (2003). Inhibition of histone deacetylase activity by butyrate. *Journal of Nutrition*, Vol. 133, No. 7 Suppl, (July 2003), pp. 2485S-2493S, ISSN 0022-3166

Doran, A.C., Meller, N., & McNamara, C.A. (2008). Role of smooth muscle cells in the initiation and early progression of atherosclerosis. *Arteriosclerosis Thrombosis and Vascular Biology*, Vol. 28, No. 5, (May 2008), pp. 812- 819, ISSN 1079-5642

Dzau, V.J., Braun-Dullaeus, R.C., & Sedding, D.G. (2002). Vascular proliferation and atherosclerosis: new perspectives and therapeutic strategies. *Nature Medicine*, Vol. 8, No. 11, (November 2002), pp. 1249-56, ISSN 1078-8956

Ekström, T.J. (2009). Epigenetic control of gene expression. *Biochemical Biophysical Acta*, Vol. 1790, No. 9, (September 2009), pp. 845–846, ISSN 0006-3002

Esteller, M. (2008). Epigenetics in cancer. *New England Journal of Medicine, Vol.* 358, No.11, (March 2008), pp. 1148–1159, ISSN 0096-6762

Fasciano, S., Patel, R.C., Handy, I. & Patel, C.V. (2005). Regulation of vascular smooth muscle proliferation by heparin. Inhibition of cyclin-dependent kinase 2 activity by p27kip1. *Journal of Biological Chemistry*, Vol. 280, No.16, (April 2005), pp. 15682-15689, ISSN 0021-9258

Feldman, L.J., & Isner, J.M. (1995). Gene therapy for vulnerable plaque. *Journal of the American College of Cardiology*, Vol. 26, No. 3, (September 1995), pp. 826-833, ISSN 0735-1097

Feng, P., Ge, L., Akyhani, N., & Liau, G. (1996). Sodium butyrate is a potent modulator of smooth muscle cell proliferation and gene expression. *Cell Proliferation*, Vol. 29, No. 5, (May 1996), pp. 231-241, ISSN 0960-7722

Ferns, G.A., Raines. E.W., Sprugel, K.H., Motani, A.S., Reidy, M.A., & Ross, R. (1991). Inhibition of neointimal smooth muscle accumulation after angioplasty by an antibody to PDGF. *Science*, Vol. 253, No. 5024, (September 1991), pp. 1129-1132, ISSN 0036-8075

Finn, A.V., Nakazawa, G., Joner, M., Kolodgie, F.D., Mont, E.K., Gold, H.K., et al. (2007). Vascular responses to drug eluting stents. Importance of delayed healing. *Arteriosclerosis Thrombosis and Vascular Biology*, Vol. 27, No. 7, (July, 2007), pp. 1500-1510, ISSN 1079-5642

Fischle, W., Wang, Y., & Allis, C.D. (2003). Histone and chromatin cross-talk. *Current Opinions in Cell Biology*, Vol. 15, No. 2, (April 2003), pp. 172-183, ISSN 0955-0674

Freeman, B.A., & Crapo, J.D. (1982). Biology of disease: free radicals and tissue injury. *Laboratory Investigation*, Vol. 47, No. 5, (November 1982), pp. 412-426, ISSN 0023-6837

Gaffney, M.M., Hynes, S.O., Barry, F., & O'Brien, T. (2007). Cardiovascular gene therapy: status and therapeutic potential. *British Journal of Pharmacology*, Vol. 152, No. 2, (September 2007), pp. 175-188, ISSN 1476-5381

Gershlick, A.H. (2002). Treating atherosclerosis: Local drug delivery from laboratory studies to clinical trials. *Atherosclerosis*, Vol. 160, No. 2, (February 2002), pp. 259-271, ISSN 0021-9150

Grossman, M., Rader, D.J., Muller, D.W., Kolansky, D.M., Kozarsky, K., Clark, B.J., et al. (1995). A pilot study of ex vivo gene therapy for homozygous familial hypercholesterolemia. *Nature Medicine*, Vol. 1, No. 11, (November 1995), pp. 1148–1154, ISSN 1078-8956

Guerin, P., Sauzeau, V., Rolli-Derkinderen, M., Al Habbash, O., Scalbert, E., Crochet, D., et al. (2005). Stent implantation activates Rho A in human arteries: Inhibitory effect of rapamycin. *Journal of Vascular Research*, Vol. 42, No. 1, (January-February 2005), pp. 21-28, ISSN 1018-1172

Habets, K.L., van Puijvelde, G.H., van Duivenvoorde, L. M., van Wanrooij, E. J., de Vos, P. Tervaert, J. W. et al. (2010). Vaccination using oxidized low-density lipoprotein-pulsed dendritic cells reduces atherosclerosis in LDL receptor-deficient mice. *Cardiovascular Research*, Vol. 85, No. 3, (February 2010), pp. 622-630, ISSN 0008-6363

Holmes, Jr. D.R. (2003). State of the art in coronary intervention. *American Journal of Cardiology*, Vol. 91, No. 3A, (February 2003), pp. 50A-53A, ISSN 1423-0135

Ito T. (2007). Role of histone modifications in chromatin dynamics. *Journal of Biochemistry*, Vol. 141, No. 5, (May 2007), pp. 609-614, ISSN 0021-924X

Jenuwein, T., & Allis, C.D. (2001). Translating the histone code. *Science*, Vol.293, No.5532, (August 2001), pp. 1074-1080, ISSN 0036-8075

Jordan, M.A., Toso, R.J., Thrower, D., & Wilson, L. (1993). Mechanism of mitotic block and inhibition of cell proliferation by taxol at low concentrations. *Proceedings of National Academy of Sciences, USA,* Vol. 90, No. 20, (October 1993), pp. 9552-9556, ISSN 0027-8424

Kawahara, K., Kawabata, H., Aratani, S., & Nakajima, T. (2003). Hypernuclear acetylation (HNA) in proliferation, differentiation and apoptosis. *Ageing Research Review*, Vol. 2, No. 3, (July 2003), pp. 287-297, ISSN 1568-1637

Kawahara, K., Watanabe, S., Ohshima, T., Soejima, Y., Oish, T., Aratani, S., et al. (1999). Hypernuclear acetylation in atherosclerotic lesions and activated vascular smooth muscle cells. *Biochemical and Biophysical Research Communications*, Vol. 266, No. 2, (December 1999), pp 417–424, ISSN 0006-291X

Kehrer, J. P. (1993). Free radicals as mediators of tissue injury and disease. *Critical Reviews in Toxicology*, Vol. 23, No. 1, (January 1993), pp. 21-48, ISSN 1040-8444

Khanna, A. (2008). Strategies and vectors for gene therapy: Its prospective therapeutic attributes against restenosis. *Journal of Clinical and Diagnostic Research*, Vol. 2, No. 3, (June 2008), pp. 871-878, ISSN 0973-709X

Kim, Y.I. (2000). AGA technical review: impact of dietary fiber on colon cancer occurrence. *Gastroenterology*, Vol. 118, No. 6, (June 2000), pp. 1235 -1257, ISSN 0016-5085

Kishore, R., & Losordo, D.W. (2007). Gene therapy for restenosis: biological solution to a biological problem. *Journal of Molecular and Cellular Cardiology*, Vol. 42, No. 3, (March 2007), pp. 461-468, ISSN 0022-2828

Kleeman, R., Zadelaar, S., & Kooistra, T. (2008). Cytokines and atherosclerosis: a comprehensive review of studies in mice. *Cardiovascular Research*, Vol. 79, No. 3, (August 2008), pp. 360-376, ISSN 0008-6363

Klingenberg, R., & Hansson, G.K. (2009). Treating inflammation in atherosclerotic cardiovascular disease: emerging therapies. *European Heart Journal*, Vol. 30, No.23, (December 2009), pp. 2838–2844, ISSN 0195-668x

Kouzarides, T. (2007). Chromatin modifications and their function. *Cell, Vol.* 128, No. 4, (February 2007), pp. 693–705, ISSN 0092-8674

Kristeleit, R., Stimson, L., Workman, P., & Aherne, W. (2004). Histone modification enzymes: novel targets for cancer drugs. *Expert Opinion Emerging Drugs*, Vol. 9, No. 1, (May 2004), pp. 135–154, ISSN 1472-8214

Kunsch, C., &, Medford, R.M. (1999). Oxidative stress as a regulator of gene expression in the vasculature. *Circulation Research*, Vol. 85, No. 8, (October 1999), pp. 753-766, ISSN 0009-7330

Li, F., Zhang, C., Schaefer, S., Estes, A., & Malik, K.U. (2005). ANG II-induced neointimal growth is mediated via cPLA2- and PLD2-activated Akt in balloon-injured rat carotid artery. *American Journal of Physiology, Heart and Circulatory Physiology*, Vol. 289, No. 6, (December 2005), pp. H2592–H2601, ISSN 0363-6135

Li, J.M., Newburger, P.E., Gounis, M.J., Dargon, P., Zhang, X., & Messina, L.M. (2010). Local arterial nanoparticle delivery of siRNA for NOX2 knockdown to prevent restenosis in an atherosclerotic rat model. *Gene Therapy*, Vol. 17, No. 10 (October 2010), 1279-1287, ISSN 0969-7128

Libby, P. (2002). Inflammation in atherosclerosis. *Nature,* Vol. 420, No. 6917, (December 2002), pp. 868-874, ISSN 0028-0836

Lindemann, R.K., Gabrielli, B., & Johnstone, R.W. (2004). Histone-deacetylase inhibitors for the treatment of cancer. *Cell Cycle,* Vol. 3, No. 6, (June 2004), pp. 779-788, ISSN 1538-4101

Lund, A.H., & van Lohuizen, M. (2004). Epigenetics and cancer. *Genes and Development,* Vol. 18, No. 19, (October 2004), pp. 2315-2335, ISSN 0890-9369

Luo, J., Nikolaev, A.Y., Imai, S., Chen, D., Su, F., Shiloh, A., et al (2001). Negative control of p53 by Sir2alpha promotes cell survival under stress. *Cell,* Vol. 107, No. 2, (October 2001), pp. 137-148, ISSN 0092-8674

Madamanchi, N.R., Vendrov, A., & Runge, M.S. (2005). Oxidative stress and vascular disease. *Arteriosclerosis Thrombosis and Vascular Biology,* Vol. 25, No. 1, (January 2005), pp. 29-38, ISSN 1079-5642

Mann, M.J., Whittemore, A.D., Donaldson, M.C., Belkin, M., Conte, M.S., Polak, J.F., et al. (1999). Ex-vivo gene therapy of human vascular bypass grafts with E2F decoy: the PREVENT single-centre, randomized, controlled trial. *Lancet,* Vol. 354, No. 9189, (October 1999), pp.1493-1498, ISSN 0099-5355

March, F., Sauty, A., Iarossi, A.S., Sukhova, G.K., Neote, K., Libby, P., etal. (1999). Differential expression of three T lymphocyte-activating CXC chemokines by human atheroma-associated cells. *Journal of Clinical Investigation,* Vol. 104, No. 8, (October 1999), pp. 1041-1050, ISSN 0021-9738

Marks, P.A., Richon, V.A., & Rifkind, R.A. (2000). Histone deacetylase inhibitors: Inducers of differentiation or apoptosis of transformed cells. *Journal of National Cancer Institute,* Vol. 92, No. 15, (August 2000), pp. 1210-1216, ISSN 0027-8874

Marmorstein, R. (2001). Structure of histone acetyltransferases. *Journal of Molecular Biology,* Vol. 311, No. 3, (August 2001), pp. 433-444, ISSN 0022-2836

Mathew, O.P., Ranganna, K., & Yatsu, F.M. (2010). Butyrate, an HDAC inhibitor, stimulates interplay between different posttranslational modifications of histone H3 and differently alters G1-specific cell cycle proteins in vascular smooth muscle cells. *Biomedicine & Pharmacotherapy,* Vol. 64, No. 10, (December 2010), pp. 733–740, ISSN 0753-3322

Matsumae, H., Yoshida, Y., Ono, K., Togi, K., Inoue, K., Furukawa, Y., et al. (2008). CCN1 knockdown suppresses neointimal hyperplasia in a rat artery balloon injury model. *Arteriosclerosis Thrombosis and Vascular Biology,* Vol. 28, No. 6 (June 2008), pp. 1077-1083, ISSN 1079-5642

Mattick, J.S., Amaral, P.P., Dinger, M.E., Mercer, T.R., & Mehler, M.F. (2009). RNA regulation of epigenetic processes. *Bioessays, Vol.* 31, No. 1, (January 2009), pp. 51-59, ISSN 1521-1878

McCarthy, M. (2001). Molecular decoy may keep bypass grafts open. *Lancet,* Vol. 358, No. 9294, (November 2001), pp. 1703, ISSN 0099-5355

McManus, K.J., & Hendzel, M.J. (2006). The relationship between histone H3 phosphorylation and acetylation throughout the mammalian cell cycle. *Biochemistry and Cell Biology,* Vol. 84, No. 4, (August 2006), pp. 640-657, ISSN 0829-8211

Melo, L.G., Pachori, A.S., Gnecchi, M., & Dzau, V.J. (2005). Genetic therapies for cardiovascular diseases. *Trends in Molecular Medicine,* Vol.11, No.5, (May 2005), pp. 240-250, ISSN 1471-4914

Morishita, R., Gibbons, G.H., Ellison, K.E., Nakajima, M., Zhang, L., Kaneda, Y., et al. (1993). Single intraluminal delivery of antisense cdc2 kinase and proliferating- cell nuclear antigen oligonucleotides results in chronic inhibition of neointimal hyperplasia. *Proceedings National Academy of Sciences, USA,* Vol. 90, No. 18, (September 1993), pp.8474-8478 ISSN 0027-8424

Natarajan, R. (2011). Drugs targeting epigenetic histone acetylation in vascular smooth muscle cells for restenosis and atherosclerosis. *Arteriosclerosis Thrombosis and Vascular Biology,* Vol. 31, No. 4, (April 2011), pp. 725-727 ISSN 1079-5642

Ng, R.K., & Gurdon, J.B. (2008). Epigenetic inheritance of cell differentiation status. *Cell Cycle,* Vol. 7, No. 9 (May 2008), pp. 1173–77, ISSN 1538-4101

O'Brien, K.D., McDonald, T.O., Chait, A., Allen, M.D., & Alpers, C.E. (1996). Neovascular expression of E-Selectin, intercellular adhesion molecule-1, and vascular cell adhesion molecule-1 in human atherosclerosis and their relation to intimal leukocyte content. *Circulation,* Vol. 93, No. 4, (February 1996), pp. 672-682, ISSN 0009-7322

Okamoto, H., Fujioka, Y., Takahashi, A., Takahashi, T., Taniguchi, T., Ishikawa, Y., etal. (2006). Trichostatin A, an inhibitor of histone deacetylase, inhibits smooth muscle cell proliferation via induction of p21 (WAF1). *Journal of Atherosclerosis and Thrombosis,* Vol. 13, No. 4, (August 2006), pp. 183-191, ISSN 1079-5642

Pons, D., de Vries, F.R., van den Elsen, P.J., Heijmans, B.T., Quax, P.H., & Jukema, J.W. (2009). Epigenetic histone acetylation modifiers in vascular remodeling: new targets for therapy in cardiovascular disease. *European Heart Journal,* Vol. 30, No. 3, (February 2009), pp. 266-277, ISSN 0195-668X

Probst, A.V., Dunleavy, E., & Almouzni, G. (2009). Epigenetic inheritance during the cell cycle. *Nature Reviews, Molecular and Cell Bioliology.* Vol. 10, No. 3, (March 2009), pp. 192–206, ISSN 1471-0072

Qian, H., Neplioueva, V., Shetty, G.A., Channon, K. M., George, S. E. (1999). Nitric oxide synthase gene therapy rapidly reduces adhesion molecule expression and inflammatory cell infiltration in carotid artery of cholesterol-fed rabbits. *Circulation,* Vol. 99, No. 23, (June 1999), pp. 2979–2982, ISSN 0009-7322

Raizner, A.E., Oesterle, S.N., Waksman, R., Serruys, P.W., Colombo, A., Lim, Y.L., et al. (2000). Inhibition of restenosis with b-emitting radiotherapy. Report of the proliferation reduction with vascular energy trial (PREVENT). *Circulation,* Vol. 102, No. 9, (August 2000), pp. 951-958, ISSN 0009-7522

Ranganna, K., Yatsu, F.M., & Hayes, B.E. (2005). Butyrate, a small pleiotropic molecule with multiple cellular and molecular actions: Its role as an anti-atherogenic agent. *Recent Research Development in Molecular Cellular Biochemistry,* Vol. 2, pp. 123-151, Research Signpost, ISBN 81-7736-294-1, Kerala, India

Ranganna, K., Yatsu, F.M., & Mathew, O.P. (2006). Insights into the pathogenesis and intervention of atherosclerosis. *Vascular Disease Prevention,* Vol. 3, No. 4, pp. 375-390, ISSN 1567-2700

Ranganna, K., Yatsu, F.M., Hayes, B.E., Milton, S.G., & Jayakumar, A. (2000). Butyrate inhibits proliferation-induced proliferating cell nuclear antigen expression (PCNA) in rat vascular smooth muscle cells. *Molecular cellular Biochemistry,* Vol. 205, No.1-2, (February 2000), pp. 149-161, ISSN 0300-8177

Ranganna, K., Yousefipour, Z., Yatsu, F.M., Milton, S.G., & Hayes, B.E. (2003). Gene expression profile of butyrate-inhibited vascular smooth muscle cell proliferation. *Molecular cellular Biochemistry,* Vol. 254, No. 1-2, (December 2003), pp. 21-36, ISSN 0300-8177

Ranganna, K., Mathew, O.P., Yousefipour, Z., Yatsu, F.M., Hayes, B.E., & Milton, S.G. (2007). Involvement of glutathione/glutathione *S*-transferase antioxidant system in butyrate-inhibited vascular smooth muscle cell proliferation. *FEBS Journal,* Vol. 274, No. 22, (November 2007), pp. 5962–5978, Online ISSN 1742 4658

Ross R. (1993). The pathogenesis of atherosclerosis: a perspective for the 1990s. *Nature,* Vol. 362, No. 6423, (April 1993), pp. 801-809, ISSN 0028-0836

Ross, R. (1995). Cell biology of atherosclerosis. *Annual Review of Physiology,* Vol. 57, (March 1995), pp. 791-804, ISSN 0066-4278

Sahar, S., Reddy, M.A., Wong, C., Meng, L., Wang, M., & Natarajan, R. (2007). Cooperation of SRC-1 and p300 with NF-kB and CREB in angiotensin II-induced IL-6 expression in vascular smooth muscle cells. *Arteriosclerosis Thrombosis and Vascular Biology,* Vol. 27, No. 7, (July 2007), pp. 1528 –1534, ISSN 1079-5642

Santini, V., Gozzini, A., & Ferrari, G. (2007). Histone deacetylase inhibitors: molecular and biological activity as a premise to clinical application. *Current Drug Metabolism,* Vol. 8, No.4, (May 2007), pp. 383–393, ISSN 1389-2002

Schreiber, S.L., & Bernstein, B.E. (2002). Signaling network model of chromatin. *Cell,* Vol. 111, No. 6, (December 2002), pp. 771-778, ISSN 0092-8674

Sharma, S., Kelly, T.K., & Jones, P.A. (2010). Epigenetics in cancer. *Carcinogenesis,* Vol. 31, No. 1, (January 2010), pp. 27–36, ISSN 0143-3334

Simons, M., Edelman, E.R., & Rosenberg, R.D. (1994). Antisense proliferating cell nuclear antigen oligonucleotides inhibit intimal hyperplasia in a rat carotid artery injury model. *Journal of Clinical Investigations,* Vol. 93, No. 6, (June 1994), pp. 2351-2356, ISSN 0021-9738

Song, S., Kang, S.W., & Choi, C. (2010). Trichostatin A enhances proliferation and migration of vascular smooth muscle cells by downregulating thioredoxin 1. *Cardiovascular Research,* Vol. 85, No. 1, (January 2010), pp. 241-249, ISSN 0008-6363

Steinberg, D., & Witztum, J.L. (2010). History of discovery. Oxidized Low-Density Lipoprotein and Atherosclerosis. *Arteriosclerosis, Thrombosis and Vascular Biology,* Vol. 30, No. 12 (December 2010), pp. 2311-2316, ISSN 1079-5642

Tangirala, R.K., Tsukamoto, K., Chun, S.H., Usher, D., Puré, E., & Rader, D.J. (1999). Regression of atherosclerosis induced by liver-directed gene transfer of apolipoprotein A-1 in mice. *Circulation,* Vol. 100, No. 17, (October 1999), pp. 1816-1822, ISSN 0009-7322

Taverna, S.D., Li, H., Ruthenburg, A.J., Allis, C.D., & Patel, D.J. (2007). How chromatin-binding modules interpret histone modifications: lessons from professional pocket pickers. *Nature Structural and Molecular Biology,* Vol.14, No. 11, (November 2007), pp. 1025–1040, ISSN 1545-9993

Teirstein, P.S., & King, S. (2003). Vascular radiation in a drug-eluting stent world: It's not over till it's over. *Circulation*, Vol. 108, No. 4, (July 2003), pp. 384-385, ISSN 0009-7322

Toshiro, M., Ueno, T., Tanaka, M., Oka, H., Miyamotq, T., Osajima, K., et al. (2005). Antiproliferative action of an angiotensin I-converting enzyme inhibitory peptide, Val-Tyr, *via* an L-type $Ca^{2+}$ channel inhibition in cultured vascular smooth muscle cells. *Hypertension Research*, Vol. 28, No. 6, (June, 2005), pp. 545–552, ISSN 1348-4214

Turner, B.M. (2003). Memorable transcription. *Nature Cell Biology*, Vol. 5, No. 5, (May 2003), pp. 390-393, ISSN 1465-7392

Turunen, M.P., Aavik, E., & Yla-Herttuala, S. (2009). Epigenetics and atherosclerosis. *Biochemical et Biophysical Acta*, Vol. 1790, No. 9, (September 2009), pp. 886-891, ISSN 0006-3002

Tzeng, E., Shears, L.L., & Robbins, P.D, Pitt, B.R., Geller, D.A., Watkins, S.C., et al. (1996). Vascular gene transfer of the human inducible nitric oxide synthase: characterization of activity and effects of myointimal hyperplasia. *Molecular Medicine*, Vol. 2, No. 2, ( March 1996), pp. 211-225, ISSN 1076-1551

Van Assche, T., Huygelen, V., & Crabtree, M.J. (2011). Targeting vascular redox biology through antioxidant gene delivery: a historical view and current prospective. *Recent Patents on Cardiovascular Drug Discovery*, Vol. 6, No. 2 , (May 2011), pp. 89-102, ISSN 1574-8901

Vinh, A., Gaspari, T.A., Liu, H.B., Dousha, L.F., Widdop, R.E., & Dear, A.E. (2008). A novel histone deacetylase inhibitor reduces abdominal aortic aneurysm formation in angiotensin II-infused apolipoprotein E-deficient mice. *Journal of Vascular Research*, Vol. 45, No. 2, (March 2008), pp. 143–152, ISSN 1018-1172

Von der Leyen, H.E., & Dzau D.J. (2001). Therapeutic potential of nitric oxide synthase gene manipulation. *Circulation*, Vol. 103, No. 22, (June 2001), pp. 2760-2765, ISSN 0009-7322

Waksman, R., Bhargava, B., White L, Chan, R.C., Mehran, R., Lansky, A.J. et al. (2000). Intracoronary b-radiation therapy inhibits recurrence of in-stent restenosis. *Circulation*, Vol. 101, No. 16, (April 25), pp. 1895-1898, ISSN 0009-7322

Waltregny, D., Gle´nisson, W., Tran, S.L., North, B.J., Verdin, E., Colige, A., etal. (2005). Histone deacetylase HDAC8 associates with smooth muscle α-actin and is essential for smooth muscle cell contractility. *FASEB J*. Vol. 19, No. 8, (June 2005), pp. 966 – 968, ISSN 0892-6638

Wilson, G. J., Polovick, J. E., Huibregtse, B.A., & Poff B. C. (2007). Overlapping paclitaxel-eluting stents: Long-term effects in a porcine coronary artery model. *Cardiovascular Research*, Vol. 76, No. 2, (November 2007), pp. 361 – 372, ISSN 0008-6363

Witztum, J.L. (1997). Immunological response to oxidized LDL. *Atherosclerosis*, Vol. 131, No. 2, (June 1997), pp. S9–S11, ISSN 0021-9150

Xu, X., Ha, C.H., Wong, C., Wang, W., Hausser, A., Pfizenmaier, K., etal. (2007). Angiotensin II stimulates protein kinase D-dependent histone deacetylase 5 phosphorylation and nuclear export lading to vascular smooth muscle cell hypertrophy. *Arteriosclerosis Thrombosis and Vascular Biology*, Vol. 27, No. 11, (November 2007), pp. 2355–2362, ISSN 1079-5642

Yan, Z.Q., Yao, Q.P., Zhang, M.L., Qi, Y.X., Guo, Z.Y., Shen, B.R., et al. (2009). Histone deacetylases modulate vascular smooth muscle cell migration induced by cyclic mechanical strain. *Journal of Biomechanics*, Vol. 42, No. 7, (May 2009), pp. 945–948, ISSN 0021-9290

Zeiffer, U., Schober, A., Lietz, M., Liehn, E.A., Erl, W., Emans, N., et al. (2004). Neointimal smooth muscle cells display a proinflammatory phenotype resulting in increased leukocyte recruitment mediated by P-selectin and chemokines. *Circulation Research*, Vol. 94, No. 6, (April 2004), pp. 776-784, ISSN 0009-7330

Zhou, X., Caligiuri, G., Hamsten, A., Lefvert, A. K., & Hansson, G.K., (2001). LDL immunization induces T-cell-dependent antibody formation and protection against atherosclerosis. *Arteriosclerosis Thrombosis and Vascular Biology*, Vol. 21, No. 1, (January 2001), pp. 108–114, ISSN 1079-5642

# 6

# Endothelial and Vascular Smooth Cell Dysfunctions: A Comprehensive Appraisal

Luigi Fabrizio Rodella and Rita Rezzani
*Anatomy Section, Department of Biomedical Sciences and Biotechnology, University of Brescia, Italy*

## 1. Introduction

Cardiovascular disease (CvDs) such as coronary artery disease, hypertension, congestive heart failure and stroke are the leading causes of death and disability in the Western World (Madamanchi et al., 2005; Thom, 1989). The majority of CvDs results from complication of atherosclerosis. Prevention of cardiovascular events is therefore urgently needed and is one of the major recent challenges of medicine. New molecular imaging approaches featuring the assessment of inflammatory processes in the vascular wall (on top of existing anatomic and functional vessel imaging procedures) could emerge as decisive tools for the understanding and prevention of cardiovascular events (Schafers et al., 2010).

## 2. Atherosclerosis

Atherosclerosis is a progressive disease, affecting medium and large-sized arteries, characterized by patchy intramural thickening of the subintimal that encroaches on the arterial lumen (Bonomini et al., 2008). The atherosclerosis plaque is characterized by an accumulation of lipid in the artery wall, together with infiltration of macrophages, T cells and mast cells, and the formation by vascular smooth muscle cells (VSMCs) of a fibrous cap composed mostly of collagen. Early lesions called "fatty streaks" consist of sub-endothelial deposition of lipid, macrophage foam cells loaded with cholesterol and T cells. Over time, a more complex lesion develops, with apoptotic as well as necrotic cells, cell debris and cholesterol crystals forming a necrotic core in the lesion. This structure is covered by a fibrous cap of variable thickness, and its "shoulder" regions are infiltrated by activated T cells, macrophages and mast cells, which produce proinflammatory mediators and enzymes (Hansson et al., 2006). Plaque growth can cause stenosis (narrowing of the lumen) that can contribute to ischemia in the surrounding tissue (Hansson & Hermansson, 2011).

Although the pathophysiological mechanisms underlying atherosclerosis are not completely understood, it is widely recognized that both inflammation and oxidative stress play important roles in all of the phases of atherosclerosis evolution (Cipollone et al., 2007).

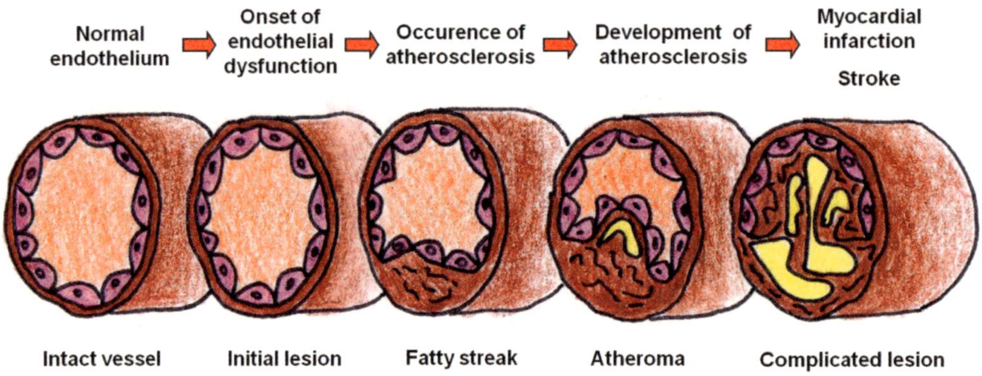


Fig. 1. Steps involved in atherosclerosis progression from endothelial dysfunction to cardiovascular complication.

### 2.1 Atherosclerosis and oxidative stress

Oxidative stress can be defined as an "imbalance between oxidants and antioxidants in favor of the oxidants, potentially leading to damage" (Sies, 1991). Age, gender, obesity, cigarette smoking, hypertension, diabetes mellitus and dyslipidemia are known atherogenic risk factors that promote the impairment of endothelial function, smooth muscle function and vessel wall metabolism. These risk factors are associated with an increased production of reactive oxygen species (ROS) (Antoniades et al., 2003). ROS play a physiological role in the vessel wall and participate as second messengers in endothelium-dependent function, in smooth muscle cells and endothelial cells (ECs) growth and survival, and in remodelling of the vessel wall. Each of these responses, when uncontrolled, contributes to vascular diseases (Fortuño et al., 2005; Griendling & Harrison, 1999; Irani, 2000; Taniyama & Griendling, 2003).

In the vasculature wall, ROS are produced by all the layers, including tunica intima, media and adventitia. ROS include superoxide anion radical ($O_2^-$), hydrogen peroxide ($H_2O_2$), hydroxyl radical (OH), nitric oxide (NO), and peroxynitrite ($ONOO^-$) (Lakshmi et al., 2009). The major vascular ROS is $O_2^-$, which inactivates NO, the main vascular relaxing factor, thus impairing relaxation (Cai & Harrison, 2000; Kojda & Harrison, 1999). Dismutation of $O_2^-$ by superoxide dismutase (SOD) produces $H_2O_2$, a more stable ROS, which, in turn, is converted to water by catalase and glutathione peroxidase. $H_2O_2$ and other peroxides appear to be important in the regulation of growth-related signalling in VSMCs and inflammatory responses in vascular lesions (Irani, 2000; Li, P.F. et al., 1997). High levels of $O_2^-$, the consequent accumulation of $H_2O_2$ and diminished NO bioavailability play a critical role in the modulation of vascular remodelling. Finally, $ONOO^-$, resulting from the reaction between $O_2^-$ and NO, constitutes a strong oxidant molecule, which is able to oxidize proteins, lipids and nucleic acids and then causes cell damage (Beckman & Koppenol, 1996; Fortuño et al., 2005).

There are several potential sources of ROS production. In cardiovascular disease the sources include xanthine oxidase, cyclooxygenase, lipooxygenase, mitochondrial respiration, cytochrome P450, uncoupled nitric oxide synthase (NOS) and NAD(P)H oxidase. They have been identified as sources of ROS generation in all type of vasculature. These sources may contribute to ROS formation, depending on cell type, cellular activation site and disease context. Numerous studies have shown that various physiological stimuli that contribute to pathogenesis of vascular disease can induce the formation of ROS (Lakshmi et al., 2009). ROS have detrimental effects on vascular function through several mechanisms. First, ROS, especially hydroxyl radicals, directly injure cell membranes and nuclei. Second, by interacting with endogenous vasoactive mediators formed in ECs, ROS modulate vasomotion and the atherogenic process. Third, ROS peroxidize lipid components, leading to the formation of oxidized lipoproteins (LDL), one of the key mediators of atherosclerosis (Bonomini et al., 2008).

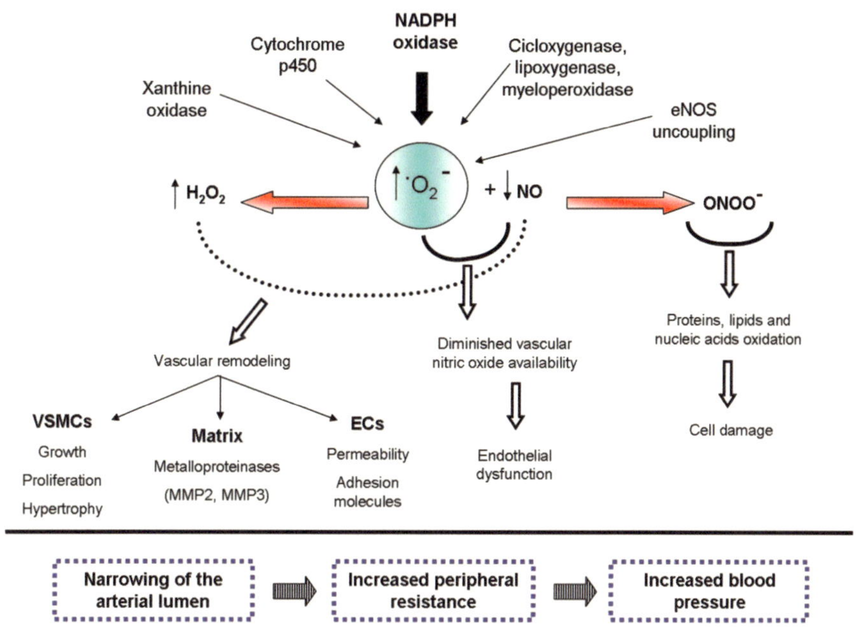


Fig. 2. Potential sources of ROS production in atherosclerosis progression.

Cholesterol is transported in the blood by LDL. These particles contain esterified cholesterol and triglycerides surrounded by a shell of phospholipids, free cholesterol and apolipoprotein B100 (ApoB100). Circulating LDL particles can accumulate in the intimal, the innermost layer of the artery. Here ApoB100 binds to proteoglycans of the extracellular matrix (ECM) through ionic interactions (Tabas et al., 2007). This is an important initiating factor in early atherogenesis (Skålen et al., 2002; Steinberg, 2009; Witztum & Steinberg, 2001). As a consequence of this subendothelial retention, LDL particles are trapped in the tunica intima, where they are prone to oxidative modifications caused by enzymatic attack of myeloperoxidase (Heinecke, 2007) and lipoxygenases, or by ROS such as hypoclorous acid (HOCl), phenoxyl radical intermediates or $ONOO^-$ generated in the intimal during inflammation and atherosclerosis (Hansson & Hermansson, 2011).

Oxidized LDL (Ox-LDL) has several biological effects (Madamanchi et al., 2005); it is pro-inflammatory; it causes inhibition of endothelial NOS (eNOS); it promotes vasoconstriction and adhesion; it stimulates cytokines such as interleukins (ILs) and increases platelet aggregation. Ox-LDL-derived products are cytotoxic and induce apoptosis. Ox-LDL can adversely affect coagulation by stimulating tissue factor and plasminogen activator inhibitor-1 (PAI-1) synthesis. Another atherogenic property of Ox-LDL is its immunogenicity and its ability to promote retention of macrophages in the arterial wall by inhibiting macrophage motility (Singh & Jialal, 2006). In addiction, Ox-LDL stimulates VSMCs proliferation (Stocker & Keaney, 2004). Thus, intimal thickening further reduces the lumen of blood vessels, leading to further potentation of hypertension and atherosclerosis (Singh & Jialal, 2006). With ongoing oxidation, the physicochemical properties gradually change, including alterations in charge, particle size, lipid content and other features. The precise nature of each of these alterations obviously depends on the oxidizing agent. For all these reasons, Ox-LDL is not a defined molecular species but is instead a spectrum of LDL particles that have undergone a variety of physicochemical changes (Hansson & Hermansson, 2011).

### 2.2 Atherosclerosis and inflammation

Inflammation participates in atherosclerosis from its inception onwards. Fatty streaks do not cause symptoms, and may either progress to more complex lesions or involute. Fatty streaks have focal increases in the content of lipoproteins within regions of the intimal, where they associate with components of the ECM such as proteoglycans, slowing their egress. This retention sequesters lipoproteins within the intimal, isolating them from plasma antioxidants, thus favoring their oxidative modification (Kruth, 2002; Packard & Libby, 2008; Skålen et al., 2002). Oxidatively modified LDL particles comprise an incompletely defined mixture, because both the lipid and protein moieties can undergo oxidative modification. Constituents of such modified lipoprotein particles can induce a local inflammatory response (Miller et al., 2003; Packard & Libby, 2008).

Vascular ECs function to prevent clotting of blood and adhesion of blood cells to the endothelial cells, in addition to playing the role of a barrier, as a cell monolayer, to prevent blood constituents from invading the vascular wall. When ECs are injured or activated by various coronary risk factors, infections or physical stimuli, adhesion molecules become expressed in ECs, and peripheral monocytes adhere to the endothelial cell surface. Adhesion molecules are broadly divided into three molecular families: integrin family, immunoglobulin family, and selectin family (L-selectin, Eselectin, P-selectin) (Yamada, 2001).

Chemoattractant factors, which include monocyte chemoattractant protein-1 (MCP-1) produced by vascular wall cells in response to modified lipoproteins, direct the migration and diapedesis of adherent monocytes (Boring et al., 1998; Packard & Libby, 2008). Monocytic cells, directly interacting with human ECs, increase several fold monocyte matrix metalloproteinase (MMP) 9 production, allowing for the subsequent infiltration of leukocytes through the endothelial layer and its associated basement membrane (Amorino & Hoover, 1998; Packard & Libby, 2008) Within the intima, monocytes mature into macrophages under the influence of macrophage colony stimulating factor (M-CSF), which is overexpressed in the inflamed intima. M-CSF stimulation also increases macrophage expression of scavenger receptors, members of the pattern-recognition receptor superfamily, which engulf modified lipoproteins through receptor-mediated endocytosis. Accumulation of cholesteryl esters in the cytoplasm converts macrophages into foam cells, i.e., lipid-laden macrophages characteristic of early-stage atherosclerosis. In parallel, macrophages proliferate and amplify the inflammatory response through the secretion of numerous growth factors and cytokines, including tumor necrosis factor α (TNFα) and IL-1β. Recent evidence supports selective recruitment of a proinflammatory subset of monocytes to nascent atheroma in mice (Packard & Libby, 2008).

A number of proinflammatory cytokines have been shown to participate in atherosclerotic plaque development, growth and rupture (Dabek, 2010; Libby et al., 2002). Nuclear factor kappa-light-chain-enhancer of activated B cells (NF-kB) seems to be a crucial transcription factor in the cross-talk among cytokines, adhesion molecules and growth factors. On one hand, NF-kB is a major transcription factor leading to cytokine synthesis, and on the other hand, the above mentioned factors keep NF-kB persistently activated in acute coronary syndromes (Dabek, 2010). In atherogenesis, NF-kB before regulates the expression of cyclooxygenases, lipooxygenases, cytokines, chemokines (i.e., MCP-1) and adhesion molecules (Dabek, 2010; Kutuk & Basaga, 2003). Later in the progression of the atherosclerotic lesion, NF-kB regulates gene expression of M-CSF, a factor stimulating infiltrating monocyte differentiation and transformation into "foamy cells", and other genes participating in the transformation (Brach et al., 1991; Dabek, 2010). As stated, atherosclerosis is an inflammatory reaction of the arterial wall. The factors IL-1β, TNF-α, IL-6, IL-12 and interferon γ (IFNγ) are involved in this reaction and their expression is coregulated by NF-kB.

Intracellular matrix degradation is an important process in both plaque development and rupture. The vital factors involved include MMPs, particularly those that are able to break down the vascular base membrane. It has been shown that NF-kB is an essential regulator of MMP gene expression, especially MMP-2 and MMP-9, which are critical in plaque rupture (Bond et al., 1998; Dabek, 2010). Thus, NF-kB regulates the expression of a wide spectrum of atherosclerosis mediating factors. On the other hand, most of these factors also up-regulate NF-kB activity. Increased NF-kB activity was found in unstable regions of atherosclerotic plaques (Brand et al., 1997; Dabek, 2010). The significance of NF-kB activity has been confirmed in some clinical studies as well. Li and colleagues reported significantly increased NF-kB activity in white blood cells from unstable angina patients *vs.* stable angina patients and *vs.* control patients (the lowest activity in the latter) (Li, J.J. et al., 2004).

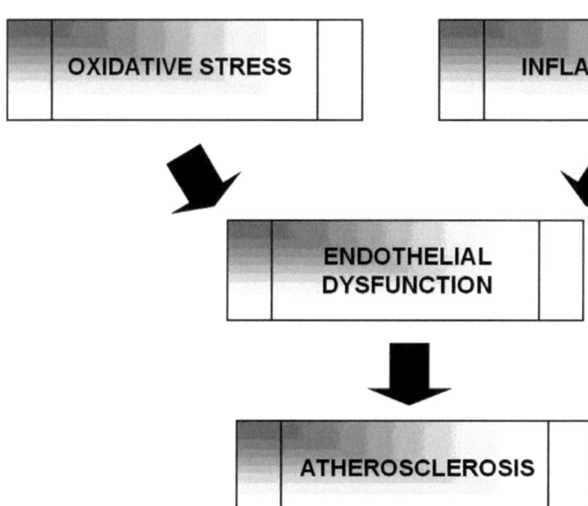


Fig. 3. Role of oxidative stress and inflammation in the early atherosclerosis.

### 3. Endothelial cells dysfunction in atherosclerosis

The endothelium is responsible for the regulation of vascular tone, the exchange of plasma and cell biomolecules, inflammation, lipid metabolism and modulation of fibrinolysis and coagulation (Andrews et al., 2010). Aging affects many pathways involved in cardiovascular functions and particularly of ECs (Barton, 2010; Virdis et al., 2010). In fact, endothelial-aging is associated with anatomical disruption, morphological abnormalities in ECs size and shape (Haudenschild et al., 1981), susceptibility to apoptosis and abnormal release of EC-derived factors (Barton, 2010). These factors, which are synthetized not only by ECs, but also by VSMCs, are now known to contribute to pathogenetic mechanisms of CVDs (Higashi et al., 2009).

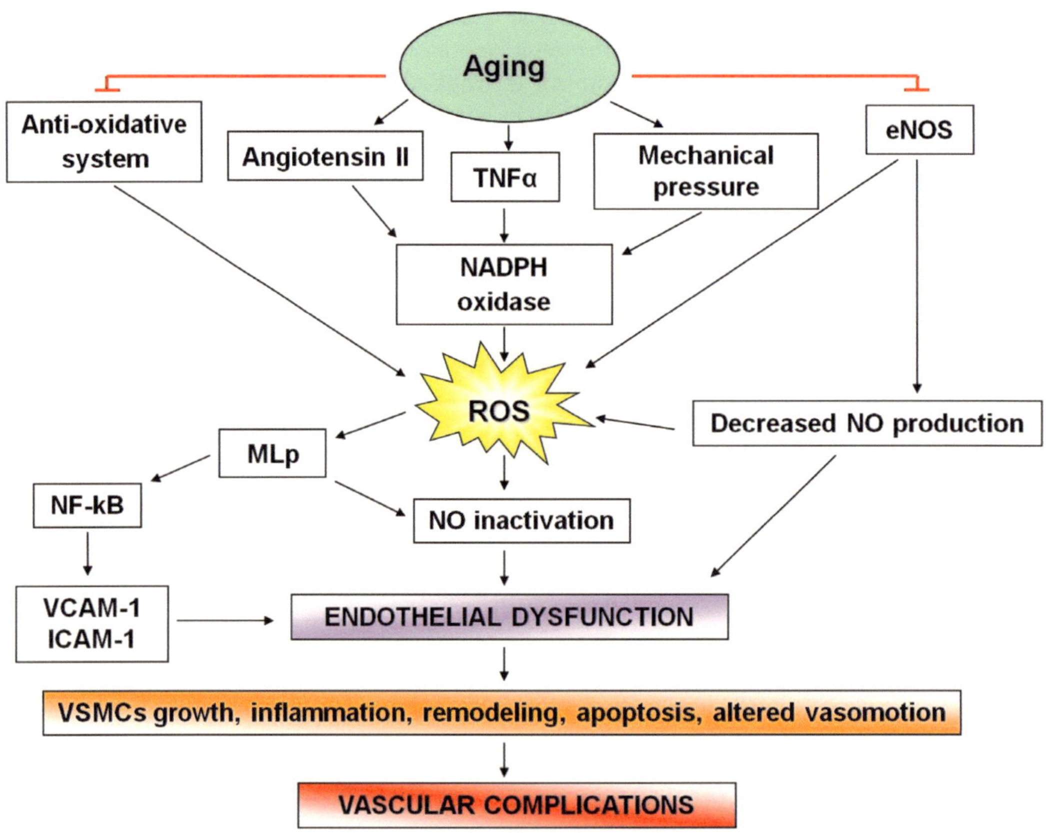


Fig. 4. Central role of ROS in inducing endothelial dysfunction in vascular diseases.

ECs dysfunction, inflammation, oxidative stress and dyslipidaemia are known to play prominent and vital roles not only in the development of atherosclerotic lesions, but also in their progression. (Andrews et al., 2010; Bai et al., 2010; Higashi et al., 2009 ; Virdis et al., 2010). Number of factors and modalities are available to interfere with age related changes in EC function (Barton, 2010; Jensen-Urstad et al., 1999). When endothelial damage compromises the normal vascular function, the intracellular dynamic balance probably leans on an athero-prone phenotype.

Growing evidence indicates that chronic and acute overproduction of ROS activates ECs as pivotal early event in atherogenesis. Oxidative stress induces cell proliferation, hypertrophy, apoptosis and inflammation through activation of various signaling cascades, redox-sensitive transcriptional factors and expression of pro-inflammatory phenotype (Higashi et al., 2009). ECs dysfunction has been shown to be associated with an increase of ROS in atherosclerotic animal models and in human subjects with atherosclerosis (Dai, D.Z. & Dai, Y., 2010; Davies et al., 2010; Higashi et al., 2009). Moreover, in APOE-deficient mice, a widely used animal model of atherosclerosis (Xu, 2009; Zhang, S.H. et al., 1992), studies have demonstrated that aged-ECs are more sensitive to apoptosis than younger ones. ECs in the areas of the artery resistant to atherosclerosis have a life span of about 12 months, whereas cells at lesion-prone sites live for few weeks and even shorter in aged animals (Xu, 2009).

### 3.1 Endothelial cell-factors

The vascular endothelium is nowadays considered to be a paracrine organ responsible for the secretion of several substances exerting atherogenic effects. The reduced bioavailability of NO as an indirect result of the effects of those factors, leads to atherosclerosis and its clinical manifestations (Muller & Morawietz, 2009; Tousoulis et al., 2010). Under normal conditions, ECs constantly produce a number of vasoactive and trophic substances that control inflammation, VSMC growth, vasomotion, platelet function and plasmatic coagulation (Barton & Haudenschild, 2001; Traupe et al., 2003).

Normal vascular activity is essential for maintaining normal function of organs, dependent on a balance of vasoconstrictive and vasodilative substances derived from the endothelium, which mainly include NO to dilate and endothelin-1 (ET-1) to constrict the cells of tunica media. Furthermore, ECs activated by ROS can regulate vascular function via the release of inflammatory mediators, such as intercellular adhesion molecule-1 (ICAM-1), vascular cell adhesion molecule (VCAM-1), MCP-1, ILs, angiotensin-II (A-II), TNFα, NF-kB and E- and P-selectin, or the release of haemostatic regulators, such as von Willebrand factor, tissue factor inhibitor and plasminogen activator, fibrinogen and NO (Sima et al., 2009; Vanhoutte, 2009).

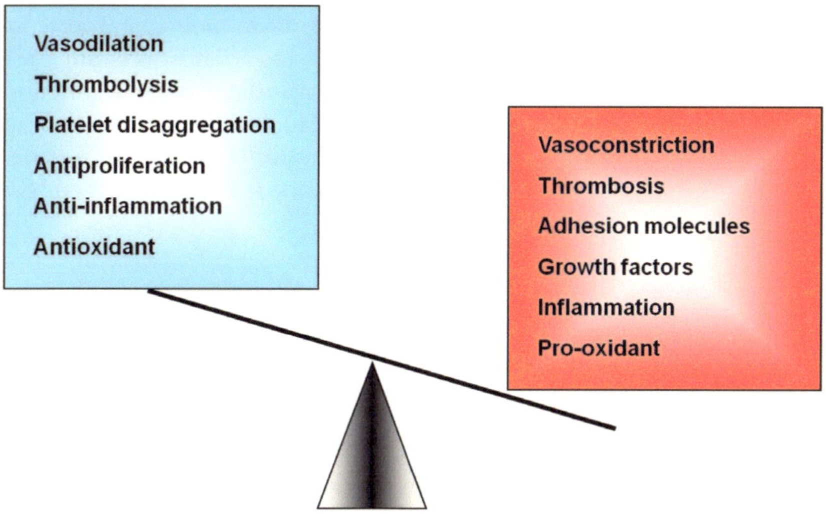


Fig. 5. Regulatory functions of the endothelium maintaining the equilibrium between antiatherogenic and atherogenic properties.

The purpose of the following paragraphs will be to provide a brief description and characterization of the main EC-factors that are synthesize and secrete after ROS stimulus during endothelial athero-susceptibility.

### 3.1.1 Angiotensin-II

A-II, a causal factor to the dysfunction of vascular endothelium, adversely stimulates the activity of the cardiovascular system (Dai, D.Z. & Dai, Y., 2010). A-II increases blood pressure by vasoconstriction and sodium and fluid retention and produces overt oxidative stress resultant from the activation of NADPH oxidase, a source of ROS in blood vessels, that promotes endothelial dysfunction, inducing cytokines, chemokines and adhesion molecules secretion and contributes to vascular remodeling (Dai, D.Z. & Dai, Y., 2010; Ferrario, 2009; Partigulova & Naumov, 2010). The A-II effects on gene expression are mediated, at least in part, through the cytoplasmic NF-kB transcription factor. Through these actions, A-II augments vascular inflammation, induces EC dysfunctions and, in so doing, enhances the atherogenic process (Sprague & Khalil, 2009).

### 3.1.2 Endothelial nitric oxide synthase

Endothelium-derived NO, formed by eNOS, (isoform 3 of NO shynthase) is known as a potent vasodilator (Barton, 2010). eNOS is also the master gene regulator used by ECs to orchestrate their own phenotype, function and survival. eNOS is modulated by shear stress (Rodella et al., 2010, a) and agonists acting on cell surface receptors; its activity is dependent on many mechanisms, including substrate availability, phosphorylation, $Ca^{2+}$ flux and protein–protein interactions (Andrews et al., 2010).

With age, a number of changes occur in the cardiovascular system that can be considered pro-atherogenic (Barton, 2010). It is widely accepted that the most important mechanism leading to endothelial dysfunction is the reduced bioavailability of NO; so the decreased bioavailability of NO is consequently regarded a critical precursor to the development of atherosclerotic plaque and has been considered as one of the factors contributing to the higher incidence of atherosclerosis, arterial hypertension and renal disease in aged individuals (Barton, 2005). Together with its role as a vasodilator, NO impedes processes that are vital for atherosclerotic progression, including vasoconstriction, VSMCs proliferation and monocyte adhesion (Napoli et al., 2006). Furthermore, with atherosclerotic conditions, eNOS can become dysfunctional as it uncouples from its dimeric state to a monomeric state, in which it is able to produce superoxide anions rather than NO (Andrews et al., 2010; Vàsquez-Vivar et al., 1998).

### 3.1.3 Endothelin-1

Endothelins are EC-derived vasoactive peptides. Since its discovery, ET-1 has been demonstrated as one of the most potent known vasoconstrictors (Barton, 2010). ET-1 is synthesized in bulk by ECs and VSMCs (Rodella et al., 2010,a) as well as by macrophages, cardiomiocytes, neurons, renal medulla and Kupffer cells (Piechota et al., 2010). Factors that stimulate the release of ET-1 include endotoxins, TNFα, IL-1, adrenaline, insulin, thrombin and A-II. ROS are involved in the modulation and activation of ET-1 that induced various signaling pathways; in fact, during the inflammation process, atherosclerosis and hypertension there are elevated levels of ET-1 (Piechota et al., 2010; Skalska et al., 2009; Teplyakov, 2004).

### 3.1.4 Tumor necrosis factor α

TNFα is crucially involved in the pathogenesis and progression of atherosclerosis, myocardial ischemia/reperfusion injury and heart failure. The TNFα-mediated vascular dysfunction involves alterations in EC metabolism and function, platelet aggregation, EC-blood cell interaction, VSMC function and proliferation (McKellar et al., 2009). It increases the expression of many pro-inflammatory, pro-coagulant, proliferative and pro-apoptotic genes involved in initiation and progression of atherosclerosis (Bergh et al., 2009). TNFα induces the rapid expression of cellular adhesion molecules (CAMs), such as VCAM-1 and ICAM-1, and E-selectin at the endothelial surface (Chandrasekharan et al., 2007; Kleinbongard et al., 2010). Endothelial dysfunction associated with TNF*a* during atherogenesis is linked to an excess in production of ROS and a decrease in NO bioavailability. The production of ROS can stimulate a cytokine cascade through NF-κB-induced transcriptional events, which then induce the expression of TNFα (Zhang, H. et al., 2009).

### 3.1.5 Cellular adhesion molecules (ICAM-1 and VCAM-1)

When ECs undergo inflammatory activation, an increase in the expression of CAMs promotes the adherence of inflammatory cells (monocytes, neutrophils, lymphocytes and macrophages) and the recruitment of additional cytokines, growth factors and MMPs into the vascular wall (Sprague & Khalil, 2009). ICAM-1 and VCAM1 are immunoglobulin-like CAMs expressed by several cell types including ECs and leukocytes. They are present in atherosclerotic lesions during their progression, because they are involved in the transendothelial migration of leukocytes, lymphocytes and antigen presenting cells to sites of inflammation (Blankenberg et al., 2001; Ho et al., 2008; Lawson & Wolf, 2009; Rodella et al., 2010,b). Nevertheless their pathological role remain still uncertain. An important stimulus for CAMs expression is the fluid shear stress, which exerts both pro-inflammatory and protective effects, depending on the type of shear.

### 3.2 Shear stress

As the regulator of vascular tone, ECs are highly sensitive to different types of shear stress caused by the complex structure of artery geometry. It is clearly observed that atherogenesis generally occurs at curved or branching points with disturbed flow. Endothelium in the regions of flow disturbances near arterial branches, bifurcations and curvatures shows an athero-prone phenotype, while laminar flow regions exhibit an athero-protective phenotype (Bai et al., 2010; Traub & Berk, 1998). When endothelial monolayer is stimulated by laminar flow, rapidly cellular responses occur, included opening of ion channels, release of vasoactive NO and activation of transcription factors and cell cycle regulators (Foteinos et al., 2008). In particular, laminar flow induces NO production through both the transcriptional up-regulation of eNOS gene expression and the posttranslational modification of eNOS protein (Jin et al., 2003; Xu, 2009). Compared with ECs under laminar flow, cells at disturbed flow show an atherogenic phenotype as alterated alignment, deformation of luminal ECs surface, accelerated proliferation and apoptosis (Bai et al., 2010; Zeng et al., 2009), higher permeability, immunoinflammation responses and more athero-prone gene expression which are proportional to risk factor severity (Foteinos et al., 2008; Xu, 2000). Oscillatory shear stress leads to continuous $O^{2-}$

production in an NADPH-oxidase-dependent manner, resulting in NF-kB-mediated monocyte adhesion.

NF-kB is an inducible transcription factor present at increased levels in the thickened intima-media of atherosclerotic lesions, whereas little or no activated NF-kB has been detected in healthy vessels (Andrews et al., 2010; Rodella et al., 2010,b). The NF-kB pathway have been implicated in athero-susceptibility for more than a decade. NF-kB is normally held inactive in the cytosol as a complex with IkB, a family of inhibitors of NF-kB. Oxidative stress by ROS production induces IkB degradation, releases of NFkB for translocation to the nucleus where it regulates pro-inflammatory genes (Davies et al., 2010). Several pro-inflammatory cytokines and growth factors found in atherosclerotic lesions, such as TNFα, ILs, MCP-1 and tissue factors, activate NF-kB signaling pathway in cultured ECs (Pennathur & Heinecke, 2007). NF-κB plays a central role in the development of inflammation through further regulation of genes encoding pro-inflammatory cytokines, CAMs, chemokines, growth factors and inducible enzymes (Andrews et al., 2010; Sprague & Khalil, 2009).

### 3.3 EC-foam cells

The formation of foam cells as a result of the lipid loading in ECs is a late event in atherosclerosis. Since the atherogenesis process is gradual, it is known that plasma hypercholesterolemia is associated with increased transcytosis of lipoproteins (Lps), leading to their accumulation within the ECs. At this location, Lps interact with proteoglycans and other matrix proteins and carry on their conversion to oxidatively modified and reassembled Lps (MLps). MLps have been identified in early intimal thickenings of human aorta and in the late atheroma (Sima et al., 2009; Tirziu et al., 1995).

It is known that, in the initial stage of atherogenesis, upon the accumulation and retention of MLp within intima, the EC lining the plaque take up MLp, which are either degraded within the cell or exocytosed into the lumen; in time, the non-regulated uptake of MLp by the EC-scavenger receptor is overwhelmed, leading to the accumulation of numerous large lipid droplets within the ECs. Concurrently, the EC shifts to a secretory phenotype, characterized by an increased number of biosynthetic organelles that correlates with the appearance of a multilayer, hyperplastic basal lamina in meshes of which MLp in accumulate large numbers. These insults lead to a dysfunctional endothelium and inflammatory process in which the EC-derived foam cells express more of new CAM and synthesize EC-factors that attract and induce migration of plasma inflammatory cells, such as monocytes and T lymphocytes to the subendothelium (Simionescu & Antohe, 2006); however, ECs maintain some of their specific attributes, such as Weibel-Palade bodies, intercellular junctions and caveolae (Sima et al., 2009). Infiltration of atherogenic Lps, monocytes and T lymphocytes within the subendothelium start the atherogenetic process both in animal models and in humans (Lawson & Wolf, 2009; Simionescu & Antohe, 2006; Williams & Tabas, 2005). In late stages of atherosclerosis, all cellular components of the plaque, ECs, VSMCs and macrophages, accumulate considerable number of lipid droplets and exhibit the foam cell characteristics (Sima et al., 2009). In the subendothelium, the monocytes become macrophage-derived foam cells, which release cytokines and factors that, within the oxidative stress process, change the cross-talk between ECs and the neighbouring VSMCs and induce migration of VSMCs from media to the developing neointima (Lawson & Wolf, 2009; Simionescu & Antohe, 2006).

## 4. The role of vascular smooth muscle cells in atherosclerosis

VSMCs are important actors in the pathogenesis of atherosclerosis. The classical "*response to injury*" hypothesis of atherosclerosis suggests that one of the major events in the development of this pathology is the intimal thickening caused by hyperplasia and migration of VSMC in the tunica intima (Ross & Glomset, 1973): the combined action of growth factors, proteolytic agents, and ECM proteins, produced by a dysfunctional endothelium and/or inflammatory cells, induces proliferation and migration of VSMCs from the tunica media into the intima (Clowes et al., 1983; Hao et al., 2003). Finally, progression of atherosclerotic lesions in the intima is characterized by the accumulation of alternating layers of dedifferentiated VSMCs and lipid-laden macrophages (Sobue et al., 1999). This model focuses on the central role of activated and proliferating VSMCs that are histologically observed in the early and late stages of atherosclerosis, thus being a key event in atherosclerosis (Dzau et al., 2002; Owens, 1995). Because of their involvement in atherosclerosis, intimal VSMCs, their origin and the mechanisms that regulate their phenotype have been the subject of numerous studies and much debate over recent years.

### 4.1 Origin of intimal VSMCs in atherosclerosis

#### 4.1.1 Phenotypic modulation of VSMCs

The long-standing dogma in the field has been that the majority of intimal VSMCs are derived from preexisting mature medial VSMCs that undergo phenotypic modulation on moving from the media to the intima (Owens et al., 2004). This hypothesis, proposed for the first time by Chamley-Campbell and colleagues (Chamley-Campbell et al., 1979) arose from a limited number of studies showing that in primary human cell cultures derived from different sources (e.g. medial cells or cells derived from atherosclerotic plaques) stable differences in phenotype could be identified. This dogma implies the potential for marked plasticity of the VSMC phenotype, with the ultimate phenotype being determined by a variety of extracellular stimuli (Bochaton-Piallat et al., 1996): numerous studies of cells cultured from different species have demonstrated that cytokines, matrix components, and mechanical stimuli can influence VSMC phenotype and behavior (Shanahan et al., 1993; Topouzis & Majesky, 1996).
VSMCs are the predominant cellular elements of the medial layer of the vascular wall, essential for good performance of the vasculature. VSMCs perform many different functions in maintaining vessel's health (Rensen et al., 2007). The VSMC is the only cell populating the normal vascular media, wherein it is uniquely responsible for maintaining vascular tone and hemodynamic stability: it is a highly specialized cell whose principal function is vasoconstriction and dilation in response to normal or pharmacologic stimuli to regulate blood vessel tone, blood pressure, and blood flow (Rzucidlo et al., 2007). Moreover, except in unusual circumstances when the adventitia may be involved, the VSMC is also the only vascular cell capable of repairing the injured vessel wall by migrating, proliferating, and elaborating an appropriate ECM. It is therefore equally essential that, when it is necessary, the VSMC can also adopt a phenotype capable of these synthetic functions (Shanahan & Weissberg, 1998). So, it is important that VSMCs retain remarkable plasticity and can undergo rather intense and reversible changes in phenotype in response to changes in local environmental cues, particularly under the influence of growth factors (Li, S. et al., 1999; Owens, 1995). In the pathogenesis of atherosclerotic lesions it is now accepted that VSMC can display at least two different phenotypes, the first characteristic of the media and the

second typical of the cells invading the intima (Shanahan & Weissberg, 1999). These phenotypes are also seen *in vitro*: an elongated spindle-shaped phenotype, with the classic "hill-and-valley" growth pattern typical of cultured contractile normal medial VSMCs and an epithelioid or rhomboid phenotype, with cells growing in a monolayer with a cobblestone morphology at confluence typical of the cells from neointima (Hao et al., 2003). In the medial layer of a mature blood vessel, VSMCs exhibit a low rate of proliferation, low synthetic activity and ECM proteins secretion, and express a unique repertoire of contractile proteins (e.g. intracellular myofilaments bundles are abundant), ion channels, and signalling molecules required for the cell's contractile function that is clearly unique compared with any other cell type (Rzucidlo et al., 2007). The dense body, the dense membrane and myofibrils (composed of thin filaments and myosin thick filaments) are well developed in differentiated VSMCs, whereas organelles (e.g. rough endoplasmic reticulum (RER), Golgi and free ribosomes) are few in number (Owens, 1995). This "contractile" state (referred also as "differentiated phenotype"), is required for the VSMC to perform its primary function. The gene expression pattern in end-differentiated VSMCs is well characterized and comprised a number of proteins involved in contraction, membrane-skeletal markers specific to smooth muscle and cell adhesion molecules and their receptors (integrins), which are important either as a structural component of the contractile apparatus or as a regulator of contraction (Owens, 1995; Rensen et al., 2007). Their expressions are regulated at the gene levels, such as at transcription and splicing: caldesmon, smooth muscle myosin heavy chain (SMM-HC), α-smooth muscle actin (α-SMA), h-caldesmon, calponin, SM22, α- and β-tropomyosins and α1 integrin genes are transcriptionally regulated; transcription of these genes (except for the α-smooth muscle actin gene) is upregulated in differentiated VSMCs, but is downregulated in dedifferentiated VSMCs (Stintzing et al., 2009). It's important to note that, although α-SMA is permanently expressed in VSMCs, it is more abundant in contractile VSMCs than in synthetic VSMCs (Lemire et al., 1994). Isoform changes of caldesmon, α-tropomyosin, vinculin/metavinculin, and SMM-HC are instead regulated by alternative splicing in a VSMC phenotype-dependent manner (Sobue et al., 1999). At present, the two marker proteins that provide the best definition of a mature contractile VSMC phenotype are SM-MHC and smoothelin. SM-MHC expression has never been detected in non-VSMCs *in vivo*, and is the only marker protein that is also VSMCs-specific during embryogenesis (Miano et al., 1994). Smoothelin complements SM-MHC as a contractile VSMC marker in that it appears to be more sensitive.

On the contrary, intimal VSMCs associated with vascular disease (as well as VSMCs involved in blood vessel formation) are phenotypically distinct from their medial counterparts (Campbell, G.R. & Campbell, J.H., 1985; Mosse et al., 1985): they resemble immature and show a typical "synthetic" state (referred also as "dedifferentiated phenotype"), characterized by an increased rate of proliferation, migration and ECM protein synthesis. Several studies by Aikawa and coworkers (Aikawa et al., 1997, 1998) demonstrated that intimal VSMCs show a synthetic phenotype including: *1*) increased DNA synthesis and expression of proliferation markers and cyclins (Gordon et al., 1990); *2*) decreased expression of smooth muscle-specific contractile markers (Layne et al., 2002); *3*) alterations in calcium handling and contractility (Hill et al., 2001); *4*) alterations in cell ultrastructure, including a general loss of myofilaments, which is replaced largely by synthetic organelles such as RER and large Golgi complex (Sobue et al., 1999), supporting its function in production and secretion of ECM components that, leading to intimal thickening and fibrosis of the vascular wall, may contribute to lesion development and/or stability (Schwartz et al., 1986, 1995). The preceding studies have been extended by Geary and colleagues (Geary et al., 2002), who completed microarray-based profiling of gene expression patterns of SMCs in the neointima. A total of 147 genes were differentially expressed in neointimal VSMCs versus normal aorta VSMCs, most genes underscoring the importance of matrix production during neointimal formation. Therefore, these VSMCs assume the proliferative activity in response to mitogens, while lose contractile ability. Markers that are upregulated in the synthetic phenotype are rare. SMemb/non-muscle myosin heavy chain isoform B (MHC-B) represents a suitable synthetic VSMCs marker, since this protein is quickly and markedly upregulated in proliferating VSMCs (Neuville et al., 1997). At last, an interesting correlation has been demonstrated, albeit occasionally, between dedifferentiated VSMC phenotype and increased LDL uptake (Thyberg, 2002) or decreased HDL binding sites (Dusserre et al., 1994). Nevertheless, the role of LDL and HDL processes in atheromatous plaque formation with respect to VSMC heterogeneity should be further investigated.

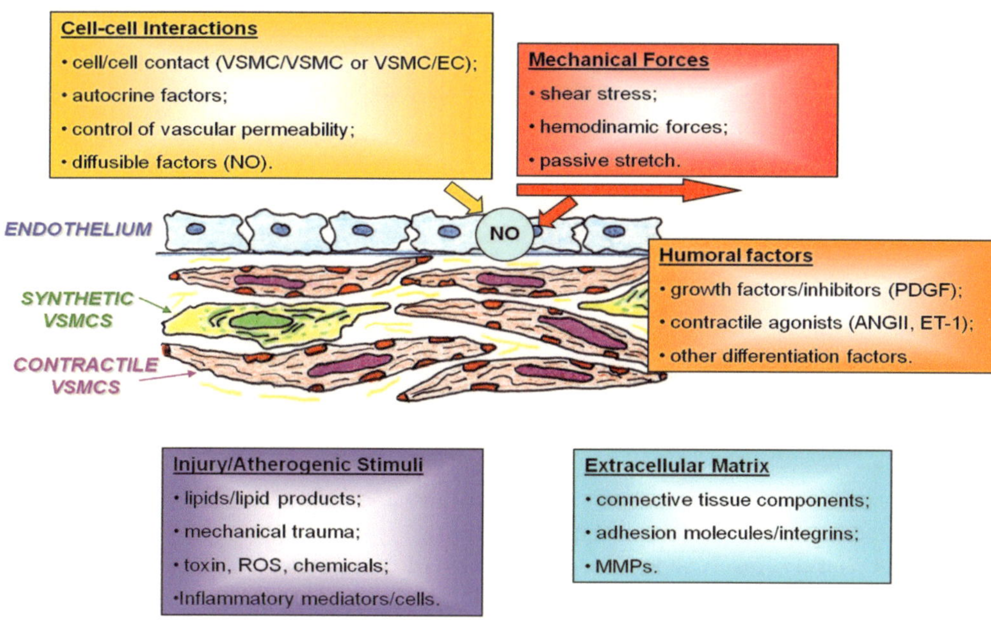


Fig. 6. Factors involved in VSMCs development, differentiation and phenotypic modulation

However, it is now recognized that a simple two-state model, based on "contractile" and "synthetic" states only, is inadequate to explain the diverse range of phenotypes that can be exhibited by the VSMCs under different physiological and pathological circumstances (Owens et al., 2004). In particular, the environmental cues that exist within atherosclerotic lesions are without doubts very different from those that exist within a normal healthy blood vessel and these change at different stages of lesion development and progression and thereby are likely to contribute to continued phenotypic switching of VSMC within the lesion. So, an heterogeneity of VSMC phenotype, ranging from contractile to synthetic, which represent the two ends of a spectrum of VSMCs with intermediate phenotypes, is nowadays considered. Not surprisingly, as the repertoire of VSMC markers has expanded, the picture that has emerged is that there is likely a wide spectrum of possible VSMC phenotypes that might exist such that it may be very artificial to assign cells to distinct subcategories. So the distinction between "contractile" and "synthetic" state of the VSMC become very difficult. The complexity of different phenotypes that may be manifested by VSMC is clearly evident not only between VSMCs of different vessels or among VSMCs within the same vessel, but there is very clear evidence that the properties of the VSMCs vary also at different stages of atherosclerosis, within different lesion types, and between VSMCs located in different regions within a given lesion (Owens et al., 2004).

### 4.1.2 Monoclonality of atheromatous lesion and heterogeneity of proliferating VSMCs

Alternative to the predominant hypothesis that all VSMCs of the media can undergo phenotypic modulation, is the concept that a predisposed VSMCs subpopulation is responsible for the production of intimal thickening. This possibility has been raised on the basis of original work by Benditt and Benditt (Benditt, E.P. & Benditt, J.M., 1973) who reported that VSMC accumulation in the atheromatous plaques is monoclonal or, at least, oligoclonal (Chung et al., 1998), implying that only a small number of "immature" cells in the vessels media and/or adventitia undergo proliferation (Holifield et al., 1996). More recent studies have questioned the origin of VSMCs comprising atherosclerosis and neointima formation. Intimal VSMCs have been proposed to originate from diverse sources, including fibroblasts of the adventitia (Zalewski et al., 2002), ECs (Gittenberger-de Groot et al., 1999) and/or circulating bone marrow-derived cells (Hillebrands et al., 2003). Whereas the gene expression pattern of differentiated VSMC is pretty well characterized (Shanahan & Weissberg, 1999), many *in vivo* and *in vitro* studies dealing with proliferating VSMC showed heterogeneous cell marker expressions of multilineage differentiation (Tintut et al., 2003). A possible explanation of the heterogeneity of VSMCs in adult vessels can be found in embryologic vascular development (Gittenberger-de Groot et al., 1999): interestingly, similar to atherosclerosis, processes of multilineage differentiation with transition states could be observed during vascular development (Slomp et al., 1997). During vasculogenesis, VSMCs originate from different sources via transdifferentiation (Liu et al., 2004) (a highly conserved phenomenon of transdifferentiation is proved by a stable cytokeratins expression in atherosclerotic lesions as well as it happens during development (Neureiter et al., 2005)) depending on the vessel type, including mesoderm, neurectoderm, epicardium (for coronary arteries) and, more rarely, endothelium (Orlandi & Bennett, 2010). It is thus possible that the various VSMC phenotypes can arise from distinct lineages. Another possibility is that local VSMC of the contractile phenotype re-obtain the embryonic potential of proliferation and migration (Bar et al., 2002) via transdifferentiation and dedifferentiation processes as a response to injury. Looking at atherosclerosis and VSMC, there is a lot of evidence that VSMC progenitor cells are essentially involved in the progression of atherosclerosis (Roberts et al., 2005).

The origin of such VSMC progenitor cells is under debate. VSMC progenitor cells have been identified in the bone marrow (multipotent vascular stem cell progenitors and mesenchymal stem cells), in the circulation (circulating VSMC progenitor cells), in the vessel wall (resident VSMC progenitor cells and mesangioblasts) and various extravascular sites (extravascular, non-bone marrow progenitor cells) (Orlandi & Bennett, 2010).

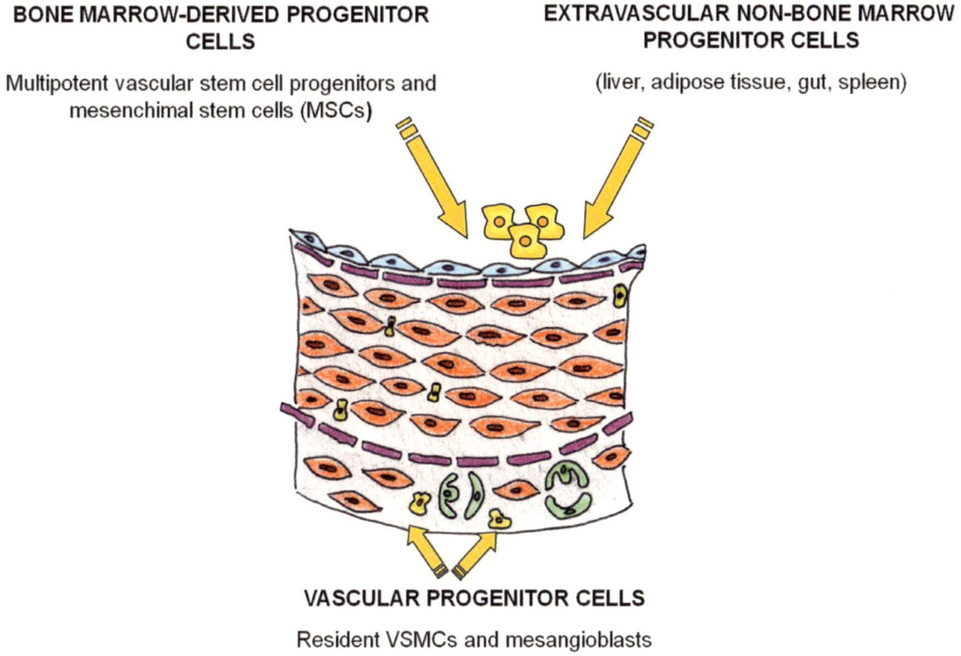


Fig. 7. Different origins of VSMCs progenitor cells.

#### 4.1.2.1 Bone marrow-derived VSMCs

Several studies have suggested that circulating bone marrow-derived cells contribute to neointima formation: one possibility is that circulating smooth muscle precursor cells of myeloid or hematopoietic lineage relocate from the blood into the neointima following vascular injury (Metharom et al., 2008) and start to proliferate giving rise to cells that express at least some properties of VSMCs (Simper et al., 2002).

Other studies, on the other hand, report no evidence for a contribution of bone marrow derived VSMCs in the neointimal layer (Hu et al., 2002; Li, J. et al., 2001). Alternatively, these circulating cells may fuse with resident VSMCs and thus show co-localization of VSMC markers and bone marrow lineage markers, although to date, no direct evidence for cell fusion in the vasculature has been shown (Owens et al., 2004).

#### 4.1.2.2 Resident VSMC progenitor cells and mesangioblasts

Inside normal vessel walls the existence of resident progenitor cells (expressing stem cell antigens) capable of contributing to neointima formation has been recently shown (Orlandi et al., 2008; Torsney et al., 2007): the number of these resident VSMCs progenitors has been shown to increase in atherosclerotic lesions (Torsney et al., 2007). These progenitor cells are different from marrow-derived smooth muscle progenitor cells, since they lack the ability to differentiate into erythroid, lymphoid, or myeloid tissue (Jackson et al., 1999). Subsequent studies examining telomere loss indicate that fibrous cap VSMCs have undergone more population doublings than cells in the normal media (Matthews et al., 2006), suggesting the existence of a resident arterial subpopulation predisposed to clonally contribute to arterial healing in response to injury (Hirschi & Majesky, 2004), so that plaques arise by selective expansion of a preexisting 'patch' of progenitor cells.

Unfortunately, against this theory, there is very limited evidence for the presence of vessel wall stem cells in human vessels. A population of $CD34^+/CD31^-$ cells has been identified in the space between the media and adventitia of large and medium-sized human arteries and veins (Pasquinelli et al., 2007), but the capacity of these cells to give rise to VSMCs was low (Zengin et al., 2006). Few other studies showed that the adventitial layer potentially harbours a population of stem cells that can also contribute to vascular remodelling. In particular, Hu and colleagues demonstrated that abundant progenitor cells in the adventitia can differentiate in VSMCs (Hu et al., 2004).

Moreover, satellite-like cells named 'mesoangioblasts' express both myogenic and EC markers (Drake et al., 1997), which can give rise to both hematopoietic and endothelial progenies (Cossu & Bianco, 2003). Gene expression profiles reveal that mesoangioblasts express genes belonging to developmental signaling pathways (such as β-catenin/Wnt signaling pathway) and are able to differentiate very efficiently into VSMCs (Tagliafico et al., 2004).

In summary, there is evidence for several distinct resident progenitor cells in different layers of the normal adult arterial wall capable of proliferating and differentiating into VSMCs. What has not yet been established is how many of these cells contribute to formation of vascular lesions and whether clonality reflects selective proliferation of one or more of these populations.

### 4.2 VSMCs: Friend or foe in atherosclerosis?

It is important to note that the exact role of VSMCs, in the progression of atherosclerosis is not clear. The functional role of VSMCs likewise is likely to vary depending on the stage of the disease. For example, at the early onset of atherosclerosis, these cells presumably plays a maladaptive role, because of their involvement in neointima formation (Rodella et al., 2011): mobilisation of these cells would therefore be predicted to promote, as a "foe", vascular disease (van Oostrom et al., 2009). On the other hand, over recent years, there has been an increasing recognition of the role played by intimal VSMCs in the formation and maintaining of a protective fibrous cap over the atherosclerotic plaque, desirable for plaque stability in the advanced atherosclerotic process (Weissberg et al., 1996). In particular, IFN-γ released by activated macrophages induces collagen synthesis by VSMCs, which is important for the stabilization of the fibrous cap (Shah et al., 1995). Moreover, injection of smooth muscle progenitor cells in a mouse model of advanced atherosclerosis reduced the progression of early atherosclerotic plaques (Zoll et al., 2008), confirming the potential benefit of VSMCs at advanced stages of atherosclerosis. Therefore, VSMCs could be beneficial in atherogenesis as a factor promoting plaque stability and can thus be considered a "friend" in vascular disease (van Oostrom et al., 2009).

Since the VSMC is the only cell capable of synthesizing the fibrous cap, failure of this vascular repair response leads to weakening of the cap and plaque rupture, with potentially fatal consequences (Weissberg et al., 1996). In diseased tissue many factors are present that substantially alter the normal balance of proliferation and apoptosis, and the apoptosis may predominate (Bennett, 2002). In particular, in plaque VSMCs an elevated level of spontaneous apoptosis and enhanced susceptibility to apoptosis induced by ROS (Li, W.G. et al., 2000) has been recently described both *in vivo* and *in vitro* (Ross, 1999). Apoptosis of VSMCs, bringing a plaque with reduced number of VSMCs, could participate in the rupture of the stability of the plaque (Rudijanto, 2007). Rupture of atherosclerotic plaques is associated with a thinning of VSMC-rich fibrous cap overlying the core (atrophic fibrous cap lesion), due to rapid replicative senescence and apoptosis of VSMCs (Schwartz et al., 2000). Rupture occurs particularly at the plaque shoulders, which exhibits lack of VSMCs and the presence of inflammatory cells (Newby et al., 1999). So, VSMCs may later contribute to plaque destabilization through apoptosis and/or activation of various protease cascades (Galis & Khatri, 2002).

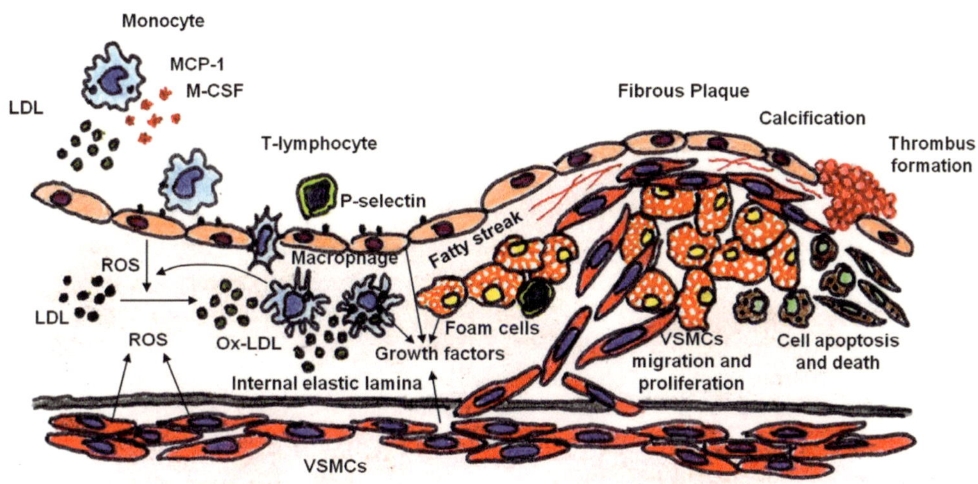


Fig. 8. Involvement of VSMCs apoptosis in fibrous plaque rupture.

However, detailed studies demonstrating whether VSMC progenitors either protect or promote vessel disease are needed before cell-based or pharmacological approaches aimed at regulating progenitor cell trafficking can be recommended.

### 4.3 VSMCs can auto-regulate their replication/migration

The contemporary paradigm explaining smooth muscle replication in the vessel wall is that dysfunctional endothelium and/or inflammatory cells produce growth factors and ECM proteins that can induce replication and migration of VSMCs from the media to the intima (van Oostrom et al., 2009). In his *"response-to injury"* hypothesis, Ross proposed that VSMCs in the wall normally exist in a quiescent state, but, when the endothelium is injured, platelets release factors that stimulate VSMCs movement into and replication within the arterial intima (Ross, 1981-1982).

Growth factors have been known to influence the differentiated state of VSMCs (Willis et al., 2004). An interesting possibility is that smooth muscle replication may be controlled by factors intrinsic to the vessel wall. One possibility comes from evidence that normal endothelium contains inhibitors of smooth muscle proliferation (Haudenschild & Schwartz, 1979). The principal factor involved in VSMCs replication is the platelet derived growth factor (PDGF), which is a potent VSMC mitogen linked to vascular homeostasis and atherogenesis (Majesky et al., 1992). This peptide not only is mitogenic for VSMCs, but is chemotactic as well (Schwartz et al., 1986): the data on PDGF and its receptor subunits

suggest, infact, a role in migration/localization of primordial VSMCs to the endothelium. This growth factor consists of two chain types, A and B, giving rise to three different PDGF subtypes (AA, AB, BB): PDGF-BB and -AB are known VMSCs chemoattractans, whereas PDGF-AA is associated with inhibition of chemotaxis (Zachary et al., 1999). PDGF binds to specific dimeric receptors (α and β) found on smooth muscle cells (Bowen-Pope & Ross, 1982) where initiates a series of events leading to DNA synthesis: receptor α can bind all PDGF subtypes, while receptor β binds only subtypes -AB and -BB. VSMCs have been determined to upregulate expression of receptor β in response to vascular injury, inducing their chemotaxis; at the same time, these cells are able to increase the PDGF-AA, acting as a paracrine or autocrine regulator of their chemotaxis. This represents the first described autoregulation pathway of VSMCs on their own proliferation/migration (Willis et al., 2004).
The second known requirement for cell cycle progression is availability of insulin-like growth factor (IGF-1), a co-factor that VSMCs require for completion of the cell cycle following stimulation with PDGF (Clemmons, 1984). Perhaps more surprising is that, as reported above, VSMCs may be able to stimulate their own growth by synthesis of both PDGF and IGF-1 (PDGF is able to stimulate smooth muscle cells to produce IGF-1).
Moreover, those VSMCs that, once migrated into the intima, retained the ability to produce mitogen, due to their dedifferentiated state (Schwartz et al., 1986), are able to sustain proliferation also after the initial stimulation of platelet and PDGF release during vascular injury. Selection of such a proliferogenic subpopulation could account for both the monoclonal phenotype of chronic human atherosclerotic lesions (Gown & Benditt, E.P., 1982) and the suggestion that monoclonality arises gradually as the human lesion evolves (Lee et al., 1985). In summary, the emerging picture of growth control in arterial smooth muscle is a complex balance of forces. In addition to exogenous stimuli to cell growth, the vessel wall is capable of synthesis of endogenous growth inhibitors (including heparin sulfates, nitric oxide (NO), and transforming growth factor (TGF)-β) and growth stimulants (such as PDGF, IGF-1, ET-1, thrombin, FGF, IFNγ, and IL-1) (Berk, 2001).

## 5. Conclusions

Atherosclerosis and its associated complications remain the primary cause of death of the 21st century in humans. Recently it has been suggested that atherosclerosis is a multifactorial, multistep disease. Clinical and histopathological studies of atherosclerotic patient groups have identified inflammatory and oxidative stress-linked mechanisms as being pathogenetically important in atherosclerosis at every step from initiation to progression. Endothelial damage is also crucial for the progress of atherosclerosis and risk factors for atherosclerosis represent crucial factors associated with endothelial dysfunction. Studies have shown that patients with cardiovascular disease are characterized by impaired endothelial function, being vascular endothelium responsible for the secretion of several substances exerting proved anti-atherogenic effects. Finally, VSMCs are an important component of atherosclerotic plaques, responsible for promoting plaque stability in advanced lesions. In contrast, VSMC apoptosis has been implicated in a number of deleterious consequences of atherosclerosis, including plaque rupture, vessel remodelling, coagulation, inflammation and calcification. A better understanding of the pathogenesis of atherosclerosis will aid in for reducing mortality. An in-depth knowledge of the various pathogenic mechanisms involved in atherosclerosis can help in formulating preventive and therapeutic strategies and devising pharmaceutical and lifestyle modifications for reducing mortality.

## 6. Acknowledgments

The Authors want to thank Dr. Favero Gaia, Dr. Foglio Eleonora and Dr. Rossini Claudia for their excellent work in writing and improving this chapter and for their contribution in realizing the figures. Moreover, the Authors thank Peroni Michele for his help in editing this chapter.

## 7. References

Aikawa, M.; Sakomura, Y.; Ueda, M.; Kimura, K.; Manabe, I.; Ishiwata, S.; Komiyama, N.; Yamaguchi, H.; Yazaki, Y. & Nagai, R. (1997). Redifferentiation of smooth muscle cells after coronary angioplasty determined via myosin heavy chain expression. *Circulation*, Vol.96, No.1, (July 1997), pp. 82-90, ISSN 0009-7322.

Aikawa, M.; Rabkin, E.; Voglic, S.J.; Shing, H.; Nagai, R.; Schoen, F.J. & Libby, P. (1998). Lipid lowering promotes accumulation of mature smooth muscle cells expressing smooth muscle myosin heavy chain isoforms in rabbit atheroma. *Circulation Research*, Vol.83, No.10, (November 1998), pp. 1015-1026, ISSN 0009-7330.

Amorino, G.P. & Hoover, R.L. (1998). Interactions of monocytic cells with human endothelial cells stimulate monocytic metalloproteinase production. *The American Journal of Pathology*, Vol.152, No.1, (January 1998), pp. 199-207, ISSN 0002-9440.

Andrews, K.L.; Moore, X.L. & Chin-Dusting, J.P. (2010). Anti-atherogenic effects of high-density lipoprotein on nitric oxide synthesis in the endothelium. *Clinical and Experimental Pharmacology and Physiology*, Vol.37, No.7, (July 2010), pp. 736-742, ISSN 0305-1870.

Antoniades, C.; Tousoulis, D.; Tentolouris, C.; Toutouzas, P. & Stefanadis, C. (2003). Oxidative stress, antioxidant vitamins, and atherosclerosis. From basic research to clinical practice. *Herz*, Vol.28, No.7, (November 2003), pp. 628-638, ISSN 0340-9937.

Bai, X.; Wang, X. & Xu, Q. (2010). Endothelial damage and stem cell repair in atherosclerosis. *Vascular Pharmacology*, Vol.52, No.5-6, (May-June 2010), pp. 224-229, ISSN 1537-1891.

Bär, H.; Wende, P.; Watson, L.; Denger, S.; van Eys, G.; Kreuzer, J. & Jahn, L. (2002). Smoothelin is an indicator of reversible phenotype modulation of smooth muscle cells in balloon-injured rat carotid arteries. *Basic Research in Cardiology*, Vol.97, No.1, (January 2002), pp. 9-16, ISSN 0300-8428.

Barton, M. (2005). Ageing as a determinant of renal and vascular disease: role of endothelial factors. *Nephrology, Dialysis, Transplantation*, Vol.20, No.3, (March 2005), pp. 485-490, ISSN 0931-0509.

Barton, M. (2010). Obesity and aging: determinants of endothelial cell dysfunction and atherosclerosis. *Pflugers archiv*, Vol.460, No.5, (October 2010), pp. 825-837, ISSN 0031-6768.

Barton, M. & Haudenschild C.C. (2001). Endothelium and atherogenesis: endothelial therapy revisited. *Journal of Cardiovascular Pharmacology*, Vol.38, No.S2, (November 2001), pp. S23-25, ISSN 0160-2446.

Beckman, J.S. & Koppenol, W.H. (1996). Nitric oxide, superoxide, and peroxynitrite: the good, the bad, and ugly. *The American Journal of Physiology*, Vol.271, No. 5Pt1, (November 1996), pp. C1424-1437, ISSN 0363-6143.

Benditt, E.P. & Benditt, J.M. (1973). Evidence for a monoclonal origin of human atherosclerotic plaques. *Proceedings of the National Academy of Sciences of the United States of America*, Vol.70, No.6, (June 1973), pp. 1753-1756, ISSN 0027-8424.

Bennett, M. (2002). Apoptosis in the cardiovascular system. *Heart*, Vol.87, No.5, (May 2002), pp. 480-487, ISSN 1355-6037.

Bergh, N.; Ulfhammer, E.; Glise, K.; Jern, S. & Karlsson, L. (2009). Influence of TNF-alpha and biomechanical stress on endothelial anti- and prothrombotic genes. *Biochemical and Biophysical Research Communications*, Vol.385, No.3, (July 2009), pp. 314-318, ISSN 0006-291X.

Berk, B.C. (2001). Vascular smooth muscle growth: autocrine growth mechanisms. *Physiological Reviews*, Vol. 81, No.3, (July 2001), pp. 999-1030, ISSN 0031-9333.

Blankenberg, S.; Rupprecht, H.J.; Bickel, C.; Peetz, D.; Hafner, G.; Tiret, L. & Meyer, J. (2001). Circulating cell adhesion molecules and death in patients with coronary artery disease. *Circulation*, Vol.104, No.12, (September 2001), pp. 1336-1342, ISSN 0009-7322.

Bochaton-Piallat, M.L.; Ropraz, P.; Gabbiani, F. & Gabbiani, G. (1996). Phenotypic heterogeneity of rat arterial smooth muscle cell clones. Implications for the development of experimental intimal thickening. *Arteriosclerosis, Thrombosis, and Vascular Biology*, Vol.16, No.6, (June 1996), pp. 815-820, ISSN 1079-5642.

Bond, M.; Fabunmi, R.P.; Baker, A.H. & Newby, A.C. (1998). Synergistic upregulation of metalloproteinase-9 by growth factors and inflammatory cytokines: an absolute requirement for transcription factor NF-kB. *FEBS Letters*, Vol.435, No.1, pp. 29–34, ISSN 0014-5793.

Bonomini, F.; Tengattini, S.; Fabiano, A.; Bianchi, R. & Rezzani, R. (2008). Atherosclerosis and oxidative stress. *Histology and Histopathology*, Vol.23, No.3, (March 2008), pp. 381-390, ISSN 1699-5848.

Boring, L.; Gosling, J.; Cleary, M. & Charo, I.F. (1998). Decreased lesion formation in CCR2-/- mice reveals a role for chemokines in the initiation of atherosclerosis. *Nature*, Vol.394, No.6696, (August 1998), pp. 894-897, ISSN 0028-0836.

Bowen-Pope, D.F. & Ross, R. (1982). Platelet-derived growth factor. II. Specific binding to cultured cells. *Journal of Biological Chemistry*, Vol.257, No.9, (May 1982), pp. 5161-5171, ISSN 0021-9258.

Brach, M.A.; Henschler, R.; Mertelsmann, R.H. & Herrmann, F. (1991). Regulation of M-CSF expression by M-CSF: role of protein kinase C and ranscription factor NF kappa B. *Pathobiology*, Vol.59, No.4, pp. 284–288, ISSN 1015-2008.

Brand, K.; Eisele, T.; Kreusel, U.; Page, M.; Page, S.; Haas, M.; Gerling, A.; Kaltschmidt, C.; Neumann, F.J.; Mackman, N.; Baeurele, P.A.; Walli, A.K. & Neumeier, D. (1997). Dysregulation of monocytic nuclear factor-kappa B by oxidized low-density lipoprotein. *Arteriosclerosis, Thrombosis and Vascular Biology*, Vol.17, No.10, (October 1997), pp. 1901–1909, ISSN 1079-5642.

Cai, H. & Harrison, D.G. (2000). Endothelial Dysfunction in Cardiovascular Diseases: The Role of Oxidant Stress. *Circulation Research*, Vol. 87, No.10, (September 2000), pp.840-844, ISSN 0009-7330.

Campbell, G.R. & Campbell, J.H. (1985). Smooth muscle phenotypic changes in arterial wall homeostasis: implications for the pathogenesis of atherosclerosis. *Experimental and Molecular Pathology*, Vol.42, No.2, (April 1985), pp. 139-162, ISSN 0014-4800.

Chamley-Campbell, J.; Campbell, G.R. & Ross, R. (1979). The smooth muscle cell in culture. *Physiological Reviews*, Vol.59, No.1, (January 1979), pp. 1-61, ISSN 0031-9333.

Chandrasekharan, U.M.; Siemionow, M.; Unsal, M.; Yang, L.; Poptic, E.; Bohn, J.; Ozer, K.; Zhou, Z.; Howe, P.H.; Penn, M. & DiCorleto, P.E. (2007). Tumor necrosis factor alpha (TNF-alpha) receptor-II is required for TNF-alpha-induced leukocyte-endothelial interaction in vivo. *Blood*, Vol.109, No.5, (March 2007), pp. 1938-1944, ISSN 0006-4971.

Chung, I.M.; Schwartz, S.M. & Murry, C.E. (1998). Clonal architecture of normal and atherosclerotic aorta: implications for atherogenesis and vascular development. *American Journal of Pathology*, Vol.152, No.4, (April 1998), pp. 913-923, ISSN 0002-9440.

Cipollone, F.; Fazia, M.L. & Mezzetti, A. (2007). Oxidative stress, inflammation and atherosclerosis plaque development. *International Congress Series*, Vol.1303, (August 2007), pp. 35-40, ISSN 0531-5131.

Clemmons, D.R. (1984). Interaction of circulating cell-derived and plasma growth factors in stimulating cultured smooth muscle cell replication. *Journal of Cellular Physiology*, Vol.121, No.2, (November 1984), pp. 425-430, ISSN 0021-9541.

Clowes, A.W.; Reidy, M.A. & Clowes, M.M. (1983). Kinetics of cellular proliferation after arterial injury. I. Smooth muscle growth in the absence of endothelium. *Laboratory Investigation*, Vol.49, No.3, (September 1983), pp. 327-333, ISSN 0023-6837.

Cossu, G. & Bianco, P. (2003). Mesoangioblasts--vascular progenitors for extravascular mesodermal tissues. *Current Opinion in Genetics and Development*, Vol.13, No.5, (October 2003), pp. 537-542, ISSN 0959-437X.

Dabek, J.; Kułach, A. & Gąsior, Z. (2010). Nuclear factor kappa-light-chain-enhancer of activated B cells (NF-κB): a new potential therapeutic target in atherosclerosis? *Pharmacological Reports*, Vol.62, No.5, (September-October 2010), pp. 778-783, ISSN 1734-1140.

Dai, D.Z. & Dai, Y. (2010). Role of endothelin receptor A and NADPH oxidase in vascular abnormalities. *Journal of Vascular Health and Risk Management*, Vol.6, (September 2010), pp. 787-794, ISSN 1178-2048.

Davies, P.F.; Civelek, M.; Fang, Y.; Guerraty, M.A. & Passerini, A.G. (2010). Endothelial heterogeneity associated with regional athero-susceptibility and adaptation to disturbed blood flow in vivo. *Seminars in Thrombosis and Hemostasis*, Vol.36, No.3, (April 2010), pp. 265-275, ISSN 0094-6176.

Drake, C.J.; Brandt, S.J.; Trusk, T.C. & Little, C.D. (1997). TAL1/SCL is expressed in endothelial progenitor cells/angioblasts and defines a dorsal-to-ventral gradient of vasculogenesis. *Developmental Biology*, Vol.192, No.1, (December 1997), pp. 17-30, ISSN 0012-1606.

Dusserre, E.; Bourdillon, M.C.; Pulcini, T. & Berthezene, F. (1994). Decrease in high density lipoprotein binding sites is associated with decrease in intracellular cholesterol efflux in dedifferentiated aortic smooth muscle cells. *Biochimica et Biophysica Acta*, Vol.1212, No.2, (May 1994), pp. 235-244.

Dzau, V.J.; Braun-Dullaeus, R.C. & Sedding, D.G. (2002). Vascular proliferation and atherosclerosis: new perspectives and therapeutic strategies. *Nature Medicine*, Vol.8, No.11, (November 2002), pp. 1249-1256, ISSN 1078-8956.

Ferrario, C. (2009). Effect of angiotensin receptor blockade on endothelial function: focus on olmesartan medoxomil. *Vascular Health and Risk Management*, Vol.5, No.1, pp. 301-314, ISSN 1176-6344.

Fortuño, A.; San José, G.; Moreno, M.U.; Díez, J. & Zalba, G. (2005). Oxidative stress and vascular remodelling. *Experimental physiology*, Vol.90, No.4, (July 2005), pp. 457-462, ISSN 0958-0670.

Foteinos, G.; Hu, Y.; Xiao, Q.; Metzler, B. & Xu, Q. (2008). Rapid Endothelial Turnover in Atherosclerosis-Prone Areas Coincides With Stem Cell Repair in Apolipoprotein E–Deficient Mice. *Circulation*, Vol.117, No.14, (March 2008), pp. 1856-1863, ISSN 0009-7322.

Galis, Z.S. & Khatri, J.J. (2002). Matrix metalloproteinases in vascular remodeling and atherogenesis: the good, the bad, and the ugly. *Circulation Research*, Vol.90, No.3, (February 2002), pp. 251-262, ISSN 0009-7330.

Geary, R.L.; Wong, J.M.; Rossini, A.; Schwartz, S.M. & Adams, L.D. (2002). Expression profiling identifies 147 genes contributing to a unique primate neointimal smooth muscle cell phenotype. *Arteriosclerosis, Thrombosis, and Vascular Biology*, Vol.22, No.12, (December 2002), pp. 2010-2016, ISSN 1079-5642.

Gittenberger-de Groot, A.C.; DeRuiter, M.C.; Bergwerff, M. & Poelmann, R.E. (1999). Smooth muscle cell origin and its relation to heterogeneity in development and disease. *Arteriosclerosis, Thrombosis, and Vascular Biology*, Vol.19, No.7, (July 1999), pp. 1589-1594, ISSN 1079-5642.

Gordon, D.; Reidy, M.A.; Benditt, E.P. & Schwartz, S.M. (1990). Cell proliferation in human coronary arteries. *Proceedings of the National Academy of Sciences of the United States of America*, Vol.87, No.12, (June 1990), pp. 4600-4604, ISSN 0027-8424.

Gown, A.M. & Benditt, E.P. (1982). Lactate dehydrogenase (LDH) isozymes of human atherosclerotic plaques. *The American Journal of Pathology*, Vol.107, No.3, (June 1982), pp. 316-321, ISSN 0002-9440.

Griendling, K.K. & Harrison, D.G. (1999). Dual role of reactive oxygen species in vascular growth. *Circulation Research*, Vol.85, No.6, (September 1999), pp.562-563, ISSN 0009-7330.

Hansson, G.K.; Robertson, A.K. & Söderberg-Nauclér, C. (2006). Inflammation and atherosclerosis. *Annual Review of Pathology*, Vol.1, pp. 297-329.

Hansson, G.K. & Hermansson, A. (2011). The immune system in atherosclerosis. *Nature Immunology*, Vol.12, No.3, (March 2011), pp. 204-212, ISSN 1529-2908.

Hao, H.; Gabbiani, G. & Bochaton-Piallat, M.L. (2003). Arterial smooth muscle cell heterogeneity: implications for atherosclerosis and restenosis development. *Arteriosclerosis, Thrombosis, and Vascular Biology*, Vol.23, No.9, (September 2003), pp. 1510-1520, ISSN 1079-5642.

Haudenschild, C.C.; Prescott, M.F. & Chobanian A.V. (1981). Aortic endothelial and subendothelial cells in experimental hypertension and aging. *Hypertension*, Vol.3, No.3 Pt 2, (May-June 1981), pp. I148-153, ISSN 0194-911X.

Haudenschild, C.C. & Schwartz, S.M. (1979). Endothelial regeneration. II. Restitution of endothelial continuity. *Laboratory Investigation*, Vol.41, No.5, (November 1979), pp. 407-418, ISSN 0023-6837.

Heinecke, J.W. (2007). The role of myeloperoxidase in HDL oxidation and atherogenesis. *Current Atherosclerosis Reports*, Vol.9, No.4, (October 2007), pp. 249-251, ISSN 1523-3804.

Higashi, Y.; Noma, K.; Yoshizumi, M. & Kihara, Y. (2009). Endothelial function and oxidative stress in cardiovascular diseases. *Circulation Journal*, Vol.73, No.3, (March 2009), pp. 411-418, ISSN 1346-9843.

Hill, B.J.; Wamhoff, B.R. & Sturek, M. (2001). Functional nucleotide receptor expression and sarcoplasmic reticulum morphology in dedifferentiated porcine coronary smooth muscle cells. *Journal of Vascular Research,* Vol.38, No.5, (September- October 2001), pp. 432-443, ISSN 1018-1172.

Hillebrands, J.L.; Klatter, F.A. & Rozing, J. (2003). Origin of vascular smooth muscle cells and the role of circulating stem cells in transplant arteriosclerosis. *Arteriosclerosis, Thrombosis, and Vascular Biology,* Vol.23, No.3, (March 2003), pp. 380-387, ISSN 1079-5642.

Hirschi, K.K. & Majesky, M.W. (2004). Smooth muscle stem cells. *The Anatomical Record. Part A, Discoveries in Molecular, Cellular, and Evolutionary Biology,* Vol.276, No.1, (January 2004), pp. 22-33, ISSN 1552-4884.

Ho, A.W.; Wong, C.K. & Lam, C.W. (2008). Tumor necrosis factor-alpha up-regulates the expression of CCL2 and adhesion molecules of human proximal tubular epithelial cells through MAPK signaling pathways. *Immunobiology,* Vol.213, No.7, pp. 533-544, ISSN 0171-2985.

Holifield, B.; Helgason, T.; Jemelka, S.; Taylor, A.; Navran, S.; Allen, J. & Seidel, C. (1996). Differentiated vascular myocytes: are they involved in neointimal formation?. *The Journal of Clinical Investigation,* Vol.97, No.3, (February 1996), pp. 814-825, ISSN 0021-9738.

Hu, Y.; Davison, F.; Ludewig, B.; Erdel, M.; Mayr, M.; Url, M.; Dietrich, H. & Xu, Q. (2002). Smooth muscle cells in transplant atherosclerotic lesions are originated from recipients, but not bone marrow progenitor cells. *Circulation,* Vol.106, No.14, (October 2002), pp. 1834-1839, ISSN 0009-7322.

Hu, Y.; Zhang, Z.; Torsney, E.; Afzal, A.R.; Davison, F.; Metzler, B. & Xu, Q. (2004). Abundant progenitor cells in the adventitia contribute to atherosclerosis of vein grafts in ApoE-deficient mice. *The Journal of Clinical Investigation,* Vol.113, No.9, (May 2004), pp. 1258-1265, ISSN 0021-9738.

Irani, K. (2000). Oxidant signaling in vascular cell growth, death, and survival : a review of the roles of reactive oxygen species in smooth muscle and endothelial cell mitogenic and apoptotic signaling. *Circulation Research,* Vol.87, No.3, (August 2000), pp.179-183, ISSN 0009-7330.

Jackson, K.A.; Mi, T. & Goodell, M.A. (1999). Hematopoietic potential of stem cells isolated from murine skeletal muscle. *Proceedings of the National Academy of Sciences of the United States of America,* Vol.96, No.25, (December 1999), pp. 14482-14486, ISSN 0027-8424.

Jensen-Urstad, K.; Bouvier, F. & Jensen-Urstad, M. (1999). Preserved vascular reactivity in elderly male athletes. *Scandinavian Journal of Medicine and Science in Sports,* Vol.9, No.2, (April 1999), pp. 88-91, ISSN 0905-7188.

Jin, Z.G.; Ueba, H.; Tanimoto, T.; Lungu, A.O.; Frame, M.D. & Berk, B.C. (2003). Ligand-independent activation of vascular endothelial growth factor receptor 2 by fluid shear stress regulates activation of endothelial nitric oxide synthase. *Circulation Research,* Vol.93, No.4, (August 2003), pp. 354-363, ISSN0009-7330.

Kleinbongard, P.; Heusch, G. & Schulz, R. (2010). TNFalpha in atherosclerosis, myocardial ischemia/reperfusion and heart failure. *Pharmacology & Therapeutics,* Vol.127, No.3, (September 2010), pp. 295-314, ISSN 0163-7258.

Kojda, G. & Harrison, D. (1999). Interactions between NO and reactive oxygen species: pathophysiological importance in atherosclerosis, hypertension, diabetes and heart failure. *Cardiovascular Research*, Vol.43, No.3, (August 1999), pp. 562-571, ISSN 0008-6363.

Kruth, H.S. (2002). Sequestration of aggregated low-density lipoproteins by macrophages. *Current Opinion in Lipidology*, Vol.13, No.5, (October 2002), pp.433-438, ISSN 0957-9672.

Kutuk, O. & Basaga, H. (2003). Inflammation meets oxidation: NF-kB as a mediator of initial lesion development in atherosclerosis. *Trends in Molecular Medicine*, Vol.9, No.12, pp. 549–557, ISSN 1471-4914.

Lakshmi, S.V.; Padmaja, G.; Kuppusamy, P. & Kutala, V.K. (2009). Oxidative stress in cardiovascular disease. *Indian Journal of Biochemistry & Biophysics*, Vol.46, No.6, (December 2009), pp. 421-440, ISSN 0301-1208.

Lawson, C. & Wolf, S. (2009). ICAM-1 signaling in endothelial cells. *Pharmacological Reports*, Vol.61, No.1, (January-February 2009), pp. 22-32, ISSN 1734-1140.

Layne, M.D.; Yet, S.F.; Maemura, K.; Hsieh, C.M.; Liu, X.; Ith, B.; Lee, M.E. & Perrella, M.A. (2002). Characterization of the mouse aortic carboxypeptidase-like protein promoter reveals activity in differentiated and dedifferentiated vascular smooth muscle cells. *Circulation Research*, Vol.90, No.6, (April 2002), pp. 728-736, ISSN 0009-7330.

Lee, K.T.; Janakidevi, K.; Kroms, M.; Schmee, J. & Thomas, W.A. (1985). Mosaicism in female hybrid hares heterozygous for glucose-6-phosphate dehydrogenase. VII. Evidence for selective advantage of one phenotype over the other in ditypic samples from aortas of hares fed cholesterol oxidation products. *Experimental and Molecular Pathology*, Vol.42, No.1, (February 1985), pp. 71-77, ISSN 0014-4800.

Lemire, J.M.; Covin, C.W.; White, S.; Giachelli, C.M. & Schwartz, S.M. (1994). Characterization of cloned aortic smooth muscle cells from young rats. *The American Journal of Pathology*, Vol.144, No.5, (May 1994), pp. 1068-1081, ISSN 0002-9440.

Li, P.F.; Dietz, R. & von Harsdorf, R. (1997). Differential effect of hydrogen peroxide and superoxide anion on apoptosis and proliferation of vascular smooth muscle cells. *Circulation*, Vol.96, No.10, (November 1997), pp.3602-3609, ISSN 0009-7322.

Li, J.; Han, X.; Jiang, J.; Zhong, R.; Williams, G.M.; Pickering, J.G. & Chow, L.H. (2001). Vascular smooth muscle cells of recipient origin mediate intimal expansion after aortic allotransplantation in mice. *The American Journal of Pathology*, Vol.158, No.6, (June 2001), pp. 1943-1947, ISSN 0002-9440.

Li, J.J.; Fang, C.H.; Chen, M.Z.; Chen, X. & Lee, S.W. (2004). Activation of nuclear factor-kappaB and correlation with elevated plasma c-reactive protein in patients with unstable angina. *Heart, Lung and Circulation*, Vol.13, No.2, (June 2004), pp.173–178, ISSN 1443-9506.

Li, S.; Sims, S.; Jiao, Y.; Chow, L.H. & Pickering, J.G. (1999). Evidence from a novel human cell clone that adult vascular smooth muscle cells can convert reversibly between non-contractile and contractile phenotypes. *Circulation Research*, Vol.85, No.4, (August 1999), pp. 338-348, ISSN 0009-7330.

Li, W.G.; Miller, F.J. Jr.; Brown, M.R.; Chatterjee, P.; Aylsworth, G.R.; Shao, J.; Spector, A.A.; Oberley, L.W. & Weintraub, N.L. (2000). Enhanced H(2)O(2)-induced cytotoxicity in "epithelioid" smooth muscle cells: implications for neointimal regression. *Arteriosclerosis, Thrombosis, and Vascular Biology*, Vol.20, No.6, (June 2000), pp. 1473-1479, ISSN 1079-5642.

Libby, P.; Ridker, P.M. & Maseri, A. (2002). Inflammation and atherosclerosis. *Circulation*, Vol.105, No.9, (March 2002), pp.1135–1143, ISSN 0009-7322.

Libby, P.; DiCarli, M. & Weissleder, R. (2010). The vascular biology of atherosclerosis and imaging targets. *Journal of Nuclear Medicine*, Vol.51, No.S1, (May 2010), pp. 33S-37S, ISSN 2159-662X.

Liu, C.; Nath, K.A.; Katusic, Z.S. & Caplice, N.M. (2004). Smooth muscle progenitor cells in vascular disease. *Trends in Cardiovascular Medicine*, Vol.14, No.7, (October 2004), pp. 288-293, ISSN 1050-1738.

Madamanchi, NR.; Vendrov, A. & Runge, MS. (2005). Oxidative stress and vascular disease. *Arteriosclerosis, Thrombosis, and Vascular Biology*, Vol.25, No.1, (January 2005), pp.29-38, ISSN 1079-5642.

Majesky, M.W.; Giachelli, C.M.; Reidy, M.A. & Schwartz, S.M. (1992). Rat carotid neointimal smooth muscle cells reexpress a developmentally regulated mRNA phenotype during repair of arterial injury. *Circulation Research*, Vol.71, No.4, (October 1992), pp. 759-768, ISSN 0009-7330.

Matthews, C.; Gorenne, I.; Scott, S.; Figg, N.; Kirkpatrick, P.; Ritchie, A.; Goddard, M. & Bennett, M. (2006). Vascular smooth muscle cells undergo telomere-based senescence in human atherosclerosis: effects of telomerase and oxidative stress. *Circulation Research*, Vol.99, No.2, (July 2006), pp. 156-164, ISSN 0009-7330.

McKellar, G.E.; McCarey, D.W.; Sattar, N. & McInnes, I.B. (2009). Role for TNF in atherosclerosis? Lessons from autoimmune disease. *Nature Reviews Cardiology*, Vol.6, No.6, (June 2009), pp. 410-417, ISSN 1759-5002.

Metharom, P.; Liu, C.; Wang, S.; Stalboerger, P.; Chen, G.; Doyle, B.; Ikeda, Y. & Caplice, N.M. (2008). Myeloid lineage of high proliferative potential human smooth muscle outgrowth cells circulating in blood and vasculogenic smooth muscle-like cells in vivo. *Atherosclerosis*, Vol.198, No.1, (May 2008), pp. 29-38, ISSN 0021-9150.

Miano, J.M.; Cserjesi, P.; Ligon, K.L.; Periasamy, M. & Olson, E.N. (1994). Smooth muscle myosin heavy chain exclusively marks the smooth muscle lineage during mouse embryogenesis. *Circulation Research*, Vol.75, No.5, (November 1994), pp. 803-812, ISSN 0009-7330.

Miller, Y.I.; Chang, M.K.; Binder, C.J.; Shaw, P.X. & Witztum, J.L. (2003). Oxidized low density lipoprotein and innate immune receptors. *Current Opinion in Lipidology*, Vol.14, No.5, (October 2003), pp. 437-445, ISSN 0957-9672.

Mosse, P.R.; Campbell, G.R.; Wang, Z.L. & Campbell, J.H. (1985). Smooth muscle phenotypic expression in human carotid arteries. I. Comparison of cells from diffuse intimal thickenings adjacent to atheromatous plaques with those of the media. *Laboratory Investigation*, Vol.53, No.5, (November 1985), pp. 556-562, ISSN 0023-6837.

Muller, G. & Morawietz, H. (2009). Nitric oxide, NAD(P)H oxidase, and atherosclerosis. *Antioxidants and Redox Signaling*, Vol.11, No.7, (July 2009), pp. 1711-1731, ISSN 1523-0864.

Napoli, C.; Williams-Ignarro, S.; de Nigris, F.; Lerman, L.O.; D'Armiento, F.P.; Crimi, E.; Byrns, R.E.; Casamassimi, A.; Lanza, A.; Gombos, F.; Sica, V. & Ignarro, L.J. (2006). Physical training and metabolic supplementation reduce spontaneous atherosclerotic plaque rupture and prolong survival in hypercholesterolemic mice. *Proceedings of National Academy of Sciences of the United States of America*, Vol.103, No.27, (July 2006), pp. 10479-10484, ISSN 0027-8424.

Neureiter, D.; Zopf, S.; Dimmler, A.; Stintzing, S.; Hahn, E.G.; Kirchner, T.; Herold, C. & Ocker, M. (2005). Different capabilities of morphological pattern formation and its association with the expression of differentiation markers in a xenograft model of human pancreatic cancer cell lines. *Pancreatology*, Vol.5, No.4-5, pp. 387-397, ISSN 1424-3903.

Neuville, P.; Geinoz, A.; Benzonana, G.; Redard, M.; Gabbiani, F.; Ropraz, P. & Gabbiani, G. (1997). Cellular retinol-binding protein-1 is expressed by distinct subsets of rat arterial smooth muscle cells in vitro and in vivo. *The American Journal of Pathology*, Vol.150, No.2, (February 1997), pp. 509-521, ISSN 0002-9440.

Newby, A.C.; Libby, P. & van der Wal, A.C. (1999). Plaque instability--the real challenge for atherosclerosis research in the next decade?. *Cardiovascular Research*, Vol.41, No.2, (February 1999), pp. 321-322, ISSN 0008-6363.

Orlandi, A.; Di Lascio, A.; Francesconi, A.; Scioli, M.G.; Arcuri, G.; Ferlosio, A. & Spagnoli, L.G. (2008). Stem cell marker expression and proliferation and apoptosis of vascular smooth muscle cells. *Cell Cycle*, Vol.7, No.24, (December 2008), pp. 3889-3897, ISSN 1551-4005.

Orlandi, A. & Bennett, M. (2010). Progenitor cell-derived smooth muscle cells in vascular disease. *Biochemical Pharmacology*, Vol. 79, No.12, (June 2010), pp.1706-1713, ISSN 0006-2952.

Owens, G.K. (1995). Regulation of differentiation of vascular smooth muscle cells. *Physiological Reviews*, Vol.75, No.3, (July 1995), pp. 487-517, ISSN 0031-9333.

Owens, G.K.; Kumar, M.S. & Wamhoff, B.R. (2004). Molecular regulation of vascular smooth muscle cell differentiation in development and disease. *Physiological Reviews*, Vol.84, No.3, (July 2004), pp. 767-801, ISSN 0031-9333.

Packard, R.R. & Libby, P. (2008). Inflammation in atherosclerosis: from vascular biology to biomarker discovery and risk prediction. *Clinical Chemistry*, Vol.54, No.1, (January 2008), pp. 24-38, ISSN 0009-9147.

Partigulova, A.S. & Naumov, V.G. (2010). Inflammation and atherosclerosis: the role of Renin-Angiotensin system and its inhibition. *Kardiologiia*, Vol.50, No.10, pp. 50-55, ISSN 0022-9040.

Pasquinelli, G.; Tazzari, P.L.; Vaselli, C.; Foroni, L.; Buzzi, M.; Storci, G.; Alviano, F.; Ricci, F.; Bonafè, M.; Orrico, C.; Bagnara, G.P.; Stella, A. & Conte, R. (2007). Thoracic aortas from multiorgan donors are suitable for obtaining resident angiogenic mesenchymal stromal cells. *Stem Cells*, Vol.25, No.7, (July 2007), pp. 1627-1634, ISSN 1948-0210.

Pennathur, S. & Heinecke, J.W. (2007). Oxidative stress and endothelial dysfunction in vascular disease. *Current Diabetes Report*, Vol.7, No.4, (August 2007), pp. 257-264, ISSN 1534-4827.

Piechota, A.; Polańczyk, A. & Goraca, A. (2010). Role of endothelin-1 receptor blockers on hemodynamic parameters and oxidative stress. *Pharmacological Reports*, Vol.62, No.1, (January-February 2010), pp. 28-34, ISSN 1734-1140.

Rensen, S.S.; Doevendans, P.A. & van Eys, G.J. (2007). Regulation and characteristics of vascular smooth muscle cell phenotypic diversity. *Netherlands Heart Journal*, Vol.15, No.3, pp. 100-108, ISSN 1568-5888.

Roberts, N.; Jahangiri, M. & Xu, Q. (2005). Progenitor cells in vascular disease. *Journal of Cellular and Molecular Medicine*, Vol.9, No.3, (July-September 2005), pp. 583-591, ISSN 1582-4934.

Rodella, L.F.; Filippini, F.; Bonomini, F.; Bresciani, R.; Reiter, R.J. & Rezzani, R. (2010), a. Beneficial effects of melatonin on nicotine-induced vasculopathy. *Journal of Pineal Research*, Vol.48, No.2, (March 2010), pp. 126-132, ISSN 0742-3098 .

Rodella, L.F.; Favero, G.; Rossini, C.; Foglio, E.; Reiter, R.J. & Rezzani, R. (2010), b. Endothelin-1 as a potential marker of melatonin's therapeutic effects in smoking-induced vasculopathy. *Life Sciences*, Vol.87, No.17-18, (October 2010), pp. 558-564, ISSN 0024-3205.

Rodella, L.F.; Rossini, C.; Favero, G., Foglio, E., Loreto, C. & Rezzani, R. (2011). Nicotine-induced morphological changes in rat aorta: the protective role of melatonin. *Cells Tissues Organs*, (April 2011, Epub ahead of print), ISSN 1422-6405.

Ross, R. & Glomset, J.A. (1973). Atherosclerosis and the arterial smooth muscle cell: Proliferation of smooth muscle is a key event in the genesis of the lesions of atherosclerosis. *Science*, Vol.180, No.93, (June 1973), pp. 1332-1339, 0036-8075.

Ross, R. (1981-1982). Atherosclerosis: a question of endothelial integrity and growth control of smooth muscle. *Harvey Lectures*, Vol.77, pp. 161-182, ISSN 0073-0874.

Ross, R. (1999). Atherosclerosis is an inflammatory disease. *American Heart Journal*, Vol.138, No.5Pt 2, (November 1999), pp. S419-420, ISSN 0002-8703.

Rudijanto, A. (2007). The role of vascular smooth muscle cells on the pathogenesis of atherosclerosis. *Acta Medica Indonesiana*, Vol.39, No.2, (April-June 2007), pp. 86-93, ISSN 0125-9326.

Rzucidlo, E.M.; Martin, K.A. & Powell, R.J. (2007). Regulation of vascular smooth muscle cell differentiation. *Journal of Vascular Surgery*, Vol.45, No.SA, (June 2007), pp. A25-32, ISSN 0741-5214.

Schäfers, M.; Schober, O. & Hermann, S. (2010). Matrix-metalloproteinases as imaging targets for inflammatory activity in atherosclerotic plaques. *The Journal of Nuclear Medicine*, Vol.51, No.5, (May 2010), pp. 663-666, ISSN 0161-5505.

Schwartz, S.M.; Campbell, G.R. & Campbell, J.H. (1986). Replication of smooth muscle cells in vascular disease. *Circulation Research*, Vol.58, No.4, (April 1986), pp. 427-444, ISSN 0009-7330.

Schwartz, S.M.; deBlois, D. & O'Brien, E.R. (1995). The intima. Soil for atherosclerosis and restenosis. *Circulation Research*, Vol.77, No.3, (September 1995), pp. 445-465, ISSN 0009-7330.

Schwartz, S.M.; Virmani, R. & Rosenfeld, M.E. (2000). The good smooth muscle cells in atherosclerosis. *Current Atherosclerosis Reports*, Vol.2, No.5, (September 2000), pp. 422-429, ISSN 1523-3804.

Shah, P.K.; Falk, E.; Badimon, J.J.; Fernandez-Ortiz, A.; Mailhac, A.; Villareal-Levy, G.; Fallon, J.T.; Regnstrom, J. & Fuster, V. (1995). Human monocyte-derived macrophages induce collagen breakdown in fibrous caps of atherosclerotic plaques. Potential role of matrix-degrading metalloproteinases and implications for plaque rupture. *Circulation*, Vol.92, No.6, (September 1995), pp. 1565-1569, ISSN 0009-7322.

Shanahan, C.M.; Weissberg, P.L. & Metcalfe, J.C. (1993). Isolation of gene markers of differentiated and proliferating vascular smooth muscle cells. *Circulation Research*, Vol.73, No.1, (July 1993), pp. 193-204, ISSN 0009-7330.

Shanahan, C.M. & Weissberg, P.L. (1998). Smooth muscle cell heterogeneity: patterns of gene expression in vascular smooth muscle cells in vitro and in vivo. *Arteriosclerosis, Thrombosis and Vascular Biology*, Vol.18, No.3, (March 1998), pp. 333-338 ISSN 1079-5642.

Shanahan, C.M. & Weissberg, P.L. (1999). Smooth muscle cell phenotypes in atherosclerotic lesions. *Current Opinion in Lipidology,* Vol.10, No.6, (December 1999), pp. 507-513, ISSN 0957-9672.

Sies, H. (1991). Oxidative stress: from basic research to clinical application. *The American Journal of Medicine,* Vol.91, No.3C, (September 1991), pp. 31S-38S, ISSN 1548-2766.

Sima, A.V.; Stancu, C.S. & Simionescu, M. (2009). Vascular endothelium in atherosclerosis. *Cell and Tissue Research,* Vol.335, No.1, (January 2009), pp. 191-203, ISSN 0302-766X.

Simionescu, M. & Antohe, F. (2006). Functional ultrastructure of the vascular endothelium: changes in various pathologies. *Handbook of Experimental Pharmacology,* No.176Pt 1, pp. 41-69, ISSN 0171-2004.

Simper, D.; Stalboerger, P.G.; Panetta, C.J.; Wang, S. & Caplice, N.M. (2002). Smooth muscle progenitor cells in human blood. *Circulation,* Vol.106, No.10, (September 2002), pp. 1199-1204, ISSN 0009-7322.

Singh, U. & Jialal, I. (2006). Oxidative stress and atherosclerosis. *Pathophysiology,* Vol.13, No.3, (August 2006), pp. 129-142, ISSN 0928-4680.

Skålén, K.; Gustafsson, M.; Rydberg, E.K.; Hultén, L.M.; Wiklund, O.; Innerarity, T.L. & Borén, J. (2002). Subendothelial retention of atherogenic lipoproteins in early atherosclerosis. *Nature,* Vol.417, No.6890, (June 2002), pp.750-754, ISSN 0028-0836.

Skalska, A.B.; Pietrzycka, A. & Stepniewski, M. (2009). Correlation of endothelin 1 plasma levels with plasma antioxidant capacity in elderly patients treated for hypertension. *Clinical Biochemistry,* Vol.42, No.4-5, (March 2009), pp. 358-364, ISSN 0009-9120.

Slomp, J.; Gittenberger-de Groot, A.C.; Glukhova, M.A.; Conny van Munsteren. J.; Kockx, M.M.; Schwartz, S.M. & Koteliansky, V.E. (1997). Differentiation, dedifferentiation, and apoptosis of smooth muscle cells during the development of the human ductus arteriosus. *Arteriosclerosis, Thrombosis and Vascular Biology,* Vol.17, No.5, (May 1997), pp. 1003-1009, ISSN 1079-5642.

Sobue, K.; Hayashi, K. & Nishida, W. (1999). Expressional regulation of smooth muscle cell-specific genes in association with phenotypic modulation. *Molecular and Cellular Biochemistry,* Vol.190, No.1-2, (January 1999), pp. 105-118, ISSN 0300-8177.

Sprague, A.H. & Khalil, R.A. (2009). Inflammatory cytokines in vascular dysfunction and vascular disease. *Biochemical Pharmacology,* Vol.78, No.6, (September 2009), pp. 539-552, ISSN 0006-2952.

Steinberg, D. (2009). The LDL modification hypothesis of atherogenesis: an update. *Journal of Lipid Research,* Vol.50S, (April 2009), pp. 376-381, ISSN 0022-2275.

Stintzing, S.; Ocker, M.; Hartner, A.; Amann, K.; Barbera, L. & Neureiter, D. (2009). Differentiation patterning of vascular smooth muscle cells (VSMC) in atherosclerosis. *Virchows Archives,* Vol.455, No.2, (August 2009), pp. 171-185, ISSN 1432-2307.

Stocker, R. & Keaney, J.F. Jr. (2004). Role of oxidative modifications in atherosclerosis. *Physiological reviews,* Vol.84, No.4, (October 2004), pp.1381-1478, ISSN 0031-9333.

Tabas, I.; Williams, K.J. & Borén, J. (2007). Subendothelial lipoprotein retention as the initiating process in atherosclerosis: update and therapeutic implications. *Circulation,* Vol.116, No.16, (October 2007), pp.1832-1844, ISSN 0009-7322.

Tagliafico, E.; Brunelli, S.; Bergamaschi, A.; De Angelis, L.; Scardigli, R.; Galli, D.; Battini, R.; Bianco, P.; Ferrari, S.; Cossu, G. & Ferrari, S. (2004). TGFbeta/BMP activate the smooth muscle/bone differentiation programs in mesoangioblasts. *Journal of Cell Science,* Vol.117, No.Pt 19, (September 2004), pp. 4377-4388, ISSN 0021-9533.

Taniyama, Y. & Griendling, K.K. (2003). Reactive oxygen species in the vasculature: molecular and cellular mechanisms. *Hypertension*, Vol.42, No.6, (December 2003), pp.1075-1081, ISSN 0194-911X.

Teplyakov, A.I. (2004). Endothelin-1 involved in systemic cytokine network inflammatory response at atherosclerosis. *Journal of Cardiovascular Pharmacology*, Vol.44, No.S1, (November 2004), pp. S274-S275, ISSN 0160-2446.

Thom T.J. (1989). International mortality from heart disease: rates and trends. *International Journal of Epidemiology*, Vol.18, No.3(S1), pp.S20-S28, ISSN 1464-3685.

Thyberg, J. (2002). Caveolae and cholesterol distribution in vascular smooth muscle cells of different phenotypes. *The Journal of Histochemistry and Cytochemistry*, Vol.50, No.2, (February 2002), pp. 185-195, ISSN 0022-1554.

Tintut, Y.; Alfonso, Z.; Saini, T.; Radcliff, K.; Watson, K.; Boström, K. & Demer, L.L. (2003). Multilineage potential of cells from the artery wall. *Circulation*, Vol.108, No.20, (November 2003), pp. 2505-2510, ISSN 0009-7322.

Tîrziu, D.; Dobrian, A.; Tasca, C.; Simionescu, M. & Simionescu, N. (1995). Intimal thickenings of human aorta contain modified reassembled lipoproteins. *Atherosclerosis*, Vol.112, No.1, (January 1995), pp. 101-114, ISSN 0021-9150.

Topouzis, S. & Majesky, M.W. (1996). Smooth muscle lineage diversity in the chick embryo. Two types of aortic smooth muscle cell differ in growth and receptor-mediated transcriptional responses to transforming growth factor-beta. *Developmental Biology*, Vol.178, No.2, (September 1996), pp. 430-445, ISSN 0012-1606.

Torsney, E.; Mandal, K.; Halliday, A.; Jahangiri, M. & Xu, Q. (2007). Characterisation of progenitor cells in human atherosclerotic vessels. *Atherosclerosis*, Vol.191, No.2, (April 2007), pp. 259-264, ISSN 0021-9150.

Tousoulis, D.; Koutsogiannis, M.; Papageorgiou, N.; Siasos, G.; Antoniades, C.; Tsiamis, E. & Stefanadis, C. (2010). Endothelial dysfunction: potential clinical implications. *Minerva Medica*, Vol.101, No.4, (August 2010), pp. 271-284, ISSN 1827-1669.

Traub, O. & Berk, B.C. (1998). Laminar shear stress: mechanisms by which endothelial cells transduce an atheroprotective force. *Arteriosclerosis, Thrombosis and Vascular Biology*, Vol.18, No.5, (May 1998), pp. 677-685, ISSN 1079-5642.

Traupe, T.; Ortmann, J.; Münter, K. & Barton, M. (2003). Endothelial therapy of atherosclerosis and its risk factors. *Current Vascular Pharmacology*, Vol.1, No.2, (June 2003), pp. 111-121, ISSN 1570-1611.

van Oostrom, O.; Fledderus, J.O.; de Kleijn, D.; Pasterkamp, G. & Verhaar, M.C. (2009). Smooth muscle progenitor cells: friend or foe in vascular disease?. *Current Stem Cell Research & Therapy*, Vol.4, No.2, (May 2009), pp. 131-140, ISSN 1574-888X.

Vanhoutte P.M. (2009). Endothelial dysfunction: The first step toward coronary arterosclerosis. *Circulation Journal*, Vol.73, No.4, (April 2009), pp. 595-601, ISSN 1346-9843.

Vásquez-Vivar, J.; Kalyanaraman, B.; Martásek, P.; Hogg, N.; Masters, B.S.; Karoui, H.; Tordo, P. & Pritchard, K.A. Jr. (1998). Superoxide generation by endothelial nitric oxide synthase: the influence of cofactors. *Proceedings of the National Academy of Sciences of the United States of America*, Vol.95, No.16, (August 1998), pp. 9220-9225, ISSN 0027-8424.

Virdis, A.; Ghiadoni, L.; Giannarelli, C. & Taddei, S. (2010). Endothelial dysfunction and vascular disease in later life. *Maturitas*, Vol.67, No.1, (September 2010), pp. 20-24, ISSN 0378-5122.

Weissberg, P.L.; Clesham, G.J. & Bennett, M.R. (1996). Is vascular smooth muscle cell proliferation beneficial?. *Lancet*, Vol.347, No.8997, (February 1996), pp. 305-307, ISSN 0140-6736.

Williams, K.J. & Tabas, I. (2005). Lipoprotein retention--and clues for atheroma regression. *Arteriosclerosis, Thrombosis and Vascular Biology*, Vol.25, No.8, (August 2005), pp. 1536-1540, ISSN 1079-5642.

Willis, A.I.; Pierre-Paul, D.; Sumpio, B.E. & Gahtan, V. (2004). Vascular smooth muscle cell migration: current research and clinical implications. *Vascular and Endovascular Surgery*, Vol.38, No.1, (January-February 2004), pp. 11-23, ISSN 1538-5744.

Witztum, J.L. & Steinberg, D. (2001). The oxidative modification hypothesis of atherosclerosis: does it hold for humans?. *Trends in Cardiovascular Medicine*, Vol.11, No.3-4, (April-May 2001), pp. 93-102, ISSN 1050-1738.

Xu, Q. (2000). Biomechanical-stress-induced signaling and gene expression in the development of arteriosclerosis. *Trends in Cardiovascular Medicine*, Vol.10, No.1, (January 2000), pp. 35-41, ISSN 1050-1738.

Xu, Q. (2009). Disturbed flow-enhanced endothelial turnover in atherosclerosis. *Trends in Cardiovascular Medicine*, Vol.19, No.6, (August 2009), pp. 191-195, ISSN 1050-1738.

Yamada, N. (2001). Atherosclerosis and oxidative stress. *Japan Medical Association Journal*, Vol.44, No.12, pp. 529-534, ISSN 1346-8650.

Zachary, I.; Servos, S. & Herren, B. (1999). Identification of novel protein kinases in vascular cells. *Methods in Molecular Medicine*, Vol. 30, pp. 111-129, ISSN 1543-1894.

Zalewski, A.; Shi, Y. & Johnson, A.G. (2002). Diverse origin of intimal cells: smooth muscle cells, myofibroblasts, fibroblasts, and beyond?. *Circulation Research*, Vol.91, No.8, (October 2002), pp. 652-655, ISSN 0009-7330.

Zeng, L.; Zampetaki, A.; Margariti, A.; Pepe, A.E.; Alam, S.; Martin, D.; Xiao, Q.; Wang, W.; Jin, Z.G.; Cockerill, G.; Mori, K.; Li, Y.S.; Hu, Y.; Chien, S. & Xu, Q. Sustained activation of XBP1 splicing leads to endothelial apoptosis and atherosclerosis development in response to disturbed flow. (2009). *Proceedings of the National Academy of Sciences of the United States of America*,Vol.106, No.20, (May 2009), pp. 8326-8331, ISSN 0027-8424.

Zengin, E.; Chalajour, F.; Gehling, U.M.; Ito, W.D.; Treede, H.; Lauke, H.; Weil, J.; Reichenspurner, H.; Kilic, N. & Ergün, S. (2006). Vascular wall resident progenitor cells: a source for postnatal vasculogenesis. *Development*, Vol.133, No.8, (April 2006), pp. 1543-1551, ISSN 0950-1991.

Zhang, S.H.; Reddick, R.L.; Piedrahita, J.A. & Maeda, N. (1992). Spontaneous hypercholesterolemia and arterial lesions in mice lacking apolipoprotein E. *Science*, Vol.258, No.5081, (October 1992), pp. 468-471, ISSN 0036-8075.

Zhang, H.; Park, Y.; Wu, J.; Chen, X.; Lee, S.; Yang, J.; Dellsperger, K.C. & Zhang, C. (2009). Role of TNF-alpha in vascular dysfunction. *Clinical Science (London)*, Vol.116, No.3, (February 2009), pp. 219-230, ISSN 1470-8736.

Zoll, J.; Fontaine, V.; Gourdy, P.; Barateau, V.; Vilar, J.; Leroyer, A.; Lopes-Kam, I.; Mallat, Z.; Arnal, J.F.; Henry, P.; Tobelem, G. & Tedgui, A. (2008). Role of human smooth muscle cell progenitors in atherosclerotic plaque development and composition. *Cardiovascular Research*, Vol.77, No.3, (February 2008), pp. 471-480, ISSN 0008-6363.

# 7

# Nutrigenomics and Atherosclerosis: The Postprandial and Long-Term Effects of Virgin Olive Oil Ingestion

Almudena Ortega, Lourdes M. Varela, Beatriz Bermudez, Sergio Lopez, Francisco J.G. Muriana and Rocio Abia

*Laboratory of Cellular and Molecular Nutrition, Instituto de la Grasa, Consejo Superior de Investigaciones Científicas, Sevilla, Spain*

## 1. Introduction

Epidemiological studies over the past 50 years have revealed numerous risk factors for atherosclerosis. They can be grouped into factors with an important genetic component and environmental factors, particularly diet, which is one of the major, constant environmental factors to which our genes are expose through life. When a gene is activated, or expressed, functionally distinct proteins are produced which can initiate a host of cellular metabolic effects. Gene expression patterns produce a phenotype, which represents the physical characteristics of an organism (e.g., hair color), or the presence or absence of a disease. Nutrition scientists realize more and more that phenotypic treats (health status) are not necessarily produce by genes alone but also by the interaction of bioactive food components on the levels of DNA, RNA, protein and metabolites (Müller & Kersten, 2003). Nutritional genomics came into being at the beginning of the 1990s. There is some confusion about the delimitation of the concept, as often the terms of nutritional genomics, nutrigenetics, and nutrigenomics, are used as synonyms. Nutritional genomics refers to the joint study of nutrition and the genome including all the other omics derived from genomics: transcriptomics (mRNA), proteomics (proteins), and metabolomics (metabolites) (Fig. 1). The terms nutritional genomics would be equivalent to the wide-ranging term of gene-diet interaction. Within the wide framework of the concept of nutritional genomics, we can distinguish 2 subconcepts: nutrigenetics and nutrigenomics. Currently, there is a wide consensus on considering nutrigenetics as the discipline that studies the different phenotypic response to diet depending on the genotype of each individual. The term nutrigenomics is subject to a greater variability in its delimitation, but it seems that there is a certain consensus in considering nutrigenomics as the discipline which studies the molecular mechanisms explaining the different phenotypic responses to diet depending on the genotype, studying how the nutrients regulate gene expression, and how these changes are interrelated with proteomics and metabolomics (Corella & Ordovas, 2009). This interpretation of the nutrigenomics concept is the one that we shall use in this Chapter.

Atherosclerosis is a complex, multifactorial disease associated with accumulation of lipids in lesions along blood vessels, leading to the occlusion of blood flow, with oxidative and inflammatory components playing major roles in its cause. Environmental factors with particular emphasis on nutrition as well as genetic factors appear to be responsible for these aberrant oxidative and inflammatory components and the lipid abnormalities associated with the disease. Diet may contribute to the atherosclerotic process by affecting lipoprotein concentration, their composition and degree of oxidation. Although certain key risk factors affecting atherosclerosis have been identified, the full molecular characterization will remain a challenge in the next century to come. As a complex biological process, the cellular and molecular details of the growth, progression and regression of the vascular lesions of atherosclerosis call for application of the newly developing omics techniques of analysis. Profiling gene expression using microarrays has proven useful in identifying new genes that may contribute to features of the atherosclerosis lesion (transcriptomics). One of the interesting challenges of modern biology is to define the diet that best fits the needs of the human species. Understanding the details of gene-nutrient interactions and of how changes in a gene or in the amount or form of a nutrient influence atherosclerosis is essential to developing insight into how to support optimal health from a nutritional perspective. There has been much interest regarding the components that contribute to the beneficial health effects of the Mediterranean diet. Recent findings suggest that bioactive components found in extra-virgin olive oil (EVOO) (oleic acid and polyphenol compounds) are endowed with several biologic activities that may contribute to the lower incidence of atherosclerosis in the Mediterranean area. This review summarizes more recent studies, including omics technologies that have lead to the development of new hypothesis concerning the cellular response to virgin olive oil (VOO) ingestion and to identify the major cellular pathways responsive to them.

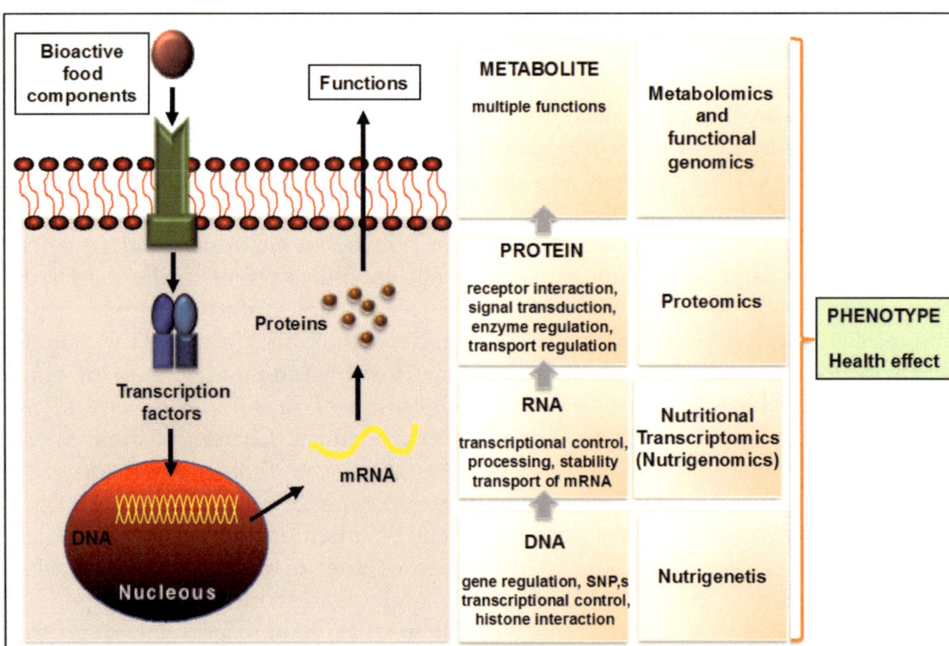


Fig. 1. Health effects of bioactive food components are related to specific interactions on a molecular level. (Adapted from Van Ommen, 2004; Müller & Kersten, 2003). SNP, single nucleotide polymorphism.

## 2. Olive oil and atherosclerosis

### 2.1 Olive oil classification according to International Olive Council

Olive oil is the main source of fat in the Mediterranean diet, and different categories of olive oils may be distinguished according to the International Olive Oil Council. Olive oil is obtained solely from the fruit of the olive tree (*Olea europaea*; family Oleaceae), and is not mixed with any other kind of oil. Olive oil extraction is the process of extracting the oil present in the olive drupes for food use. The oil is produced in the mesocarp cells, and is stored in a particular type of vacuole called a lipovacuole; every cell within an olive contains a tiny olive oil droplet. Olive oil extraction is defined as the process of separating the oil from the other fruit contents (vegetative extract liquid and solid material) and extracting the oil present in the drupes for food use. This separation is attained only by physical procedures under thermal conditions that do not alter the oil.

Several different types of oil can be oil extracted from the olive fruit and are classified as follows:

**Virgin** indicates that the oil was extracted by physical procedures only with no chemical treatment, and is in essence crude oil.

**Refined** indicates that the oil has been chemically treated to neutralise strong tastes (which are characterized as defects) and neutralise the acid content (free fatty acids). Refined oil is commonly regarded as a lower quality than virgin oil.

**Pomace olive oil** indicates oil that has been extracted from the pomace (ground flesh and pits left after pressing olives) using chemical solvents (typically hexane) and by heat.

Oil can be classified into different grades as follow:

**Extra-virgin olive oil** is the highest quality of olive oils and is produced by cold extraction of the olives; the oil has a free acidity of no more than 0.8 grams of oleic acid per 100 grams (0.8% acidity), and is often thought to have a superior taste. There can be no refined oil in extra-virgin olive oil.

**Virgin olive oil** has an acidity of less than 2%, and is often thought to have a good taste. There can be no refined oil in virgin olive oil.

**Olive oil.** Oils labelled as Olive oil are usually a blend of refined olive oil and one of the above two categories of virgin olive oil; typically, these blends contain less than or equal to 1.5% acidity. This grade of oil commonly lacks a strong flavour. Different blends are produced by adding more or less virgin oil to achieve different tastes.

**Olive-pomace oil** is a blend of refined pomace olive oil and possibly some virgin oil. This oil is safe to consume, but it may not be called olive oil.

**Lampante oil** is olive oil that is not used for consumption; lampante comes from olives that have strong physico-chemical and organoleptic defects and contain greater than 3,3% of acidity.

### 2.2 Olive oil composition

VOO is composed mainly of TGs (98-99 % of the total oil weight) and contains small quantities of free fatty acids (FFAs), and more than 230 chemical compounds such as aliphatic and triterpenic alcohols, sterols, hydrocarbons, volatile compounds and antioxidants. TGs are the major energy reserve for plants and animals. Chemically speaking, these are molecules derived from the natural esterification of three fatty acid molecules with a glycerol molecule. The glycerol molecule can simplistically be seen as an "E-shaped" molecule, with the fatty acids in turn resembling longish hydrocarbon chains, varying (in the case of olive oil) from about 14 to 24 carbon atoms in length (Fig. 2). The fatty acid composition of olive oil varies widely depending on the cultivar, maturity of the fruit, altitude, climate, and several other factors. A fatty acid has the general formula: CH3(CH2)nCOOH where n is typically an even number between 12 and 22. If no double bonds are present the molecules are called saturated fatty acids (SFAs). If a chain contains double bonds, it is called an unsaturated fatty acid. A single double bond makes monounsaturated fatty acids (MUFAs). More than one double bond makes polyunsaturated fatty acids (PUFAs). The major fatty acids in olive oil triglycerides are: oleic acid (C18:1), a monounsaturated omega-9 fatty acid. It makes up 55 to 83% of olive oil. Linoleic acid (C18:2), a polyunsaturated omega-6 fatty acid that makes up about 3.5 to 21% of olive oil. Palmitic acid (C16:0), a SFA that makes up 7.5 to 20% of olive oil. Stearic acid (C18:0), a SFA that makes up 0.5 to 5% of olive oil (Fig. 2). Linolenic acid (C18:3) (specifically alpha-Linolenic acid), a polyunsaturated omega-3 fatty acid that makes up 0 to 1.5% of olive oil. In the triglycerides the main fatty acids are represented by monounsaturates (oleic acid), with a slight amount of saturates (palmitic and stearic acids) and an adequate presence of polyunsaturates (linoleic and α-linolenic acid) (Bermudez et al., 2011). Most prevalent in olive oil is the oleic-oleic-oleic (OOO) triglyceride, followed, in order of incidence, by palmitic-oleic-oleic (POO), oleic-oleic-linoleic (OOL), palmitic-oleic-linoleic (POL), and stearic-oleic-oleic (SOO).

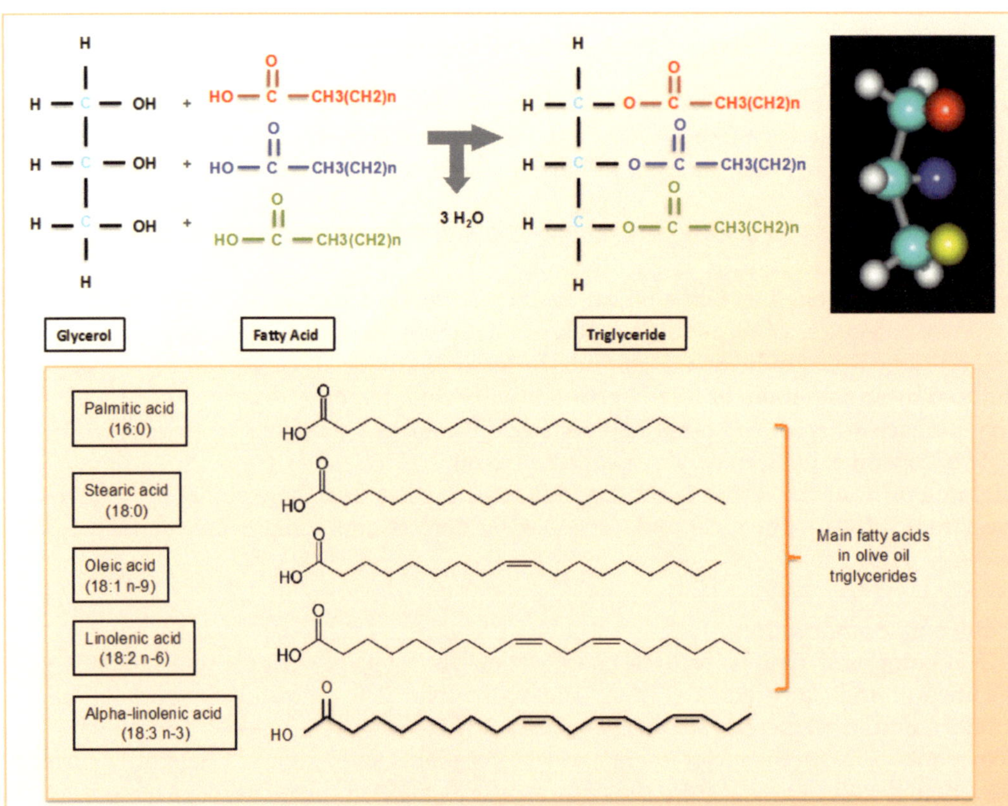


Fig. 2. Structure of triglycerides and main fatty acids in olive oil triglycerides.

The minor components of VOO are α-tocopherol, phenol compounds, carotenoids (β-carotene and lutein), squalene, pytosterols, and chlorophyll (in addition to a great number of aromatic substances). The factor that can influence the composition of VOO, especially in regard to its minor components, are the type of cultivar, the characteristics of the olive tree growing soil, climatic factors, fruit ripening stage, time of harvesting and degree of technology used in its production. The main antioxidants of VOO are phenols represented by lipophilic and hydrophilic phenols. Carotenes, on the contrary are contained in small concentrations. The lipophilic phenols, such as tocopherols and tocotrienols, can be found in other vegetable oils. In VOO more than 90% of total concentration of tocopherols is constituted by α-tocopherol. The VOO hydrophilic phenols constitute a group of secondary plant metabolites showing peculiar organoleptic and healthy properties. They are not generally present in other oils and fats (Servili et al., 2009). VOO contains four major classes of phenolic compounds: flavonoids, lignans, simple phenolics and secoiridois (Table 1). Although some cultivars contain flavonoids, the content in olive oil is low compared to other fruits and vegetables. Lignans are present at more significant

| **Phenolic alcohols (simple phenolics)** | **Phenolic acids and derivatives** |
|---|---|
| (3,4-Dihydroxyphenil) ethanol (3,4 DHPEA) (HY) | Vanillic acid |
| | Syringic acid |
| (4-Hydroxyphenil) ethanol (p-HPEA) (TYR) | p-Coumaric acid |
| (3,4-Dyhydroxyphenyl) ethanol-glucoside | o-Coumaric acid |
| Flavones | Gallic acid |
| Apigenin | Caffeic acid |
| Luteolin | Protocatechuic acid |
| Rutin | p-Hydroxibenzoic acid |
| Lignans | Ferulic acid |
| (+)-Acetoxypinoresinol | Cinnamic acid |
| (+)-Pinoresinol | 4-(acetoxyithil)-1,2-Dihydroxybenzene |
| (+)-Hydroxypinoresinol | Benzoic acid |
| | **Hydroxy-isocromas** |
| | Phenyl-6,7-dihydroxi-isochroman |
| **Secoiridoids** | |
| Dialdehydic form of decarboxymethyl elenolic acid linked to 3,4-DHPEA (3,4 DHPEA-EDA) | |
| Dialdehydic form of decarboxymethyl elenolic acid linked to p-HPEA (p-HPEA-EDA) | |
| Oleuropein aglycon (3,4 DHPEA-EA) | |
| Ligstroside aglycon | |
| Oleuropein | |
| p-HPEA-derivative | |
| Dialdehydic form of oleuropein aglycon | |
| Dialdehydic form of ligstroside aglycon | |

Table 1. Phenolic composition of a Virgin Olive Oil.

amounts. The levels of secoiridoids and simple phenolics, many of which are exclusive to VOO, are the major phenolics found in olive oil. The simple phenolics present in VOO are predominantly hydroxytyrosol (HT) (3,4-dihydroxyphenylethanol) and tyrosol (TYR) (4-hydroxyphenylethanol) whilst the secoiridoids are derived from the glusosides of oleuropein and ligstroside forms, they contain in their chemical structure an HT (oleuropein derivatives) or TYR (ligstroside derivatives) moiety linked to elenolic acid (Corona et al., 2009). After ingestion, olive oil polyphenols can be partially modified in the acidic environment of the stomach, aglycone secoiridoids are subject to hydrolysis leading to approximate 5-fold increase in the amount of free HT and 3-fold increase in free TYR. If the ingested secoiridoid is glucosylated it appears not to be subject to gastric hydrolysis, meaning that phenolics such as glucosides of oleuropein enter the small intestine unmodified, along with high amount of free HT and TYR and remaining secoiridoid aglycones. The major site for the absorption of olive oil polyphenols is the small intestine, HT and TYR are dose-dependently absorbed and they are metabolized primarily to O-glucuronidated conjugates. HT also undergoes O-methylation by the action of catechol-O-methyl-transferase, and both homovanillic acid and homovanillyl alcohol have been detected in human and animal plasma and urine after the oral administration of either VOO or pure HT and TYR. Studies have also demonstrated that secoiridoids, which appear not to be absorbed in the small intestine, undergo bacterial catabolism in the large intestine with oleuropein undergoing rapid degradation by the colonic microflora producing HT as the major end product (Corona, et al., 2006). The intense interest in VOO polyphenols and their metabolites can be attributed to the association of such substances with several biological activities; these include antioxidant activity as well as other important healthy properties that will be discussed later. For this reason, olive polyphenols are recognized as potential nutraceutical targets for food and pharmaceutical industries.

### 2.3 Atherosclerosis and virgin olive oil

Atherosclerosis underlies the leading cause of death in industrialised societies (Lloyd-Jones et al., 2010). The key-initiating step of early stages of atherosclerosis is the subendothelial accumulation of apolipoprotein B-containing lipoproteins. These lipoproteins are produced by the liver and the intestinal cells and consist of a core of neutral lipids, mainly cholesteryl esters and triglycerides (TGs), surrounded by a monolayer of phospholipids and proteins. Hepatic apoB-lipoproteins are secreted as very-low density lipoproteins (VLDL), and they are converted to atherogenic low-density lipoproteins (LDL) during the circulation; in contrast, the intestinal apoB-lipoproteins are secreted as chylomicrons. The VLDL and chylomicrons can be converted into atherogenic remnant lipoproteins by lipolysis. The VLDL, chylomicrons and their remnants, which are known as triglyceride-rich lipoproteins (TRLs), appear in the blood after a high-fat meal (postprandial state) and are considered to be highly atherogenic (Havel, 1994; Zilversmith, 1979). In fact, chylomicronemia causes atherosclerosis in mice (Weinstein et al., 2010) and decreasing the TRLs level reduces the progression of coronary artery disease to the same degree as decreasing the LDL-cholesterol level (Hodis et al., 1999). TRLs comprise a large variety of nascent and metabolically modified lipoprotein particles that vary in size and density, as well as lipid and apolipoprotein composition. Studies have indicated that the size and the specific structural arrangement of lipids and apolipoproteins are associated with atherogenicity. Morover, studies have consistently shown that there is an inverse relationship between the lipoprotein particle size and the ability to enter the arterial wall. Small TRLs and their remnants can enter the arterial wall and are independently associated with the presence, severity, and progression of atherosclerosis (Hodis, 1999). Short-term intake of the Mediterranean diet and the acute intake of an olive oil meal could favour the lower cardiovascular risk in Mediterranean countries by secreting a reduced number and higher-size TRLs particles compared with other fat sources (Perez-Martinez et al., 2011). Recent studies suggest that lipoproteins may also contribute to atherogenesis by affecting the mechanisms of the control of gene expression. Many lipoproteins-gene interactions have only been investigated under fasting conditions, Lopez et al., 2009 nicely reviews the emerging importance of gene-nutrient interactions at the postprandial state, which impacts ultimately on atherosclerosis risk.

A large body of knowledge exists from epidemiological, clinical, experimental animal models and in vitro studies that have indicated that olive oil can be regarded as functional food for its anti-atherogenic properties. Diets enriched with olive oil prevent the development and progression of atherosclerosis (Aguilera et al., 2002; Kanrantonis et al., 2006) and may also play an important role in atherosclerosis regression (Mangiapane et al., 1999; Tsalina et al., 2007, 2010). These and recent reports have suggested that the beneficial effects of olive oil on atherosclerosis may be influenced by the high oleic acid content and the minor fraction of the oil; potential benefitial microconstituents include tocopherols, phenolic compounds, phytosterols, triterpenoids and unusual glycolipids that exert an antagonistic effect on PAF (1-O-hexadecyl-2-acetyl-sn-glycero-3-phosphocholine). There are several mechanisms by which olive oil affects the development of atherosclerosis. Theses mechanisms have been nicely reviewed by Carluccio et al., 2007, and include the following: 1) regulation of cholesterol levels as olive oil decreases LDL-cholesterol and increases HDL-cholesterol; 2) decreased susceptibility of human LDL to oxidation, because of the lower susceptibility of its MUFAs content and to the ability of its polyphenol fraction to scavenge free radicals and reduce oxidative stress; 3) both, oleic acid and olive oil antioxidant polyphenols inhibit endothelial activation and monocyte recruitment during early atherogenesis; 4) decreased macrophage production of inflammatory cytokines, eicosanoid inflammatory mediators derived from arachidonic acids and increased nitric oxide (NO) production, which improves vascular stability; 5) decreased macrophages matrix-metalloproteinases (MMPs) production, which improves plaque stability; 6) oleic acid and olive oil polyphenols are associated with a reduced risk of hypertension; 7) oleic acid and olive oil polyphenols also affect blood coagulation and fibrinolytic factors, thereby reducing the risk of acute thrombotic cardiovascular events; and 8) a decreased rate of oxidation of DNA (Machowetz et al., 2007); human atherosclerosis is associated with DNA damage in both circulating cells and cells that comprise the vessel wall.

EVOO is therefore becoming more important due to its beneficial effects on human health. EVOO has proven effective in controlling atherosclerotic lesions, mainly within the framework of a Mediterranean-type diet (low cholesterol). An animal model that reproduces the processes taking place in the development of human atherosclerosis has been crucial to obtaining these conclusions, and this has been provided by the apoE-deficient mouse. Using this model, it has been proved that EVOO possesses beneficial antiatherogenic effects, and its enrichment with polyphenols (Rosenblat et al., 2008) and with long chain n-3 PUFAs (Eilertsen et al., 2011) further improves these effects, leading to the attenuation of atherosclerosis development. Feeding these mice with various olive oils rich in different minor components or with these components in isolation has made it possible to assess the contribution of those molecules to the beneficial effect of this food, these effects have been review by Guillen et al., 2009 and include the following: 1) increase of small, dense HDL enriched with apo A-IV tightly bound to paraoxonase; these apolipoprotein A-IV-enriched particles were very effective in inactivating the peroxides present in the low-density lipoproteins (LDL) which are thought to initiate atherosclerosis; 2) minor components decrease plasma triglycerides and LDL-colesterol and very low density lipoprotein cholesterol (VLDL-colesterol), as well as 3) parameters of oxidative stress, such as isoprostane (8-iso-prostaglandin F2a); 4) EVOO acts against oxidative stress, which occurs primarily through a direct antioxidant effect as well as through an indirect mechanism that involves greater expression and activity of certain enzymes with antioxidant activities such as catalase and glutathione peroxidase-1 (Oliveras-Lopez et al., 2008). Among the antioxidants from EVOO, phenolic compounds have received the most attention. Oleuropein derivatives, especially HT, have been shown to have protective effects against markers associated with the atherogenic process (González-Santiago et al., 2006; Zrelli et al., 2011), some studies (Acin et al., 2006), however, have shown opposite results with HT administration in the atherosclerotic process. Given the anti-atherogenic properties of EVOO evident in animal models fed a Western diet, clinical trials are needed to establish whether these oils are a safe and effective means of treating atherosclerosis.

## 3. Nutrigenomics of olive oil

### 3.1 Gene-diet interactions after acute ingestion of olive oil

In addition to the mechanisms described above, olive oil components can exert an anti-atherogenic affect by acting at the genomic level. Nearly all evidence for the impact of olive oil on gene expression is derived from research using animal or human cells in culture. Carefully designed human clinical studies to establish a cause-and-effect relationship between olive oil affecting gene expression and the atherosclerotic process are scare and will be review here. Recent in vivo studies have shown that sustained consumption of VOO influence peripheral blood mononuclear cells (PBMNCs) gene expression (nutritional transcriptomics) (Table 2). PBMNCs are often used to asses changes in gene expression in vivo because the leucocytes recruitment from the circulation to the vessel wall for subsequent migration into the sub-endothelial layer is a critical step in atherosclerotic plaque formation; additionally, PBMNCs can be easily obtained from volunteers through simple blood draws. Previous studies have shown that in healthy individuals, a 3-week consumption of VOO as a principal fat source in a diet low in natural antioxidants (Khymenets et al., 2009) up-regulated the expression of genes associated with DNA repair proteins such as, the excision repair cross complementation group (ERCC-5) and the X-ray repair complementing defective repair Chinese hamster cells 5 (XRCC-5). VOO consumption also up-regulated aldehyde dehydrogenase 1 family, member A1 (ALDH1A1) and LIAS (lipoic acid synthetase) gene expression. ALDH1A1 is a gene encoding protein which protect cells from the oxidative stress induced by lipid peroxidation; the LIAS protein plays an important role in α-(+)-lipolitic acid (LA) synthesis. LA is an important antioxidant that has been shown to inhibit atherosclerosis in mouse models of human atherosclerosis due to its anti-inflammatory, antihyperglyceridemic and weight-reducing effects. Morover, apoptosis-related genes such as, BIRC-1 (baculoviral IAP repeat-containing protein 1) and TNSF-10 (tumor necrosis factor (ligand) superfamily, member 10), were also upregulated. BIRC-1 inhibits apoptosis while TNSF-10 promotes macrophages and lymphocytes apoptosis. VOO ingestion also modified OGT gene expression (O-linked N-acetylglucosamine (GlcNAc) transferase). Nuclear and cytoplasmic protein glycosylation is a widespread and reversible posttranslational modification in eukaryotic cells; intracellular glycosylation via the addition of N-acetylglucosamine to serine and threonine is catalysed by OGT. Thus, OGT plays a significant role in modulating protein stability, protein-proteins interactions, transactivation processes, and the enzyme activity of target proteins; moreover OGT plays a critical role in regulating cell function and survival in the cardiovascular system. VOO consumption also profoundly impacted the expression of the USP-48 (ubiquitin specific peptidase-48) gene. USP-48 is a member of the ubiquitin proteasome system that removes damaged, oxidized and /or misfolded proteins; it also plays a role in inflammation, proliferation and apoptosis. PPARBP (peroxisome proliferator-activated receptor-binding protein), which is an essential transcriptional mediator of adipogenesis, lipid metabolism, insulin sensitivity and glucose homeostasis via peroxisome proliferator-activated receptor-γ (PPAR-γ) regulation, and ADAM-17 (a disintegrin and metalloproteinase domain 17), a membrane -anchored metalloprotease, were also upregulated. ADAM-17 is a candidate gene of atherosclerosis susceptibility in mice models of atherosclerosis (Holdt et al., 2008), it mediates the release of several cell-signaling and cell adhesion molecules such as vascular endothelial (VE)-cadherin, vascular cell adhesion molecule-1 (VCAM-1), intercellular adhesion molecule-1 (ICAM-1) or L-selectin affecting endothelial permeability and leukocyte transmigration. According with this study, Reiss et al. 2011, have recently show that unsaturated FFA increase ADAM-mediated substrate cleavage, with corresponding functional consequences on cell proliferation, cell migration, and endothelial permeability, events of high significance in atherogenesis.

LLorent-Cortes et al. 2010, have also concluded that a Mediterranean-type diet in a high-risk cardiovascular population impacts the expression of genes involved in inflammation, vascular foam cell formation and vascular remodelling in human monocytes. Inflammation plays a role in the onset and development of atherosclerosis. In this study, VOO ingestion prevented an increase in cyclo-oxygenase-2 (COX-2) expression and decreased monocyte chemotactic protein-1 (MCP-1) gene expression compared with a traditional Mediterranean diet (TMD) with nuts or a low fat diet. COX-2 is a pro-inflammatory enzyme that increases prostanoid levels (thromboxane A2; TXA2 and prostaglandine E2; PGE2); bioactive molecules present in VOO such as 1-hydroxityrosol and phenyl-6,7-dihydroxi-isochroman which is an ortho-diphenol present in EVOO, down-regulate COX-2 synthesis by preventing nuclear factor-kappaB (NF-kB) activation in macrophages and monocytes (Maiuri et al., 2005; Trefiletti et al., 2011). MCP-1 is a potent regulator of leucocyte trafficking, and animal studies have shown that a VOO diet can reduce neutrophil accumulation and decreases the MCP-1 blood levels (Leite et al., 2005); again, these data support the hypothesis that VOO is anti-inflammatory. Morover, the dietary intervention with VOO specifically prevented low density lipoprotein receptor-related protein-1 (LRP-1) overexpression in the high cardiovascular risk population. LRP-1 plays a major role in macrophage-foam cell formation and migration; additionally, LRP-1 is also a key receptor for the prothrombotic transformation of the vascular wall. Morover, VOO dietary intervention prevented an increase in the expression of genes involved in intracellular lipid accumulation in macrophages and monocytes (e.g., CD36 antigen; CD36) and in the process of thrombosis (e.g., tissue factor pathway inhibitory, FFPI) compared to a TMD enriched with nuts (high in PUFAs).

| Reference | Subjects | Study design | Intervention | Gene Expression | Function |
|---|---|---|---|---|---|
| Khyments et al., 2009 | Healthy men (6) and women (4) | | Virgin olive oil in a diet low in antioxidants (1 wk washout, 3 wk 25ml VOO) | XRCC5, ERCC5<br>ALDH1A1, LIAS<br>OGT,<br>BIRC1, TNFSF-10<br>PPARBP,<br>USP48,<br>ADAM17. | DNA repair<br>Oxidative stress<br>Protein stability<br>Apoptosis<br>PPAR-ϒ regulation<br>Tissue remodelling<br>Endothelial permeability |
| Llorente-Cortes et al., 2010 | Asymptomatic high cardiovascular-risk subjects (type 2 diabetes, hypertension, hypercholesterolemia, low HDL-cholesterol) (23 men, 26 women) | Randomized, controlled | Virgin olive oil or nuts in the context of a traditional Mediterranean diet (3 mo). | COX-2, MCP-1,<br>TFPI,<br>LRP1, CD36. | Inflammation<br>Thrombosis<br>Lipid accumulation |
| Konstantinidou et al., 2010 | Healthy men and women (90) | Randomized, parallel, controlled | Virgin olive oil or washed virgin olive oil (without polyphenols) in the context of a traditional Mediterranean diet. | IFNγ, ARHGAP15, IL7R<br>ADRB2<br>POLK | Inflammation<br>Oxidative stress<br>DNA repair |

Table 2. Changes in gene expression of atherosclerotic-related genes after acute ingestion of virgin olive oil in human studies.

The last two nutritional interventions, suggest that the benefits associated with a TMD and VOO consumption can reduce cardiovascular risk via nutrigenomic effects; however, these studies could not distinguish between the effects elicited by minor components of VOO and those promoted by the fat content of the oil. A recent study by Konstantinidou et al, 2010 indicated that olive oil polyphenols play a significant role in the down-regulation of pro-atherogenic genes in human PBMNCs after 3 months of a dietary intervention with a TMD+VOO and TMD+WOO (washed virgin olive oil which has the same characteristics as VOO except for a lower polyphenol content). The dietary intervention decreased the expression of genes related to inflammation (e.g., interferon-γ, IFN-γ; Rho GTPase activating protein-15, ARHGAP-15; and Interleukin 7 receptor, IL7R) oxidative stress (e.g., adrenergic β-2 receptor surface, ADRB2) and DNA damage (e.g., polymerase DNA directed k, POLK). Changes in the expression of all of these genes, except POLK, were particularly observed when VOO, rich in polyphenols, was present in the TMD. The decrease in gene expression associated with inflammatory that was observed in this study agrees with previous studies that have reported a decrease in systemic inflammatory markers and oxidative stress due to the ingestion of polyphenols from olive oil and olive leaf extract (Poudyal et al., 2010; Puel et al., 2008). IFN-γ is considered to be a key inflammatory mediator and the release of this cytokine is regulated by polyphenols from red wine and dietary tea polyphenols (Deng et al., 2010; Magrone et al., 2008). ARHGAP-15 encodes for a Rho GTPase-activating protein that regulates the activity of GTPases. To date, little is known about the physiological role of ARHGAP-15, however, recent studies by Costa et al., 2011 have shown that this protein is associated with the selective regulation of multiple neutrophil functions. The protein encoded by the IL7R gene is a receptor for IL-7, which is associated with inflammation; interestingly, olive oil consumption has been shown to reduce the IL-7 serum concentration in patients with the metabolic syndrome (Esposito et al., 2004). POLK is a DNA repair gene that copies undamaged DNA templates. Previous studies have indicated that down-regulation of POLK is not associated with polyphenol content of VOO. Thus, the protective effect of VOO associated with DNA repair is related to the fat content (MUFA) and other minor oil components. ADRB2 has previously been associated with body composition (Bea et al., 2010), overexpression of the receptor that enhances reactive oxygen species (ROS) signalling (Di Lisa et al., 2011), and ADRB2 inhibition, which reduces macrophage cytokine production. Down-regulation of the ADRB2 gene, particularly in the TDM+VOO intervention group, along with an improvement in the oxidative status of the volunteers, may indicate that olive oil polyphenols protect against oxidative stress. Collectively, these studies support the hypothesis that olive oil polyphenol consumption in the context of a TMD may protect against cardiovascular disease by modulating the expression of atherosclerosis-related genes.

### 3.2 Influence of olive oil on gene-diet interaction at the postprandial state

Humans that reside in industrialised societies spend most of the daytime in a non-fasting state that is influence by meal consumption patterns and the amounts of food ingested. Postprandial lipaemia is characterised by an increase in TGs, specifically in the form of TRLs. Over 25 years ago, Zilversmit, 1979 proposed that atherogenesis was a postprandial phenomenon because high concentrations of lipoproteins and their remnants following food ingestion could deposit on the arterial wall and accumulate in atheromatous plaques. In postprandial studies, subjects usually receive a fat-loading test meal with a variable composition according to the nutrient to be tested. In these studies, both, the amount and the type of fat ingested influence postprandial lipaemia. Although, controversial results have been obtained for comparing an olive oil fat meal with other dietary fats, some studies have shown that VOO intake decreases the postprandial TGs concentration and results in a faster TRLs clearance from the blood in normolipidemic subjetcs (Abia et al., 2001). The amount of fat ingested influences the results as small doses of olive oil (25 ml) did not promote postprandial lipaemia, whereas larger doses (40 and 50 ml) of any type of olive oil promoted lipaemia (Fitó et al., 2002; Covas et al., 2006). Olive oil is considered to be an optimal fat for the modulation of extrinsic cardiovascular risk factors in the postprandial state. The influence of olive oil on postprandial insulin release and action, endothelial function, blood pressure, inflammatory processes and hemostasis has been recently review by Bearmudez et al., 2011.

### 3.2.1 Postprandial effect of olive oil in PBMNCs

Early in vivo postprandial human studies have shown that VOO activates PBMCs immediately after ingestion and may induce changes in gene expression (Bellido et al., 2004). Postprandial studies have shown that high-fat meals can induce β cell dysfunction and insulin resistance in healthy individuals, as well as in subjects with type 2 diabetes or the metabolic syndrome. However, postprandial olive oil (MUFAs) can buffer β cell hyperactivity and insulin intolerance compared to butter (SFAs) in subjects with high fasting triglyceride concentrations (Lopez et al., 2011). Moreover, changes in expression of insulin sensitivity related genes occur in human PBMNCs after an oral fat load of VOO (Konstantinidou et al., 2009) (Table 3). In this study, the expression of genes such as OGT, arachidonate 5-lipoxygenase-activating protein (ALOX5AP), LIAS, PPARBP, ADBR2 and ADAM-17 were up-regulated at 6 h after VOO ingestion. LIAS and PPARBP regulate insulin sensitivity by activating and co-activating PPARγ, respectively. PPARγ is a nuclear hormone receptor that plays a crucial role in adipogenesis and insulin sensitisation. The authors hypothesised that the up-regulation of both of these genes may be one feed back mechanism that counteracts the postprandial oxidative stress that plays a role in the development of insulin resistance. The ADRB2 gene encodes for a major lipolytic receptor in human fat cells that modulates insulin secretion and protects against oxidative stress. Because insulin signaling activates the OGT gene, the authors attributed the increase in OGT expression with the several feedback mechanisms that serve to attenuate sustained insulin signalling. CD36 is an integral membrane glycoprotein expressed on the surface of cells active in fatty acid metabolism (adipocytes, muscle cells, platelets, monocytes, heart and intestine cells). This protein plays diverse functions, including uptake of long-chain fatty acids and oxidized low-density lipoproteins. CD36 deficiency underlies insulin resistance, defective fatty acid metabolism and hypertriglyceridemia in spontaneously hypertensive rats (SHRs), furthermore, lipid-induced insulin resistant has been associated with atherogenesis through mechanisms mediated by the expression of scavenger receptor CD36 (Kashyap et al., 2009). CD36 gene expression was modulated during the postprandial period after VOO ingestion (Konstantinidou et al., 2009), however the authors did not find a relationship between in CD36 gene expression and insulin levels in the subjects. Rather, they found an association with a postprandial increase in plasma fatty acids and the satiety response after VOO ingestion. ADAM-17 is considered to be an attractive target for controlling insulin resistance. It also regulates tumor necrosis factor (TNF-α), major negative regulator of the

| Reference | Subjects | Study design | Intervention | Gene Expression | Function |
|---|---|---|---|---|---|
| Jimenez-Gomez et al., 2009 | Healthy men (20) | Randomized, crossover Postprandial | Three diet intervention period of 4 wks [SFA (butter), MUFA (VOO) and PUFA (walnut)] followed by fat-load rich in either SFA, MUFA , or PUFA (60% fat) | TNF-α, IL-6 | Inflammation |
| Konstantinidou et al., 2009 | Healthy men (11) | Postprandial | Virgin olive oil (1 wk washout, followed by 50mL fat-load). | LIAS, PPARBP, ADRB2, ADAM17<br>OGT, ALOX5AP<br>CD36 | Insulin-sensitivity<br><br>Scavenger receptor, satiety |
| Konstantinidou et al., 2009 | Healthy men (6) | Postprandial | Virgin olive oil (1 wk washout, followed by 50mL fat-load). | IL-10, IFN-Y<br>DCLRE1C, POLK<br>OGT, ADAM17<br>USP48,<br>ABCA7 | Inflammation<br>DNA repair<br>Oxidative stress<br>Tissue remodelling<br>Apolipoprotein-dependent formation of HDL |
| Camargo et al., 2010 | 20 patiens (9 men, 11 women ) suffering metabolic syndrome | Double-blinded, randomized, crossover postprandial | Virgin olive oil-based breakfast with high and low content of phenolic compounds. (1 wk washout period, followed by 40 mL fat-load) | CCL3, CXCL1, CXCL2, CXCL3, CXCR4<br>PTGS2<br>ILB1, IL6<br>SGK1, NFKBIA<br>DUSP1, DUSP2, TRIB1 | Leucocyte infiltration<br><br>Prostaglandin biosynthesis<br>Inflammation<br>NF-kB activation<br>Migration<br>Proliferation, chemotaxis. |

Table 3. Changes in gene expression of atherosclerotic-related genes after the ingestion of virgin olive oil in human studies during the postprandial period.

insulin receptor pathway, at posttranscriptional level. PPARBP may also increase insulin sensitivity by down-regulating the expression of TNF-α. The consumption of an olive oil-enriched breakfast decreases postprandial expression of TNF-α mRNA compared with a breakfast rich in butter and walnuts (Jimenez-Gomez et al., 2009). Correspondingly, acute consumption of EVOO decreased the circulating levels of soluble TNF-α in young healthy individuals (Papageorgiou et al., 2011). TNF-α activates a cytokine production cascade and thereby has a crucial role in the inflammatory process that is associated with atherogenesis; thus, dietary modification of TNF-α may prevent atherosclerosis.

In human interventional studies, an acute intake of olive oil increased the HDL cholesterol level, decreased inflammation, decreased lipid oxidation and decreased DNA oxidative damage. Studies by Konstantinidow et al. 2009, showed that there was a postprandial increase in the expression of PBMNCs genes related to DNA-repair (DNA-cross-link repair 1C, DCLRE1C and POLK) and inflammation (interleukin-10, IL-10; IFN-γ) 6h after ingestion of 50 mL of VOO. IL-10 is an anti-inflammatory cytokine that inhibits the production of interleukin-6 (IL-6), which is considered to be the most important inflammatory mediator. Il-6 release from rat adipocytes is regulated by the dietary fatty acid composition, and lower values of IL-6 are released with an olive oil diet (Garcia-Escobar et al., 2010); however, the postprandial change in plasma IL-6 concentrations does not seem to be altered by VOO ingestion (Teng et al., 2011; Manning et al., 2008). Postprandial VOO down-regulated IFN-γ gene expression. IFN-γ is a key pro-atherogenic cytokine that induces expression of adhesion molecules in endothelium and recruit leucocytes (Zhang et al., 2011), induces the expression of genes that have been implicated in atherosclerosis, promotes uptake of modified LDL (N. Li et al., 2010), and regulates macrophage foam cell formation and plaque stability, which are essential steps that mediate the pathogenesis of atherosclerosis. ATP-binding cassette, subfamily A, member 7 (ABCA7) is a protein that mediates the biogenesis of HDL with cellular lipids and helical apolipoproteins. In agreement with this, an increase in ABCA7 gene expression was observed in the postprandial studies after VOO ingestion.

The authors also observed up-regulation of several oxidative stress related genes and genes that may regulate NF-kB activation such as USP48 and a-kinase anchor protein-13 (AKAP-13). NF-kB regulates numerous processes in the cardiovascular system, including inflammation, cell survival, differentiation, proliferation and apoptosis. In vascular cells, NF-kB activation is mediated by diverse extracellular signals including Ang II, oxLDL, TRLs, advanced glycation end-products, and inflammatory cytokines. NF-kB activation by circulating cytokines has been linked to atherosclerosis and thrombosis and a number of NF-kB-regulated pro-inflammatory proteins are relevant for the initiation and progression of atherosclerosis. The induction of NF-κB signalling, results in transcriptional regulation of pro-inflammatory genes, including cytokines, chemokines, adhesion molecules, antioxidants, transcription factors, growth factors, and apoptosis and angiogenesis regulators (van der Heiden et al., 2010). The data showed so far, suggest that olive oil ingestion may protective during the postprandial by altering gene expression changes. However, the authors could not distinguish whether the protective effect was caused by the minor components of olive oil or to the fat content.

To adress this problem, Camargo et al., 2010 performed postprandial studies with two VOO based breakfast, with a high and low phenolic compounds content, administered to patients suffering form metabolic syndrome. The phenol fraction of VOO repressed the expression of several PBMNCs genes that are involved in inflammation processes mediated by cytokine-cytokine receptor interactions, arachidonic acid metabolism, mitogen-activated protein kinases (MAPKs) and transcription factor NF-kB/AP-1, such as the SGK1 (serum/glucocorticoid-regulated kinase-1) and the NFKBIA (nuclear factor of kappa light chain gene enhancer in B cells inhibitor, alpha) genes. SGK1 encodes a serum/glucocorticoid-regulated kinase that enhances nuclear NF-kB activity by phosphorylating the inhibitory kinase IKKα. The NFKBIA gene, encodes the IkBα protein,which is a member of an inhibitory IkB protein family that sequesters NF-kB into the cytoplasm. As NF-kB binds to the IKBα promoter to activate its transcription, a decrease in NFKBIA expression should be associated with a decrease in NF-kB activation. The hypothesis that olive oil polyphenols decreases NF-kB activation is supported by in vivo studies, which showed that VOO ingestion reduces inflammatory response of PMBSCs mediated by transcription factor NF-kB when compared to, butter and walnut-enriched diets during the postprandial state (Bellido et al., 2004). The study also showed the VOO consumption decreased the expression of PTGS2 (prostagladin-endoperoxide synthase-2), interleukin 1- β (IL-1β) and IL-6. The PTGS2 gene encodes for COX-2, which is an inducible isozyme that mediates prostaglandin biosynthesis from the substrate arachidonic acid. Pro-inflammatory cytokines, prostaglandins and NO, which are produced by monocytes and activated macrophages, play critical roles in inflammatory diseases such as atherosclerosis. VOO and hydrolysed olive vegetation water (Bitler et al., 2005) exhibit anti-inflammatory activities in the human monocytic leukemia cell line (THP-1). Previous studies have shown that, HT down-regulates iNOS and COX-2 gene expression in THP-1 cells (Zhang et al., 2009) and in murine macrophages by preventing NF-kB, STAT-1alpha (signal transducer and activator of transcription-1) and IRF-1 (interferon regulatory factor-1) activation (Maiuri et al., 2005). In vitro studies by Graham et al., 2011 have recently shown that TRLs, isolated from healthy volunteers after ingestion of VOO and pomace olive oil, enriched in minor components, produces a decrease in IL-6 and IL-1B secretion along with a down-regulation of COX-2 mRNA in macrophages. IL-6 is a pro-inflammatory cytokines that may contribute to the development of atherosclerosis by promoting insulin resistance, dyslipidaemia and endothelial dysfunction (Wilson, 2008). IL-6 synthesis is stimulated by IL-1β, which is another pro-inflammatory cytokine that regulates endothelial cell proliferation and the expression of adhesion molecules on the arterial wall (Andreotti et al., 2002). Studies, with a high-fat diet induced insulin-resistant animal model, showed that the ingestion of green tea polyphenols decreased IL-1β and IL-6β mRNA expression in cardiac muscle (Qin et al., 2010).

Circulating monocytes are components of innate immunity, and many pro-inflammatory cytokines and adhesion molecules facilitate monocyte adhesion and migration to the vascular endothelial wall. Monocyte migration is a key event in the pathogenesis of atherosclerosis. Therefore, modulating PMBCs activity and creating a less deleterious inflammatory profile may decrease leucocytes recruitment from the circulation to the vessel wall, important process in the initiation of atherosclerosis. According to this, Camargo et al., 2010 observed a decreased expression of chemokine, cc motif, ligand-3 (CCL3), chemokine, cxc motif, ligan-1 (CXCL1), chemokine, cxc motif, ligan-2 (CXCL2), chemokine, cxc motif, ligan-3 (CXCL3) and chemokine, cxc motif, receptor-4 (CXCR4) after acute-intake of phenol-rich olive oil. The CCL3 gene, which encodes for macrophage inflammatory protein-1 (MIP-1) has been implicated in inducing leucocyte-endothelial cell interactions and leucocyte recruitment in vivo (Gregory et al., 2006). CXCL1, CXCL2 and CXCL3, regulate leucocytes cell trafficking. CXCR4 have been shown to mediate bone mesenchymal stem cells migration through the endothelium in response to ox-LDL (M. Li et al., 2010). Dual-specificity phosphatase-1 (DUSP-1), dual-specificity phosphatase-2 (DUSP-2) and tribbes homology-1 (TRIB-1), gene expression were decreased by phenol-rich olive oil. DUSP-1 is actively involved in atherosclerosis and a chronic deficiency of DUSP-1 in ApoE(-/-) mice leads to decreased atherosclerosis via mechanisms involving impaired macrophage migration and defective extracellular signal-regulated kinase signalling (Shen et al., 2010). TRBIR1 is also involved in MAPK signalling and is up-regulated in vascular smooth muscle cells (SMCs) of human atherosclerotic plaques; TRBIR1 expression levels are key for modulating the extent of vascular SMCs proliferation and chemotaxis (Sung et al., 2007). Extracellular matrix degradation occurs in several pathological conditions such as atherosclerosis. Among the circulating cells, activated monocytes may directly contribute to atherosclerosis by expressing MMPs. In particular, monocytes express matrix metalloproteinase-9 (MMP-9), which is a member of the MMPs family that acts on the extracellular matrix, facilitates the migration of recruited monocytes to the sub-endothelial layer and acts on precursors of inflammatory cytokines, thereby amplifying the inflammatory response. In vitro studies showed that oleuropein aglycone, which a typical olive oil polyphenol, prevented an increase in MMP-9 expression and secretion in THP-1 cells (Dell´Agli et al., 2010); these data provide further evidence regarding the mechanisms by which olive oil reduces inflammation during atherosclerosis.

### 3.2.2 Postprandial effect of olive oil on the endothelium

Low-grade inflammation is often associated with endothelial dysfunction, which is associated with the development of atherosclerosis. Moreover, remnant like-lipoproteins have been associated with endothelial dysfunction and coronary artery disease in subjects with metabolic syndrome (Nakamura et al., 2005). A large number of genes are regulated after endothelial cells are exposed to TRLs with the net effect reflecting receptor and non-receptor mediated pathways that are activated or inhibited depending on the fatty acid type, lipid and apolipoprotein composition of TRLs and the presence or absence of lipoprotein lipase (Williams et al., 2004). TRLs have been shown to induce pro- and anti-inflammatory responses in the endothelium, and TRL composition plays a key role in determining these responses. TRLs that were isolated after a meal enriched in SFAs induced E-selectin, VCAM-1 and lectin-like oxidised-LDL receptor-1 (LOX-1) gene expression to a higher extent compared to TRLs that were isolated after a meal enriched in MUFAs and PUFAs (Williams et al., 2004); similarly, chylomicrons separated after ingestion of safflower oil, which is rich in polyunsaturated linoleic acid, induced a higher expression level of adhesion molecules compared with chylomicrons that were separated after ingestion of olive oil, rich in monounsaturated oleic acid (Jagla & Schrezenmeir, 2001). The effects of lipoproteins on vasoactive substances may also play a role in endothelial dysfunction. The endothelium-derived relaxing factor NO has gained wide attention because the current data suggests that it may protect against hypertension and atherosclerosis. In general, high-fat meals have often been associated with a loss of postprandial vascular reactivity compared to low fat meals. However several studies have shown that differences in food composition and the fatty acid content of meals may contribute to the observed effects on vascular reactivity via postprandial lipoproteins modifications. Thus, meals that contain MUFAs and eicosapentaenoic/docosahexaenoic acids (EPA/DHA) can attenuate the endothelial function impairment likely by reducing the most atherogenic postprandial lipoprotein subclass containing apolipoproteins B and C (Hilpert et al., 2007). Olive oil polyphenols can also inhibit endothelial adhesion molecule expression through NF-kB inhibition (Carluccio et al., 2003). In endothelial cell models, oleic acid (Carluccio et al., 1999) and phenolic extracts from EVOO, strongly reduced the gene expression of the vascular wall cell adhesion molecules (ICAM-1, VCAM-1), being HT, oleuropein and oleuropein aglycone the main polyphenols responsible for these effects (Dell´Agli et al., 2006; Carluccio et al., 2003)

### 3.2.3 Postprandial effect of olive oil in smooth muscle cells

SMCs are essential for proper vasculature function. SMCs contract and relax to alter the luminal diameter, which enables the blood vessels to maintain an appropriate blood pressure. However, vascular SMCs can also proliferate and migrate and synthesise large amounts of extracellular matrix (ECM) components. Thus, SMCs plays an important role in atherogenesis. TRLs induce the SMCs proliferation and migration via MAPKs activation, G protein-coupled receptor (GPCR)-dependent or independent protein kinase C (PKC) activation, epidermal growth factor receptor (EGF) transactivation and heparing-binding EGF-like growth factor shedding. TRLs can exert their effects on SMCs by acting at the genomic level (Lopez et al., 1999). TRL up-regulates the expression of genes involved in proliferation (e.g., cycin D1, CCND1; cyclin E, CCNE1; proliferating cell nuclear antigen, PCNA), inflammation (e.g., interleukin-8, IL-8; IL-1B; COX-2; suppressor of cytokine signaling 5, SOCS-5), signal transduction (e.g., mitogen-activated protein kinase 1, MAP3K-1; mitogen-activated protein kinase phosphatase-3, MKP-3; dual-specificity tyrosine phosphorylation-regulated kinase 1A, DYRK1A), oxidative stress (e.g., stress-activated protein kinase-3, SAPK-3 and stress-activated protein kinase-2A, SAPK-2A) and cytoskeleton function and motility (e.g., vimentin, VIM; keratin 19, KRT-19; fibrillin, FBN; tubulin beta, TUBB) (Bermudez et al., 2008). Furthermore, increasing evidence has shown that the pathophysiological contribution of TRLs to atherosclerosis development of plaque stability depends on the fatty acid composition of TRLs. The same study showed that TRLs obtained after the ingestion of olive oil produced a less deleterious pro-atherogenic profile compared to TRLs obtained after ingestion of butter (SFAs) or a mix of vegetable and fish oils (PUFAs). Since the olive oil contained no minor components, the effects were mainly attributed to oleic acid. However, oleic acid is not the sole component of olive oil that confers health benefits. In that sense, oleanolic acid, which is a natural triterpenoid that is present in pommace olive oil, induces prostaglandine I2 (PGI2) production through a mechanism that involves COX-2 mRNA upregulation via MAPKs signalling pathways ( Martinez-Gonzalez et al., 2008).

## 4. Conclusions

Nutrigenomic analyses directly asseses the influence of bioactive food compounds on gene expression. An increasing amount of data indicate that the fatty acids and polyphenols present in EVOO modulate the expression of key atherosclerotic-related genes, in vascular (macrophages, endothelial and smooth muscle cells) and peripheral blood mononuclear cells, towards a less-atherogenic gene profile. These compounds exert an effect after acute ingestion of the oil and during the postprandial state, and may provide protection during several stages of atherosclerosis. These data presented here, suggest that the traditional Mediterranean diet (rich in VOO) is optimal for both healthy and high-risk cardiovascular populations for the prevention of atherosclerosis plaque progression. The current literature suggests that EVOO, with its adequate PUFAs content, being poor in SFAs, high in MUFAs, and rich in antioxidants, is the best dietary fat for the prevention of atherosclerotic disease and ischemic cardiopathy. The ultimate goal in the prevention and treatment of coronary atherosclerosis is to reduce the risk of new heart attacks and reduce the mortality associated with cardiovascular failure. Thus, identification of an optimal diet may aid in the prevention of disease development and decrease the risk of associated cardiovascular events.

## 5. Abbreviations

ABCA-7 = ATP-binding cassette, subfamily A, member-7
ADAM-17 = A disintegrin and metalloproteinase domain-17
ADRB2 = Adrenergic β-2 receptor surface
ARHGAP-15 = Rho GTPase activating protein-15
BIRC-1 = Baculoviral IAP repeat-containing protein-1
CCL3 = Chemokine, cc motif, ligand-3
CD36 = CD36 antigen
COX-2 = Cyclo-oxygenase-2
CXCL1 = Chemokine, cxc motif, ligan-1
CXCL2 = Chemokine, cxc motif, ligan-2
CXCL3 = Chemokine, cxc motif, ligan-3
CXCR4 = Chemokine, cxc motif, receptor-4
DUSP-1 = Dual-specificity phosphatase-1
DUSP-2 = Dual-specificity phosphatase-2
EVOO = Extra-virgin olive oil
FFA = Free fatty acids
HDL = High density lipoprotein
HT = Hydroxytyrosol
IFN-γ = Interferon-γ
ICAM-1 = Intercellular adhesion molecule-1
IL-1β = Interleukin 1-β
IL-6 = Interleukin-6
IL7R = Interleukin 7 receptor
IL-10 = Interleukin 10
LA = α-(+)-Lipolitic acid
LDL = Low-density lipoproteins
LIAS = Lipoic acid synthetase
LRP-1 = Lipoprotein receptor-related protein-1
MCP-1 = Monocyte chemotactic protein-1
MMPs = Matrix-metalloproteinases
MMP-9 = Matrix metalloproteinase-9
MUFAs = Monounsaturated fatty acids
NF-κB = Nuclear factor-kappaB
NFKBIA = Nuclear factor of kappa light chain gene enhancer in B cells inhibitor, alpha
NO = Nitric oxide
OGT = O-linked N-acetylglucosamine (GlcNAc) transferase

PBMNCs = Peripheral blood mononuclear cells
POLK = Polymerase DNA directed k
PPARBP = Peroxisome proliferator-activated receptor-binding protein
PPAR-γ = Peroxisome proliferator-activated receptor-γ
PTGS2 = Prostagladine-endoperoxide synthase-2
PUFAs = Polyunsaturated fatty acids
SFAs = Saturated fatty acids
SGK-1 = Serum/glucocorticoid-regulated kinase-1
SMCs = Smooth muscle cells
TGs = Triglycerides
TMD = Traditional Mediterranean diet
TNF-α = Tumor necrosis factor
TNSF-10 = Tumor necrosis factor (ligand) superfamily, member 10
TRIB-1 = Tribbes homology-1
TRLs = Triglyceride-rich lipoproteins
TYR = Tyrosol
USP-48 = Ubiquitin specific peptidase- 48
VCAM-1=Vascular cell adhesion molecule-1
VLDL = Very-low density lipoproteins
VOO = Virgin olive oil

## 6. Acknowledgements

This work has been supported by grant (AGL2008-02811) from the Spanish Ministry of Innovation and Science and Marie Curie grant PERG07-GA-2010-268413.
AO, LMV, BB, SL contributed equally to this work.

## 7. References

Abia, R; Pacheco, YM; Perona, JS; Montero, E; Muriana, FJ. & Ruiz-Gutiérrez, V. (2001). The metabolic availability of dietary triacylglycerols from two high oleic oils during the postprandial period does not depend on the amount of oleic acid ingested by healthy men. *Journal of Nutrition,* Vol.131, No.1, pp. 59-65.

Acín, S; Navarro, MA; Arbonés-Mainar, JM; Guillén, N; Sarría, AJ; Carnicer, R; Surra, JC; Orman, I; Segovia, JC; Torre, R; Covas, MI; Fernández-Bolaños, J; Ruiz-Gutiérrez, V. & Osada J. Hydroxytyrosol administration enhances atherosclerotic lesion development in apo E deficient mice. *Journal of Biochemistry,* Vol.140, No.3, pp. 383-391.

Aguilera, CM; Ramirez-Tortosa, MC; Mesa, MD; Ramirez-Tortosa, CL. & Gil, A. (2002). Sunflower, virgin-olive and fish oils differentially affect the progression of aortic lesions in rabbits with experimental atherosclerosis. *Atherosclerosis,* Vol.162, no.2, pp. 335-344.

Andreotti, F; Porto, I; Crea, F. & Maseri, A. (2002). Inflammatory gene polymorphisms and ischaemic heart disease: review of population association studies. *Heart,* Vol.87, pp. 107–112.

Bea, JW; Lohman, TG; Cussler, EC; Going, SB. & Thompson, PA. (2010). Lifestyle modifies the relationship between body composition and adrenergic receptor genetic polymorphisms, ADRB2, ADRB3 and ADRA2B: a secondary analysis of a randomized controlled trial of physical activity among postmenopausal women. *Behavior Genetics*, Vol.40, No.5, pp. 649-659.

Bellido, C; López-Miranda, J; Blanco-Colio, LM; Pérez-Martínez, P, Muriana, FJ; Martín-Ventura, JL, Marín, C; Gómez, P; Fuentes, F; Egido, J. & Pérez-Jiménez, F. (2004). Butter and walnuts, but not olive oil, elicit postprandial activation of nuclear transcription factor kappaB in peripheral blood mononuclear cells from healthy men. *American Journal of Clinical Nutrition*, Vol.80, No.6, pp. 1487-1491.

Bermudez, B; Lopez, S; Ortega, A; Varela, LM; Pacheco, YM; Abia, R. & Muriana FJ. (2011). Oleic acid in olive oil: from a metabolic framework toward a clinical perspective. *Current Pharmacology Design*, Vol.17, No.8, pp. 831-843.

Bermúdez, B; López, S; Pacheco, YM; Villar, J; Muriana, FJ; Hoheisel, JD, Bauer, A. & Abia, R. (2008). Influence of postprandial triglyceride-rich lipoproteins on lipid-mediated gene expression in smooth muscle cells of the human coronary artery. *Cardiovascular Research*, Vol.79, No.2, pp. 294-303.

Bitler, CM; Viale, TM; Damaj, B. & Crea, R. (2005). Hydrolyzed olive vegetation water in mice has anti-inflammatory activity. *Journal of Nutrition*, Vol.135, No.6, pp. 1475-1479.

Camargo, A; Ruano, J; Fernandez, JM; Parnell, LD; Jimenez, A; Santos-Gonzalez, M; Marin, C; Perez-Martinez, P; Uceda, M; Lopez-Miranda, J. & Perez-Jimenez, F. (2010). Gene expression changes in mononuclear cells in patients with metabolic syndrome after acute intake of phenol-rich virgin olive oil. *BMC Genomics*, Vol.11, No.253, pp. 1-11.

Carluccio, MA; Massaro, M; Bonfrate, C; Siculella, L, Maffia, M; Nicolardi, G; Distante, A; Storelli, C. & De Caterina, R. (1999). Oleic acid inhibits endothelial activation : A direct vascular antiatherogenic mechanism of a nutritional component in the mediterranean diet. *Arteriosclerosis Thrombosis and Vascular Biology*, Vol.19, No.2, pp. 220-228.

Carluccio, MA; Massaro, M; Scoditti, E. & De Caterina, R. (2007). Vasculoprotective potential of olive oil components. *Molecular Nutrition Food Research*, Vol.51, No.10, pp. 1225-1234.

Carluccio, MA; Siculella, L; Ancora, MA; Massaro, M; Scoditti, E; Storelli, C; Visioli, F; Distante, A. & De Caterina, R. (2003). Olive oil and red wine antioxidant polyphenols inhibit endothelial activation: antiatherogenic properties of Mediterranean diet phytochemicals. *Arteriosclerosis Thrombosis and Vascular Biology*, Vol.23, No.4, pp. 622-629.

Corella, D. & Ordovas, JM. (2009). Nutrigenomics in cardiovascular medicine. *Circulation: Cardiovascular Genetics*, Vol.2, No.6, pp. 637-651.

Corona, G; Tzounis, X; Assunta Dessì, M; Deiana, M; Debnam, ES; Visioli, F. & Spencer, JP. (2006). The fate of olive oil polyphenols in the gastrointestinal tract: implications of gastric and colonic microflora-dependent biotransformation. *Free Radical Research*, Vol.40, No.6, pp. 647-658.

Corona, G; Spencer, JP. & Dessì MA. (2009) Extra virgin olive oil phenolics: absorption, metabolism, and biological activities in the GI tract.Toxicology and Industrial Health, Vol. 25, No.(4-5), pp. 285-293.

Costa, C; Germena, G; Martin-Conte, EL; Molinaris, I; Bosco, E; Marengo, S; Azzolino, O; Altruda, F, Ranieri, VM. & Hirsch, E. (2011). The RacGAP ArhGAP15 is a master negative regulator of neutrophil functions. *Blood,* (ahead of publication)

Covas, MI; de la Torre, K; Farré-Albaladejo, M, Kaikkonen, J; Fitó, M; López-Sabater, C; Pujadas-Bastardes, MA; Joglar, J; Weinbrenner, T; Lamuela-Raventós, RM. & de la Torre, R. (2006). Postprandial LDL phenolic content and LDL oxidation are modulated by olive oil phenolic compounds in humans. *Free Radical Biology and Medicine,* Vol.40, No.4, pp. 608-616.

Dell'Agli, M; Fagnani, R; Mitro, N; Scurati, S; Masciadri, M; Mussoni, L; Galli, GV; Bosisio, E; Crestani, M; De Fabiani, E, Tremoli, E. & Caruso D. (2006). Minor components of olive oil modulate proatherogenic adhesion molecules involved in endothelial activation. *Journal of Agricultural and Food Chemistry,* Vol.54, No.9, pp. 3259-3264.

Dell'Agli, M; Fagnani, R; Galli, GV; Maschi, O; Gilardi, F; Bellosta, S; Crestani, M; Bosisio, E; De Fabiani, E. & Caruso, D. (2010). Olive oil phenols modulate the expression of metalloproteinase 9 in THP-1 cells by acting on nuclear factor-kappaB signaling. *Journal of Agricultural and Food Chemistry,* Vol.58, No.4, pp. 2246-2252.

Deng, Q; Xu, J; Yu, B; He, J; Zhang, K; Ding, X. & Chen, D. (2010). Effect of dietary tea polyphenols on growth performance and cell-mediated immune response of post-weaning piglets under oxidative stress. *Archives of Animal Nutrition,* Vol.64, No.1, pp. 12-21.

Di Lisa, F; Kaludercic, N. & Paolocci, N. (2011). $\beta_2$-Adrenoceptors, NADPH oxidase, ROS and p38 MAPK: another 'radical' road to heart failure?. *British Journal of Pharmacology,* Vol.162, No.5, pp, 1009-1011.

Eilertsen, KE; Mæhre, HK; Cludts, K; Olsen, JO. & Hoylaerts, MF. (2011). Dietary enrichment of apolipoprotein E-deficient mice with extra virgin olive oil in combination with seal oil inhibits atherogenesis. Lipids in Health and Disease, Vol.3, No.10, 41-49.

Esposito, K; Marfella, R; Ciotola, M; Di Palo, C; Giugliano, F; Giugliano, G; D'Armiento, M; D'Andrea, F. & Giugliano, D. (2004). Effect of a mediterranean-style diet on endothelial dysfunction and markers of vascular inflammation in the metabolic syndrome: a randomized trial. *JAMA,* Vol.292, No.12, pp. 1440-1446.

Fitó, M; Gimeno, E; Covas, MI; Miró, E; López-Sabater, Mdel C; Farré M. & Marrugat J. (2002). Postprandial and short-term effects of dietary virgin olive oil on oxidant/antioxidant status. *Lipids,* Vol.37, No.3, pp. 245-251.

García-Escobar, E; Rodríguez-Pacheco, F; García-Serrano, S; Gómez-Zumaquero, JM; Haro-Mora, JJ; Soriguer, F. & Rojo-Martínez, G. (2010). Nutritional regulation of interleukin-6 release from adipocytes. *International Journal of Obesity (London),* Vol.34, No.8, pp. 1328-1332.

González-Santiago, M; Martín-Bautista, E; Carrero, JJ; Fonollá, J; Baró, L; Bartolomé, MV; Gil-Loyzaga, P. & López-Huertas E. (2006). One-month administration of hydroxytyrosol, a phenolic antioxidant present in olive oil, to hyperlipemic rabbits improves blood lipid profile, antioxidant status and reduces atherosclerosis development. *Atherosclerosis,* Vol.188, No.1, pp. 35-42.

Graham, VS; Lawson, C; Wheeler-Jones, CP; Perona, JS; Ruiz-Gutierrez, V. & Botham, KM. (2011). Triacylglycerol-rich lipoproteins derived from healthy donors fed different olive oils modulate cytokine secretion and cyclooxygenase-2 expression in macrophages: the potential role of oleanolic acid. *European Journal of Nutrition,* (ahead of publication).

Gregory, JL; Morand, EF; McKeown, SJ; Ralph, JA; Hall, P; Yang, YH; McColl, SR. & Hickey, MJ. (2006). Macrophage migration inhibitory factor induces macrophage recruitment via CC chemokine ligand 2. *Journal of Immunology,* Vol.177, No.11, pp. 8072-8079.

Guillén, N; Acín, S; Navarro, MA; Surra, JC; Arnal, C; Lou-Bonafonte, JM; Muniesa, P; Martínez-Gracia, MV. & Osada, J. (2009). Knowledge of the biological actions of extra virgin olive oil gained from mice lacking apolipoprotein E. *Revista Española de Cardiologia,* Vol.62, No.3, pp.294-304.

Havel, RJ. (1994). Postprandial hyperlipidemia and remnant lipoproteins. *Current Opinion of Lipidology,* Vol. 5, No.2, pp. 102–119.

Hilpert, KF; West, SG; Kris-Etherton, PM; Hecker, KD; Simpson, NM. & Alaupovic, P. (2007). Postprandial effect of n-3 polyunsaturated fatty acids on apolipoprotein B-containing lipoproteins and vascular reactivity in type 2 diabetes. *American Journal of Clinical Nutrition,* Vol.85, No.2, pp. 369-376.

Hodis, HN; Mack, WJ; Krauss, RM. & Alaupovic, P. (1999). Pathophysiology of triglyceride-rich lipoproteins in atherothrombosis: clinical aspects. *Clinical Cardiology,* Vol.22, No.6 Suppl, pp. 15-20.

Hodis, HN. (1999). Triglyceride-rich lipoprotein remnant particles and risk of atherosclerosis. *Circulation.* Vol. 99, No. 22, pp. 2852-2854.

Holdt, LM; Thiery, J; Breslow, JL. & Teupser, D. (2008). Increased ADAM17 mRNA expression and activity is associated with atherosclerosis resistance in LDL-receptor deficient mice. *Arteriosclerosis Thrombosis and Vascular Biology,* Vol.28, No.6, pp. 1097-1103.

Jagla, A. & Schrezenmeir, J. (2001). Postprandial triglycerides and endothelial function. *Experimental and Clinical Endocrinology and Diabetes,* Vol.109, No.4, pp. S533-547.

Jiménez-Gómez, Y; López-Miranda, J; Blanco-Colio, LM; Marín, C; Pérez-Martínez, P; Ruano, J; Paniagua, JA; Rodríguez, F; Egido, J. & Pérez-Jiménez, F. (2009). Olive oil and walnut breakfasts reduce the postprandial inflammatory response in mononuclear cells compared with a butter breakfast in healthy men. *Atherosclerosis,* Vol.204, No.2, pp. e70-76.

Karantonis, HC; Antonopoulou, S; Perrea, DN; Sokolis, DP; Theocharis, SE; Kavantzas N; Lliopoulos, DG. &Demopoulos, CA. (2006). In vivo antiatherogenic properties of olive oil and its constituent lipid classes in hyperlipidemic rabbits. *Nutrition, Metabolism and Cardiovascular Disease,* Vol.16, No.3, pp 174-185.

Kashyap, SR; Loachimescu, AG; Gornik, HL; Gopan, T; Davidson, MB; Makdissi, A; Major, J; Febbraio, M. & Silverstein, RL. (2009). Lipid-induced insulin resistance is associated with increased monocyte expression of scavenger receptor CD36 and internalization of oxidized LDL. *Obesity (Silver Spring),* Vol.17, No.12, pp. 2142-8.

Khymenets, O; Fitó, M; Covas, MI; Farré, M; Pujadas, MA, Muñoz, D; Konstantinidou, V. & de la Torre, R. (2009). Mononuclear cell transcriptome response after sustained virgin olive oil consumption in humans: an exploratory nutrigenomics study. *OMICS*, Vol.13, No.1, pp. 7-19.

Konstantinidou, V; Covas, MI; Muñoz-Aguayo, D; Khymenets, O; de la Torre, R; Saez, G; Tormos Mdel, C; Toledo, E; Marti, A; Ruiz-Gutiérrez, V; Ruiz Mendez, MV. & Fito, M. (2010). In vivo nutrigenomic effects of virgin olive oil polyphenols within the frame of the Mediterranean diet: a randomized controlled trial. *FASEB Journal*, Vol.24, No.7, pp. 2546-2557.

Konstantinidou, V; Khymenets, O; Covas, MI; de la Torre, R; Muñoz-Aguayo, D; Anglada, R; Farré, M. & Fito, M. (2009). Time course of changes in the expression of insulin sensitivity-related genes after an acute load of virgin olive oil. *OMICS*. Vol.13, No.5, pp. 431-438.

Leite, MS; Pacheco, P; Gomes, RN; Guedes, AT; Castro-Faria-Neto, HC; Bozza, PT. & Koatz, VL. (2005). Mechanisms of increased survival after lipopolysaccharide-induced endotoxic shock in mice consuming olive oil-enriched diet. *Shock*, Vol.23, No.2, pp. 173-178.

Lopez, S; Bermudez, B; Ortega, A; Varela, LM; Pacheco, YM; Villar, J; Abia, R. & Muriana, FJ. (2011). Effects of meals rich in either monounsaturated or saturated fat on lipid concentrations and on insulin secretion and action in subjects with high fasting triglyceride concentrations. *American Journal of Clinical Nutrition*, Vol.93, No.3, pp. 494-499.

Lopez, S; Ortega, A; Varela, LM; Bermudez, B; Muriana, FJ. & Abia, R. (2009). Recent advances in lipoprotein and atherosclerosis: a nutrigenomics approach. *Grasas y Aceites*, Vol.60, No.1, pp.33-40.

Li, M; Yu, J; Li, Y; Li, D; Yan, D; Qu, Z. & Ruan, Q. (2010). CXCR4 positive bone mesenchymal stem cells migrate to human endothelial cell stimulated by ox-LDL via SDF-1alpha/CXCR4 signaling axis. *Experimental Molecular Pathology*, Vol.88, No.2, pp. 250-255.

Li, N; McLaren, JE; Michael, DR; Clement, M; Fielding, CA. & Ramji, DP. (2010). ERK is integral to the IFN-γ-mediated activation of STAT1, the expression of key genes implicated in atherosclerosis, and the uptake of modified lipoproteins by human macrophages. *Journal of Immunology*, Vol.185, No.5, pp. 3041-3048.

Llorente-Cortés, V; Estruch, R; Mena, MP; Ros, E; González, MA; Fitó, M; Lamuela-Raventós, RM. & Badimon, L. (2010). Effect of Mediterranean diet on the expression of pro-atherogenic genes in a population at high cardiovascular risk. *Atherosclerosis*, Vol.208, No.2, pp. 442-450.

Lloyd-Jones, D; Adams, RJ; Brown, TM; Carnethon, M; Dai, S; De Simone, G; Ferguson, TB; Ford, E; Furie, K; Gillespie, C; Go, A; Greenlund, K; Haase, N; Hailpern, S; Ho, PM; Howard, V; Kissela, B; Kittner, S; Lackland, D; Lisabeth, L; Marelli, A; McDermott, MM; Meigs, J; Mozaffarian, D; Mussolino, M; Nichol, G; Roger, VL; Rosamond, W; Sacco, R; Sorlie, P; Stafford, R; Thom, T; Wasserthiel-Smoller, S; Wong, ND. & Wylie-Rosett, J. (2010). Executive summary: heart disease and stroke statistics-2010 update: a report from the American Heart Association. American Heart Association

Statistics Committee and Stroke Statistics Subcommittee. *Circulation,* Vol.121, No.7, pp 948-954.

Machowetz, A; Poulsen, HE; Gruendel, S; Weimann, A; Fitó, M; Marrugat, J; de la Torre, R; Salonen, JT; Nyyssönen, K; Mursu, J; Nascetti, S; Gaddi, A; Kiesewetter, H; Bäumler, H; Selmi, H; Kaikkonen, J; Zunft, HJ; Covas, MI. & Koebnick, C. (2007). Effect of olive oils on biomarkers of oxidative DNA stress in Northern and Southern Europeans. *FASEB Journal*, Vol.21, No.1, pp. 45-52.

Magrone, T; Candore, G; Caruso, C; Jirillo, E. & Covelli, V. (2008). Polyphenols from red wine modulate immune responsiveness: biological and clinical significance. *Current Pharmaceutical Design*, Vol.14, No.26, pp. 2733-2748.

Mangiapane, EH; McAteer, MA; Benson, GM; White, DA. & Salter, AM. (1999). Modulation of the regression of atherosclerosis in the hamster by dietary lipids: comparison of coconut oil and olive oil. *British Journal of Nutrition,* Vol.82, No.5, pp. 401-419.

Maiuri, MC; De Stefano, D; Di Meglio, P; Irace, C; Savarese, M; Sacchi, R; Cinelli, MP. & Carnuccio, R. (2005). Hydroxytyrosol, a phenolic compound from virgin olive oil, prevents macrophage activation. *Naunyn-Schmiedebergs Archives of Pharmacology,* Vol. 371, No.6, pp. 457-465.

Manning, PJ; Sutherland, WH; McGrath, MM; de Jong, SA; Walker, RJ. & Williams, MJ. (2008). Postprandial cytokine concentrations and meal composition in obese and lean women. *Obesity (Silver Spring),* Vol.16, No.9, pp. 2046-2052.

Martínez-González, J; Rodríguez-Rodríguez, R; González-Díez, M, Rodríguez, C, Herrera, MD, Ruiz-Gutierrez, V. & Badimon, L. (2008). Oleanolic acid induces prostacyclin release in human vascular smooth muscle cells through a cyclooxygenase-2-dependent mechanism. *Journal of Nutrition,* Vol.138, No.3, pp. 443-448.

Müller, M. & Kersten S. (2003). Nutrigenomics: goals and strategies. *Nature Reviews. Genetics,* Vol.4, No.4, pp. 315-22.

Nakamura, T; Takano, H; Umetani, K; Kawabata, K; Obata, JE; Kitta, Y; Kodama, Y; Mende, A; Ichigi, Y; Fujioka, D; Saito, Y. & Kugiyama, K. (2005). Remnant lipoproteinemia is a risk factor for endothelial vasomotor dysfunction and coronary artery disease in metabolic syndrome. *Atherosclerosis,* Vol. 181, No.2, pp. 321-327.

Oliveras-López, MJ; Berná, G; Carneiro, EM; López-García de la Serrana, H; Martín, F. & López, MC. (2008). An extra-virgin olive oil rich in polyphenolic compounds has antioxidant effects in OF1 mice. Journal of Nutrition, Vol.138, No.6, pp. 1074-1078.

Papageorgiou, N; Tousoulis, D; Psaltopoulou, T; Giolis, A; Antoniades, C; Tsiamis, E; Miliou, A; Toutouzas, K; Siasos, G. & Stefanadis C. (2011). Divergent anti-inflammatory effects of different oil acute consumption on healthy individuals. *European Journal Clinical Nutrition*, Vol.65, No.4, pp. 514-519.

Perez-Martinez, P; Ordovas, JM; Garcia-Rios, A; Delgado-Lista, J; Delgado-Casado, N; Cruz-Teno, C; Camargo, A; Yubero-Serrano, EM; Rodriguez, F; Perez-Jimenez, F. & Lopez-Miranda J. (2011). Consumption of diets with different type of fat influences triacylglycerols-rich lipoproteins particle number and size during the postprandial state. *Nutrition, Metabolism & Cardiovascular Diseases*, Vol.21, pp. 39-45.

Poudyal, H; Campbell, F. & Brown, L. (2010). Olive leaf extract attenuates cardiac, hepatic, and metabolic changes in high carbohydrate-, high fat-fed rats. *Journal of Nutrition,* Vol.140, No.5, pp. 946-53.

Puel, C; Mardon, J; Agalias, A; Davicco, MJ; Lebecque, P; Mazur, A; Horcajada, MN; Skaltsounis, AL. & Coxam, V. (2008). Major phenolic compounds in olive oil modulate bone loss in an ovariectomy/inflammation experimental model. *Journal of Agricultural and Food Chemistry,* Vol.56, No.20, pp. 9417-9422.

Qin, B; Polansky, MM; Harry, D. & Anderson, RA. (2010). Green tea polyphenols improve cardiac muscle mRNA and protein levels of signal pathways related to insulin and lipid metabolism and inflammation in insulin-resistant rats. *Molecular Nutrition and Food Research,* Vol.54, Suppl 1, pp. S14-23.

Reiss, K; Cornelsen, I; Husmann, M; Gimpl, G. & Bhakdi S. (2011). Unsaturated fatty acids drive ADAM-dependent cell adhesion, proliferation and migration by modulating membrane fluidity. *Journal Biological Chemistry,* (ahead of print).

Rosenblat, M; Volkova, N; Coleman, R; Almagor, Y. and Aviram, M. (2008). Antiatherogenicity of extra virgin olive oil and its enrichment with green tea polyphenols in the atherosclerotic apolipoprotein-E-deficient mice: enhanced macrophage cholesterol efflux. *Journal of Nutritional Biochemistry,* Vol.19, No.8, pp. 514-523.

Servili, M; Esposto, S; Fabiani, R; Urbani, S; Taticchi, A; Mariucci, F; Selvaggini, R. & Montedoro GF. (2009). Phenolic compounds in olive oil: antioxidant, health and organoleptic activities according to their chemical structure. *Inflammopharmacology,* Vol.17, No.2, 76-84.

Shen, J; Chandrasekharan, UM; Ashraf, MZ; Long, E; Morton, RE; Liu, Y; Smith, JD. & DiCorleto, PE. (2010). Lack of mitogen-activated protein kinase phosphatase-1 protects ApoE-null mice against atherosclerosis. *Circulation Research,* Vol.106, No.5, pp. 902-910.

Sung, HY; Guan, H; Czibula, A; King, AR; Eder, K; Heath, E; Suvarna, SK; Dower, SK; Wilson, AG; Francis, SE; Crossman, DC. & Kiss-Toth, E. (2007). Human tribbles-1 controls proliferation and chemotaxis of smooth muscle cells via MAPK signaling pathways. *Journal of Biological Chemistry,* Vol.282, No.25, pp. 18379-18387.

Teng, KT; Nagapan, G; Cheng, HM. & Nesaretnam, K. (2011). Palm olein and olive oil cause a higher increase in postprandial lipemia compared with lard but had no effect on plasma glucose, insulin and adipocytokines. *Lipids,* Vol.46, No.4, pp. 381-388.

Trefiletti, G; Rita Togna, A; Latina, V; Marra, C; Guiso, M. & Togna, GI. (2011). 1-Phenyl-6,7-dihydroxy-isochroman suppresses lipopolysaccharide-induced pro-inflammatory mediator production in human monocytes. *British Journal of Nutrition,* Vol.106, No.1, pp. 33-36.

Tsantila, N; Karantonis, HC; Perrea, DN; Theocharis, SE; Iliopoulos, DG; Antonopoulou, S. & Demopoulos CA. (2007). Antithrombotic and antiatherosclerotic properties of olive oil and olive pomace polar extracts in rabbits. *Mediators of Inflammation,* Vol.2007, No. 36204, pp.1-11.

Tsantila, N; Karantonis, HC; Perrea, DN; Theocharis, SE; Iliopoulos, DG; Iatrou, C; Antonopoulou, S. & Demopoulos, CA. (2010) Atherosclerosis regression study in rabbits upon olive pomace polar lipid extract administration. *Nutrition, Metabolism and Cardiovascular Disease,* Vol. 20, No. 10, pp. 740-747.

Van der Heiden, K; Cuhlmann, S; Luong, Le A; Zakkar, M. & Evans, PC. (2010). Role of nuclear factor kB in cardiovascular health and disease. *Clinical Sciences (London),* Vol.118, No.10, pp. 593-605.

Van Ommen, B. (2004). Nutrigenomics: exploiting systems biology in the nutrition and health arenas. *Nutrition,* Vol.20, No.1, pp. 4-8.

Weinstein, MM; Yin, L; Tu, Y; Wang, X; Wu, X; Castellani, LW; Walzem, RL; Lusis, AJ; Fong, LG; Beigneux, AP. & Young, SG. (2010). Chylomicronemia elicits atherosclerosis in mice--brief report. *Arteriosclerosis Thrombosis and Vascular Biology,* Vol.30, No.1, pp. 20-23.

Williams, CM; Maitin, V. & Jackson, KG. (2004). Triacylglycerol-rich lipoprotein-gene interactions in endothelial cells. *Biochemical Society Transations,* Vol.32, No.6, pp. 994-998.

Wilson, PW. (2008). Evidence of systemic inflammation and estimation of coronary artery disease risk: a population perspective. *American Journal of Medicine,* Vol.121, No.10 Supple1, pp. S15–S20.

Zhang, J; Alcaide, P; Liu, L; Sun, J; He, A; Luscinskas, FW. & Shi, GP. (2011). Regulation of endothelial cell adhesion molecule expression by mast cells, macrophages, and neutrophils. *PLoS One,* Vol.6, No.1, pp. e14525.

Zhang, X; Cao, J. & Zhong, L. (2009). Hydroxytyrosol inhibits pro-inflammatory cytokines, iNOS, and COX-2 expression in human monocytic cells. *Naunyn-Schmiedebergs Archives of Pharmacology,* Vol.379, No.6, pp. 581-586.

Zilversmit, DB. (1979). Atherogenesis: a postprandial phenomenon. *Circulation,* Vol. 60, No.3, pp, 473–485.

Zrelli, H; Matsuoka, M; Kitazaki, S; Zarrouk, M. & Miyazaki, H. (2011). Hydroxytyrosol reduces intracellular reactive oxygen species levels in vascular endothelial cells by upregulating catalase expression through the AMPK-FOXO3a pathway. European Journal of Pharmacology. Vol.660, No.(2-3), pp. 275-282.

# Molecular Understanding of Endothelial Cell and Blood Interactions with Bacterial Cellulose: Novel Opportunities for Artificial Blood Vessels

Helen Fink[1], Anders Sellborn[2] and Alexandra Krettek[3,4]
[1]*Dept of Chemical and Biological Engineering, Chalmers University of Technology*
[2]*Dept of Surgery, Inst. of Clin. Sciences, Sahlgrenska Acad. at University of Gothenburg*
[3]*Dept of Intern. Med., Inst. of Medicine, Sahlgrenska Acad. at University of Gothenburg*
[4]*Nordic School of Public Health*
*Sweden*

## 1. Introduction

Cardiovascular disease (CVD) is the main cause of death or invalidism in high-income countries today. Moreover, worldwide demographic changes are aiding CVD's rapid progression towards the number one killer in middle- and low-income countries. The World Health Organisation estimates that if current trends are allowed to continue, about 20 million people will die from CVD by 2015. This group of disorders, which affect the heart and blood vessels, includes coronary heart disease, cerebrovascular disease and peripherial arterial disease, deep vein thrombosis and pulmonary embolism.

The main cause of these acute life-threatening conditions is atherosclerosis. Atherosclerotic plaques and restenosis can result in severe occlusions of peripheral and coronary arteries. Current treatments include drug therapy and bypass surgery, and depend on the severity of the disease. All treatments require molecular understanding of the processes that govern atherosclerosis. This is especially important when introducing artificial graft materials *in vivo*.

Generally, the first choice for vascular replacement graft material is the patient's own vessels, i.e., autologous vessels. If these are in shortage supply or do not exhibit sufficient quality due to, e.g., other diseases or previous surgery, artificial alternatives become necessary. Today, clinics use biomaterials such as expanded polytetrafluorethylene (ePTFE) and polyethylene terephtalate fibre (Dacron®) as prosthetic grafts for reconstructive vascular surgery. However, their performance is dismal in small diameter vessels (>6 mm) like coronary arteries and peripheral arteries below the knee, resulting in early thrombosis and intimal hyperplasia. Therefore, about 10% of patients with CVD are left untreated due to the lack of replacement material for small vessels.

Considering the large number of patients who need replacement vessels, the substantial demand for alternative small-caliber grafts is urgent, driving scientists to search for and develop new materials. Recently, this has even led to the use of completely biological vessels. However, the growth of such requires months, rendering them unsuitable for acute situations such as heart infarction, which demand a substitute vessel immediately.

## 2. What is the ideal vascular graft?

Several issues demand consideration when constructing a vascular graft: the mechanical properties of the graft must resemble those of a native blood vessel, and the graft must be biocompatible with its host. One important factor is compliance, i.e., how well the vessel withstands pressure from the bloodstream and whether it can maintain systemic pressure in the vascular system. Vascular grafts should also be "invisible" to the immune system and possess non-thrombogenic properties.

One interesting option is bacterial cellulose (BC), whose unique properties (strength, good integration into host tissue and flexibility that allows production in various shapes and sizes) make it an exciting candidate for vascular graft material. The most abundant biopolymer on earth, cellulose is insoluble in water and degradable by microbial enzymes. Several organisms such as plants, algae and bacteria can produce BC. Some members of the bacterial genus Acetobacter, especially *Gluconacetobacter xylinum*, synthesize and secrete cellulose extracellularly. The network structure of cellulose fibrils resembles that of collagen in the extracellular matrix (ECM).

This chapter describes how BC interacts with human endothelial cells (EC) and blood. Specifically, we will evaluate whether surface modifications could promote adhesion of EC and also whether BC's thrombogenic properties compare favorably with conventional graft materials. These properties are critical because materials intended as vascular grafts must satisfy many important features, including blood compatibility, cell interactions and mechanical properties.

## 3. Tissue engineering of blood vessels

Tissue engineering is a relatively new scientific discipline that combines cells, engineering and materials to improve or replace biological functions. Langer and Vacanti, two pioneers in the field, describe tissue engineering as an interdisciplinary area that applies the principles of engineering and life sciences to the development of biological substitutes that restore, maintain or improve tissue formation (Langer & Vacanti, 1993).

The basic concept of tissue engineering includes a physical support (3D-scaffold) composed of synthetic polymers or natural materials (collagen, elastin or fibrin). This support mimicks ECM and initially serves as a scaffold or template on which cells can organize and mature *in vitro* prior to implantation at the appropriate location.

Initial research in the mid-20th century focused on developing bioinert materials, eliciting a minimal host response characterized by passive blood transport and minimal interactions with blood and tissues. Although widely available, these industrial materials, including Teflon and silicone, were not developed specifically for medical applications. Later, the production of completely non-reactive substances became unrealistic.

Today, other biomaterials are being developed to stimulate reactions between proteins and cells at the molecular level in a highly precise and controllable manner. The key concept underpinning development of such biomaterials is that the scaffold should contain chemical or structural information that mimicks cell-cell communication and controls tissue formation, such as growth factors, the adhesion peptide Arg–Gly–Asp (RGD) and other molecules that mimic ECM components. RGD is the minimal sequence in basement membrane proteins such as fibronectin, fibrinogen and von Willebrand Factor, all required for cell adhesion (Pierschbacher & Ruoslahti, 1984).

A successful tissue engineered blood vessel must: be biocompatible, i.e., noninflammatory, nontoxic, nonimmunogenic and noncarcinogenic; infection-resistant and nonthrombogenic. It also must have appropriate mechanical properties, e.g., tensile strength, burst strength, good suture retention and compliance, and possess appropriate vasoactive physiological properties, including contraction or relaxation in response to neural or chemical stimuli and more.

The feasibility of constructing and using tissue engineered blood vessels was first demonstrated in landmark studies by L'Heureux (L'Heureux et al., 1998) and Niklason (Niklason et al., 1999). The vessels, which were produced using different in vitro techniques, had very good mechanical properties and functioned well in experimental animals. Although *in vitro* and experimental techniques have been developed since then, no clinical implantations have been made until now.

### 3.1 Biomaterials/biomaterial scaffolds

Williams defines biomaterial as any natural or man-made material that comprises the whole or part of a living structure or biomedical device that performs, augments, or replaces a natural function (Williams, 1999).

Many different materials have been investigated for biomaterial applications. They can be divided into natural materials, i.e., collagen (Weinberg & Bell, 1986; L'Heureux et al., 1998); fibrin (Cummings et al., 2004; Kumar & Krishnan, 2002); hyaluronic acid (Remuzzi et al., 2004; Turner et al., 2004); silk fibroin (Zhang et al., 2009) and BC (Backdahl et al., 2006; Klemm et al., 2001; Bodin et al., 2007; Fink et al., 2010)) and synthetic polymers, i.e., polyglycolic acid (PGA) (Niklason et al., 1999; McKee et al., 2003), polyethylene terephthalate (PET) (Sharefkin et al., 1983; Herring et al., 1984) and ePTFE (Zilla et al., 1987; Meinhart et al., 2005). The required properties for biomaterials vary with cell type, implantation site and strategy for tissue formation. Common demands for all biomaterials include biocompatibility, e.g., avoiding foreign body reactions, capsule formation and chronic inflammatory reactions. Additionally, materials intended to be in contact with blood require evaluation for thrombogenicity. Mechanical properties are important and depend on the target tissue. Since biomaterials used as vascular grafts must withstand blood pressure, they must be investigated for burst pressure, compliance, suture strength and fatigue before using them as implants.

A recent and popular approach involves electrospinning different materials to create nanofibre constructs. Both electrospun synthetic polymers and native ECM proteins have been used for cell seeding to construct vascular grafts (Hashi et al., 2007; Huang et al., 2001; Boland et al., 2004; Kenawy el et al., 2003).

### 3.2 Materials for vascular grafts

Jaboulay and Briau performed the first arterial transplantation in 1896, but imperfect anastomoses resulted in thrombosis (Jaboulay & Briau, 1896). Since then, more sophisticated techniques have been developed. The search for arterial vascular grafts began in 1952, when Voorhees discovered Vinyon N (nylon), the first fabric graft (Voorhees et al., 1952). A few years later, DeBakey discovered Dacron® in 1958 (Nose, 2008). Today, arterial and even especially venous autografts are used routinely in surgery, creating bypasses for patients with peripheral or coronary occlusive vascular diseases. However, autograft availability is limited, particularly for arteries.

Dacron® and ePTFE are still widely used as arterial replacements. Despite their success in replacing large diameter (>6 mm) high-flow vessels, these materials show thrombogenicity and compliance mismatch in low-flow or small-diameter vessels. Sophisticated techniques have been evaluated to enhance patency, including chemical modifications, coatings and seeding of the surface with different cells. In contrast to natural materials, synthetics often lack adhesion sites. Although passive materials can reproduce sufficient physiological mechanical strength, proper metabolic function and cellular signalling requires intact cellular machinery.

BC is an attractive material for biomaterial applications. Its structure resembles that of collagen, the component in arteries and veins that gives the blood vessel its strength. BC's manufacturing process allows versatility in shape and size, including tubes. Studies have shown successful growth of cardiac rat-derived myocytes and fibroblasts (Entcheva et al., 2004), rat-derived hepatocytes (Kino et al., 1998; Yang et al., 1994) and osteoprogenitor cells (Takata et al., 2001) from mice on cellulose-based materials. However, these matrices are based not on natural cellulose but rather on derivatives such as cellulose acetate and regenerative cellulose.

Although BC is biocompatible, it generally does not promote cell growth (Watanabe et al., 1993a). Thus, BC must be modified to support EC adherence. Modification of wet state BC is challenging because fibre structure and strength must be maintained. This is especially important for vascular grafts, which must withstand blood pressure.

## 4. Different approaches to engineered blood vessels

### 4.1 Collagen-based blood vessel model

Weinberg and colleagues developed a collagen-based blood vessel model (Weinberg et al., 1986). Improvement of the construct's mechanical properties is ongoing due to poor mechanical integrity.

### 4.2 Cell self-assembly model

The cell self-assembly model is made using intact layers of human vascular cells grown to overconfluence to form visible sheets of cells and ECM (L'Heureux et al., 1993, 1998). A sheet of smooth muscle cells (SMCs) is rolled around a mandrel to form the medial layer. Similarly, a sheet of fibroblasts is rolled over the SMC sheet media, forming an adventitial layer. Finally, ECs seeded onto the lumen of the matured vessel form a confluent monolayer. These constructs withstood more than 2000 mmHg pressure before bursting.

### 4.3 Cell-seeded polymeric scaffold–hybrid graft

This graft was developed by Niklason (Niklason et al., 1999). Vascular cells were seeded into a biodegradable scaffold (PGA) and cultured for 8 weeks under pulsatile radial stress (165 beats per minute and 5% radial strain). ECs seeded onto the lumen of the construct formed a confluent monolayer. Cultured under pulsatile conditions, the histological structure of the constructs resembled that of native arteries. Due to high collagen content, the constructs had a burst pressure greater than 2000 mmHg and they could contract. *In vivo* studies of tissue engineered blood vessels in Yucatan miniature pigs were promising.

With degradable material such as PGA, it is critical to ensure adequate strength of ECM (collagen, elastin) produced by the vascular cells. Degradation products may be toxic to the cells. Non-degradable scaffolds offer durable support, but tissue acceptance is mandatory. Ideally, the scaffold should be compliant, similar to native vessels.

### 4.4 Acellularized construct

A rolled small intestinal submucosa (SIS) has been used as a small diameter vascular graft. A cell-free, 100-µm-thick collagen layer derived from small intestine, SIS is compliant, making it an interesting candidate for vascular implantation and requiring investigation (Roeder et al., 1999, Huynh et al., 1999).

### 4.5 Artificial artery generated in the peritoneal cavity

In the peritoneal cavity, artificial arteries are generated on silastic tubes. The arteries are lined by nonthrombogenic, mesothelial (endothelial-like) cells. The feasibility of this approach in humans is a matter of debate.

## 5. Bacterial synthesized cellulose as biomaterial

Cellulose, the most abundant biopolymer on earth, is insoluble in water and degradable by microbial enzymes. Several organisms, e.g., plants, algae and bacteria can produce cellulose, and the bacteria *Gluconacetobacter xylinum* can synthesize and secret cellulose extracellularly (Brown et al., 1976). BC is composed of linear nanosized fibrils of D-glucose molecules (Ross et al., 1991). The network structure of cellulose fibrils resembles that of collagen in the ECM of native connective tissue (Fig. 1) (Backdahl et al., 2006).

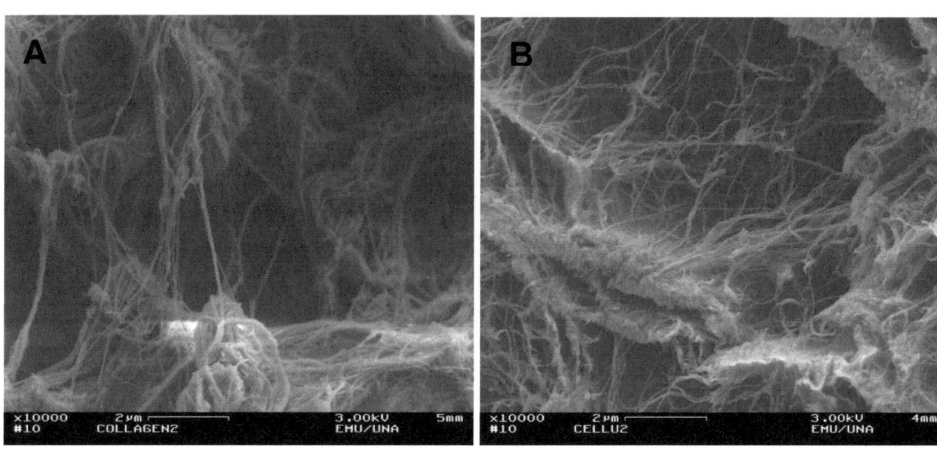


Fig. 1. SEM images of (A) collagen and (B) BC reprinted with permission from Backdahl et al., 2006. Copyright Elsevier 2006.

Although BC is not a hydrogel in the true sense of the meaning, it is often referred to as such because of its high water content, insolubility in water and highly hydrophilic nature. Since BC consists of a highly entangled network of fibrils, it also provides strong mechanical properties that ensure the ability of tissue engineered blood vessels to withstand mechanical forces and prevent rupture. BC can be designed and shaped into three dimensional structures such as tubes or sheets (Backdahl et al., 2006). A major advantage of using BC rather than cellulose produced by any other organism is that BC is completely free of biogenic compounds such as lignin, pectin and arabinan found in, e.g., plant cellulose. During the production process, it is also possible to modify several other properties including pore size, surface properties and layering of the material (Backdahl et al., 2008).

BC is used in various areas including food matrix (nata de coco), dietary fibres, acoustic or filter membranes and ultra-strength paper. In addition, BC has been suggested as a potential material for tissue engineering in several areas, e.g., as scaffold for tissue engineering of cartilage, blood vessels (BASYC®) and successful treatment of second and third degree burns, stomach ulcers and other situations that require a temporary skin substitute (Biofill®, Gengiflex®, XCell®) or to recover periodontal tissue (Gengiflex®) (Czaja et al., 2006; Svensson et al., 2005; Fontana et al., 1990).

### 5.1 Structure and morphology

Beginning with the water-soluble monosaccharide D-glucose, cellulose synthesis is produced extracellularly as pellicles at the air/liquid interface. Glucan chains of BC are extruded from several enzyme complexes and aggregated by van der Waals forces to form sub-fibrils, approximately 1.5 nm wide. BC sub-fibrils crystallise into microfibrils and then into bundles, which form a dense reticulated structure stabilized by hydrogen bonding. In culture medium, the bundles assemble into ribbons, forming a network of cellulose. This network of cellulose nanofibrils provides BC with high mechanical strength and a water retention capacity of about 99% (Iguchi et al., 2000).

The macroscopic morphology of BC varies with different culture conditions. In static conditions, BC accumulates on the surface of nutrient-rich culture medium, at the oxygen-rich air-liquid interface. Statically cultured BC has lower crystallinity than BC fermented during agitation.

Our molecular studies on EC-blood interactions with BC used BC synthesized by *Gluconacetobacter xylinum* (ATCC 1700178, American Type Culture Collection). Cellulose tubes were grown in corn steep liquid media at 30°C for 7 days. The cellulose was then purified by boiling, first in 0.1 M NaOH at 60°C for 4h and then in Millipore™ water. Finally, the cellulose was sterilised by autoclaving for 20 minutes. Due to the production process, BC consists of two distinctly different layers: one side has a compact network of fibrils with few if any pores, and the other side has a porous network structure. A density gradient arises between the sides.

### 5.2 Mechanical properties

The optimal scaffold is a biocompatible biomaterial that provides proper mechanical and physical properties, thus promoting cell adhesion and tissue formation. Prior to implantation into animals, BC tubes undergo extensive mechanical testing (burst strength, compliance and tensile strength). Films or sheets of BC show remarkable mechanical strength, due to high crystallinity, high planar orientation of the ribbons, ultrafine structure and a complex network (Iguchi et al., 2000). The mechanical properties of BC tubes are similar to those of pig carotid arteries (Backdahl et al., 2006). BC's compliance curve resembles that of a native artery more than any other synthetic material on the market, which is advantageous. Material density can be altered by varying the culture conditions or by post-culture modifications.

### 5.3 Biocompatibility

Integration of a material with the host tissue is essential for the success of tissue engineered blood vessels. According to Williams, the biocompatibility of a material is defined as "the ability of a material to perform with an appropriate host response in a specific application" (Williams, 1999). Therefore, an appropriate host response would involve a biomaterial that induces a very low inflammatory and foreign body response in the host tissue.

A study by Helenius et al. showed that BC is well integrated into the host tissue and does not induce inflammatory or foreign body responses (Helenius et al., 2006). They implanted BC pieces subcutaneously in rats and explanted them after 1, 4 and 12 weeks. Incorporation of the implant in the host tissue made it difficult to distinguish a clear interface between the implant and the host tissue (Helenius et al., 2006). These results are supported by another *in vivo* study, where BC tubes were implanted into the carotid arteries in pigs (Wippermann et al., 2009). Therefore, BC clearly has good biocompatibility and shows promising potential as scaffold material.

### 5.4 Surface modification

One challenge in the field of vascular grafts involves promoting EC attachment and spreading, since many biomaterials similar to BC exhibit limited support for cellular adhesion (Watanabe et al., 1993b). Over the years, many strategies have been developed to modify material surfaces.

To optimize cell-biomaterial interactions, manufacturers coat synthetic scaffolds with cell adhesive proteins such as collagen, fibronectin or laminin (Seeger & Klingman, 1988; Kaehler et al., 1989). However, varying protein composition results in a biofilm with passive protein adsorption, and that composition can modify over time (Vroman, 1987). Additionally, protein adsorption to BC is very low.

Much attention has focused on cell adhesion peptide RGD and its derivatives as possible alternative for stimulating reproducible and predictable cell adhesion (D'Souza et al., 1991; Hersel et al., 2003; Walluscheck et al., 1996; Gabriel et al., 2006). Most RGD modifications occur via covalent binding to the material (Massia & Hubbell, 1990). Although cellulose contains reactive hydroxyl groups that can be chemically modified, these very same hydroxyl groups participate in hydrogen bonding, which holds the cellulose fibre network together. Disruption of these bonds associates with loss of fibre ultrastructure (Sassi & Chanzy, 1995; Sassi et al., 2000). Dry films of BC have been modified with carboxymethyl and acetyl groups (Kim et al., 2002). However, surface modifications to wet state BC remain incompletely understood. Thus, modification of a BC hydrogel is especially challenging, since solvent exchange and cellulose modification typically destroy the hydrogel morphology.

Modification of a BC hydrogel is especially challenging because solvent exchange and cellulose modification typically destroy hydrogel morphology. Thus far, most modifications have been performed on dried BC. Consequently, a new method is needed to increase cell attachment without altering the structure of the BC network.

#### 5.4.1 Xyloglucan

Xyloglucan (XG), the most abundant hemicellulose, is present in the primary wall of many plants. In contrast to cellulose, XG is water-soluble and interacts strongly with cellulose fibres (Hanus & Mazeau, 2006). We have taken advantage of these properties, which provide an elegant means of introducing cell adhesion peptide RGD with XG as a carrier molecule to BC.

BC and cotton linters, as reference material, were modified with XG and XG bearing a GRGDS pentapeptide (Bodin et al., 2007). Compared with organic solvents, modification in the water phase was clearly advantageous for preserving the morphology, as observed with SEM (Fig. 2). XG adsorption increased the wettability only to a minor extent, possibly explaining the decreased or undetectable adsorption of adhesive proteins shown by QCM-D. QCM-D studies further revealed that fibrinogen antibodies do not bind to BC, leading to the conclusion that cell enhancement would result from the presence of RGD epitopes, not from unspecific protein adsorption, e.g., fibronectin, from the cell culture medium. XG also enhances hepatocyte adhesion (Seo et al., 2004), and modification of BC with XG does not adversely affect ECs.

#### 5.4.1.1 Increased cell spreading and adhesion on XGD-modified BC

XG-RGD-modification increased cell adhesion by 20%, and also increased the metabolism of seeded ECs as compared with unmodified BC. In contrast, the proliferation rate was less affected, presumably due to biological variation between cell donors. Our results (Fink et al., 2011a) concur with studies on RGD-grafted regenerated cellulose, which showed that an adhesion peptide enhances adhesion by approximately 20% (Bartouilh de Taillac et al., 2004). Another study showed that cellulose binding proteins bound to different adhesion peptides improve adhesion and spreading of human microvascular cells to cellulose (Andrade et al., 2010). In our study, the absence of serum negatively influenced cell adhesion on unmodified BC but did not act similarly in modified BC, further indicating that increased adhesion is peptide specific.

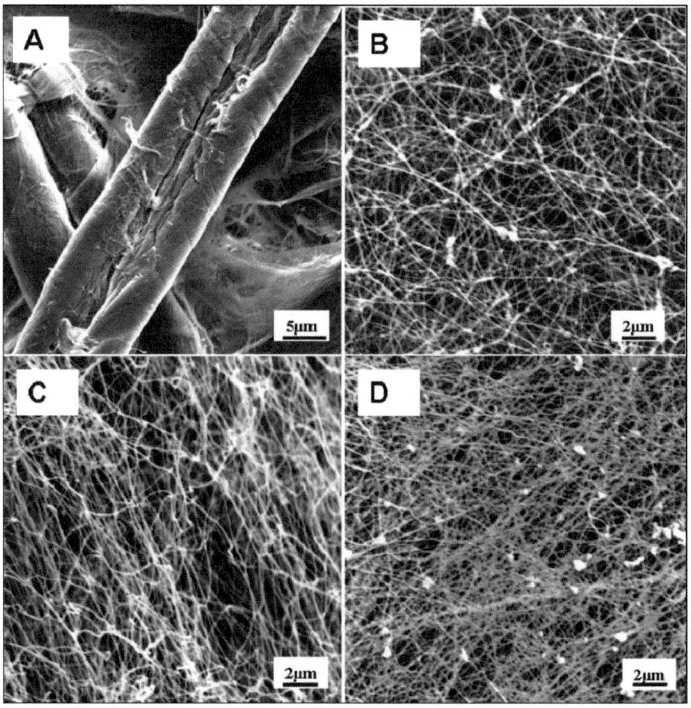


Fig. 2. SEM micrograph of BC morphology of (A) cotton linter, (B) unmodified BC, (C) XG-RGD modified BC and (D) acetone treated BC. Reprinted with permission from Bodin et al., 2007. Copyright American Chemical Society 2007.

Initial cell attachment is crucial to subsequent behaviour such as spreading, proliferation and cell differentiation on substrates. The extent of cell spreading is an important parameter for the biocompatibility of materials. EC adhesion to the ECM proteins is normally followed by cell spreading, a process in which cells reorganize the f-actin cytoskeleton, resulting in flattening and spreading of the cell. These polymerised actin filaments attach the cells to the substrate via focal adhesions. Cells grown on RGD-modified BC spread out, displaying a well-organized actin cytoskeleton with prominent f-actin fibres. They also grow in clusters, which we believe is a step towards achieving a confluent monolayer.

## 6. Endothelial cells as cellular source for graft lining

The endothelium is composed of a monolayer of squamous epithelial cells that line the inside of blood vessels in a confluent layer, with a total area of 350-1000 $m^2$ and a weight of 0.5-1.5 kg (Pries et al., 2000; Jaffe, 1987). The morphology of these cells is flat, resembling a cobblestone pattern. This morphology is essential to maintaining good blood flow without turbulence. ECs function not only as a physiological barrier, separating the blood from surrounding tissues, but also as a dynamic layer of cells that displays antithrombotic properties in its resting state. This is achieved by physically preventing elements in the blood from contacting prothrombotic elements in the subendothelium and by active synthesis of various mediators. Endothelial functions help maintain blood vessel function.

The endothelium upholds delicate balances in the vasculature, i.e., vasoconstriction/vasodilatation, anticoagulant/procoagulant properties, blood cell adherence/nonadherence and growth promotion/inhibition. It regulates vascular tone, maintains hemostasis, controls vascular structure and mediates inflammatory and immunological responses.

The endothelium responds to inflammatory conditions by regulating its own permeability and releasing a variety of substances. It mediates inflammation with pro-inflammatory mediators including cytokines such as the interleukins (IL) (e.g., IL-1β, IL-6, IL-8), platelet-activating factor (PAF) and also by expressing endothelial cell leukocyte adhesion molecule-1 (ELAM-1) and intercellular adhesion molecule 1 (ICAM-1), inflammatory mediators that control the interaction between EC and circulating blood cells and leukocytes, leading to extravasation of leukocytes.

During an inflammatory response, adhesion molecule P-selectin is expressed on ECs after exposure to leukotrine B4 or histamine, which are produced by mast cells. Tumor necrosis factor alpha (TNF-α) and lipopolysaccharides (LPS) induce P-selectin expression and the synthesis of E-selectin, another selectin that appears a few hours after the inflammatory process begins. Because the interactions between these selectins and their corresponding glycoprotein ligands (sialyl-Lewis$^x$ moiety) on leukocytes are relatively weak and reversible, leukocytes are unable to attach firmly to the endothelium. Instead, they "roll" along the surface of the vessel wall. The interactions are enhanced as other integrins are induced on the endothelium.

Leukocyte integrins LFA-1 and Mac-1 normally adhere only weakly to leukocytes. On the other hand, IL-8 and other chemokines bound to the endothelial surface trigger a conformational change in LFA-1 and Mac-1 on the rolling leukocytes, increasing adhesiveness and consequently firmly anchoring the leukocytes to the endothelium. Rolling is arrested and the leukocytes squeeze between the ECs into the subendothelial tissue, a process known as diapedesis.

### 6.1 Angiogenesis and vessel remodeling

ECs regulate vessel structure by producing both growth promoting and growth inhibiting factors. SMC growth is stimulated by platelet-derived growth factor (PDGF), fibroblast growth factor (FGF), transforming growth factor alpha (TGF-$\alpha$), endothelin and angiotensin II. Growth is inhibited by nitric oxide (NO), prostacylin ($PGI_2$), some FGFs, insulin-like growth factor 1 (IGF-1) and thrombospondin.

Angiogenesis is regulated by a variety of growth factors. Hypoxia and inflammatory cytokines such as FGF increase vascular endothelial growth factor-A (VEGF-A) levels through autocrine and paracrine mechanisms. VEGF-A, an endothelial-specific growth factor that consists of a heparin-binding homodimer, is a major regulator of EC function and angiogenesis. VEGF-A activates several EC functions, e.g., proliferation, migration and NO-release, processes that participate importantly in new blood vessel formation. VEGF-A also increases vessel wall permeability. Both VEGF and FGF induce EC production of proteases such as matrix metalloproteinases (MMPs) and plasminogen activator (PA). At least twenty MMPs participate in angiogenesis (Kroll & Waltenberger, 2000; Lamalice et al., 2007).

Proteases digest the basement membrane, allowing ECs to invade surrounding tissue, where they proliferate and migrate to form a sprout. The sprout elongates and the ECs differentiate to form a lumen. ECs in the newly formed vessel produce PDGF-BB, which attracts mural cells (pericytes to capillaries/SMC to larger arteries and veins) and stabilises the vessel. Expressed on ECs, heparin sulphate proteoglycans and their glycosaminoglycans (GAG) side-chains play an important role in angiogenesis because they bind circulating growth factors like VEGF (Kroll & Waltenberger, 2000).

### 6.2 Regulation of vascular tone

ECs regulate vessel tone and, consequently, local blood flow by managing the communication between the blood and the underlying SMCs, and by releasing substances that influence SMCs to relax or contract. In addition, ECs synthesise both vasodilating and vasoconstricting agents.

Vasodilatation is mediated through $PGI_2$ and (NO/endothelium-derived relaxing factor (EDRF) and endothelium-derived hyperpolarizing factor (EDHF), where NO plays a central role. Vasoconstricting agents released by ECs include endothelin, angiotensin II and thromboxane $A_2$ ($TXA_2$).

Shear stress, bradykinin, thrombin, serotonin and various drugs stimulate ECs to release prostacyklin, thus stimulating adenylate cyclase, which increases cyclic adenosine monophosphate (cAMP) in SMCs. NO is synthesized from L-arginine by NO synthase and diffuses to SMCs, where it activates guanylate cyclase to produce cyclic guanosine monophosphate (cGMP). This leads to decreased intracellular calcium and muscle relaxation. Sensing mechanical changes in the environment, f-actin mediates mechanical induction of NO, leading to signal transduction into the cell.

The eNOS gene contains a shear stress regulatory element (SSRE) that increases or decreases eNOS activity (Balligand et al., 2009). Acetylcholine stimulation of M1 muscarinic receptors releases endothelium-derived hyperpolarizing factor (EDHF), changing membrane potential (Pagliaro et al., 2000). Endothelin consists of three isoforms, ET-1, ET-2 and ET-3. ECs produce endothelin-1, the most potent mediator of vasoconstriction. Two endothelin receptors are found in the vasculature: $ET_A$ on SMCs and $ET_B$ on ECs. Binding of endothelin-

1 to the $ET_A$-receptor results in signal transduction and smooth muscle relaxation. On the other hand, activation of $ET_B$ on ECs stimulates NO and $PGI_2$ production. In contrast, angotensin II is a much weaker vasoconstrictor. Renin cleaves angiotensinogen to angiotensin I, which is then converted to angiotensin by endothelial angiotensin-converting enzyme (ACE) (Nordt & Bode, 2000).

## 7. Blood compatibility of biomaterials is a challenge

A nonthrombogenic surface is the key to a successful vascular graft. Non-thrombogenicity can be achieved by various surface modifications. Since ECs could provide a nonthrombogenic surface, intense investigation has focussed on endothelialisation in this context. In our studies, we used ECs passage 4 from non-diseased human saphenous veins, by-products of coronary bypass surgery.

The thrombogenicity of a biomaterial is an essential factor for any material that will be in contact with blood. Although the thrombogenic property of cellulose has been extensively researched as it has been used for haemodialysis membranes (Fushimi et al., 1998; Mao et al., 2004), the thrombogenicity of BC remains undetermined because it is a relatively new material for vessel grafts. Therefore, one of our studies focussed on delineating the blood compatibility of BC in comparison with ePTFE and PET vascular grafts, which are both used clinically as graft material (Fink et al., 2011b).

The endothelium's most important function in relation to biomaterials is hemostatic control. Under normal physiological conditions, ECs express thrombo-resistant molecules, but they must be able to switch to a procoagulant state upon injury to initiate coagulation and clot formation. Since blood is transported under high pressure, minimization of blood loss requires a rapid response. Some molecules are continuously secreted by ECs while others are only produced upon stimulation. Molecules can be expressed on the surface or secreted into the blood stream. The different endothelial anti- and procoagulant factors are discussed below in their biological context.

### 7.1 Primary hemostasis – Platelet adhesion, activation and aggregation

Prostacylin $I_2$ ($PGI_2$), nitric oxide (NO) and adenosine diphosphatase (ADPase) suppress platelet activation, aggregation and platelet-wall-interaction. Both NO and $PGI_2$ are secreted and act in a paracrine manner, whereas ADPase is expressed on the EC surface. Platelet inhibition by $PGI_2$ is mediated through a guanosine nucleotide binding receptor. This receptor-mediated signal transduction increases cAMP levels and inhibits platelet activation and the release of proaggregatory compounds such as $TXA_2$ (Moncada, 1982). $PGI_2$ production is stimulated by diverse agonists such as thrombin, histamine and bradykinin, and synthesised via arachidonic acid (AA) and prostaglandin ($PGG_2$) (Wu, 1995).

ECs produce EDRFs, which are responsible for acetylcholine-induced vasorelaxation. The most important EDRF is NO, which synthesises nitric oxide synthase (NOS) by converting L-arginine. NO is a small molecule, so it diffuses easily. When NO enters platelets, it inhibits their adhesion and activation via guanylyl cyclise (Radomski et al., 1987c). $PGI_2$ and NO have synergistic effects on inhibition of platelet adhesion, activation and aggregation and also reverse platelet aggregation (Radomski et al., 1987a; b)

### 7.2 Secondary hemostasis – Coagulation

The endothelium physically separates coagulation factor VIIa from tissue factor (TF) and prevents platelet exposure to collagen and von Willebrandt factor (vWF) (Fig. 3).

Thrombomodulin (TM) is expressed on the surface of ECs. Thrombin binds to TM, thereby undergoing a conformational change that results in enhanced affinity for protein C. Thrombin is the only enzyme capable of activating protein C. Activated protein C cleaves and inactivates clotting factors Va and VIIIa (Esmon, 1993). The thrombin-TM complex, effectively removes thrombin from the blood and internalises it, leading to its degradation. The TM molecule can also bind FXa, thus inhibiting prothrombin activation (Thompson & Salem, 1986). Protein S, also synthesised by ECs, binds to the endothelial surface and protein Ca to form a complex, thus enhancing FVa and FVIIIa inhibition (Fig. 3).

The endothelium expresses heparin sulphate proteoglycans with anticoagulant activity on its surface. Heparin is a cofactor for antithrombin III, a plasma protein present that can inhibit thrombin, IXa, FXa and XIIa. The complex binding of thrombin to antithrombin III occurs slowly. This process is accelerated by the interaction with heparin, which has many binding sites for antithrombin, and serves to localise and increase its activity more than a thousand-fold. The β-isoform of antithrombin is more highly effective than the α-isoform. Moreover, the β-isoformis effectively inhibits thrombin-induced SMC proliferation (Swedenborg, 1998). Synthesised in the liver and also by ECs, tissue factor pathway inhibitor (TFPI) forms a complex with Xa and inactivates the VIIa-tissue factor complex by binding to it.

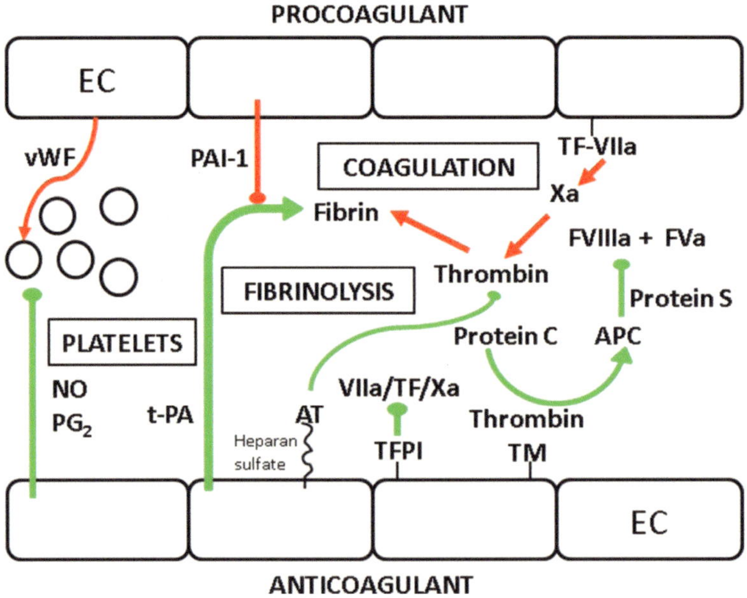


Fig. 3. Schematic illustration of the regulation of coagulation by ECs.

#### 7.2.1 Procoagulation factor

The endothelium also participates importantly in the initiation of coagulation, which arrests bleeding. It expresses a variety of procoagulant factors, including vWF, coagulation factors V and VII, TF and high molecular weight kininogen (HMWK).

ECs synthesise vWF, a platelet adhesion molecule that secretes following stimulation by thrombin, and stores it in vesicles (Weibel-Palade bodies). vWF possesses binding sites for coagulation factor VIII, collagen (exposed after injury) and platelets (GPIb- XI-V), and acts as a bridging molecule in platelet aggregation and activation (Ruggeri, 1994). Importantly, the absence of vWF leads to severe bleeding disorders.

ECs also secrete TF, which is found mainly in the subendothelium at sites not normally exposed to the bloodstream. The basal production of TF is low in comparison with the underlying SMCs and fibroblasts, but it can increase 10- to 40-fold upon stimulation. In addition, ECs have binding sites for factor VII, IX, IXa, X and Xa. Binding to factor IXa inhibits EC decay in the presence of factors VIII and X, which provide an additional feedback mechanism for cell-bound procoagulant activity (Jaffe, 1987; Vane et al., 1990).

### 7.2.2 Fibrinolysis

The endothelium also helps regulated fibrinolysis (Fig. 3). The degradation of fibrin requires plasmin. Plasminogen binds to the cell surface and facilitates plasmin conversion by two PAs, tissue type plasminogen activator (tPA) and urokinase (uPA) (van Hinsbergh). Physiologically, the most important PA in vascular fibrinolysis is tPA. Indeed, tPA enhances the conversion of plasminogen 100-fold when it binds to fibrin. The release of tPA is either constitutively or pathway-mediated. Thrombin, FVa, bradykinin, PAF and shear stress all induce the synthesis and release of tPA from ECs (Emeis, 1992; Giles et al., 1990; Brown et al., 1999). When tPA binds to the EC surface, it is protected from degradation by the two PA inhibitors (PAI), PAI-1 and PAI-2, which are also released by ECs. PAI-1 requires vitronectin, present in ECM, to maintain its activity; it is the main inhibitor to tPA. Recombinant t-PA (rt-PA) is the most frequently used substance for inducing thrombolysis by pharmacological means (Noble et al., 1995; Bennett et al., 1991).

### 7.2.3 Biomaterial-induced coagulation

Evaluation of coagulation induced by biomaterials is mostly studied in terms of platelet adhesion, partial thromboplastin time (PTT), protein adsorption by QCM-D or ellipsometry (Liu et al., 2009; Mao et al., 2004;van Oeveren et al., 2002; Keuren et al., 2003). The QCM-D method is surface-sensitive, but the distance from the surface to where measurement is possible is limited. Currently, it is not possible to attach BC to quartz crystals. Therefore, cellulose other than BC must be used. However, this material could be used for QCM-D measurements as a model surface, complementing other studies. Because ellipsometry is an optical method, it is not possible to use native BC for this assay either. Automated calibrated thrombin generation is very sensitive and has become a widespread method for quantitative analysis of coagulation kinetics in blood plasma (van Oeveren et al., 2002; Gerotziafas et al., 2005; Hemker et al., 2003). Thrombin generation is also considered the most sensitive method to assay thrombogenicity.

Since BC is used in a wet state, finding appropriate analysis techniques has been challenging. To our knowledge, ours is the first study to investigate the thrombogenic properties of BC compared with other graft materials (Fink et al., 2011b). We also developed a modified automated calibrated thrombin generation assay (Fink et al., 2010). This makes it possible to follow thrombin generation, in the presence of a material, in real time rather than using an endpoint assay. Our assay has led to new insights into the kinetics of thrombin generation induced by a material surface, which otherwise would have been missed.

Most methods that study the coagulation process measure coagulation in the bulk without regards to where it began or the kinetics describing the propagation from the initiation point. Our method (Fink et al., 2011b) makes it possible to visualize the exact initiation point of coagulation and determine how coagulation propagates (Kantlehner et al., 2000). The captured images are used to calculate the coagulation time of the plasma at the surface (surface coagulation time) and into the bulk (propagation). Such factors are highly relevant to the study of material interactions with blood.

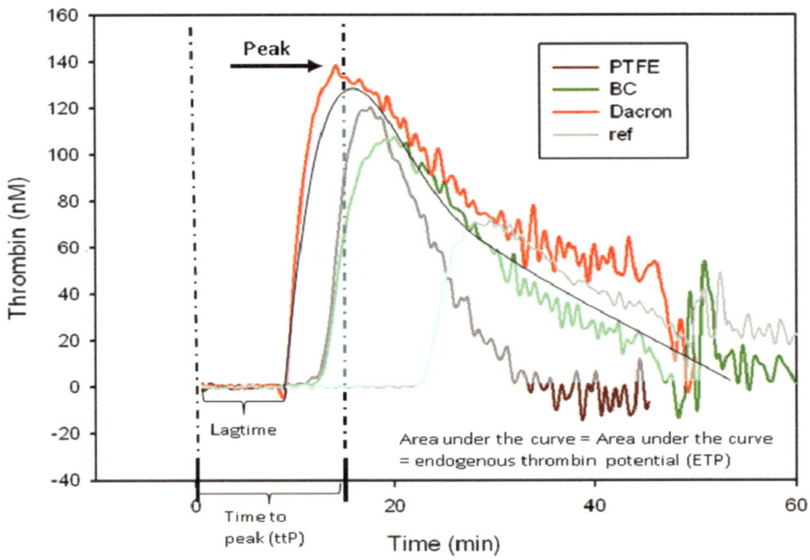


Fig. 4. Thrombogram generated from thrombin generation assay displaying lagtime, time to peak (ttPeak), peak and endogenous thrombin potential (ETP).

We measured the levels of thrombin and factor XIIa using calibrated automated thrombography, which displays the concentration of thrombin and factor XIIa, respectively, in clotting plasma with or without platelets (platelet-rich plasma/platelet-free plasma, PRP/PFP). The splitting of a fluorogenic substrate is monitored for either thrombin or factor XIIa and compared with a known thrombin or factor XIIa activity, respectively, in a parallel non-clotting sample. To evaluate thrombin and factor XIIa generation exclusively induced by the biomaterial surfaces, we fixed material samples with heparinised O-rings and analysed them by calculating the average rate of fluorescence increase over a period of 60 min.

#### 7.2.3.1 Biomaterial induced coagulation of biological cellulose

We compared biomaterial-induced coagulation of BC with clinically used graft materials, i.e., ePTFE and PET. In addition, we visualised coagulation propagation at the material surfaces and into the plasma bulk.

Thrombin generation experiments revealed dramatic differences between the tested materials (Fink et al., 2010). Both ePTFE and BC generate longer lagtimes and time to Peak (ttPeak) values than PET (Fig. 4). Furthermore, BC generates the lowest 'Peak', indicating a slower coagulation process at the surface. These results are also supported by the measurements of factor XIIa generation and analysis of surface coagulation times, where BC had the lowest FIIa generation and slowest propagation of coagulation into the bulk (Fig. 5). Compared with PET, thrombin generation in the whole blood Chandler-Loop system depicted the same response, yielding decreased accumulation of thrombin-antithrombin III complex (TAT) on both BC and ePTFE. Since the measurements are performed after one hour and not continuously, the difference in coagulation speed cannot be observed. On the other hand, this assay is performed in whole blood during flow conditions that more closely resemble an *in vivo* situation compared to measurements in platelet-free plasma during static conditions. It is interesting and promising that these two systems show similar results.

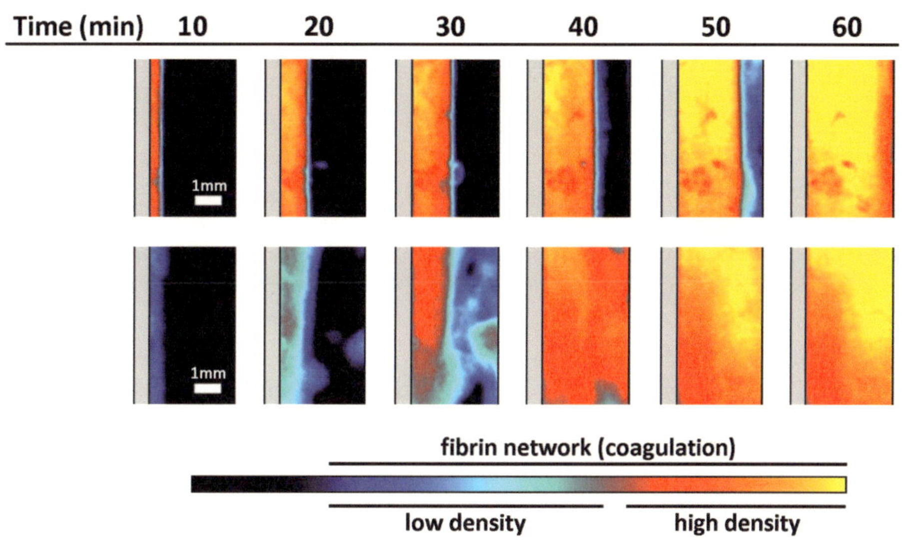


Fig. 5. Representative time-lapse images from a comparative experiment in the imaging of coagulation setup. Graft material samples are attached along the left wall in the images. The colour represents the density of the formed fibrin network (Courtesy of Lars Faxälv, PhD).

Hypothetically, the slower coagulation process on BC (Fig. 5) could be an advantage when blood contacts biomaterial applications, because it would provide time for the blood flow to divert and dilute activated coagulation products. The whole blood model also shows that 4 mm BC tubes perform well regarding anti-thrombogenic properties and perform better compared with ePTFE than 6 mm tubes. Measurements of thrombin generation correlate very well with the XIIa generation assay and visualisation of propagation. Together these methods potentially could provide fast screening methods for evaluating the thrombogenicity of biomaterials.
The amount of TAT generated depends on blood velocity (e.g., shear rate) in the loop system. Higher velocities associate with increased TAT generation. Shear rates are higher in the 4 mm loop system compared with the 6 mm system, and the narrower material also exhibits greater coagulation activation. Interestingly, however, platelet consumption does not increase, suggesting platelet activation. The amount of TAT generated on ePTFE increased 18-fold on 4 mm tubes as compared with 6 mm tubes, but we detected only a 3-fold increase for BC tubes. In comparison with the other tested materials, the platelet

consumption of BC is remarkably low, especially compared with heparinised polyvinyl chloride (PVC), which is known to have low thrombogenic properties (Johnell et al., 2005). In addition, cellulose showed no visible sign of clotting following one hour of incubation with whole blood containing only small amounts of soluble heparin.

### 7.3 Complement system

The immune complement system (CS) is part of the innate immune system. Its main task is to protect the body from pathogenic agents like bacteria, viruses and fungi. On contact with a foreign surface, e.g., a bacterial surface, the CS activates in a cascade that either destroys the bacterial surface or releases bioactive degradation products, or both, causing inflammatory reactions in the surrounding tissue.

Consisting of more than 30 different cell-bound and soluble proteins that circulate as inactive zymogens under nonpathological conditions, the immune CS is present in blood and serum. Its most important factor is complement factor 3 (C3). Cleavage of C3 by C3 convertase creates C3a and C3b, causing a cascade of further cleavage and activation events. Three different pathways lead to the creation of C3 convertase: the classical pathway, the alternative pathway and the mannose-binding lectin pathway. The classical complement pathway typically requires antibodies for activation, whereas the alternative and lectin pathways can be activated by C3 hydrolysis or antigens without the presence of antibody.

#### 7.3.1 Classical pathway

Classical convertase is initiated when antibodies bind to a surface such as a bacterium. When factor C1 binds to an antibody, it cleaves is cleaved and binds to additional factors forming the classical convertase (C4b2a) (Kinoshita, 1991).

#### 7.3.2 Alternative pathway

The alternative pathway is triggered by either spontaneous C3 hydrolysis, which forms C3a and C3b, or covalent binding of C3b from the classical and lectin pathways to a surface. The C3b molecule is capable of covalently binding to a pathogenic membrane surface in its vicinity. If there is no pathogen in the blood, the C3a and C3b protein fragments will deactivate when they rejoin with each other. Upon binding with a cellular membrane, C3b is binds to factor Ba and P, forming the alternative pathway C3-convertase (C3bBbP). A characteristic feature of the alternative pathway is a feedback mechanism that leads to accelerated C3 activation. Such mechanisms are not present in the classical pathway (Medicus et al., 1976; Rother et al., 1998).

#### 7.3.3 Mannose-binding lectin pathway

A variant of the classical pathway, the Mannose-binding lectin pathway does not require antibodies. Activation of this pathway occurs when mannose-binding lectin (MBL) binds to mannose residues on the pathogen surface. Subsequently, the MBL complex can split C4 and C2, generating C3-convertase, as in the classical pathway (Petersen et al., 2001). This pathway will not be discussed further in this chapter.

The convertases from both the classical and alternative pathways cleave C5 into C5a and C5b. The C5b molecule associates with C6, C7, C8, and C9, forming the C5b-9 membrane attack complex (MAC), which is inserted into the cell membrane and initiates cell lysis. The C5b-9, also called the terminal complement complex (TCC), may exist as a soluble active form denoted sC5b-9. This soluble form can be measured to assess complement activation . The C5a and C3a fragments are anaphylatoxins that participate in the recruitment of inflammatory cells and trigger mast cell degranulation. Therefore, these anaphylatoxins participate in many forms of acute and chronic inflammation including sepsis (Guo et al., 2004; Ward, 2008).

### 7.3.4 Complement activation

Extracorporal treatments such as haemodialysis and cardiopulmonary bypass activate the CS. Contact between blood and biomaterials may generate degradation fragments of complement C3a and C5a and soluble C5b-9. These fragments result in chemotaxis of leukocytes, cytokine release and generation of prostaglandins, resulting in a life-threatening condition termed "whole body" inflammation. Biomaterial induced CS is activated by both the classical and alternative pathways (Nilsson et al., 2007).

The Chandler-Loop system was also used to assess CS activation. The complement activation parameters (C3a and C5b-9) were much higher for BC compared with the other materials, for both 4 and 6 mm tubes. Cellulose is known to induce complement activation in hemodialysis membranes (Frank et al., 2001). The mechanisms underlying these results for BC are still unclear and require further investigation. Bacterial fragments could still be present in the material. However, endotoxin values are well within the limit for cardiovascular devices. It is also possible that exposed hydroxyl groups induce complement activation through the alternative pathway (Arima et al., 2009; Toda et al., 2008). The physiological significance *in vivo* of this complement activation remains undetermined. Interestingly, platelet activation is low even when complement activation is high. According to the literature, platelet consumption and complement activation are closely related (Fushimi et al., 1998; Hamad et al., 2008; Peerschke et al., 2006; Gyongyossy-Issa et al., 1994).

## 8. What are the future therapeutic possibilities?

This chapter has presented possible approaches to modifying BC that enhance EC growth *in vitro*. The XG method, an easy one-step procedure carried out in water, is an elegant technique for modifying BC to promote EC. Its advantage is the preservation of the fibre structure, thus maintaining its strength. The modification of BC with the XG technique is far from limited to the RGD peptide. Different peptide sequences or other active groups and growth factors could be attached to the XG molecule. Platelets could potentially adhere to exposed RGD peptides. Therefore, other peptides, more specific to ECs, or different combinations of peptides should be explored.

Measurements of thrombin generation correlated well with the XIIa generation assay and visualisation of the propagation of coagulation. Together, these methods could offer potential fast screening methods for evaluating the thrombogenicity of biomaterials and future surface modifications.

BC could be used for vascular grafts in two different approaches: (i) implantation as a tube without cells or (ii) seeding prior to implantation. The ideal BC modification would provide an initial nonthrombogenic surface and promote long-term endothelialisation. Future modifications of BC could include heparinisation or combinations of surface modifications, e.g., different peptides or coatings. Heparin is a potent antithrombotic agent that functions by binding antithrombin. In recent years, heparinised ePTFE grafts (Propaten®) have been developed (Losel-Sadee & Alefelder, 2009). Although encouraging outcomes for below-knee bypass are reported, the compliance mismatch of ePTFE grafts still remains. However, this is an exciting modification and preliminary studies on heparinised BC tubes show considerably lower amounts of thrombin on the hep-BC surface.

Our studies show that modification of BC with the adhesion-promoting peptide RGD results in increased EC adhesion, metabolism and spreading. Furthermore, BC induces slower coagulation than clinically available materials such as Gore-Tex® and Dacron® and induces the least contact activation as evaluated by Factor XIIa generation. In addition, BC consumes low quantities of platelets and generates low thrombin values as compared with Dacron® and Gore-Tex®.

## 9. Conclusion

Our work demonstrates that it is possible to introduce an adhesion peptide to BC that enhances EC adhesion without altering the fibre network or mechanical properties. The anti-thrombogenic properties of BC, especially 4 mm tubes, are promising as compared with conventional graft materials. Therefore, BC emerges as a promising, novel vascular graft material for small-caliber grafts. Molecular studies confirm that BC exhibits low thrombogenicity and extensive EC adhesion, which are beneficial when introducing artificial materials *in vivo* during by-pass surgery. Together with the modification methods presented in this chapter, BC has the potential to become a material for artificial vessels, thus underlining the importance of increasing molecular understanding of EC and BC interactions to create novel opportunities for artificial blood vessels.

## 10. Acknowledgements

The Authors thank Karen Williams for editorial expertise.

## 11. References

Andrade, F. K., et al. 2010. Improving bacterial cellulose for blood vessel replacement: Functionalization with a chimeric protein containing a cellulose-binding module and an adhesion peptide. *Acta Biomater,* 6, 4034-41.

Arima, Y., et al. 2009. Complement Activation by Polymers Carrying Hydroxyl Groups. *ACS Applied Materials & Interfaces.*

Backdahl, H., et al. 2008. Engineering microporosity in bacterial cellulose scaffolds. *J Tissue Eng Regen Med,* 2, 320-30.

Backdahl, H., et al. 2006. Mechanical properties of bacterial cellulose and interactions with smooth muscle cells. *Biomaterials,* 27, 2141-9.

Balligand, J. L., et al. 2009. eNOS activation by physical forces: from short-term regulation of contraction to chronic remodeling of cardiovascular tissues. *Physiol Rev,* 89, 481-534.

Bartouilh De Taillac, L., et al. 2004. Grafting of RGD peptides to cellulose to enhance human osteoprogenitor cells adhesion and proliferation. *Composites Science and Technology,* 64, 827-837.

Bennett, W. F., et al. 1991. High resolution analysis of functional determinants on human tissue-type plasminogen activator. *J Biol Chem,* 266, 5191-201.

Bodin, A., et al. 2007. Modification of nanocellulose with a xyloglucan-RGD conjugate enhances adhesion and proliferation of endothelial cells: Implications for tissue engineering. *Biomacromolecules,* 8, 3697-3704.

Boland, E. D., et al. 2004. Electrospinning collagen and elastin: preliminary vascular tissue engineering. *Front Biosci,* 9, 1422-32.

Brown, N. J., et al. 1999. Bradykinin stimulates tissue plasminogen activator release in human vasculature. *Hypertension,* 33, 1431-5.

Brown, R. M., Jr., et al. 1976. Cellulose biosynthesis in Acetobacter xylinum: visualization of the site of synthesis and direct measurement of the in vivo process. *Proc Natl Acad Sci U S A,* 73, 4565-9.

Cummings, C. L., et al. 2004. Properties of engineered vascular constructs made from collagen, fibrin, and collagen-fibrin mixtures. *Biomaterials,* 25, 3699-706.

Czaja, W., et al. 2006. Microbial cellulose--the natural power to heal wounds. *Biomaterials,* 27, 145-151.

D'Souza, S. E., et al. 1991. Arginyl-glycyl-aspartic acid (RGD): a cell adhesion motif. *Trends Biochem Sci,* 16, 246-50.

Emeis, J. J. 1992. Regulation of the acute release of tissue-type plasminogen activator from the endothelium by coagulation activation products. *Ann N Y Acad Sci,* 667, 249-58.

Entcheva, E., et al. 2004. Functional cardiac cell constructs on cellulose-based scaffolding. *Biomaterials,* 25, 5753-62.

Esmon, C. T. 1993. Molecular events that control the protein C anticoagulant pathway. *Thromb Haemost,* 70, 29-35.

Fink, H., et al. 2010. Real-time measurements of coagulation on bacterial cellulose and conventional vascular graft materials. *Acta Biomaterialia,* 6, 1125-1130.

Fink, H., et al. 2011a. Bacterial cellulose modified with xyloglucan bearing the adhesion peptide RGD promotes endothelial cell adhesion and metabolism—a promising modification for vascular grafts. Journal of Tissue Engineering and Regenerative Medicine, 5, 454-463.

Fink, H., et al. 2011b. An in vitro study of blood compatibility of vascular grafts made of bacterial cellulose in comparison with conventionally-used graft materials. *Journal of Biomedical Materials Research Part A,* 97A, 52-58.

Fontana, J., et al. 1990. Acetobacter cellulose pellicle as a temporary skin substitute. *Applied Biochemistry and Biotechnology,* 24-25, 253-264.

Frank, R. D., et al. 2001. Role of contact system activation in hemodialyzer-induced thrombogenicity. *Kidney Int,* 60, 1972-81.

Fushimi, F., et al. 1998. Platelet adhesion, contact phase coagulation activation, and C5a generation of polyethylene glycol acid-grafted high flux cellulosic membrane with varieties of grafting amounts. *Artif Organs,* 22, 821-6.

Gabriel, M., et al. 2006. Direct grafting of RGD-motif-containing peptide on the surface of polycaprolactone films. *J Biomater Sci Polym Ed,* 17, 567-77.

Gerotziafas, G. T., et al. 2005. Towards a standardization of thrombin generation assessment: the influence of tissue factor, platelets and phospholipids concentration on the normal values of Thrombogram-Thrombinoscope assay. *Thromb J,* 3, 16.

Giles, A. R., et al. 1990. The fibrinolytic potential of the normal primate following the generation of thrombin in vivo. *Thromb Haemost,* 63, 476-81.

Guo, R. F., et al. 2004. Role of C5a-C5aR interaction in sepsis. *Shock,* 21, 1-7.

Gyongyossy-Issa, M. I., et al. 1994. Complement activation in platelet concentrates is surface-dependent and modulated by the platelets. *J Lab Clin Med,* 123, 859-68.

Hamad, O. A., et al. 2008. Complement activation triggered by chondroitin sulfate released by thrombin receptor-activated platelets. *J Thromb Haemost,* 6, 1413-21.

Hanus, J. & Mazeau, K. 2006. The xyloglucan-cellulose assembly at the atomic scale. *Biopolymers,* 82, 59-73.

Hashi, C. K., et al. 2007. Antithrombogenic property of bone marrow mesenchymal stem cells in nanofibrous vascular grafts. *Proc Natl Acad Sci U S A,* 104, 11915-20.

Helenius, G., et al. 2006. In vivo biocompatibility of bacterial cellulose. *J Biomed Mater Res A,* 76, 431-8.

Hemker, H. C., et al. 2003. Calibrated automated thrombin generation measurement in clotting plasma. *Pathophysiol Haemost Thromb,* 33, 4-15.

Herring, M., et al. 1984. Endothelial seeding of Dacron and polytetrafluoroethylene grafts: the cellular events of healing. *Surgery,* 96, 745-55.

Hersel, U., et al. 2003. RGD modified polymers: biomaterials for stimulated cell adhesion and beyond. *Biomaterials,* 24, 4385-415.

Huang, L., et al. 2001. Engineered collagen-PEO nanofibers and fabrics. *J Biomater Sci Polym Ed,* 12, 979-93.

Iguchi, M., et al. 2000. Bacterial cellulose—a masterpiece of nature's arts. *Journal of Materials Science,* 35, 261-270.

Jaboulay, M. & Briau, E. 1896. Recherches experimentales sur la suture et al greffe arterielle. *Lyon Med,* 81, 97.

Jaffe, E. A. 1987. Cell biology of endothelial cells. *Hum Pathol,* 18, 234-9.

Johnell, M., et al. 2005. The influence of different heparin surface concentrations and antithrombin-binding capacity on inflammation and coagulation. *Biomaterials,* 26, 1731-9.

Kaehler, J., et al. 1989. Precoating substrate and surface configuration determine adherence and spreading of seeded endothelial cells on polytetrafluoroethylene grafts. *J Vasc Surg,* 9, 535-41.

Kantlehner, M., et al. 2000. Surface coating with cyclic RGD peptides stimulates osteoblast adhesion and proliferation as well as bone formation. *Chembiochem,* 1, 107-14.

Kenawy El, R., et al. 2003. Electrospinning of poly(ethylene-co-vinyl alcohol) fibers. *Biomaterials,* 24, 907-13.

Keuren, J. F. W., et al. 2003. Thrombogenicity of polysaccharide-coated surfaces. *Biomaterials,* 24, 1917-1924.

Kim, D.-Y., et al. 2002. Surface acetylation of bacterial cellulose. *Cellulose,* 9, 361-367.

Kino, Y., et al. 1998. Multiporous cellulose microcarrier for the development of a hybrid artificial liver using isolated hepatocytes. *J Surg Res,* 79, 71-6.

Kinoshita, T. 1991. Biology of complement: the overture. *Immunol Today,* 12, 291-5.

Klemm, D., et al. 2001. Bacterial synthesized cellulose -- artificial blood vessels for microsurgery. *Progress in Polymer Science,* 26, 1561-1603.

Kroll, J. & Waltenberger, J. 2000. [Regulation of the endothelial function and angiogenesis by vascular endothelial growth factor-A (VEGF-A]. *Z Kardiol,* 89, 206-18.

Kumar, T. R. & Krishnan, L. K. 2002. A stable matrix for generation of tissue-engineered nonthrombogenic vascular grafts. *Tissue Eng,* 8, 763-70.

L'Heureux, N., et al. 1998. A completely biological tissue-engineered human blood vessel. *FASEB J,* 12, 47-56.

Lamalice, L., et al. 2007. Endothelial cell migration during angiogenesis. *Circ Res,* 100, 782-94.

Langer, R. & Vacanti, J. P. 1993. Tissue engineering. *Science,* 260, 920-6.

Liu, P. S., et al. 2009. Grafting of zwitterion from cellulose membranes via ATRP for improving blood compatibility. *Biomacromolecules,* 10, 2809-16.

Losel-Sadee, H. & Alefelder, C. 2009. Heparin-bonded expanded polytetrafluoroethylene graft for infragenicular bypass: five-year results. *J Cardiovasc Surg (Torino),* 50, 339-43.

Mao, C., et al. 2004. Various approaches to modify biomaterial surfaces for improving hemocompatibility. *Advances in Colloid and Interface Science,* 110, 5-17.

Massia, S. P. & Hubbell, J. A. 1990. Covalent surface immobilization of Arg-Gly-Asp- and Tyr-Ile-Gly-Ser-Arg-containing peptides to obtain well-defined cell-adhesive substrates. *Anal Biochem,* 187, 292-301.

Mckee, J. A., et al. 2003. Human arteries engineered in vitro. *EMBO Rep,* 4, 633-8.

Medicus, R. G., et al. 1976. Alternative pathway of complement: recruitment of precursor properdin by the labile C3/C5 convertase and the potentiation of the pathway. *J Exp Med,* 144, 1076-93.

Meinhart, J. G., et al. 2005. Enhanced endothelial cell retention on shear-stressed synthetic vascular grafts precoated with RGD-cross-linked fibrin. *Tissue Eng,* 11, 887-95.

Moncada, S. 1982. Prostacyclin and arterial wall biology. *Arteriosclerosis,* 2, 193-207.

Niklason, L. E., et al. 1999. Functional Arteries Grown in Vitro. *Science,* 284, 489-493.

Nilsson, B., et al. 2007. The role of complement in biomaterial-induced inflammation. *Mol Immunol,* 44, 82-94.

Noble, S., et al. 1995. Enoxaparin. A reappraisal of its pharmacology and clinical applications in the prevention and treatment of thromboembolic disease. *Drugs,* 49, 388-410.

Nordt, T. K. & Bode, C. 2000. [Endothelium and endogenous fibrinolysis]. *Z Kardiol,* 89, 219-26.

Nose, Y. 2008. Dr. Michael E. DeBakey and his contributions in the field of artificial organs. September 7, 1908-July 11, 2008. *Artif Organs,* 32, 661-6.

Pagliaro, P., et al. 2000. The endothelium-derived hyperpolarizing factor: does it play a role in vivo and is it involved in the regulation of vascular tone only? *Ital Heart J,* 1, 264-8.

Peerschke, E. I., et al. 2006. Blood platelets activate the classical pathway of human complement. *J Thromb Haemost,* 4, 2035-42.

Petersen, S. V., et al. 2001. The mannan-binding lectin pathway of complement activation: biology and disease association. *Mol Immunol,* 38, 133-49.

Pierschbacher, M. D. & Ruoslahti, E. 1984. Cell attachment activity of fibronectin can be duplicated by small synthetic fragments of the molecule. *Nature,* 309, 30-3.

Pries, A. R., et al. 2000. The endothelial surface layer. *Pflügers Archiv European Journal of Physiology,* 440, 653-666.

Radomski, M. W., et al. 1987a. The anti-aggregating properties of vascular endothelium: interactions between prostacyclin and nitric oxide. *Br J Pharmacol,* 92, 639-46.

Radomski, M. W., et al. 1987b. Comparative pharmacology of endothelium-derived relaxing factor, nitric oxide and prostacyclin in platelets. *Br J Pharmacol,* 92, 181-7.

Radomski, M. W., et al. 1987c. The role of nitric oxide and cGMP in platelet adhesion to vascular endothelium. *Biochem Biophys Res Commun,* 148, 1482-9.

Remuzzi, A., et al. 2004. Vascular smooth muscle cells on hyaluronic acid: culture and mechanical characterization of an engineered vascular construct. *Tissue Eng,* 10, 699-710.

Ross, P., et al. 1991. Cellulose biosynthesis and function in bacteria. *Microbiol Rev,* 55, 35-58.

Rother, K., et al. 1998. *The complement system,* Berlin, Springer.

Ruggeri, Z. M. 1994. Glycoprotein Ib and von Willebrand factor in the process of thrombus formation. *Ann N Y Acad Sci,* 714, 200-10.

Sassi, J.-F. & Chanzy, H. 1995. Ultrastructural aspects of the acetylation of cellulose. *Cellulose,* 2, 111-127.

Sassi, J.-F., et al. 2000. Relative susceptibility of the Iα and Iβ phases of cellulose towards acetylation. *Cellulose,* 7, 119-132.

Seeger, J. M. & Klingman, N. 1988. Improved in vivo endothelialization of prosthetic grafts by surface modification with fibronectin. *J Vasc Surg,* 8, 476-82.

Seo, S. J., et al. 2004. Xyloglucan as a synthetic extracellular matrix for hepatocyte attachment. *J Biomater Sci Polym Ed,* 15, 1375-87.

Sharefkin, J. B., et al. 1983. Seeding of Dacron vascular prostheses with endothelium of aortic origin. *J Surg Res,* 34, 33-43.

Swedenborg, J. 1998. The mechanisms of action of alpha- and beta-isoforms of antithrombin. *Blood Coagul Fibrinolysis,* 9 Suppl 3, S7-10.

Svensson, A., et al. 2005. Bacterial cellulose as a potential scaffold for tissue engineering of cartilage. *Biomaterials,* 26, 419-431.

Takata, T., et al. 2001. Migration of osteoblastic cells on various guided bone regeneration membranes. *Clin Oral Implants Res,* 12, 332-8.

Thompson, E. A. & Salem, H. H. 1986. Inhibition by human thrombomodulin of factor Xa-mediated cleavage of prothrombin. *J Clin Invest,* 78, 13-7.

Toda, M., et al. 2008. Complement activation on surfaces carrying amino groups. *Biomaterials,* 29, 407-417.

Turner, N. J., et al. 2004. A novel hyaluronan-based biomaterial (Hyaff-11) as a scaffold for endothelial cells in tissue engineered vascular grafts. *Biomaterials,* 25, 5955-64.

Walluscheck, K. P., et al. 1996. Endothelial cell seeding of de-endothelialised human arteries: improvement by adhesion molecule induction and flow-seeding technology. *Eur J Vasc Endovasc Surg,* 12, 46-53.

Van Hinsbergh, V. W. Regulation of the synthesis and secretion of plasminogen activators by endothelial cells.

Van Oeveren, W., et al. 2002. Comparison of coagulation activity tests in vitro for selected biomaterials. *Artif Organs,* 26, 506-11.

Van Oeveren, W., et al. 2002. Comparison of Coagulation Activity Tests In Vitro for Selected Biomaterials. *Artificial Organs,* 26, 506-511.

Vane, J. R., et al. 1990. Regulatory functions of the vascular endothelium. *N Engl J Med,* 323, 27-36.

Ward, P. A. 2008. Sepsis, apoptosis and complement. *Biochem Pharmacol,* 76, 1383-8.

Watanabe, K., et al. 1993a. A new bacterial cellulose substrate for mammalian cell culture. *Cytotechnology,* 13, 107-114.

Watanabe, K., et al. 1993b. A new bacterial cellulose substrate for mammalian cell culture. *Cytotechnology* 13, 107-114.

Weinberg, C. B. & Bell, E. 1986. A blood vessel model constructed from collagen and cultured vascular cells. *Science,* 231, 397-400.

Williams, D. F. 1999. *The Williams dictionary of biomaterials,* Liverpool, Liverpool Univ. Press.

Wippermann, J., et al. 2009. Preliminary results of small arterial substitute performed with a new cylindrical biomaterial composed of bacterial cellulose. *Eur J Vasc Endovasc Surg,* 37, 592-6.

Voorhees, A. B., Jr., et al. 1952. The use of tubes constructed from vinyon "N" cloth in bridging arterial defects. *Ann Surg,* 135, 332-6.

Vroman, L. 1987. Methods of investigating protein interactions on artificial and natural surfaces. *Ann N Y Acad Sci,* 516, 300-5.

Wu, K. K. 1995. Molecular regulation and augmentation of prostacyclin biosynthesis. *Agents Actions Suppl,* 45, 11-7.

Yang, M. B., et al. 1994. Hollow fibers for hepatocyte encapsulation and transplantation: studies of survival and function in rats. *Cell Transplant,* 3, 373-85.

Zhang, X., et al. 2009. Dynamic culture conditions to generate silk-based tissue-engineered vascular grafts. *Biomaterials,* 30, 3213-23.

Zilla, P., et al. 1987. Endothelial cell seeding of polytetrafluoroethylene vascular grafts in humans: a preliminary report. *J Vasc Surg,* 6, 535-41.

# Part 2

# Macrophages and Inflammation in Atherosclerosis

# 9

# Atherogenesis, Inflammation and Autoimmunity – An Overview

Katja Lakota et al.*
*University Medical Centre-Ljubljana, Rheumatology, Ljubljana,*
*University of Primorska, FAMNIT, Koper,*
*Slovenia*

## 1. Introduction

In the 16th century, Leonardo Da Vinci had described "the narrowing of the passage of blood vessels, thickening of the coats of these vessels and hardening of arteries" in his work (Boon, 2009). This is the first known documentation of atherosclerosis (AS). Today, our understanding of atherogenesis as a process of a chronic inflammatory disease has been greatly promoted by many theories, such as, the cellular cycle of cholesterol and hypercholesterolemia, dysfunction of endothelial cells, oxidized lipoproteins, discovery of scavenger receptors and response to injury theory, among others. The factors leading to the elucidation of atherogenesis are still not all known, since AS can persist silently (subclinically) without showing any serious symptoms for a longer period. That, together with the fact that AS is not limited to warm-blooded vertebrates and the occurrence of intimal thickening of coronary arteries in rabbitfish (Duran et al., 2010), as well as evidence of coronary AS in salmonids (Farrell, 2002), brings proof that AS is still a largely elusive, complicated and multi-component disease.

AS is not a modern world disease as determined by recent images obtained from coronary arteries and the aorta of ancient mummies. Atheromatous lesions, as well as aortic AS were identified in an Aleutian mummy from Alaska originating from ~400 AD (Zimmerman, 1998). In 2009, images generated by computer tomography of vascular calcifications in examined Egyptian mummies found that 16 out of the 22 examined mummies had identifiable cardiovascular tissue, with definite AS present in 5 and AS found in additional 4 mummies (together 56% of total) (Allam et al., 2009). This study was recently expanded to 52 ancient Egyptian mummies from the Middle Kingdom to the Greco-Roman period and identified cardiovascular structures in 44 mummies, with 20 of these showing either definite AS (n=12, as defined by calcification within the wall of an identifiable artery) or probable AS (n=8, as defined by calcifications along the expected course of an artery) (Allam et al., 2011).

---

*Andrej Artenjak[1], Sasa Cucnik[1], Jana Brguljan-Hitij[2], Borut Cegovnik[2],
Barbara Salobir[2], Rok Accetto[2], Borut Bozic[1,3], Blaz Rozman[1] and Snezna Sodin-Semrl[1,4]
[1]*University Medical Centre-Ljubljana, Rheumatology, Ljubljana, Slovenia*
[2]*University Medical Centre-Ljubljana, Hypertension, Ljubljana, Slovenia*
[3]*University of Ljubljana, Faculty of Pharmacy, Clinical Biochemistry, Ljubljana, Slovenia*
[4]*University of Primorska, FAMNIT, Koper, Slovenia*

The calcifications were located in the aorta, as well as coronary, carotid, iliac, femoral and peripheral arteries. The 20 mummies with definite and probable AS were significantly older at time of death (mean age 45.1 ± 9.2 years) as compared to mummies that had cardiovascular tissue identified without AS (mean age 34.5 ± 11.8 years). Since social status (mummies were usually of higher status, than others in the population), diet (mainly wildlife and grains) and tobacco (not yet known) were not risk factors in the life of ancient Egyptians, they could not contribute to the development of AS in this population. Age, however has been re-affirmed with these studies, as one of the most important independent systemic risk factors for AS.

## 2. Brief clinical characterization of the disease

AS is a chronic, multifocal immunoinflammatory, fibroproliferative disease and is the most common form of arteriosclerosis. AS is a disease of the arterial wall, which often starts in young people. In middle-aged individuals, AS can start to appear in clinically recognizable forms, such as coronary artery disease (CAD), cerebral vascular or peripheral artery disease. It can affect all large and medium-sized arteries including the coronary, carotid, cerebral arteries, the aorta, its branches and main arteries of the extremities. Areas of non-laminar blood flow are highly susceptible to plaque formation.

The clinical endpoints of AS may result as a consequence of several mechanisms, such as:

1. artery-to-artery embolism of thrombus formed on an atherosclerotic plaque,
2. atheroembolism of cholesterol crystals or other atheromatous debris,
3. acute thrombotic occlusion resulting from plaque rupture,
4. structural disintegration of the arterial wall resulting from dissection or subintimal hematoma, and
5. reduced perfusion resulting from critical stenosis or occlusion caused by progressive plaque growth

Ultrasound is one of the most commonly used noninvasive examinations for assessment of early and advanced atherosclerotic vascular changes, also of the carotid intima media thickness. However, ultrasound has limited diagnostic and prognostic value, and for pre-operative procedures, arteriographies and other methods of the involved vessels are necessary.

AS is considered to be the leading cause of death and loss of disability adjusted life-years worldwide, particularly in the developed countries, according to United States Statistical Update from 2011 (Roger et al., 2011). CAD accounted for ≅ 1 of every 6 deaths and stroke ≅ 1 of 18 deaths in 2007. Recently, peripheral artery disease was reported to be present in 12% of United States citizens (Beers et al., 2006).

## 3. Inflammation and the involvement of cells/molecules in atherosclerosis

Inflammation contributes to the formation and progression of AS (Libby, 2002; Moubayed et al., 2007). Since AS represents a chronic inflammatory state, levels of C-reactive protein (CRP) are important, and were found to be an independent predictor of cardiovascular disease (CVD) (Fruchart et al., 2004), although other studies have not been able to confirm this (Kullo & Ballantyne, 2005). Serum amyloid A (SAA) has been reported to also play a role in atherosclerosis (King et al., 2011) which has been supported by animal models (Chait et al., 2005; Hua et al., 2009; Malle & De Beer, 1996). In human primary coronary artery endothelial cells, SAA was reported to induce the release of interleukin-6 (IL-6), IL-8 and stimulate the expression and release of soluble intercellular adhesion molecule (sICAM) and soluble vascular adhesion molecule (sVCAM), as well as E-selectin synthesis. The data indicated greater susceptibility of coronary artery endothelial cells (in comparison to human umbilical vein endothelial cells) to SAA (Lakota et al., 2007) which indicated the potential role of SAA in CAD. Studies for fibrinogen consistently link this factor, which is involved in both inflammation and thrombosis, with AS burden and risk of coronary heart disease (CHD) (Kullo & Ballantyne, 2005). Lipoprotein-associated phospholipase A2 (Lp-PLA2) is a novel biomarker of vascular-specific inflammation providing information about atherosclerotic plaque inflammation and stability. Elevated levels of serum Lp-PLA2 are indicative of rupture-prone plaques and a strong independent predictor of cardiovascular risk (Colley et al., 2011). Most recently, Herder et al. reported on biomarkers associated with prediction of incident coronary events (Herder, Karakas, et al., 2011). The group mentioned the following markers: IL-6, IL-8, IL-18, macrophage migration inhibitory factor (MIF), monocyte chemotactic protein-1, interferon-γ inducible protein-10, transforming growth factor-β1 (TGF-β1), sE-selectin and sICAM (Herder, Baumert, et al., 2011). The data showed that the combination of blood biomarkers could improve the prediction of cardiovascular outcome above the traditional ones used.

Some infectious diseases represent an independent initiator of vascular inflammation which can contribute to atherogenesis and progression of AS. Bacteria and viruses can upregulate cytokines, chemokines and acute phase reactants, such as CRP and SAA, which lead to endothelial dysfunction. Overall, expression of Toll-like receptors in the atheroma, mouse model experiments and the role of genetic polymorphisms, all currently suggest microbe activation of inflammation in plaques and AS progression (Vallejo, 2011). Infection is also known to convert a lipidogenic profile into a pro-atherogenic one (Khovidhunkit et al., 2000).

Infections important in association with AS were shown in many studies and include the following infectious agents *Herpes virus, C. pneumonie, P. gingivitis, H. pylori, among others (Kowalski et al., 2006; Ludewig et al., 2004; Ross, 1999). There was also presence of bacterial antigens reported in atheroma (Ott et al., 2006).* The latter finding raises the question of single antigen importance versus total infectious burden in accelerating AS (Gabrielli et al., 2002).

Presence of antibodies against infectious agents represent a risk factor for CVD. In terms of specific antigen involvement in AS, the following (among others) have been reported: *H.pylori* heat shock protein (HSP)-60 elicited antibodies can crossreact with endogenous molecules, stress-related endothelial HSP-60 and the presence of HSP-60-specific T lymphocytes in the circulation, may increase the risk of AS (Ayada et al., 2007). Occurrence of antiphospholipid antibodies after certain infections is also common and can lead to initial endothelial dysfunction (Altman, 2003). Latency and intracellular infection importance stays an open ended question (especially in *C.pneumonie, Cytomegalovirus*). Long term effects of infections on AS progression are unclear, however statistics show undoubtedly more cases of stroke and myocardial infarction in the first 3 days following an acute urinary/respiratory infection with declining numbers in following weeks (Graham et al., 2007).

A unifying view of the pathophysiology of AS proposes that inflammation has a key role by transducing the effects of many known risk factors of the disease. Although the combined experimental and clinical evidence may convince some, the chicken and egg problem about causality, remains unsolved (Libby et al., 2011).

### 3.1 Initial injury

Endothelial cells provide a physical barrier layer between the circulatory system and the intima, however the cells also actively synthesize molecules responsible for the maintenance of circulatory homeostasis and participate in plaque development.

The initial process in the development of AS is isolated endothelium injury and subsequent endothelial activation followed by expression of different pro-inflammatory cytokines, chemokines and adhesive molecules resulting in monocyte attraction, the rolling mechanism and their migration into the tunica intima (Jan et al., 2010; Ross, 1999). Monocytes transform into macrophages, the activation of which leads to the hallmark of plaque development or foam cell formation. An important molecule in this process is oxidized low density lipoproteins (oxLDL), which originates from retained LDLs in the tunica intima. Molecules of oxLDL and their binding to scavanger receptors on macrophages stimulates the accumulation of lipids in the cells and the formation of foam cells (Hansson, 2005).

When inflammatory cells (such as leukocytes, monocytes and macrophages) migrating into the intima, start to accumulate subendothelial lipid, particularly oxidized lipid, this exacerbates the initial, local inflammatory reaction and maintains activation of the overlying endothelium. This results in continued expression of adhesion molecules and pro-inflammatory cytokines and chemokines perpetuating cell activation. Normally, the endothelium shows anti-adhesive, anti-thrombotic and vasoregulatory properties. Thus, stress conditions, mechanical damage or patho-physiological stimulation can cause modified endothelial cell characteristics (Stoltz et al., 2007). Endothelial injury can be different based on the different original vascular beds the cells arise from. Their physiological roles in coagulation, hemodynamics and susceptibility to patho-physiological stimuli can also differ depending on the vascular bed origin and the influence of the microenviroment (Aird, 2007; Cines et al., 1998; Lacorre et al., 2004; Luu et al., 2010; Yano et al., 2007). For example, differences in endothelial cell responses were described for activation with tumour necrosis factor $\alpha$ (TNF-$\alpha$) (Lehle et al., 2007; Methe et al., 2007; Viemann et al., 2006), SAA and IL-1$\beta$ (Lakota et al., 2007; Lakota et al., 2009) and oxLDL (Deng et al., 2006). Recently, endothelial damage has been reported as being able to be repaired with endothelial progenitor cells (Bai et al., 2010).

Endothelial cells seem to be involved prevalently in the earlier stages of atherogenesis, leading to initial vascular injury, as well as in later stages, when they detach in response to injury and enter the circulation. Circulating endothelial cells can be used as a marker of vascular injury. Their number increase is associated with CVD, as well as they can serve as an accurate predictor of major adverse events following myocardial infarction. They also inversely correlate with flow-mediated dilatation and positively correlate with markers of endothelial injury (such as von Willebrand factor, tissue plasminogen activator inhibitor, E-selectin) and prothombotic state (tissue factor). They are rarely found in healthy individuals, but are increased and correlate with disease activity in different vasculitides, in systemic lupus erythematosus (SLE) and systemic sclerosis (SSc) (Boos et al., 2006). Interestingly, Mutin et al. showed increased circulating endothelial cells in acute myocardial infarction and unstable angina without increased levels of markers of activation (ICAM, VCAM, E-selectin) and no apoptosis (Mutin et al., 1999).

### 3.2 Progression of atherosclerotic plaques

Early atherosclerotic lesions called fatty streaks involve a growing extracellular lipid core within the atherosclerotic plaques. The next stage of atherosclerotic plaque formation involves the proliferation and migration of smooth muscle cells into the tunica intima, accumulation of collagen and fibrous cap formation (Hansson, 2005; Libby, 2002). T lymphocytes with a prevailing Th1 response, together with smooth muscle cell proliferation and deposition of collagenous fibers contribute to the fibrous cap formation. Fibrosis and collagen accumulation have a patho-physiological parallel in other chronic inflammatory diseases such as rheumatoid arthritis (RA), cirrhosis and pulmonary fibrosis, among others, where monocytes and lymphocytes are also the active players. In later stages of AS plaque development, expression of proteases increases (i.e. matrix metalloproteinases (MMPs)) leading to degradation of collagen.

During the development of AS plaques, monocyte-derived macrophages and T-lymphocytes that invade evolving atherosclerotic lesions produce soluble inflammatory mediators (cytokines and chemokines) which are very important in the perpetuation of the disease. Certain cytokines and chemokines (i.e. IL-1, IL-12, IL-18, TNF- α, MIF, interferon-γ (IFN-γ) , and granulocyte macrophage colony stimulating factor (GM-CSF) have explicit pro-atherogenic characteristics, others (i.e. IL-10 and probably IL-5) have anti-atherogenic properties, while IL-4, IL-6, and GM-CSF can have both pro- or anti-atherogenic properties. Several of the pro-atherogenic cytokines affect plasma cholesterol levels, indicating that inflammation and lipid metabolism are interlinked processes in AS (Kleemann et al., 2008).

Fatty streaks do not necessarily progress into advanced lesions. Certainly the progression of plaques is not linear (Figure 1) and depends largely on the microenvironment. Plaques can be clinically silent for years. Almost all adolescent children may already show some evidence of fatty streaks (Kumar et al., 2007).

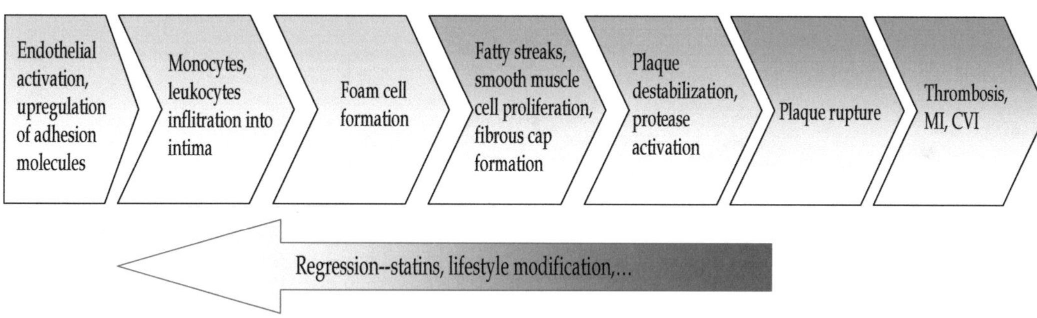


Fig. 1. Simplified putative scheme of progression/regression of atherosclerosis at the cellular and molecular levels. MI, myocardial infarction; CVI, cerebrovascular insult

Clinical prognosis is determined by the biological nature of the atherosclerotic plaque. Atheroma with active inflammatory processes are most prone to ruptures (Libby, 2002; Ross, 1999) and inflammation largely accounts for progression of stable to unstable angina (J.T. Wu & L.L. Wu, 2005). Rupture prone/unstable plaques are the ones with a large lipid core, many inflammatory cells and a thin fibrous cap (Gziut & Gil, 2008; Krone & Muller-Wieland, 1999).

There are three typical types of cellular/molecular influences of plaque rupture, among others:

a. desquamation of the endothelium (due to proinflammatory mediators, MMPs, T cells which attack the basal membrane of the endothelium) which uncovers the collagen and thrombosis can occur. Although desquamation is common and often asymptomatic it accounts for ¼ of fatal coronary thromboses (Libby, 2002). Mast cells contribute to endothelial erosions by releasing proteases that degrade cadherin and fibronectin (Mayranpaa et al., 2006)

b. disruption of neo-angiogenic blood vessels, growing in the atheroma full of growth factors. This leads to thrombin activation, collagen expression and smooth muscle cell proliferation (Libby, 2002)
c. fibrous cap rupture is the most common of plaque rupture and is due to inflammation in the lipid core, MMPs and tissue factor release from plaques. TGF-β and vascular endothelial growth factor released for the purpose of wound healing of the ruptures causes additional fibroses which narrow further the lumen of the vessel and can cause ischemia.

Major clinical complications and subclinical events are presented in Figure 2.

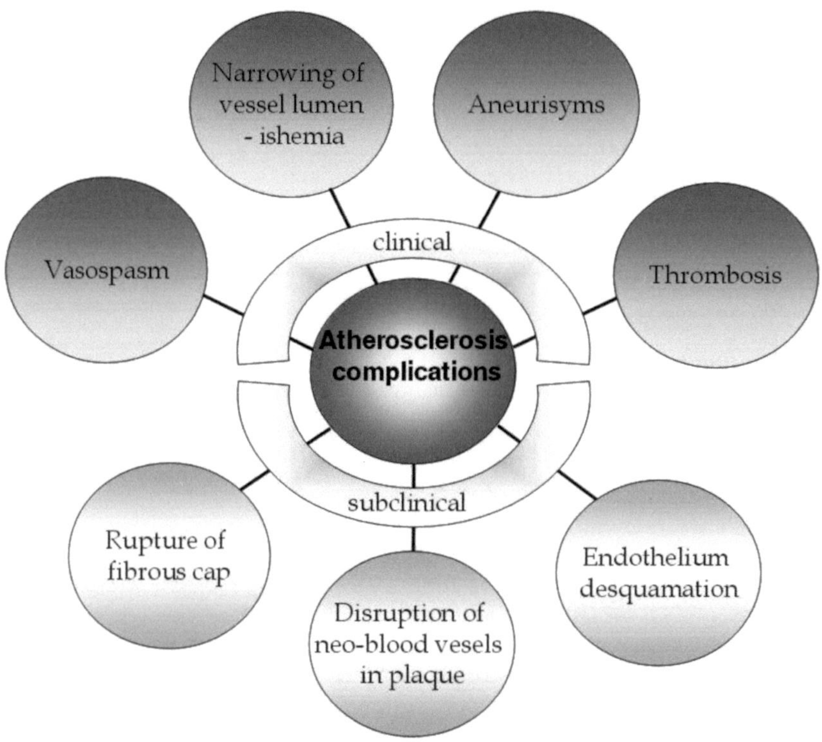


Fig. 2. Some clinical and subclinical atherosclerosis complications

### 3.3 Regression of atherosclerotic plaques

Previously, AS was thought to be reversible in early stages with changes of lifestyle and dietary modifications, as shown on animal models (J.J. Badimon et al., 1990; Malinow, 1983) and was believed to be reversible only to the stages before fatty streak formation. Currently, however, it is accepted that later stages can also be reversible as well. Some important regressions of even necrotic lesions and foam cell disappearance were achieved with injections of cholesterol-free phosphocholine liposomes which lower total cholesterol and mobilize cholesterol from plaques in animals (Williams et al., 2008). In regression of AS,

endothelium-dependent relaxation improves, as well as hypersensitivity of blood vessels, however maximal vasodilator activity/capacity does not improve (presumably due to fibrosis of arteries) (Heistad et al., 1990).
There are some problems occurring with evaluating the extent of AS, as well as in extrapolating animal studies to humans (Vilahur et al., 2011). The evaluation of AS regression presents a problem especially because the probability of cardiovascular events is stochastic and not only dependent on size of the plaque. Due to this, interpreting clinical studies in a manner of regression can also be difficult.

## 4. Autoimmunity and atherogenesis

Our understanding of AS has been crucially changed from a simply degenerative disorder to one that is a complex, inflammatory and autoimmune disease, in which all branches of immune system are involved. The role of autoimmunity has been shown in clinical and experimental models. Active immunization with HSP-60 or β2-GPI induces autoantibodies and accelerates AS. The transfer of lymphocytes from β2-GPI-immunized mice to other mice resulted in advanced AS (Sherer & Shoenfeld, 2006).
The AS process may be magnified and accelerated in patients with autoimmune diseases. Autoimmunity-related risk factors according to Bijl et al. include the presence of anti-cardiolipid antibodies (aCL), antibodies against oxLDL, antibodies against endothelial cells, antibodies against neutrophil cytoplasm antigens, antibodies against ribonuclear proteins and antibodies against lipoprotein lipase (Bijl, 2003). Additional risk factors recorded by Ronda and Meroni included anti-HSP-60/70 antibodies and anti-β2-glycoprotein (β2-GPI) antibodies (Ronda & Meroni, 2008). It must be pointed out however, that HSP-70 antigen itself is protective for AS (Frostegard, 2005).
The acceleration of AS in patients with autoimmune disease is due to the underlying immune system dysfunction, the presence of systemic inflammation and endothelial activation with the effects of chronic therapies (Ronda & Meroni, 2008). Accelerated and premature AS is associated specifically with autoimmune rheumatic diseases of inflammatory nature, most markedly with SLE (Roman et al., 2003; Salmon & Roman, 2008) and antiphospholipid syndrome (APS) (Jara et al., 2007), but also with RA (Salmon & Roman, 2008) and SSc (Shoenfeld et al., 2005), certain forms of vasculitis (Shoenfeld et al., 2005) and Sjogren's Syndrome (Gerli et al., 2010; Vaudo et al., 2005). For SSc however, the data are still inconsistent (Zinger et al., 2009).
Many components of the immune system are involved in AS and all arms of the immune system are engaged in atherogenesis with different cells (such as monocytes, macrophages, T lymphocytes) and different molecules involving both the cellular and humoral, innate and adaptive immunity. Certain important mechanisms for AS in autoimmune diseases are proposed below. One of them postulates that pre-existing adaptive and innate immunity involving HSP-60 exposed on the arterial endothelial cells could lead to the development of an initial inflammatory stage of atherogenesis. The progress of AS depends on the expression and accessibility of atherogenic HSP-60 epitopes on endothelial cells. Since low level of autoimmunity to HSP-60 is evolutionary present in all individuals, the development of AS depends mainly or even exclusively, on the condition of the endothelial cells (Wick & et al., 2006). β2-GPI is another autoantigen expressed within subendothelial regions and intimal-medial border of human atherosclerotic plagues, suggested to be involved in atherogenesis. It is targeted by anti-

β2-GPI antibodies, which results in increased amounts of colocalized CD4+ lymphocytes in the endothelia (Ronda & Meroni, 2008; Shoenfeld et al., 2001). These antibodies can also induce a pro-inflammatory and procoagulant phenotype (Harats & George, 2001). β2-GPI can also form complexes with oxLDL, which stimulate the immune system to produce autoantibodies to these oxLDL/β2-GPI complexes. Such immune complexes are uptaken by macrophages. Complexes, together with autoantibodies, have been described in patients with SLE and/or APS, indicating another mechanism of accelerated AS in patients with underlaying autoimmune disease (Matsuura et al., 2009). Further data is emerging that IgG anti-oxLDL/β2-GPI antibodies have been associated with pro-atherogenic functions, whereas IgM anti-oxLDL/β2-GPI have been considered to be anti-atherogenic (Narshi et al., 2011). In our recent study of 70 RA female patients, which were followed for 5.5 years, neither antibodies against β2-GPI, nor rheumatoid factor or CRP contributed to AS progression, as measured by carotid intima media thickness and number of plaques (Holc et al., 2011).

The increased risk of AS in patients with autoimmune rheumatic diseases is explained only in part by traditional AS risk factors, such as those from the Framingham study (Lloyd-Jones et al., 2004; Tegos et al., 2001), for example autoimmune patients commonly have dislipidemias. The process of inflammation (as a nontraditional risk factor) can aggravate atherosclerosis via different mechanisms secondary to autoimmunity and infectious diseases. Increased levels or presence of inflammatory markers: CRP, SAA, fibrinogen, IL-6, cluster differentiation markers CD40/CD40L and adhesion molecules have been reported (Shoenfeld et al., 2005).

Peroxidation of LDLs is low in the blood, but is extensive in the intima. Oxygen radicals and oxidizing enzymes modify proteins and lipids of the LDL, which activate endothelial cells to express vascular cell adhesion molecules (L. Badimon et al., 2011). OxLDL is a target of the immune system resulting in the production of autoantibodies (R. Wu & Lefvert, 1995), which could be, on one hand, an enhancer of oxLDL uptake by macrophages, inflammation and atherogenesis (Ronda & Meroni, 2008) or, on the other hand, may contribute to oxLDL clearance in healthy persons (Cerne et al., 2002). Antibodies against HDL have also been implicated in AS. Cross-reactivity is thought to exist between aCL, anti-HDL and anti-ApoA-I IgG antibodies in patients with SLE and primary APS and can lead to the diminishing HDL's protective role (Delgado Alves et al., 2003; Shoenfeld et al., 2005; Tincani et al., 2006).

A representative compilation of autoimmune diseases with accelerated AS is provided below (Figure 3).

Possible risk factors for AS in autoimmune diseases also represent frequently accompanying renal involvement. Questions were raised if plaques are more prone to rupture due to the fact that they are also qualitatively different in autoimmune diseases. Since systemic autoimmune disease patients are on drug therapy for life, there is a need to stress the influence of some common drugs. For instance, corticosteroids increase triglyceride levels, while methotrexate increases the levels of serum homocysteine (Frostegard, 2005).

Vaccination represents an attractive approach to induce long–term protective immunity. Atherosclerosis was reduced by vaccination with oxLDL or HSP-60 in animal experiments (Hansson, 2005) that could be due to the induction of protective antibodies or T cells.

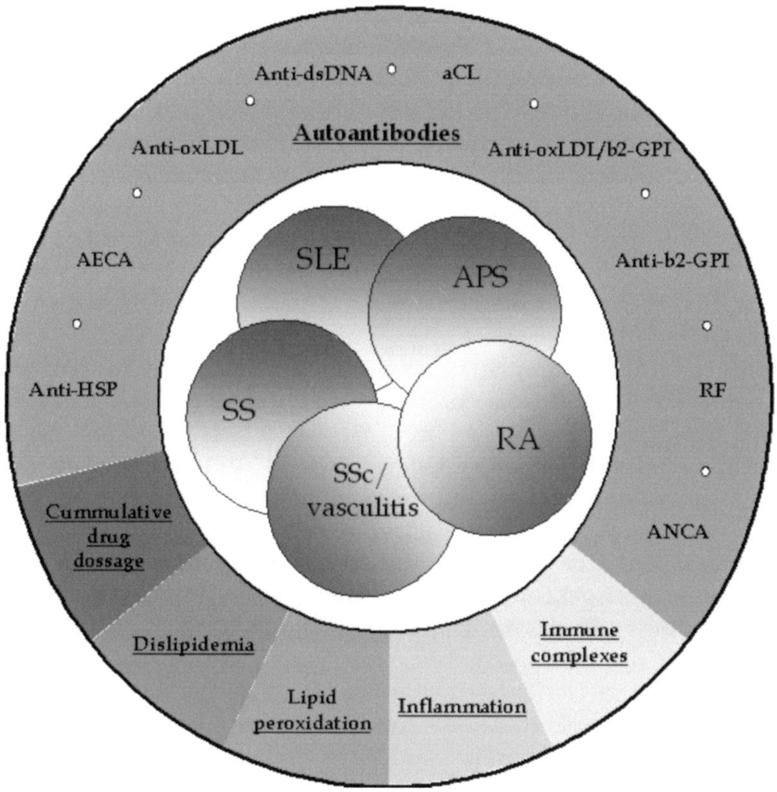


Fig. 3. Representative compilation of autoimmune diseases with accelerated AS with the processes and autoantibodies indicated. aCL, antibodies against cardiolipin; AECA, anti-endothelial cell antibodies; ANCA, anti-neutrophil cytoplasmic antibodies; Anti-β2-GPI, antibodies against β2-glycoprotein I; Anti-dsDNA, antibodies against double stranded DNA; Anti-HSP, antibodies against heat-shock protein antibodies; Anti-oxLDL, antibodies against oxidized LDL; Anti-oxLDL/β2-GPI, antibodies against oxidized LDL/β2-glycoprotein I complexes; RF, rheumatoid factor; APS, antiphospholipid syndrome; RA, rheumatoid arthritis; SLE, systemic lupus erythematosus; SS, Sjogren's syndrome; SSc, systemic sclerosis

## 5. Antiinflammatory atheroprotective effects and therapies in atherosclerosis

A growing body of evidence indicates that inflammation not only provides the baseline for future atherosclerotic events, but is a necessity for coronary plaque formation. The unique responsiveness of human coronary artery endothelial cells could account for the greater susceptibility of coronary arteries to inflammation and atherogenesis leading to cardiovascular pathology. Both black tea extract and resveratrol have been shown to significantly inhibit IL-1$\beta$-induced IL-6 and tissue factor expression and activity responses in human coronary artery endothelial cells (Lakota et al.., 2009).

The downregulation of TNF-alpha induced by skeletal muscle derived IL-6 may also participate in mediating the atheroprotective effect of physical activity (Szostak & Laurant, 2011).

Powerful anti-inflammatory agents could represent treatments for acute coronary syndrome (Hansson, 2005; Libby, 2002; Nilsson et al., 2005). Eicosanoid-modulating anti-inflammatory compounds, such as the cyclooxygenase-2 inhibitor rofecoxib are inappropriate in patients with CVD, since enzymes inhibited by them, are important in both the production of pro- and anti-thrombotic eicosanoids, depending on the cells effected. Lipid-lowering statins also have anti-inflammatory properties, likely stemming from the ability of statins to inhibit the formation of mevalonic acid, effecting cholesterol, as well as several isoprenoid intermediates used by lipids to attach to different intracellular signaling molecules. In certain studies, the reduction of inflammation (reflected by CRP levels) through statin therapy improved the clinical outcome of CAD, independently of the reduction in serum cholesterol levels (Hansson, 2005).

When macrophages are appropriately activated they can secrete anti-inflammatory cytokines and synthesize matrix repair proteins that stabilize vulnerable plaques (Wilson, 2010). There are also many results from mice studies which show that modulating the activity of selected cytokines (either systemically or locally) can prevent or retard the development of atherosclerotic lesions and could significantly contribute to early detection and treatment of AS or in combination with established hypolipidaemic and antihypertensive treatment. The activity of the cytokines of interest can be modulated by different techniques such as genetic deletion, overexpression, immunoneutralization, or *in vivo* administration of the cytokines or their receptors or inhibitors (Kleemann et al., 2008).

*Chlamydia pneumoniae* (Cp) infection has been associated with AS, and beneficial effects of antibiotic therapy on future cardiovascular events have been described. For example, a dramatic reduction in endpoints (cardiovascular death, hospital admission with unstable angina or acute myocardial infarction or need for revascularization) in a small number of high risk patients with CAD suggested the potential of azithromycin therapy in preventing future acute cardiac events (Mehta et al., 1998). The reduced intima media thickness progression after roxithromycin therapy in Cp seropositivity may be explained by several beneficial effects of antibiotic treatment on atherosclerotic plaque formation, such as those attributable to a reduced smooth muscle cell proliferation or a decreased smooth muscle cell migration from the media and adventitia into the intima, a reduced lipid accumulation, an improvement of endothelial function, and diminished inflammatory activity (Sander et al., 2002). The group reported a significant reduction of CRP in the Cp-positive group of patients with ischemic stroke treated with roxithromycin in a two year follow-up study. In contrast, there was no significant change of CRP in the placebo-treated Cp-positive group. Reductions in CRP and other inflammatory markers were also observed in previous antibiotic trials (Gurfinkel et al., 1999; Muhlestein et al., 2000).

## 6. Conclusion

Taken together, AS is a complex, multi-component, inflammatory, as well as autoimmune disease. Balancing pro- and anti-inflammatory mediators, destructive and protective antibodies can be one approach to maintaining homeostasis. Serum markers of inflammation have emerged as an important component of cardiovascular risk factor burden. On the other hand, some current reports indicate that detection of novel inflammatory marker levels (i.e. using microchips or multi-marker panels) are adding only minimally to the ability of traditional risk factors to predict cardiovascular outcome. However, discovering novel detection methods for different types of markers may be a way to help clinicians in identifying/clarifying which patients are at borderline risk and require drug therapy earlier. Fine-tuning the stage of disease progression using appropriate medication can lead to AS regression. Clinicians need more information to support their optimal judgment in this crucial decision-making process. Further directions suggest more predictive and personalized multi-marker medicine and appropriate earlier risk intervention. In addition, more preventive care and participatory feedback are necessary.

## 7. References

Aird, W.C. (2007). Phenotypic heterogeneity of the endothelium: I. Structure, function, and mechanisms. *Circ Res*, Vol.100, No.2, (February 2007), pp. 158-173, ISSN 1524-4571

Allam, A.H.; Thompson, R.C.; Wann, L.S.; Miyamoto, M.I.; Nur El-Din Ael, H.; El-Maksoud, G.A., et al. (2011). Atherosclerosis in ancient Egyptian mummies: the Horus study. *JACC Cardiovasc Imaging*, Vol.4, No.4, (April 2011), pp. 315-327, ISSN 1876-7591

Allam, A.H.; Thompson, R.C.; Wann, L.S.; Miyamoto, M.I. & Thomas, G.S. (2009). Computed tomographic assessment of atherosclerosis in ancient Egyptian mummies. *JAMA*, Vol.302, No.19, (November 2009), pp. 2091-2094, ISSN 1538-3598

Altman, R. (2003). Risk factors in coronary atherosclerosis athero-inflammation: the meeting point. *Thromb J*, Vol.1, No.1, (July 2003), pp. 4, ISSN 1477-9560

Ayada, K.; Yokota, K.; Kobayashi, K.; Shoenfeld, Y.; Matsuura, E. & Oguma, K. (2007). Chronic infections and atherosclerosis. *Ann N Y Acad Sci*, Vol.1108, (June 2007), pp. 594-602, ISSN 0077-8923

Badimon, J.J.; Badimon, L. & Fuster, V. (1990). Regression of atherosclerotic lesions by high density lipoprotein plasma fraction in the cholesterol-fed rabbit. *J Clin Invest*, Vol.85, No.4, (April 1990), pp. 1234-1241, ISSN 0021-9738

Badimon, L.; Storey, R.F. & Vilahur, G. (2011). Update on lipids, inflammation and atherothrombosis. *Thromb Haemost*, Vol.105 Suppl 1, (May 2011), pp. S34-42, ISSN 0340-6245

Bai, X.; Wang, X. & Xu, Q. (2010). Endothelial damage and stem cell repair in atherosclerosis. *Vascul Pharmacol*, Vol.52, No.5-6, (May-Jun 2010), pp. 224-229, ISSN 1879-3649

Beers, M.H.; Porter, S.R.; Jones, V.T.; Kaplan, L.J. & Berkwits, M., Eds. (2006). *The Merck manual of diagnosis and therapy*, Merck Research Laboratories, Division of Merck & Co., INC., ISBN 0-911910-18-2, Whitehouse Station, NJ

Bijl, M. (2003). Endothelial activation, endothelial dysfunction and premature atherosclerosis in systemic autoimmune diseases. *Neth J Med*, Vol.61, No.9, (September 2003), pp. 273-277, ISSN 0300-2977

Boon, B. (2009). Leonardo da Vinci on atherosclerosis and the function of the sinuses of Valsalva. *Neth Heart J*, Vol.17, No.12, (December 2009), pp. 496-499, ISSN 1876-6250

Boos, C.J.; Lip, G.Y. & Blann, A.D. (2006). Circulating endothelial cells in cardiovascular disease. *J Am Coll Cardiol*, Vol.48, No.8, (October 2006), pp. 1538-1547, ISSN 1558-3597

Cerne, D.; Jurgens, G.; Ledinski, G.; Kager, G.; Greilberger, J. & Lukac-Bajalo, J. (2002). Relationship between the sialic acid content of low-density lipoprotein (LDL) and autoantibodies to oxidized LDL in the plasma of healthy subjects and patients with atherosclerosis. *Clin Chem Lab Med*, Vol.40, No.1, (January 2002), pp. 15-20, ISSN 1434-6621

Chait, A.; Han, C.Y.; Oram, J.F. & Heinecke, J.W. (2005). Thematic review series: The immune system and atherogenesis. Lipoprotein-associated inflammatory proteins:

markers or mediators of cardiovascular disease? *J Lipid Res*, Vol.46, No.3, (March 2005), pp. 389-403, ISSN 0022-2275

Cines, D.B.; Pollak, E.S.; Buck, C.A.; Loscalzo, J.; Zimmerman, G.A.; McEver, R.P., et al. (1998). Endothelial cells in physiology and in the pathophysiology of vascular disorders. *Blood*, Vol.91, No.10, (May 1998), pp. 3527-3561, ISSN 0006-4971

Colley, K.J.; Wolfert, R.L. & Cobble, M.E. (2011). Lipoprotein associated phospholipase A(2): role in atherosclerosis and utility as a biomarker for cardiovascular risk. *EPMA J*, Vol.2, No.1, (March 2011), pp. 27-38, ISSN 1878-5085

Delgado Alves, J.; Kumar, S. & Isenberg, D.A. (2003). Cross-reactivity between anti-cardiolipin, anti-high-density lipoprotein and anti-apolipoprotein A-I IgG antibodies in patients with systemic lupus erythematosus and primary antiphospholipid syndrome. *Rheumatology (Oxford)*, Vol.42, No.7, (July 2003), pp. 893-899, ISSN 1462-0324

Deng, D.X.; Tsalenko, A.; Vailaya, A.; Ben-Dor, A.; Kundu, R.; Estay, I., et al. (2006). Differences in vascular bed disease susceptibility reflect differences in gene expression response to atherogenic stimuli. *Circ Res*, Vol.98, No.2, (February 2006), pp. 200-208, ISSN 1524-4571

Duran, A.C.; Rodriguez, C.; Gil de Sola, L.; Fernandez, B.; Arque, J.M. & Sans-Coma, V. (2010). Intimal thickening of coronary arteries in the rabbitfish, Chimaera monstrosa L. (Chondrichthyes: Holocephali). *J Fish Dis*, Vol.33, No.8, (August 2010), pp. 675-682, ISSN 1365-2761

Farrell, A.P. (2002). Cardiorespiratory performance in salmonids during exercise at high temperature: insights into cardiovascular design limitations in fishes. *Comp Biochem Physiol A Mol Integr Physiol*, Vol.132, No.4, (August 2002), pp. 797-810, ISSN 1095-6433

Frostegard, J. (2005). Atherosclerosis in patients with autoimmune disorders. *Arterioscler Thromb Vasc Biol*, Vol.25, No.9, (September 2005), pp. 1776-1785, ISSN 1524-4636

Fruchart, J.C.; Nierman, M.C.; Stroes, E.S.; Kastelein, J.J. & Duriez, P. (2004). New risk factors for atherosclerosis and patient risk assessment. *Circulation*, Vol.109, No.23 Suppl 1, (June 2004), pp. III15-19, ISSN 1524-4539

Gabrielli, M.; Santarelli, L. & Gasbarrini, A. (2002). Role for chronic infections in atherosclerosis? *Circulation*, Vol.106, No.7, (August 2002), pp. e32; author reply 32, ISSN 1524-4539

Gerli, R.; Vaudo, G.; Bocci, E.B.; Schillaci, G.; Alunno, A.; Luccioli, F., et al. (2010). Functional impairment of the arterial wall in primary Sjogren's syndrome: combined action of immunologic and inflammatory factors. *Arthritis Care Res (Hoboken)*, Vol.62, No.5, (May 2010), pp. 712-718, ISSN 2151-4658

Graham, I.; Atar, D.; Borch-Johnsen, K.; Boysen, G.; Burell, G.; Cifkova, R., et al. (2007). European guidelines on cardiovascular disease prevention in clinical practice: executive summary: Fourth Joint Task Force of the European Society of Cardiology and Other Societies on Cardiovascular Disease Prevention in Clinical Practice (Constituted by representatives of nine societies and by invited experts). *Eur Heart J*, Vol.28, No.19, (October 2007), pp. 2375-2414, ISSN 0195-668X

Gurfinkel, E.; Bozovich, G.; Beck, E.; Testa, E.; Livellara, B. & Mautner, B. (1999). Treatment with the antibiotic roxithromycin in patients with acute non-Q-wave coronary syndromes. The final report of the ROXIS Study. *Eur Heart J*, Vol.20, No.2, (January 1999), pp. 121-127, ISSN 0195-668X

Gziut, A.I. & Gil, R.J. (2008). Coronary aneurysms. *Pol Arch Med Wewn*, Vol.118, No.12, (December 2008), pp. 741-746, ISSN 0032-3772

Hansson, G.K. (2005). Inflammation, atherosclerosis, and coronary artery disease. *N Engl J Med*, Vol.352, No.16, (April 2005), pp. 1685-1695, ISSN 1533-4406

Harats, D. & George, J. (2001). Beta2-glycoprotein I and atherosclerosis. *Curr Opin Lipidol*, Vol.12, No.5, (October 2001), pp. 543-546, ISSN 0957-9672

Heistad, D.D.; Armstrong, M.L. & Lopez, J.A. (1990). What causes spasm of atherosclerotic arteries? Is regression of plaques beneficial? *Trans Am Clin Climatol Assoc*, Vol.101, 1990), pp. 103-110; discussion 110-113, ISSN 0065-7778

Herder, C.; Baumert, J.; Zierer, A.; Roden, M.; Meisinger, C.; Karakas, M., et al. (2011). Immunological and Cardiometabolic Risk Factors in the Prediction of Type 2 Diabetes and Coronary Events: MONICA/KORA Augsburg Case-Cohort Study. *PLoS One*, Vol.6, No.6, (June [online] 2011), pp. e19852, ISSN 1932-6203

Herder, C.; Karakas, M. & Koenig, W. (2011). Biomarkers for the prediction of type 2 diabetes and cardiovascular disease. *Clin Pharmacol Ther*, Vol.90, No.1, (July 2011), pp. 52-66, ISSN 1532-6535

Holc, I.; Hojs, R.; Cikes, N.; Ambrozic, A.; Cucnik, S.; Kveder, T., et al. (2011). Antiphospholipid antibodies and atherosclerosis: Insights from Rheumatoid arthritis - a five-year follow-up study. *Rheumatology (Oxford)*, ([no date] 2011), pp. [article in press],

Hua, S.; Song, C.; Geczy, C.L.; Freedman, S.B. & Witting, P.K. (2009). A role for acute-phase serum amyloid A and high-density lipoprotein in oxidative stress, endothelial dysfunction and atherosclerosis. *Redox Rep*, Vol.14, No.5, (October 2009), pp. 187-196, ISSN 1743-2928

Jan, M.; Meng, S.; Chen, N.C.; Mai, J.; Wang, H. & Yang, X.F. (2010). Inflammatory and autoimmune reactions in atherosclerosis and vaccine design informatics. *J Biomed Biotechnol*, Vol.2010, (n.d. 2010), pp. ID 459798, ISSN 1110-7251

Jara, L.J.; Medina, G. & Vera-Lastra, O. (2007). Systemic antiphospholipid syndrome and atherosclerosis. *Clin Rev Allergy Immunol*, Vol.32, No.2, (April 2007), pp. 172-177, ISSN 1080-0549

Khovidhunkit, W.; Memon, R.A.; Feingold, K.R. & Grunfeld, C. (2000). Infection and inflammation-induced proatherogenic changes of lipoproteins. *J Infect Dis*, Vol.181 Suppl 3, (June 2000), pp. S462-472, ISSN 0022-1899

King, V.L.; Thompson, J. & Tannock, L.R. (2011). Serum amyloid A in atherosclerosis. *Curr Opin Lipidol*, Vol.22, No.4, (Aug 2011), pp. 302-307, ISSN 1473-6535

Kleemann, R.; Zadelaar, S. & Kooistra, T. (2008). Cytokines and atherosclerosis: a comprehensive review of studies in mice. *Cardiovasc Res*, Vol.79, No.3, (August 2008), pp. 360-376, ISSN 0008-6363

Kowalski, M.; Pawlik, M.; Konturek, J.W. & Konturek, S.J. (2006). Helicobacter pylori infection in coronary artery disease. *J Physiol Pharmacol*, Vol.57 Suppl 3, (September 2006), pp. 101-111, ISSN 1899-1505

Krone, W. & Muller-Wieland, D. (1999). Lipid lowering therapy and stabilization of atherosclerotic plaques. *Thromb Haemost*, Vol.82 Suppl 1, (September 1999), pp. 60-61, ISSN 0340-6245

Kullo, I.J. & Ballantyne, C.M. (2005). Conditional risk factors for atherosclerosis. *Mayo Clin Proc*, Vol.80, No.2, (February 2005), pp. 219-230, ISSN 0025-6196

Kumar, V.; Abbas, A.K.; Fausto, N. & Mitchell, R.N., Eds. (2007). *Robbins Basic Pathology* Saunders/Elsevier, ISBN 978-1-4160-2973-1, Philadelphia

Lacorre, D.A.; Baekkevold, E.S.; Garrido, I.; Brandtzaeg, P.; Haraldsen, G.; Amalric, F., et al. (2004). Plasticity of endothelial cells: rapid dedifferentiation of freshly isolated high

endothelial venule endothelial cells outside the lymphoid tissue microenvironment. *Blood*, Vol.103, No.11, (June 2004), pp. 4164-4172, ISSN 0006-4971
Lakota, K.; Mrak-Poljsak, K.; Rozman, B.; Kveder, T.; Tomsic, M. & Sodin-Semrl, S. (2007). Serum amyloid A activation of inflammatory and adhesion molecules in human coronary artery and umibilical vein endothelial cells. *European Journal of Inflammation*, Vol.5, No.2,(2007), pp. 73-81, ISSN 1721-727X
Lakota, K.; Mrak-Poljsak, K.; Rozman, B. & Sodin-Semrl, S. (2009). Increased responsiveness of human coronary artery endothelial cells in inflammation and coagulation. *Mediators Inflamm*, Vol.2009, (2009), pp. 146872, ISSN 1466-1861
Lehle, K.; Kunz-Schughart, L.A.; Kuhn, P.; Schreml, S.; Birnbaum, D.E. & Preuner, J.G. (2007). Validity of a patient-derived system of tissue-specific human endothelial cells: interleukin-6 as a surrogate marker in the coronary system. *Am J Physiol Heart Circ Physiol*, Vol.293, No.3, (September 2007), pp. H1721-1728, ISSN 0363-6135
Libby, P. (2002). Inflammation in atherosclerosis. *Nature*, Vol.420, No.6917, (December 2002), pp. 868-874, ISSN 0028-0836
Libby, P.; Ridker, P.M. & Hansson, G.K. (2011). Progress and challenges in translating the biology of atherosclerosis. *Nature*, Vol.473, No.7347, (May 2011), pp. 317-325, ISSN 1476-4687
Lloyd-Jones, D.M.; Wilson, P.W.; Larson, M.G.; Beiser, A.; Leip, E.P.; D'Agostino, R.B., et al. (2004). Framingham risk score and prediction of lifetime risk for coronary heart disease. *Am J Cardiol*, Vol.94, No.1, (July 2004), pp. 20-24, ISSN 0002-9149
Ludewig, B.; Krebs, P. & Scandella, E. (2004). Immunopathogenesis of atherosclerosis. *J Leukoc Biol*, Vol.76, No.2, (August 2004), pp. 300-306, ISSN 0741-5400
Luu, N.T.; Rahman, M.; Stone, P.C.; Rainger, G.E. & Nash, G.B. (2010). Responses of endothelial cells from different vessels to inflammatory cytokines and shear stress: evidence for the pliability of endothelial phenotype. *J Vasc Res*, Vol.47, No.5, (August 2010), pp. 451-461, ISSN 1423-0135
Malinow, M.R. (1983). Experimental models of atherosclerosis regression. *Atherosclerosis*, Vol.48, No.2, (August 1983), pp. 105-118, ISSN 0021-9150
Malle, E. & De Beer, F.C. (1996). Human serum amyloid A (SAA) protein: a prominent acute-phase reactant for clinical practice. *Eur J Clin Invest*, Vol.26, No.6, (June 1996), pp. 427-435, ISSN 0014-2972
Matsuura, E.; Kobayashi, K. & Lopez, L.R. (2009). Atherosclerosis in autoimmune diseases. *Curr Rheumatol Rep*, Vol.11, No.1, (February 2009), pp. 61-69, ISSN 1534-6307
Mayranpaa, M.I.; Heikkila, H.M.; Lindstedt, K.A.; Walls, A.F. & Kovanen, P.T. (2006). Desquamation of human coronary artery endothelium by human mast cell proteases: implications for plaque erosion. *Coron Artery Dis*, Vol.17, No.7, (November 2006), pp. 611-621, ISSN 0954-6928
Mehta, J.L.; Saldeen, T.G. & Rand, K. (1998). Interactive role of infection, inflammation and traditional risk factors in atherosclerosis and coronary artery disease. *J Am Coll Cardiol*, Vol.31, No.6, (May 1998), pp. 1217-1225, ISSN 0735-1097
Methe, H.; Balcells, M.; Alegret Mdel, C.; Santacana, M.; Molins, B.; Hamik, A., et al. (2007). Vascular bed origin dictates flow pattern regulation of endothelial adhesion molecule expression. *Am J Physiol Heart Circ Physiol*, Vol.292, No.5, (May 2007), pp. H2167-2175, ISSN 0363-6135
Moubayed, S.P.; Heinonen, T.M. & Tardif, J.C. (2007). Anti-inflammatory drugs and atherosclerosis. *Curr Opin Lipidol*, Vol.18, No.6, (December 2007), pp. 638-644, ISSN 0957-9672

Muhlestein, J.B.; Anderson, J.L.; Carlquist, J.F.; Salunkhe, K.; Horne, B.D.; Pearson, R.R., et al. (2000). Randomized secondary prevention trial of azithromycin in patients with coronary artery disease: primary clinical results of the ACADEMIC study. *Circulation*, Vol.102, No.15, (October 10 2000), pp. 1755-1760, ISSN 1524-4539

Mutin, M.; Canavy, I.; Blann, A.; Bory, M.; Sampol, J. & Dignat-George, F. (1999). Direct evidence of endothelial injury in acute myocardial infarction and unstable angina by demonstration of circulating endothelial cells. *Blood*, Vol.93, No.9, (May 1999), pp. 2951-2958, ISSN 0006-4971

Narshi, C.B.; Giles, I.P. & Rahman, A. (2011). The endothelium: an interface between autoimmunity and atherosclerosis in systemic lupus erythematosus? *Lupus*, Vol.20, No.1, (January 2011), pp. 5-13, ISSN 1477-0962

Nilsson, J.; Hansson, G.K. & Shah, P.K. (2005). Immunomodulation of atherosclerosis: implications for vaccine development. *Arterioscler Thromb Vasc Biol*, Vol.25, No.1, (January 2005), pp. 18-28, ISSN 1524-4636

Ott, S.J.; El Mokhtari, N.E.; Musfeldt, M.; Hellmig, S.; Freitag, S.; Rehman, A., et al. (2006). Detection of diverse bacterial signatures in atherosclerotic lesions of patients with coronary heart disease. *Circulation*, Vol.113, No.7, (February 2006), pp. 929-937, ISSN 1524-4539

Roger, V.L.; Go, A.S.; Lloyd-Jones, D.M.; Adams, R.J.; Berry, J.D.; Brown, T.M., et al. (2011). Heart disease and stroke statistics--2011 update: a report from the American Heart Association. *Circulation*, Vol.123, No.4, (February 2009 2011), pp. e18-e209, ISSN 1524-4539

Roman, M.J.; Shanker, B.A.; Davis, A.; Lockshin, M.D.; Sammaritano, L.; Simantov, R., et al. (2003). Prevalence and correlates of accelerated atherosclerosis in systemic lupus erythematosus. *N Engl J Med*, Vol.349, No.25, (December 2003), pp. 2399-2406, ISSN 1533-4406

Ronda, N. & Meroni, P.L. (2008). Accelerated Atherosclerosis in Autoimmune diseases, In. *Diagnostic Criteria in Autoimmune Diseases*, Shoenfeld, Y.; Cervera, R.& Gershwin, M. E., 383-388, Humana Press, ISBN 978-1-60327-284-1, Totowa

Ross, R. (1999). Atherosclerosis--an inflammatory disease. *N Engl J Med*, Vol.340, No.2, (January 1999), pp. 115-126, ISSN 0028-4793

Salmon, J.E. & Roman, M.J. (2008). Subclinical atherosclerosis in rheumatoid arthritis and systemic lupus erythematosus. *Am J Med*, Vol.121, No.10 Suppl 1, (October 2008), pp. S3-8, ISSN 1555-7162

Sander, D.; Winbeck, K.; Klingelhofer, J.; Etgen, T. & Conrad, B. (2002). Reduced progression of early carotid atherosclerosis after antibiotic treatment and Chlamydia pneumoniae seropositivity. *Circulation*, Vol.106, No.19, (November 5 2002), pp. 2428-2433, ISSN 1524-4539

Sherer, Y. & Shoenfeld, Y. (2006). Mechanisms of disease: atherosclerosis in autoimmune diseases. *Nat Clin Pract Rheumatol*, Vol.2, No.2, (February 2006), pp. 99-106, ISSN 1745-8382

Shoenfeld, Y.; Gerli, R.; Doria, A.; Matsuura, E.; Cerinic, M.M.; Ronda, N., et al. (2005). Accelerated atherosclerosis in autoimmune rheumatic diseases. *Circulation*, Vol.112, No.21, (November 2005), pp. 3337-3347, ISSN 1524-4539

Shoenfeld, Y.; Sherer, Y. & Harats, D. (2001). Artherosclerosis as an infectious, inflammatory and autoimmune disease. *Trends Immunol*, Vol.22, No.6, (June 2001), pp. 293-295, ISSN 1471-4906

Stoltz, J.F.; Muller, S.; Kadi, A.; Decot, V.; Menu, P. & Bensoussan, D. (2007). Introduction to endothelial cell biology. *Clin Hemorheol Microcirc*, Vol.37, No.1-2, (June 2007), pp. 5-8, ISSN 1386-0291

Szostak, J. & Laurant, P. (2011). The forgotten face of regular physical exercise: a 'natural' anti-atherogenic activity. *Clin Sci (Lond)*, Vol.121, No.3, (August 2011), pp. 91-106, ISSN 1470-8736

Tegos, T.J.; Kalodiki, E.; Sabetai, M.M. & Nicolaides, A.N. (2001). The genesis of atherosclerosis and risk factors: a review. *Angiology*, Vol.52, No.2, (February 2001), pp. 89-98, ISSN 0003-3197

Tincani, A.; Rebaioli, C.B.; Taglietti, M. & Shoenfeld, Y. (2006). Heart involvement in systemic lupus erythematosus, anti-phospholipid syndrome and neonatal lupus. *Rheumatology (Oxford)*, Vol.45 Suppl 4, (October 2006), pp. iv8-13, ISSN 1462-0332

Vallejo, J.G. (2011). Role of toll-like receptors in cardiovascular diseases. *Clin Sci (Lond)*, Vol.121, No.1, (July 2011), pp. 1-10, ISSN 1470-8736

Vaudo, G.; Bocci, E.B.; Shoenfeld, Y.; Schillaci, G.; Wu, R.; Del Papa, N., et al. (2005). Precocious intima-media thickening in patients with primary Sjogren's syndrome. *Arthritis Rheum*, Vol.52, No.12, (December 2005), pp. 3890-3897, ISSN 0004-3591

Viemann, D.; Goebeler, M.; Schmid, S.; Nordhues, U.; Klimmek, K.; Sorg, C., et al. (2006). TNF induces distinct gene expression programs in microvascular and macrovascular human endothelial cells. *J Leukoc Biol*, Vol.80, No.1, (July 2006), pp. 174-185, ISSN 0741-5400

Vilahur, G.; Padro, T. & Badimon, L. (2011). Atherosclerosis and thrombosis: insights from large animal models. *J Biomed Biotechnol*, Vol.2011, (n.d. 2011), pp. ID 907575, ISSN 1110-7251

Wick, G. & et al. (2006). Atherosclerosis: autoimmunity to heat-shock proteins, In. *The autoimmune diseases*, Rose, N. R.& Mackay, I. R., 889-897, Academic Press, ISBN-13 978-0-12-595961-2, San Diego

Williams, K.J.; Feig, J.E. & Fisher, E.A. (2008). Rapid regression of atherosclerosis: insights from the clinical and experimental literature. *Nat Clin Pract Cardiovasc Med*, Vol.5, No.2, (February 2008), pp. 91-102, ISSN 1743-4300

Wilson, H.M. (2010). Macrophages heterogeneity in atherosclerosis - implications for therapy. *J Cell Mol Med*, Vol.14, No.8, (August 2010), pp. 2055-2065, ISSN 1582-4934

Wu, J.T. & Wu, L.L. (2005). Association of soluble markers with various stages and major events of atherosclerosis. *Ann Clin Lab Sci*, Vol.35, No.3, (Summer 2005), pp. 240-250, ISSN 0091-7370

Wu, R. & Lefvert, A.K. (1995). Autoantibodies against oxidized low density lipoproteins (oxLDL): characterization of antibody isotype, subclass, affinity and effect on the macrophage uptake of oxLDL. *Clin Exp Immunol*, Vol.102, No.1, (October 1995), pp. 174-180, ISSN 0009-9104

Yano, K.; Gale, D.; Massberg, S.; Cheruvu, P.K.; Monahan-Earley, R.; Morgan, E.S., et al. (2007). Phenotypic heterogeneity is an evolutionarily conserved feature of the endothelium. *Blood*, Vol.109, No.2, (January 2007), pp. 613-615, ISSN 0006-4971

Zimmerman, M.R. (1998). Aleutian and Alaskan mummies, In. *Mummies, Disease and Ancient Cultures*, Cockburn, A.; Cockburn, E.& Reyman, T. A., 138-141, University Press, ISBN-13 9780521589543, Cambridge

Zinger, H.; Sherer, Y. & Shoenfeld, Y. (2009). Atherosclerosis in autoimmune rheumatic diseases-mechanisms and clinical findings. *Clin Rev Allergy Immunol*, Vol.37, No.1, (August 2009), pp. 20-28, ISSN 1559-0267

# 10

# Mechanisms of Leukocyte Recruitment Into the Aorta During Atherosclerosis

Matthew J. Butcher and Elena Galkina
*Eastern Virginia Medical School*
*United States of America*

## 1. Introduction

Atherosclerosis continues to be the leading cause of cardiovascular disease. Atherosclerotic lesion progression depends on chronic inflammation in the aorta and the immune response is involved in this process (Galkina & Ley, 2009; Hansson & Hermansson, 2011). While it is now generally accepted that chronic inflammation of the arterial wall, precipitated by an immune response targeting modified low density lipoproteins, heat shock protein 60, β2-glycoprotein I, and other self-antigens, underlies the pathophysiology of atherosclerosis, this notion was met with scepticism historically.

The term atherosclerosis was first introduced by the French surgeon and pathologist Jean Lobstein in 1829. Within a few years the associated cellular immune alterations in the arteries of atherosclerotic cadavers were described by two schools of pathology yielding two theories on the pathology atherosclerosis. Carl von Rokitansky proposed that initial injury of the aorta preceded the cellular inflammatory changes, suggesting a secondary role for aortic leukocytes. In contrast, Rudolf Virchow postulated an initiating role for aortic cellular conglomerates (Methe & Weis, 2007; Mayerl et al., 2006). However, despite these observations, the response-to- injury model of atherosclerosis prevailed in the literature until the early 1980s. In 1979, the presence of monocytes adhering to the endothelial layer of porcine and human atheroma was demonstarted (Gerrity & Naito, 1980). In 1980, expression of HLA-DR by vascular endothelial cells was reported (Hirschberg et al., 1980). It was also found that interferon-γ (IFN-γ) potently induced MHC-II expression on cultured endothelial cells, suggesting that T cell-derived cytokines may play an important role in the vasculature (Pober et al., 1983). In 1985 and 1986, the presence of HLA-$DR^+$ cells, $CD4^+$ and $CD8^+$ T cells in carotid entarterectomy specimens was reported, further implicating that a cellular immune response occurs in atherosclerosis (Jonasson et al., 1985; Jonasson et al., 1986). Since these initial findings a plethora of recent papers have further highlighted the presence of multiple subsets of leukocytes in aortas, and demonstrated the importance of the immune system during atherogenesis. The occurrence of inflammatory cells in the aorta depends on the dynamics of their recruitment and possibly egress, as well as the balance between proliferation, survival, and apoptosis within the aorta. To date, several adhesion molecules and chemokines, which support subset-specific leukocyte homing into the aorta, have been identified, but questions concerning the role of the adventitial vasa vasorum in leukocyte homing, kinetics and the specific mechanisms of migration of different cell subsets including B cells, T cells, mast cells, Treg and Th17 cells remain to be answered.

## 2. Multiple steps of the adhesion cascade

Peripheral blood leukocytes are programmed to constitutively home to secondary lymphoid organs in search of possible antigens, in order to mount an appropriate immune response against infections. It has also been recognized that a small subset of leukocytes home into non-lymphoid tissues as a part of constitutive homing in order to sample antigens in local tissues. In line with this notion, leukocytes are found within normal/non-inflamed aortas and recent studies have demonstrated that these cells constitutively migrate into the aorta. The migration of leukocytes into non-lymphoid sites where injury, infection or inflammation has occurred is also highly specific. To date, there are several examples of immune-mediated chronic diseases such as rheumatoid arthritis, Type 1 diabetes mellitus, psoriasis, and multiple sclerosis that have marked adhesion molecule-mediated homing of leukocytes into the site of inflammation. It is now appreciated that atherosclerosis-prone conditions activate aortic vascular cells, upregulate adhesion molecules, and chemokines; thereby supporting leukocyte homing into the aorta (Galkina & Ley, 2007a) – a key step in the pathology of atherosclerosis.

### 2.1 Steps of the adhesion cascade

#### 2.1.1 Selectins and rolling

The adhesion cascade is defined as series of overlapping and synergistic interactions among adhesion molecules and chemokines. There are several major steps of the leukocyte adhesion cascade including selectin–dependent tethering and rolling, selectin or arrest chemokine-dependent activation, integrin-dependent arrest, firm adhesion and diapedesis, which are closely interconnected and regulate cell-specific migration. The first steps of the adhesion cascade consist of tethering, capture, and rolling, which are initiated via selectin-carbohydrate ligand interactions along the endothelium (McEver, 2002). L-selectin is expressed by all leukocytes, mediates leukocyte rolling and can also participate in secondary capture, defined as leukocyte capture by adherent leukocytes (reviewed in (Ley et al., 2007)). P- and E-selectin are expressed by the activated endothelium and serve as rolling molecules for most leukocytes (McEver, 2002). Activated platelets also express P-selectin. P-selecin binds PSGL-1 expressing neutrophils, monocytes, and lymphocytes (Ley & Kansas, 2004). E-selectin binds PSGL-1, CD44, E-selectin ligand-1(ESL-1) on myeloid cells and CD43 on T-helper 1 lymphocytes (reviewed in (Ley et al., 2007)). Selectins tightly control leukocyte rolling velocity via regulation of the rapid formation and dissociation of bonds between selectins and their ligands (Alon et al., 1997). L- and P-selectin support rolling at relatively fast velocities, while E-selectin supports leukocyte rolling at very slow velocities (Kunkel & Ley, 1996). Evidence suggests that selectin ligation by endothelial ligands can induce activation of integrins, and provide a link between rolling and the subsequent integrin-mediated firm adhesion (Zarbock et al., 2007).

#### 2.1.2 Integrins, arrest chemokines, and firm adhesion

Following the steps of tethering and rolling, leukocyte integrins initiate slowing rolling, and induce further firm adhesion. The integrin family consists of $\alpha$ and $\beta$ subunits that form heterodimers yielding a total of 24 integrins (Hynes, 2002). All leukocytes express leukocyte function-associated molecule (LFA-1, CD11a/CD18, or $\alpha$-L$\beta$2), while myeloid cells predominately express Mac-1. Endothelial ligands for LFA-1 and Mac-1 include intercellular adhesion molecule 1 (ICAM-1) and ICAM-2. The $\alpha_4\beta_1$ (VLA-4) integrin is a member of the $\alpha_4$

subfamily and is mostly expressed on extralymphoid monocytes and on lymphocytes (Luster et al., 2005). Vascular cell adhesion molecule-1 (VCAM-1) (Kinashi, 2007) and the CS-1 peptide of fibronectin (Guan & Hynes, 1990) serve as ligands for VLA-4. VCAM-1 is not constitutively expressed in most tissues, but is upregulated after stimulation with TNF-$\alpha$ and IL-1. Chemokines support migration via the formation of chemotactic gradients from emigrated leukocytes and resident tissue cells. Endothelial cells synthesize and present chemokines on the luminal surface. Most chemokines can be also immobilized by extracellular matrix components, including heparan sulfate and glycosaminoglycans, and presented to leukocytes (Ley et al., 2007). Several members of a specialized group of arrest chemokines play an essential role in integrin activation and firm adhesion.

### 2.1.3 JAMs, PECAM-1, VE-Cadherin and transmigration

Increased time of firm leukocyte adhesion reduces rolling velocities, and initiates cell crawling or locomotion in order to find an appropriate site for transmigration/diapedesis. There are two principal mechanisms of transmigration: via intercellular junctions or through the endothelial cell body (Carman & Springer, 2004; Shaw et al., 2004). To date, it is unclear which parameters preferentially affect the pathways of transmigration. CD99-related antigen (CD99L2), endothelial cell-selective adhesion molecule (ESAM) and junctional adhesion molecules (JAMs) are important regulators of diapedesis. JAMs belong to the members of immunoglobulin superfamily, which are localized to intercellular junctions of polarized endothelial and epithelial cells, but are also expressed on circulating leukocytes and platelets (Mandell & Parkos, 2005). JAMs participate in homophilic and heterophilic cell interactions, and thus, support the extravasation of leukocytes into tissues. JAM-A binds to LFA-1, JAM-B to VLA-4, and JAM-C to Mac-1 (Vestweber, 2007). VE-cadherin is expressed between endothelial cells and serves as a barrier for extravasating leukocytes *in vivo* (Lampugnani et al., 1992). ICAM-1 and ICAM-2 can also participate in leukocyte transmigration through the development of the specific structures that surround leukocytes during transmigration (Carman & Springer, 2004), and/or form ring-like clusters of LFA-1 at the interface between the transmigrating leukocyte and endothelial junctions (Shaw et al., 2004). Platelet endothelial cell adhesion molecule-1 (PECAM-1) is a member of the immunoglobulin superfamily that is expressed on leukocytes, platelets, and interendothelial junctions. PECAM-1 promotes leukocyte transmigration as an adhesion molecule (Newman, 1997), but can also serve as a signaling receptor (Vestweber, 2007).

## 3. Regulators of adhesion molecule expression in atherogenesis

Many inflammatory factors such as multiple cytokines, 5-lipoxygenase, 12/15-lipoxygenase, heme oxygenase-1, paraoxonases, C-reactive protein, reactive oxygen species, advanced glycation end products (AGE), oxidized-LDL, and blood flow conditions (reviewed by (Tedgui & Mallat, 2006; Galkina & Ley, 2009), play crucial roles during atherogenesis. One of the many essential functions of these factors is the induction and the regulation of the expression of adhesion molecules and chemokines. As these factors have been reviewed in depth elsewhere (Galkina & 2009; Tedgui & Mallat, 2006), we will focus briefly only on some inflammatory molecules and conditions that have been demonstrated to affect the expression of adhesion molecules and chemokines within the vasculature.

### 3.1 Effects of cytokines on the expression of aortic adhesion molecules and chemokines

#### 3.1.1 TNFα and the TNFα superfamily

The pro-inflammatory effects of TNF-α in atherogenesis are well established. TNF-α upregulates a variety of adhesion proteins, including LFA-1, VCAM-1, and ICAM-1 on human endothelial cells *in vitro* (Sprague & Khalil, 2009). Cleavage, but not the membrane bound form of TNF-α, is required for TNFα's pro-atherogenic properties. Mast-cell-, MΦ-, and neutrophil-derived TNF-α and IL-6 similarly promote the expression of several adhesion molecules, including VCAM-1, ICAM-1, P- and E-selectin, in endothelial cells and further support the adherence of neutrophils under physiological shear stress conditions (Zhang et al., 2011). Another member of the TNF superfamily, Lymphotoxin-β (LTβ), can similarly promote CXCL13 and CCL21 induction in medial smooth muscle cells (Grabner et al., 2009). In addition, further investigation into the mechanisms behind LTβ-receptor mediated production of CXCL13 and CCL21 by smooth muscle cells revealed a synergistic interaction between TNF-α and LTβ-β mediated activation of the NF-κB pathway that led in elevated expression of multiple chemokines in smooth muscle cells (Lötzer, et al. 2010).

#### 3.1.2 The interleukin-17 family

Recently, several studies have demonstrated the presence of Th17 and other IL-17A$^+$ cells within murine and human atherosclerotic tissues (Ait-Oufella et al., 2011). Th17 and other IL-17A$^+$ T cells play critical roles in the defence against extracellular bacteria and fungi, but also promote inflammation in multiple autoimmune disorders through the production of several chemokines by IL-17 receptor expressing resident epithelial, endothelial cells, and fibroblasts. IL-17A may similarly be involved in atherogenesis through the production of multiple chemokines and adhesion molecules; however, the exact role of this cytokine is currently contested.

### 3.2 The effect of other inflammatory factors and flow conditions on the expression of adhesion molecules and chemokines

#### 3.2.1 Modified LDL

In addition to oxLDL's antigenic properties and its ability to induce foam cell formation and endothelial cell dysfunction, several studies have demonstrated that modified LDL may also directly affect the expression of adhesion molecules, and thereby affect the recruitment of leukocytes to the aorta. OxLDL can be trapped beneath the subendothelial matrix via heparin sulphate-dependent binding *in vivo* (Pillarisetti et al., 1997) and thus, locally affect vascular cells. OxLDL promotes P-selectin expression in activated human aortic endothelial cells (Gebuhrer et al., 1995), and monocyte transmigration through human umbilical vein endothelial cell layers (Hashimoto et al., 2007). Similarly, modified (Keiper et al., 2005; Parhami et al., 1993) or enzymatically degraded LDL (Klouche et al., 1999) induces CCL2, CXCL1, ICAM-1, PECAM-1, JAM-C, P- and E-selectin in endothelial cells *in vitro.* Several studies have demonstrated that lysophosphatidylcholine (LysoPTdCho), a component of oxidized LDL, functions as a chemotactic factor for monocytes (Quinn et al. 1988), and neutrophils (Murugesan et al. 2003), both directly (Quinn et al. 1987), and via regulation of endothelial VCAM-1, ICAM-1 (Kume et al. 1992), CCL2, and IL-8 (Murugesan et al. 2003).

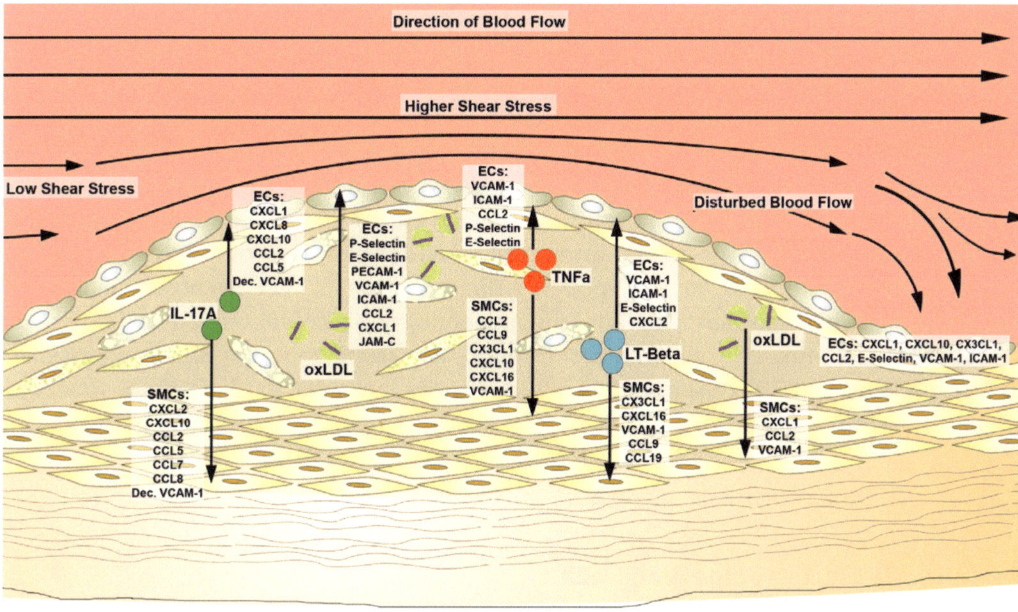


Fig. 1. Regulators of adhesion molecule expression.

Several factors that may affect the expression of adhesion molecules during atherogenesis are shown. Multiple cytokines upregulate adhesion molecule expression in endothelial and smooth muscle cells. In addition, other pro-inflammatory conditions such as low shear stress, oscillatory blood flow (arrows, right), modified LDL, ROS and AGE (not shown) regulate endothelial and smooth muscle cell adhesion molecules. "Dec." denotes adhesion molecules that have been demonstrated to be down regulated.

### 3.2.2 Flow conditions

Flow conditions at branching points of the vasculature may also affect the expression of adhesion molecules and account for anatomical variations in the sites of atherogenesis (VanderLaan et al., 2004). Shear stress, the force that acts on the endothelium as a result of blood flow, plays a critical role in the development of endothelial dysfunction and atherosclerosis. Areas of coronary arties that exhibit low shear stress or areas where shear stress is oscillatory frequently contain atherosclerotic plaques (Davies et al., 2002; Pedersen et al., 1999). There are multiple lines of evidence indicating that the areas of low shear stress or oscillatory flow conditions display changes in the expression of adhesion molecules. Indeed, human aortic endothelial cell culture with oscillatory flow conditions *in vitro* upregulate VCAM-1 and ICAM-1 (Brooks et al., 2002). Similarly, in an *in vivo* model of oscillatory flow using a common carotid artery cast in *Apoe*$^{-/-}$ mice, several chemokines were upregulated in areas of low shear stress (CCL2, CXCL1, CXCL10, and CX3CL1) and oscillatory shear stress (CCL2, and CXCL1) (Cheng et al., 2007). Furthermore, in a study examining the response of endothelial cells to changes in shear stress, HAECs pre-stimulated with TNF-α and simultaneously exposed to a linear gradient of shear stress (0-16 dyne/cm$^2$) resulted in the upregulation of VCAM-1, E-Selectin under lower shear stress conditions and ICAM-1 under high shear stress conditions (Tsou et al., 2008).

### 3.3 Soluble adhesion molecules and atherosclerosis

Multiple studies have demonstrated that soluble adhesion molecules, including sE-Selectin, sP-Selectin, sL-Selectin, sVCAM-1, sICAM-1, sCD40, and sCD40L, are elevated within the plasma of coronary artery disease patients and are associated with the severity of stenosis, as well as, several atherosclerotic disease risk factors including smoking, obesity, diabetes, hypertension, etc (reviewed in Roldan, et al. 2003). However, the functional relevance of these soluble adhesion molecules is currently unclear. Increased levels of soluble adhesion molecules may arise from cytokine-stimulated shedding, enzymatic cleavage, loss of membrane integrity, necrosis, and/or apoptosis (Pigot et al., 1992; Leeuwenbern, et al. 1992; Newman, et al., 1993), and may play a role in antagonizing leukocyte recruitment (Tu, et al. 2001) or promote leukocyte recruitment through the formation of cellular aggregates. Ultimately, additional mechanistic studies will be required in order to pinpoint the functions of these soluble forms *in vivo.*

## 4. Leukocyte migration into aortas

### 4.1 Monocytes

#### 4.1.1 Monocyte homing to the aortic wall

Monocytes play a key role in atherosclerosis (reviewed in (Galkina & Ley, 2009; Hansson & Hermansson, 2011)). Monocytes migrate into the sub-endothelial space of the aortic intima, where they differentiate into MΦ (Gerrity and Naito, 1980; Jonasson et al., 1986), and dendritic cells (Bobryshev and Lord, 1998). Although it has not been shown directly, some data suggest that environmental signals within the blood and aortas determine the differentiation programs that give rise to MΦ or dendritic cells in the aorta. Monocyte accumulation is progressive and proportional to the extent of atherosclerosis (Swirski et al., 2006). Monocyte-derived cells are found in both the aortic adventitia and in atherosclerotic lesions. Similar frequencies of adoptively transferred allelic CD45 isoform monocytes and recipient monocytes were found within the carotid lesions, but not the adventitia of recipients; suggesting that MΦ-derived foam cells arise mainly from blood-derived monocytes rather than resident MΦ (Lessner et al., 2002). Whether or not adventitial MΦ include a self-renewing pool remains unclear. The spleen can also serve as a reservoir of monocytes (Swirski et al., 2009). The role of splenic monocytes in atherosclerosis remains to be determined.

P-selectin was one of the first adhesion molecules that clearly showed its involvement in monocyte recruitment into the aorta. Blockade of P-selectin resulted in reduced monocyte rolling and attachment to the carotid endothelium (Ramos et al., 1999). Further experiments demonstrated that P-selectin deficiency caused a decrease in fatty streaks and reduction in MΦ numbers within the plaques (Table I). E-selectin expression is elevated within atherosclerotic aortas, and E-selectin deficiency causes slightly reduced plaque burden (Collins et al., 2000). There is a functional overlap between E-selectin and P-selectin as combined deficiency in E- and P-selectin decreases atherosclerosis by 80% (Dong et al., 1998). Recently, a potential role for β2 and β3 integrins and an intracellular protein-thrombopspondin (TSP)-4 in monocyte migration was proposed. Deficiency in TSP-4 lead to reduced number of lesional MΦ, and decreased β2 and β3 integrin-dependent MΦ adhesion and migration *in vitro* (Frolova et al., 2010).

VCAM-1 is a central adhesion molecule that supports slow rolling and tight adhesion of monocytes to the atherosclerotic endothelium. Blockade of VCAM-1 or $\alpha_4$ integrins resulted in increased rolling velocity and attenuated adhesion of monocytes in *ex vivo* models of isolated perfused carotid arteries (Huo et al., 2000; Ramos et al., 1999). Blockade of $\alpha_4$ integrin using blocking Abs showed reduced influx of MΦ into plaques (Patel et al., 1998). Since VCAM-1-deficient mice are not viable, mice in which the fourth Ig domain of VCAM-1 was disrupted (*Vcam-1*$^{D4D/D4D}$) were generated (Cybulsky et al., 2001). Reduced levels of VCAM-1 resulted in the reduction of atherogenesis in *Vcam1*$^{D4D/D4D}$*Ldlr*$^{-/-}$ mice (Cybulsky et al., 2001). VCAM-1 levels affect plaque formation, since *Vcam-1*$^{D4D/+}$*Apoe*$^{-/-}$ mice showed a gene-dosage dependent influx of monocytes and plaque burden (Dansky et al., 2001).

Evidence suggests that several arrest chemokines expressed on the endothelium initiate integrin activation and firm leukocyte adhesion. CXCL1 (Huo et al., 2001) and CCL5 (Huo et al., 2003) either alone or as a heterodimer with CXCL4 (von Hundelshausen et al., 2005) have been discovered as aortic arrest chemokines for monocyte adhesion. CXCL1 and CCL5 and their receptors CXCR2 and CCR5 promote monocyte arrest on the atherosclerotic endothelium in the flow chamber system (Huo et al., 2001; Huo et al., 2003; Weber et al., 1999). CXCL7 also efficiently triggers monocyte arrest to the inflamed endothelium under flow conditions (Baltus et al., 2005). Migration inhibitory factor (MIF) regulates monocyte arrest via the interaction of the CXCR2/CD74 complex expressed on monocytes with MIF-expressing atherosclerotic endothelium (Bernhagen et al., 2007). Additionally, MIF deficiency or the blockade of MIF with anti-MIF Abs resulted in reduced lipid deposition, intimal thickening and MΦ infiltration in the aorta (Pan et al., 2004; Burger-Kentischer et al., 2006).

CCL2 is one of the key chemokines in monocyte biology. Classical CCR2$^{+}$ monocytes exit the bone marrow in a CCL-2-dependent manner, and both CCL2 and CCL7 maintain monocyte homeostasis in the circulation (Serbina & Pamer, 2006; Tsou et al., 2007). Several studies suggest that the CCL2/CCR2 axis participates in atherogenesis by the modulation of monocyte recruitment into the aorta (Boring et al., 1998; Dawson et al., 1999; Gosling et al., 1999; Gu et al., 1998). Interestingly, since CCL2 has no effects on monocyte arrest on the early atherosclerotic endothelium (Huo et al., 2001), CCL2 may function as a regulator of monocytes egress from bone marrow or chemokine that regulates monocyte transmigration.

Deficiency of JAM-A reduces monocyte arrest and transmigration on activated JAM-A-deficient endothelial cells under flow conditions *in vitro*, and attenuates neointimal formation (Zernecke et al., 2006). In line with this notion, JAM-A is involved in monocyte adhesion to isolated perfused *Apoe*$^{-/-}$ carotid arteries (Ostermann et al., 2005). JAM-C blockade decreases neointimal MΦ content and reduces neointimal hyperplasia indicating a potential role of JAM-C in the regulation of monocyte transmigration (Shagdarsuren et al., 2009). Inactivation of ESAM-1 leads to diminished transmigration of THP-1 cells in *in vitro* assays, and ESAM-deficient *Apoe*$^{-/-}$ mice display attenuated atherosclerosis (Inoue et al., 2010). It is interesting that not only the adhesion molecules, but also one of the scavenger receptors – CD36 regulates MΦ migration. CD36 signaling in response to oxLDL alters cytoskeletal dynamics and inhibits the migration of MΦs. This may be one of the mechanisms of MΦ accumulation in aortic lipid-rich areas (Park et al., 2009).

| Leukocyte type | Adhesion molecules, chemokine receptors | Effects | References |
|---|---|---|---|
| Monocytes, selectins | P-selectin (rolling) | Reduced rolling and attachment with anti-P-selectin or PSGL-1 Abs (an ex vivo model of isolated carotid arteries).<br>Reduced lesion size and MΦ content (Selp$^{-/-}$ mice on C57BL/6, Ldlr$^{-/-}$, and Apoe$^{-/-}$ background). | (Ramos et al., 1999)<br>(Collins et al., 2000; Dong et al., 2000; Johnson et al., 1997; Nageh et al., 1997) |
| | E-selectin (rolling) | Slightly reduced lesions (Sele$^{-/-}$Apoe$^{-/-}$ mice).<br>Reduced lesions for all stages of atherogenesis (Selp$^{-/-}$Sele$^{-/-}$Ldlr$^{-/-}$ mice). | (Collins et al., 2000)<br>(Dong et al., 1998) |
| Monocytes, integrins | VCAM-1/VLA-4 (adhesion) | Increased rolling velocities with anti-VCAM-1 or anti-$\alpha_4$ integrin Abs. Increased rolling velocities and decrease adhesion by blocking of VLA-4 binding to both VCAM-1 and fibronectin connecting segment-1 (both, an ex vivo model of isolated perfused carotid arteries). Blockade of VLA-4 with anti-VLA-4 Abs decreases monocyte migration in vivo.<br>Reduced early atherosclerotic lesions (Vcam-1$^{D4D/D4D}$Ldlr$^{-/-}$ mice).<br>Gene-dosage dependent influx of monocytes and lesion development (Vcam-1$^{D4D/+}$ Apoe$^{-/-}$ mice). | (Huo et al., 2000; Ramos et al., 1999)<br>(Patel et al., 1998)<br>(Cybulsky et al., 2001)<br>(Dansky et al., 2001) |
| | ICAM-1 (adhesion) | Decreased short-term monocyte migration into plaques by blocking Abs to ICAM-1 (Apoe$^{-/-}$ mice). Reduced lesions in Itgb2$^{-/-}$ and Icam-1$^{-/-}$Itgb2$^{-/-}$ (C57BL/6 mice on WD). | (Patel et al., 1998)<br>(Nageh et al., 1997) |
| Monocytes, chemokines | migration/arrest<br>CXCL1, CCL5<br>CCL5/CXCL4<br>CXCL7<br>MIF | Monocyte arrest in the flow chamber assay.<br>Interactions via CXCL2/CD74 complex induce integrin activation.<br>MIF deficiency reduces lipid deposition, and MΦ infiltration in the aorta.<br>Reduced MΦ content in Apoe$^{-/-}$ mice that received neutralizing Abs to MIF. | (Huo et al., 2001; Weber et al., 1999; von Hundelshausen et al., 2005)<br>(Bernhagen et al., 2007b), (Pan et al., 2004; Burger-Kentischer et al., 2006) |
| Monocytes<br>JAM-A (transmigration)<br>JAM-C (transmigration)<br>CD36 | JAMs<br>CD36 | Reduced monocyte arrest and transmigration on activated F11r$^{-/-}$/Apoe$^{-/-}$ endothelial cells in the flow chamber assays; wire injury of carotid artery .<br>JAM-C Ab blockade decreases neointimal MΦ after wire injury of carotid arteries.<br>Regulate oxLDL-induced cytoskeletal dynamics to inhibit migration and enhance MΦ spreading. Adhesion and migration assays with Cd36$^{-/-}$ monocytes in vitro. | (Zernecke et al., 2006)<br>(Shagdarsuren et al., 2009)<br>(Park et al., 2009) |
| Inflammatory and Patrolling monocytes | CCR5<br>CCR2, CX3CR1, CCR5 | CCR5 blockade with neutralizing Abs, Ccr2$^{-/-}$ and Cx3cr1$^{-/-}$monocytes in the homing experiments using latex beads technology to distinguish between monocyte subsets. | (Swirski et al., 2007; Tacke et al., 2007) |
| Possible egress | CCR7 | Blockade of CD68$^{+}$ cell regression by blocking Abs to CCL19 and CCL21 or CCR7 deficiency in transplantational model of atherosclerosis. | (Feig et al., 2010; Trogan et al., 2006) |
| T cells | L-selectin (Rolling) | Reduced migration of Sele$^{-/-}$ T cells into aortas of C57BL/6 and Apoe$^{-/-}$ mice (adoptive transfers). L-selectin deficiency reduces primary and secondary capture (intravital microscopy of femoral arteries). | (Galkina et al., 2006)<br>(Eriksson et al., 2001) |
| | CCL5 (adhesion/migration) | Reduced content of CD4 and Th1-related Tim3 expression in Ccr5$^{-/-}$Apoe$^{-/-}$ mice. | (Braunersreuther et al., 2007; Feig et al., 2010)<br>(Heller et al., 2006) |
| | CXCL10 (adhesion/migration) | Cxcl10$^{-/-}$/Apoe$^{-/-}$ T cells into aortas were significantly reduced. | (Galkina et al., 2007; Aslanian & Charo, 2006) |
| | CXCR6<br>CXCL16 (adhesion/migration) | Reduced migration of Cxcr6$^{-/-}$ T cells into atherosclerotic aortas. But increased atherogenesis in Cxcl16$^{-/-}$Apoe$^{-/-}$ mice. | |
| | MIF (adhesion/migration) | Blockade of MIF with neutralizing Abs resulted in diminished number of T cells within the aortas and reduction of atherosclerosis in Apoe$^{-/-}$ mice. | (Bernhagen et al., 2007a) |
| | CCR7 (entry/egress) | Ccr7$^{-/-}$Ldlr$^{-/-}$ mice have reduced number of T cells in atherosclerotic lesions. | (Luchtefeld et al., 2010) |
| B cells | L-selectin (rolling) | Reduced homing of adoptively transferred L-selectin-deficient B cells into normal and atherosclerotic aortas. | (Galkina et al., 2006) |
| Neutrophils | CXCL12/CXCR4 (migration/adhesion) | Blockade of CXCL12/CXCR4 by a small-molecule agonist, CxcR4 deficiency results in leukocytosis and increased neutrophil content in the plaques of Ldlr$^{-/-}$ mice. | (Zernecke et al., 2008) |
| | CCL2, CCL5 (migration/adhesion) | Impaired migration of Ccr1, CCr2, CCr5 and Cxcr2-deficient neutrophils into atherosclerotic plaques of Apoe$^{-/-}$ mice. | (Drechsler et al., 2010) |

Table 1. Adhesion molecules and chemokine receptors that are involved in the recruitment of leukocytes into the aortic wall. (Adapted from (Galkina & Ley, 2007))

Two subsets of human monocytes representing $CD14^{high}$ and $CD14^{+}CD16^{+}$ cells have been described (Passlick et al., 1989), and a new additional subset of $CD14^{dim}$ human monocytes that patrols blood vessels has been added (Cros et al., 2010). Similarly, there are two distinct subsets of blood circulating murine monocytes: $Ly6C^{high}/CCR2^{+}/CX3CR1^{low}$ inflammatory monocytes and $Ly6C^{low}/CCR2^{-}/CX3CR1^{high}$ monocytes (Geissmann et al., 2003). Both circulate through lymphoid and non-lymphoid organs under homeostatic conditions (Geissmann et al., 2003; Tacke et al., 2007). Hypercholesterolemia induces monocytosis in *Apoe*$^{-/-}$ mice with a predominant increase in the numbers of $Ly6C^{high}$ monocytes (Swirski et al., 2007; Tacke et al., 2007). As different repertoires of chemokine receptors and adhesion molecules are expressed by each monocyte subset, these cells use different mechanisms to traffic into the aorta. $Ly6C^{low}$ monocytes enter the atherosclerotic wall in a CCR5-dependent manner, but do not require CX3CR1 or CCR2 (Tacke et al., 2007). Surprisingly, $Ly6C^{high}/CCR2^{+}$ monocytes require not only CCR2, but also CX3CR1 and CCR5 for their recruitment into the aorta (Tacke et al., 2007). Monocyte subsets also differently express several adhesion molecules, which can affect their homing capacity. L-selectin is expressed by $Ly6C^{high}$ monocytes and likely provides primary and secondary capture of monocytes to the endothelium. $Ly6C^{low}$ monocytes express low levels of L-selectin and CD54, but elevated levels of CD43 (Sunderkotter et al., 2004). Endothelial E-selectin may provide initial rolling of $Ly6C^{low}$ monocytes on endothelium. Further understanding of the pathways that govern the recruitment of monocyte subsets into atherosclerotic aorta is crucial to advance our efforts to reduce the frequency of aortic pro-inflammatory monocytes/macrophages and thus, further aortic chronic inflammation.

### 4.1.2 Egress of macrophages and dendritic cells from atherosclerotic aortas

Elevated levels of monocyte-derived cells in atherosclerotic plaques could be the result of several processes including: 1) hyperlipidemia-induced monocytosis and increased monocyte recruitment, 2) increased proliferation, 3) altered balance of survival/apoptosis/clearance, 4) attenuated egress from the aorta. Evidence suggests that reduced numbers of plaque MFs orchestrate the regression of atherosclerosis repression; however, the cellular and molecular mechanisms underlying this process are not well understood. One of the first studies that focused on the potential mechanisms of MΦ and dendritic cell egress from atherosclerotic plaques were performed using a surgical model of plaque regression. In this model, plaque-bearing aortas from *Apoe*$^{-/-}$ donor mice were transplanted into *C57BL/6* mice with low levels of circulating cholesterol, such that the surgically transferred segment became a functional segment of the recipient's aorta (Llodra et al., 2004). Significant migration of $CD68^{+}$ cells out of the plaque was detected in *C57BL/6* recipients, whereas little emigration was detected from progressive plaques in *Apoe*$^{-/-}$ recipients (Llodra et al., 2004). Further experiments determined a role of the chemokine receptor CCR7 (Trogan et al., 2006). Liver X receptor α (LXRα) and LXRβ— are nuclear hormone receptors that play key roles in maintaining cholesterol homeostasis in MΦ, primarily by regulating multiple components of the reverse cholesterol transport pathway (Bradley & Tontonoz, 2005). Interestingly, emigrated $CD68^{+}$ cells expressed LXRα mRNA in foam cells in the regression environment (Trogan et al., 2006). LXR increases expression of CCR7 on CD68+ cells, and thus supports CCR7-dependent regression of CD68+ cells from the aorta (Feig et al., 2010). In line with this notion, beneficial effects of

HDL on aortic Mφ egress were observed in a model of atherosclerosis regression. Transplantation of advanced atherosclerotic segments from *Apoe*$^{-/-}$ donors to recipient mice bearing different levels of HDL cholesterol levels revealed that normalization of HDL decreases plaque burden and emigration of CD68$^{+}$ cells from aortas. Thus, these data establish that HDL can serve as a regulator of *in vivo* egress of CD68$^{+}$ cells from the plaque (Feig et al., 2011). It is likely that the balance of "In and Out" processes regulates MΦ and dendritic cells cellularity in the plaque. New data also suggest that normalization of cholesterol can correct monocyte recruitment into the aorta and additionally, lead to decreased MΦ content in atherosclerotic aortas. Treatment of *Apoe*$^{-/-}$ with apoE-encoding adenoviral vectors induced plaque regression, and attenuated CCR7-independent aortic MΦ content (Potteaux et al., 2011). Thus, interfering with monocyte recruitment into and possible egress from atherosclerotic plaques may be therapeutically beneficial, in parallel with aggressive lipid lowering therapies, to maintain and reinforce the reduction in monocyte recruitment to the aorta.

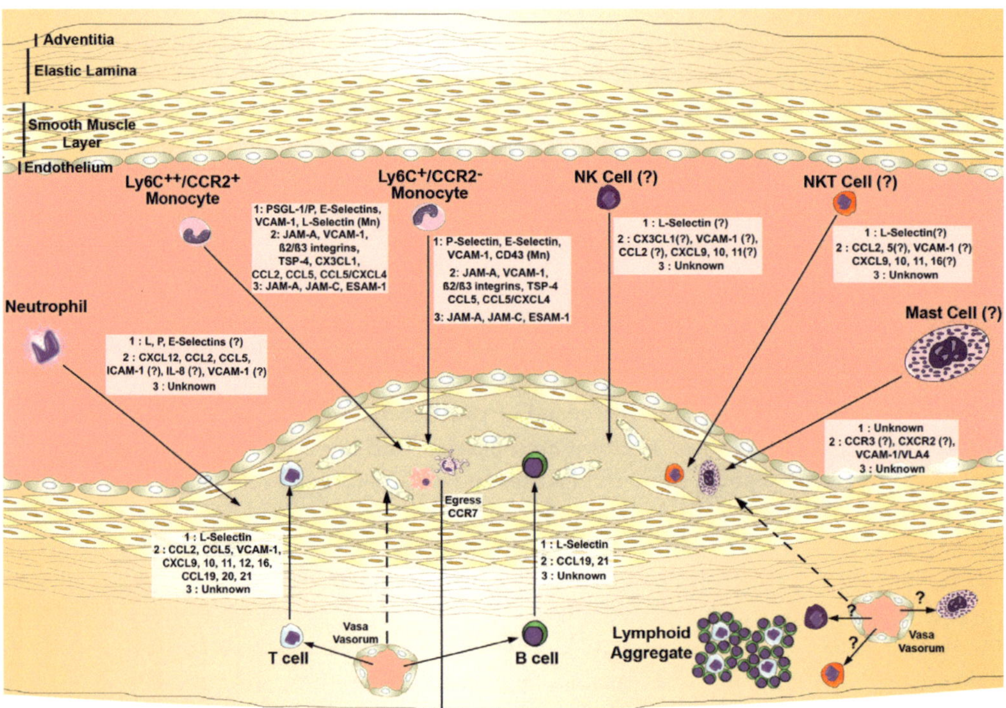


Fig. 2. Mechanisms of leukocyte recruitment in atherosclerosis
Different steps of the adhesion cascade and adhesion molecules control the recruitment of leukocytes to atherosclerotic plaques. The aortic adventitia, elastic laminia, smooth muscle, endothelial layers, as well as tertiary lymphoid aggregates and vasa vasorum are shown. The adhesion proteins and chemokines involved in the rolling and tethering (1), arrest and firm adhesion (2), and transmigration (3) of leukocytes to the endothelium are shown. Factors that play a role in the recruitment of leukocyte subsets in atherogenesis are denoted by question marks. While neutrophils and monocytes are known to be recruited from the lumen, it is not clear if NK, NKT, and mast cells are recruited from the lumen as well.

### 4.2 T cell recruitment

#### 4.2.1 Naive and effector T cell homing

Initially T cells were found within human atherosclerotic plaques, predominantly in the regions of fibrous cap (Jonasson et al., 1986). Interestingly, $CD8^+$ T cells were almost as frequent as $CD4^+$ T cells in the plaques; this differs from the CD4/CD8 ratio normally seen in the blood or other peripheral lymphoid tissue (Jonasson et al., 1986). Even at the earlier stages of atherogenesis, activated T cells have been discovered within the intimal fatty streaks of the human aortic wall (Munro et al., 1987). Importantly, T cells were also detected in non-diseased young aortas (Wick et al., 1997). Leukocytes are distributed at the site-specific areas around the ostia of intercostal arteries of grossly normal aorta (Kishikawa et al., 1993). T cells also reside in the aortic adventitia of *C57BL/6* (Galkina et al., 2006) and *Apoe*$^{-/-}$ mice (Galkina et al., 2006; Moos et al., 2005). Adoptive transfer of T cells into *C57BL/6* mice revealed that T cells preferentially migrate into the aortic adventitia and to a lesser extent into the aortic layers of normal aortas. Indirect evidence suggests that T cell migration occurs likely through the vasa vasorum (Galkina et al., 2006). T cells also preferentially migrate into the adventitia of *Apoe*$^{-/-}$ mice, indicating that T cells use similar routes of homing to the atherosclerotic and healthy aorta (Galkina et al., 2006).

There are many examples of tissue-specific sets of adhesion molecules that provide selective recruitment (reviewed in (Ley et al., 2007)). Little is known about lymphocyte recruitment into the aorta, and it is unclear whether a specific set of adhesion molecules and chemokines are responsible for the influx of the different types of leukocytes into healthy and atherosclerosis-prone aortas. At least one of the selectins, L-selectin, supports the migration of T cells into the aorta (Galkina et al., 2006). L-selectin might not only directly interact with aortic endothelium, but rather provide secondary capture through L-selectin/PSGL-1 interactions (Eriksson et al., 2001; Kunkel et al., 1998). In support of this notion, L-selectin-dependent secondary capture was observed by intravital microscopy in the femoral artery and abdominal aorta (Eriksson et al., 2001).

Evidence demonstrates that different subsets of T cells, including naïve, Tregs, Th1 and Th17 cells are present within the atherosclerotic aortas. Although we are still far from understanding how these different populations accumulate in aortas, some mechanistic details have been already shown. CCL5 is expressed on the luminal surface of carotid arteries, and platelet-dependent CCL5 deposition has been reported (Huo et al., 2003; von Hundelshausen et al., 2001). Deficiency in CCR5 reduced aortic $CD4^+$ cells in parallel with attenuated atherosclerosis in *Ccr5*$^{-/-}$*Apoe*$^{-/-}$ mice (Braunersreuther et al., 2007), indicating the importance of the CCL5/CCR5 axis for T cell migration into aortas. Naïve T cells express CCR7, which plays important functions in T cell recruitment into secondary lymphoid tissues and sites of inflammation. Importantly, CCR7 deficiency attenuates atherosclerosis via the regulation of T cell egress (Luchtefeld et al., 2010). The ligand for CCR7, CCL19 is expressed by SMCs and MΦ in the plaques (Reape et al., 1999). CXCL9, CXCL11 (Mach et al., 1999; Ranjbaran et al., 2006), and CXCL12 (Bi-Younes et al., 2000), are also detected in the lesions. CXCL10 and CXCL9 mediate the CXCR3-dependent rapid shear-resistant arrest of T cells on stimulated EC (Piali et al., 1998). It was also shown that CXCL10 participates in T cell homing into atherosclerotic aortas (Heller et al., 2006).

CXCL16 is detected in human and mouse atherosclerosis-prone tissues and serves in the membrane-bound form as a scavenger receptor and in the soluble form as a chemokine. CXCL16 protects against atherosclerosis, likely through a benefit of CXCL16 as a scavenger receptor (Aslanian and Charo, 2006). Subsets of $T_{EFF}$ cell express CXCR6, a chemokine receptor for CXCL16 (Matloubian et al., 2000). The absence of CXCR6 in *Cxcr6*$^{-/-}$*Apoe*$^{-/-}$ mice leads to reduced homing of CXCR6$^{+}$ T cells into atherosclerotic aortas (Galkina et al., 2007). CXCR2 and CXCR4 were recently identified as functional receptors for macrophage migration inhibition factor (MIF) (Bernhagen et al., 2007b). Blockade of MIF resulted in a diminished number of monocytes/MΦ and T cells within the aortas.

Tregs play an important role in the maintenance of the immunological tolerance (review in (Sakaguchi et al., 2008)). Induction of a regulatory T cell type 1 (Treg type 1) responses and adoptive transfer of naturally arising CD4$^{+}$CD25/$^{+}$ T regs reduce atherosclerosis in *Apoe*$^{-/-}$ mice (Mallat et al., 2003; Ait-Oufella et al., 2006). Foxp3$^{+}$ cells in human atherosclerotic lesions colocalize with the Treg-associated chemokine receptor CCR4 and its ligand, CCL17 (Heller et al., 2006). The molecular mechanisms that regulate homing of Treg cells into aortas are not well understood.

Th17 cells are a new lineage of CD4$^{+}$ T cells that play important roles in acute inflammation and autoimmune diseases (Bettelli et al., 2007). Expression of CCR6 and CCR4 characterizes a unique subset of IL-17$^{+}$ human peripheral blood T cells (Costa-Rodriguez et al., 2007). Th17 cells also express homeostatic CCR7 and CXCR5 and share some chemokine receptors with other T cell lineages. Although IL-17A$^{+}$ cells are less abundant than Th1 cells, IL-17A$^{+}$ T cells are present in both atherosclerotic human and mouse arteries. While the mechanisms of Th17 cell homing into aortas are unclear, some ligands such as CCL2, CCL20, and CCL21 are expressed within the plaques and could be used by Th17 and other IL-17+ cells to home to aortas.

### 4.3 B cell influx

In 1981, B cells were discovered within the adventitia (Parums & Mitchinson, 1981), and immunoglobulin-positive cells were detected within the subendothelial intima of atherosclerotic and non-atherosclerotic rabbits (Hansson et al., 1980). CD22$^{+}$ B cells were also detected in atherosclerotic plaques of *Apoe*$^{-/-}$ mice (Zhou & Hansson, 1999). B cells reside in the adventitia of *C57BL/6* aortas as a consequence of constitutive L-selectin-dependent homing to the aorta (Galkina et al., 2006). The phenotype of B cells within the aorta and surrounding adventitia is unclear, and further studies are needed to characterize adhesion molecule and chemokine receptor repertoire of aortic B cells. Recently, a role for smooth muscle cells (SMCs) in the regulation of lymphocyte homing was suggested. SMCs induce the production of CCL7, CCL9, CXCL13, CCL19, CXCL16, VCAM-1, and ICAM-1 (Lotzer et al., 2010). Supernatants of TNF receptor superfamily member 1A (TNFR-1) and LTβ-receptor-activated SMC markedly supported migration of B cells in vitro (Lotzer et al., 2010). It remains unclear whether elevated levels of endothelial homeostatic chemokines lead to accelerated recruitment of B cells into atherosclerosis-prone vessels.

### 4.4 Neutrophil recruitment in atherosclerosis

Despite a clear association between neutrophilia, neutrophil activation, and coronary artery disease (Baetta & Corsini, 2010; Mazzone et al., 1993), neutrophils are relatively low in abundance within human atherosclerotic plaques (Baetta & Corsini, 2010). While neutrophils in atherosclerosis have been understudied to date, several lines of evidence suggest that neutrophil recruitment occurs during atherogenesis. CXCR4 and its ligand CXCL12 are involved in the efflux of neutrophils from bone marrow and in the regulation of neutrophil recruitment to atherosclerotic plaques (Zernecke et al., 2008). In addition, neutrophils were shown to adhere to the endothelium on the shoulder regions of atherosclerotic plaques (Rotzius et al., 2010). CXCR4 blockade-induced neutrophilia resulted in elevated plaque neutrophil content. In addition, as neutrophil chemotaxis to atherosclerotic plaques was impaired in CCR1, CCR2, CCR5, and CXCR2 deficient *Apoe*$^{-/-}$ mice, CCL2 and platelet-derived CCL5 supported neutrophil recruitment to carotid arteries. Based on several studies, neutrophils might migrate to developing plaques in a CCR1- and CCR5-dependent manner where they participate in promoting atherogenesis by supporting monocyte recruitment (Soehnlein et al., 2009) and inflammation (Nicholls & Hazen, 2009).

### 4.5 Mast cells in atherogenesis

While vascular mast cells are rare, they are nonetheless present within the adventitia and shoulder regions of atherosclerotic plaques (Lindstedt et al., 2007). Mast cell deficient *Kit*$^{W\text{-}sh/W\text{-}sh}$ mice display alterations in ApoE and ApoAII-dependent cholesterol efflux (Lee et al., 2002). Interestingly *Kit*$^{W\text{-}sh/W\text{-}sh}$ mice on the *Ldlr*$^{-/-}$ background demonstrated increased collagen content, fibrous cap development and reduced plaque T cell and MΦ cellularity (Sun et al., 2007). Mast cell activation correlated with MΦ and endothelial cell apoptosis, vascular leakage, CXCR2 and VLA-4-mediated recruitment of leukocytes to atheroma (Bot, et al., 2007). Mast cells play a pro-inflammatory role in atherogenesis; however, little is known about the recruitment of mast cells during atherosclerosis. Lesional mast cells express CCR3, suggesting that mast cells may utilize eotaxin, which is expressed by vascular smooth muscle cells, to migrate toward atherosclerotic plaques (Haley et al., 2000).

### 4.6 Natural killer (NK) cell recruitment in atherogenesis

NK cells are found within the shoulder regions of early and advanced human atherosclerotic lesions. While there is currently no NK-deficient mouse model of atherosclerosis, there are several lines of evidence to suggest that NK cells play a role during atherosclerosis (reviewed in Galkina & Ley, 2007, 2009). However, little is known about NK cell recruitment during atherogenesis. NK cells express a variety of adhesion molecules, including L-selectin, PSGL-1, β2 and α4 integrins, and chemokine receptors, including CXCR3, CCR2, and CX3CR1 (Galkina & Ley, 2007). Further studies are necessary. Further studies are necessary to identify the players in the migration cascade of NK cells to atherosclerotic aortas.

### 4.7 Natural killer T (NKT) cell recruitment in atherogenesis

Several lines of evidence support the pro-atherogenic nature of NKT-cells during the development of atherosclerosis in both humans and mice (Galkina and Ley, 2009). As glycolipid antigens can be presented by CD1 to CD1-restricted T cells, NKT cells possibly play an important role in responding to lipid antigen presentation within the aortic wall. NKT cells express receptors for inflammation-related chemokines, including CCR2, CCR5, CXCR3, and CXCR6 and CCL2. Thus, NKT cells likely use CCL5, CXCL9-11 and CXCL16 chemokines to migrate to atherosclerotic plaques.

## 5. Leukocyte recruitment during experimental atherosclerosis: Luminal “inside-out” migration vs extra-luminal “outside-in” recruitment

Traditionally, leukocyte migration during atherosclerosis has been considered to occur in an "inside-out" manner, focusing on monocyte adhesion to the endothelium on the luminal side of the artery and transmigration through the endothelium to arrive at the developing atherosclerotic plaque. Several lines of evidence support this model. Rolling and firm adherence of monocytes to the endothelium was demonstrated to occur in *ex vivo* carotid artery adhesion models as well as *in vivo* models (reviewed in (Galkina & Ley, 2007b; Zernecke and Weber, 2010)). However at present, there is no direct intravital microscopic evidence to support direct lymphocyte recruitment from the arterial lumen. Adoptive transfers of lymphocytes into *Apoe*$^{-/-}$ mice demonstrated that lymphocytes accumulate within the associated arterial adventitia suggesting a possible route of migration via adventitial vasa vasorum. Interestingly, the inhibition of plaque neovascularisation reduces MΦ accumulation and the progression of advanced atherosclerosis (Moreno et al., 2006). Recent studies have also revealed that the vasa vasorum can penetrate the media, enter atheroma, and come close to the arterial lumen (Moreno et al., 2006; Ritman & Lerman, 2007; Mulligan-Kehoe, 2010). Furthermore, administration of growth factors in acid gelatine hydrogel microspheres around the periaortic area in 10-11 week old male *Apoe*$^{-/-}$ mice strongly promoted vasa vasorum neovascularisation of the aorta and corresponded with larger atherosclerotic plaques (Tanaka et al., 2011). Recently three studies have further implicated adventitial inflammation in the pathogenesis of atherosclerosis. Several reports have demonstrated that T and B cell aggregates accumulate within the aortic adventitia in atherosclerotic aortas (Galkina et al., 2003; Moos et al., 2005; Zhao et al., 2004). LTβ was required for the formation of aortic tertiary lymphoid organs within the adventitia (Grabner, et. al. 2009). Interestingly, these tertiary lymphoid structures were characterized by distinct clusters of germinal centers, proliferating T cells, and elevated production of the lymphorganogenic chemokines CXCL13 and CCL21. Mechanistic experiments utilizing LTβ-receptor deficient smooth muscle cells revealed that TNF-α and LTβ-dependent activation of the NF-κB pathway was sufficient to induce the expression of multiple chemokines, including CCL2, CCL5, CXCL1, CX3CL1, CCL7, CCL9, CXCL13, CCL19, and CXCL16 (Lötzer, et al. 2010). Together, these studies suggest that the adventitia plays an important structural role as the site of antigen presentation. In addition, neovascularisation from the adventitia to the arterial medial layer may provide a route of access for adventitial leukocytes to migrate to the media. Further studies will be necessary to truly determine the spatio-temporal relationship between the vasa vasorum, aortic tertiary lymphoid structures, and atherogenesis; and how these activities relate to leukocyte recruitment.

## 6. Conclusions

Our understanding of the mechanisms of leukocyte recruitment during atherogenesis has progressed notably since the early 1980s. The mechanisms of monocyte subset migration have been thoroughly studied; however, there are still many fundamental questions that remain to be investigated. To date, it is unclear what mechanisms are responsible for the recruitment of neutrophils, B cells, mast cells, NKT and NK cells into the aorta. In addition, while the recruitment of monocytes and neutrophils has been demonstrated to occur in an arterial lumen-to-plaque fashion, the directions of lymphocyte and mast cell recruitment in atherogenesis has yet to be defined. While several studies have highlighted the importance of the vasa vasorum and adventitial lymphoid structures, the effects of these anatomical structures on leukocyte recruitment have yet to be explored. With progress in tissue-specific drug targeting, one potential alternative approach to halting the progression of atherosclerosis would be to develop blocking agents against crucial adhesion molecules within the aorta that play critical roles in aoritc leukocyte recruitment at the different stage of atherosclerosis.

## 7. Acknowledgments

This work was supported by American Heart Association Pre-doctoral Fellowship grant 11PRE7520041 (to Matthew Butcher) and by the NHLBI RO1 HL107522 (to Elena Galkina). Due to space constraints we were unable to cite all of the relevant research articles and reviews. We apologize to the authors whose work could not be included.

## 8. References

Ait-Oufella,H., Salomon,B.L., Potteaux,S., Robertson,A.K., Gourdy,P., Zoll,J., Merval,R., Esposito,B., Cohen,J.L., Fisson,S., Flavell,R.A., Hansson,G.K., Klatzmann,D., Tedgui,A., & Mallat,Z. (2006). Natural regulatory T cells control the development of atherosclerosis in mice. *Nat. Med. 12*, 178-180, ISSN 1078-8956.

Ait-Oufella,H., Taleb,S., Mallat,Z., & Tedgui,A. (2011). Recent advances on the role of cytokines in atherosclerosis. *Arterioscler. Thromb. Vasc. Biol. 31*, 969-979, ISSN 1524-4636.

Alon,R., Chen,S., Puri,K.D., Finger,E.B., & Springer,T.A. (1997). The kinetics of L-selectin tethers and the mechanics of selectin-mediated rolling. *J. Cell Biol. 138*, pp. 1169-1180, ISSN 0021-9525.

Aslanian,A.M. & Charo,I.F. (2006). Targeted disruption of the scavenger receptor and chemokine CXCL16 accelerates atherosclerosis. *Circulation 114*, pp. 583-590, ISSN 1524-4539.

Baetta,R. & Corsini,A. (2010). Role of polymorphonuclear neutrophils in atherosclerosis: current state and future perspectives. *Atherosclerosis 210*, pp. 1-13, ISSN 1879-1484.

Baltus,T., von Hundelshausen P., Mause,S.F., Buhre,W., Rossaint,R., & Weber,C. (2005). Differential and additive effects of platelet-derived chemokines on monocyte arrest on inflamed endothelium under flow conditions. *J. Leukoc. Biol. 78*, pp. 435-441, ISSN 0741-5400.

Bernhagen,J., Krohn,R., Lue,H., Gregory,J.L., Zernecke,A., Koenen,R.R., Dewor,M., Georgiev,I., Schober,A., Leng,L., Kooistra,T., Fingerle-Rowson,G., Ghezzi,P., Kleemann,R., McColl,S.R., Bucala,R., Hickey,M.J., & Weber,C. (2007). MIF is a noncognate ligand of CXC chemokine receptors in inflammatory and atherogenic cell recruitment. *Nat. Med.*, pp. 587-96, ISSN 1078-8956.

Bettelli,E., Korn,T., & Kuchroo,V.K. (2007). Th17: the third member of the effector T cell trilogy. *Curr. Opin. Immunol. 19*, 652-657, ISSN 0952-7915.

Bi-Younes,S., Sauty,A., Mach,F., Sukhova,G.K., Libby,P., & Luster,A.D. (2000). The stromal cell-derived factor-1 chemokine is a potent platelet agonist highly expressed in atherosclerotic plaques. *Circ. Res. 86*, 131-138, ISSN 1524-4571.

Bobryshev,Y.V. & Lord,R.S. (1998). Detection of vascular dendritic cells accumulating calcified deposits in their cytoplasm. *Tissue Cell 30*, 383-388, ISSN 0040-8166.

Boring,L., Gosling,J., Cleary,M., & Charo,I.F. (1998). Decreased lesion formation in CCR2-/- mice reveals a role for chemokines in the initiation of atherosclerosis. *Nature 394*, 894-897, ISSN 0028-0836.

Bot,I.; de Jager,S.C.; Zernecke,A.; Lindstedt,K.A.; van Berkel,T.J.; Weber,C.; Biessen,E.A. (2007). Perivascular mast cells promote atherogenesis and induce plaque destabilization in apolipoprotein E-deficient mice. *Circulation,*115, 2516-25, ISSN 1524-4539.

Bradley,M.N. & Tontonoz,P. (2005). Lesion macrophages are a key target for the antiatherogenic effects of LXR agonists. *Arterioscler. Thromb. Vasc. Biol. 25*, 10-11, ISSN 1524-4636.

Braunersreuther,V., Zernecke,A., Arnaud,C., Liehn,E.A., Steffens,S., Shagdarsuren,E., Bidzhekov,K., Burger,F., Pelli,G., Luckow,B., Mach,F., & Weber,C. (2007). Ccr5 but not Ccr1 deficiency reduces development of diet-induced atherosclerosis in mice. *Arterioscler. Thromb. Vasc. Biol. 27*, 373-379, ISSN 1524-4636.

Brooks,A.R., Lelkes,P.I., & Rubanyi,G.M. (2002). Gene expression profiling of human aortic endothelial cells exposed to disturbed flow and steady laminar flow. *Physiol Genomics 9*, 27-41, ISSN 1531-2267.

Burger-Kentischer,A., Gobel,H., Kleemann,R., Zernecke,A., Bucala,R., Leng,L., Finkelmeier,D., Geiger,G., Schaefer,H.E., Schober,A., Weber,C., Brunner,H., Rutten,H., Ihling,C., & Bernhagen,J. (2006). Reduction of the aortic inflammatory response in spontaneous atherosclerosis by blockade of macrophage migration inhibitory factor (MIF). *Atherosclerosis 184*, 28-38, ISSN 0021-9150.

Carman,C.V. & Springer,T.A. (2004). A transmigratory cup in leukocyte diapedesis both through individual vascular endothelial cells and between them. *J. Cell Biol. 167*, 377-388, ISSN 0021-9525.

Cheng,C., Tempel,D., van,H.R., de Boer,H.C., Segers,D., Huisman,M., van Zonneveld,A.J., Leenen,P.J., van der,S.A., Serruys,P.W., de,C.R., & Krams,R. (2007). Shear stress-induced changes in atherosclerotic plaque composition are modulated by chemokines. *J. Clin. Invest 117*, 616-626, ISSN 0021-9738.

Collins,R.G., Velji,R., Guevara,N.V., Hicks,M.J., Chan,L., & Beaudet,A.L. (2000). P-Selectin or intercellular adhesion molecule (ICAM)-1 deficiency substantially protects against atherosclerosis in apolipoprotein E-deficient mice. *J. Exp. Med. 191*, 189-194, ISSN 0022-1007.

Costa-Rodriguez,E.V., Rivino,L., Geginat,J., Jarrossay,D., Gattorno,M., Lanzavecchia,A., Sallusto,F., & Napolitani,G. (2007). Surface phenotype and antigenic specificity of human interleukin 17-producing T helper memory cells. *Nat. Immunol. 8*, 639-646, ISSN 1529-2908.

Cros,J., Cagnard,N., Woollard,K., Patey,N., Zhang,S.Y., Senechal,B., Puel,A., Biswas,S.K., Moshous,D., Picard,C., Jais,J.P., D'Cruz,D., Casanova,J.L., Trouillet,C., &

Geissmann,F. (2010). Human CD14dim monocytes patrol and sense nucleic acids and viruses via TLR7 and TLR8 receptors. *Immunity. 33*, 375-386, ISSN 1097-4180.

Cybulsky,M.I., Iiyama,K., Li,H., Zhu,S., Chen,M., Iiyama,M., Davis,V., Gutierrez-Ramos,J.C., Connelly,P.W., & Milstone,D.S. (2001). A major role for VCAM-1, but not ICAM-1, in early atherosclerosis. *J. Clin. Invest 107*, 1255-1262, ISSN 0021-9738.

Dansky,H.M., Barlow,C.B., Lominska,C., Sikes,J.L., Kao,C., Weinsaft,J., Cybulsky,M.I., & Smith,J.D. (2001). Adhesion of monocytes to arterial endothelium and initiation of atherosclerosis are critically dependent on vascular cell adhesion molecule-1 gene dosage. *Arterioscler. Thromb. Vasc. Biol. 21*, 1662-1667, ISSN 1524-4636.

Davies,P.F., Polacek,D.C., Shi,C., & Helmke,B.P. (2002). The convergence of haemodynamics, genomics, and endothelial structure in studies of the focal origin of atherosclerosis. *Biorheology 39*, 299-306, ISSN 0006-355X.

Dawson,T.C., Kuziel,W.A., Osahar,T.A., & Maeda,N. (1999). Absence of CC chemokine receptor-2 reduces atherosclerosis in apolipoprotein E-deficient mice. *Atherosclerosis 143*, 205-211, ISSN 0021-9150.

Dong,Z.M., Brown,A.A., & Wagner,D.D. (2000). Prominent role of P-selectin in the development of advanced atherosclerosis in ApoE-deficient mice. *Circulation 101*, 2290-2295, ISSN 1524-4539.

Dong,Z.M., Chapman,S.M., Brown,A.A., Frenette,P.S., Hynes,R.O., & Wagner,D.D. (1998). The combined role of P- and E-selectins in atherosclerosis. *J. Clin. Invest 102*, 145-152, ISSN 0021-9738.

Eriksson,E.E., Xie,X., Werr,J., Thoren,P., & Lindbom,L. (2001). Importance of primary capture and L-selectin-dependent secondary capture in leukocyte accumulation in inflammation and atherosclerosis in vivo. *J. Exp. Med. 194*, 205-218, ISSN 0022-1007.

Feig,J.E., Pineda-Torra,I., Sanson,M., Bradley,M.N., Vengrenyuk,Y., Bogunovic,D., Gautier,E.L., Rubinstein,D., Hong,C., Liu,J., Wu,C., van,R.N., Bhardwaj,N., Garabedian,M., Tontonoz,P., & Fisher,E.A. (2010). LXR promotes the maximal egress of monocyte-derived cells from mouse aortic plaques during atherosclerosis regression. *J. Clin. Invest 120*, 4415-4424, ISSN 1558-8238.

Feig,J.E., Rong,J.X., Shamir,R., Sanson,M., Vengrenyuk,Y., Liu,J., Rayner,K., Moore,K., Garabedian,M., & Fisher,E.A. (2011). HDL promotes rapid atherosclerosis regression in mice and alters inflammatory properties of plaque monocyte-derived cells. *Proc. Natl. Acad. Sci. U. S. A 108*, 7166-7171, ISSN 1091-6490.

Frolova,E.G., Pluskota,E., Krukovets,I., Burke,T., Drumm,C., Smith,J.D., Blech,L., Febbraio,M., Bornstein,P., Plow,E.F., & Stenina,O.I. (2010). Thrombospondin-4 regulates vascular inflammation and atherogenesis. *Circ. Res. 107*, 1313-1325, ISSN 1524-4571.

Galkina,E., Harry,B.L., Ludwig,A., Liehn,E.A., Sanders,J.M., Bruce,A., Weber,C., & Ley,K. (2007). CXCR6 promotes atherosclerosis by supporting T-cell homing, interferon-gamma production, and macrophage accumulation in the aortic wall. *Circulation 116*, 1801-1811, ISSN 1524-4539.

Galkina,E., Kadl,A., Sanders,J., Varughese,D., Sarembock,I.J., & Ley,K. (2006). Lymphocyte recruitment into the aortic wall before and during development of atherosclerosis is partially L-selectin dependent. *J. Exp. Med. 203*, 1273-1282, ISSN 1524-4539.

Galkina,E. & Ley,K. (2007a). Leukocyte influx in atherosclerosis. *Curr. Drug Targets. 8*, 1239-1248, ISSN 0022-1007.

Galkina,E. & Ley,K. (2007b). Vascular adhesion molecules in atherosclerosis. *Arterioscler Thromb Vasc Biol 27*, 2292-2301, ISSN 1524-4636.

Galkina,E. & Ley,K. (2009). Immune and inflammatory mechanisms of atherosclerosis (*). *Annu. Rev. Immunol. 27*, 165-197, ISSN 0732-0582.

Gebuhrer,V., Murphy,J.F., Bordet,J.C., Reck,M.P., & McGregor,J.L. (1995). Oxidized low-density lipoprotein induces the expression of P-selectin (GMP140/PADGEM/CD62) on human endothelial cells. *Biochem. J. 306 ( Pt 1)*, 293-298, ISSN 0264-6021.

Geissmann,F., Jung,S., & Littman,D.R. (2003). Blood monocytes consist of two principal subsets with distinct migratory properties. *Immunity. 19*, 71-82, ISSN 1074-7613.

Gerrity,R.G. & Naito,H.K. (1980). Ultrastructural identification of monocyte-derived foam cells in fatty streak lesions. *Artery 8*, 208-214, ISSN 0098-6127.

Gosling,J., Slaymaker,S., Gu,L., Tseng,S., Zlot,C.H., Young,S.G., Rollins,B.J., & Charo,I.F. (1999). MCP-1 deficiency reduces susceptibility to atherosclerosis in mice that overexpress human apolipoprotein *B. J. Clin. Invest 103*, 773-778, ISSN 0021-9738.

Grabner,R., Lotzer,K., Dopping,S., Hildner,M., Radke,D., Beer,M., Spanbroek,R., Lippert,B., Reardon,C.A., Getz,G.S., Fu,Y.X., Hehlgans,T., Mebius,R.E., van der,W.M., Kruspe,D., Englert,C., Lovas,A., Hu,D., Randolph,G.J., Weih,F., & Habenicht,A.J. (2009). Lymphotoxin beta receptor signaling promotes tertiary lymphoid organogenesis in the aorta adventitia of aged ApoE-/- mice. *J. Exp. Med. 206*, 233-248, ISSN 1540-9538.

Gu,L., Okada,Y., Clinton,S.K., Gerard,C., Sukhova,G.K., Libby,P., & Rollins,B.J. (1998). Absence of monocyte chemoattractant protein-1 reduces atherosclerosis in low density lipoprotein receptor-deficient mice. *Mol. Cell 2*, 275-281, ISSN 1097-2765.

Guan,J.L. & Hynes,R.O. (1990). Lymphoid cells recognize an alternatively spliced segment of fibronectin via the integrin receptor alpha 4 beta 1. *Cell 60*, 53-61, ISSN 0092-8674.

Haley,K.J., Lilly,C.M., Yang,J.H., Feng,Y., Kennedy,S.P., Turi,T.G., Thompson,J.F., Sukhova,G.H., Libby,P., & Lee,R.T. (2000). Overexpression of eotaxin and the CCR3 receptor in human atherosclerosis: using genomic technology to identify a potential novel pathway of vascular inflammation. *Circulation 102*, 2185-2189, ISSN 1524-4539.

Hansson,G.K., Bondjers,G., Bylock,A., & Hjalmarsson,L. (1980). Ultrastructural studies on the localization of IgG in the aortic endothelium and subendothelial intima of atherosclerotic and nonatherosclerotic rabbits. *Exp. Mol. Pathol. 33*, 302-315, ISSN 0014-4800.

Hansson,G.K. & Hermansson,A. (2011). The immune system in atherosclerosis. *Nat. Immunol. 12*, 204-212, ISSN 1529-2916.

Hashimoto,K., Kataoka,N., Nakamura,E., Tsujioka,K., Kajiya,F. (2007). Oxidized LDL specifically promotes the initiation of monocyte invasion during transendothelial migration with upregulated PECAM-1 and downregulated VE-cadherin on endothelial junctions. *Atherosclerosis* 194, e9-e17, ISSN 1879-1484.

Heller,E.A., Liu,E., Tager,A.M., Yuan,Q., Lin,A.Y., Ahluwalia,N., Jones,K., Koehn,S.L., Lok,V.M., Aikawa,E., Moore,K.J., Luster,A.D., & Gerszten,R.E. (2006). Chemokine CXCL10 promotes atherogenesis by modulating the local balance of effector and regulatory T cells. *Circulation 113*, 2301-2312, ISSN 1524-4539.

Hirschberg,H., Bergh,O.J., & Thorsby,E. (1980). Antigen-presenting properties of human vascular endothelial cells. *J. Exp. Med. 152*, 249s-255s, ISSN 0022-1007.

Huo,Y., Hafezi-Moghadam,A., & Ley,K. (2000). Role of vascular cell adhesion molecule-1 and fibronectin connecting segment-1 in monocyte rolling and adhesion on early atherosclerotic lesions. *Circ. Res. 87*, 153-159, ISSN 0009-7330.

Huo,Y., Schober,A., Forlow,S.B., Smith,D.F., Hyman,M.C., Jung,S., Littman,D.R., Weber,C., & Ley,K. (2003). Circulating activated platelets exacerbate atherosclerosis in mice deficient in apolipoprotein *E. Nat. Med. 9*, 61-67, ISSN 1078-8956.

Huo,Y., Weber,C., Forlow,S.B., Sperandio,M., Thatte,J., Mack,M., Jung,S., Littman,D.R., & Ley,K. (2001). The chemokine KC, but not monocyte chemoattractant protein-1, triggers monocyte arrest on early atherosclerotic endothelium. *J. Clin. Invest 108*, 1307-1314, ISSN 0021-9738.

Hynes,R.O. (2002). Integrins: bidirectional, allosteric signaling machines. *Cell 110*, 673-687, ISSN 0092-8674.

Inoue,M., Ishida,T., Yasuda,T., Toh,R., Hara,T., Cangara,H.M., Rikitake,Y., Taira,K., Sun,L., Kundu,R.K., Quertermous,T., & Hirata,K. (2010). Endothelial cell-selective adhesion molecule modulates atherosclerosis through plaque angiogenesis and monocyte-endothelial interaction. *Microvasc. Res. 80*, 179-187, ISSN 1095-9319.

Johnson,R.C., Chapman,S.M., Dong,Z.M., Ordovas,J.M., Mayadas,T.N., Herz,J., Hynes,R.O., Schaefer,E.J., & Wagner,D.D. (1997). Absence of P-selectin delays fatty streak formation in mice. *J. Clin. Invest 99*, 1037-1043, ISSN 0021-9738.

Jonasson,L., Holm,J., Skalli,O., Bondjers,G., & Hansson,G.K. (1986). Regional accumulations of T cells, macrophages, and smooth muscle cells in the human atherosclerotic plaque. *Arteriosclerosis 6*, 131-138, ISSN 0276-5047.

Jonasson,L., Holm,J., Skalli,O., Gabbiani,G., & Hansson,G.K. (1985). Expression of class II transplantation antigen on vascular smooth muscle cells in human atherosclerosis. *J. Clin. Invest 76*, 125-131, ISSN 0021-9738.

Keiper,T., Al-Fakhri,N., Chavakis,E., Athanasopoulos,A.N., Isermann,B., Herzog,S., Saffrich,R., Hersemeyer,K., Bohle,R.M., Haendeler,J., Preissner,K.T., Santoso,S., & Chavakis,T. (2005). The role of junctional adhesion molecule-C (JAM-C) in oxidized LDL-mediated leukocyte recruitment. *FASEB J. 19*, 2078-2080, ISSN 1530-6860.

Kinashi,T. (2007). Integrin regulation of lymphocyte trafficking: lessons from structural and signaling studies. *Adv. Immunol. 93*, 185-227, ISSN 0065-2776.

Kishikawa,H., Shimokama,T., & Watanabe,T. (1993). Localization of T lymphocytes and macrophages expressing IL-1, IL-2 receptor, IL-6 and TNF in human aortic intima. Role of cell-mediated immunity in human atherogenesis. *Virchows Arch. A Pathol. Anat. Histopathol. 423*, 433-442, ISSN 0174-7398.

Klouche,M., May,A.E., Hemmes,M., Messner,M., Kanse,S.M., Preissner,K.T., & Bhakdi,S. (1999). Enzymatically modified, nonoxidized LDL induces selective adhesion and transmigration of monocytes and T-lymphocytes through human endothelial cell monolayers. *Arterioscler. Thromb. Vasc. Biol. 19*, 784-793, ISSN 1079-5642.

Kume,N., Cybulsky,M.I., Gimbrone Jr.,M.A. (1992) Lysophosphatidylcholine, a component of atherogenic lipoproteins, induces mononuclear leukocyte adhesion molecules in cultured human and rabbit arterial endothelial cells. *J. Clin. Invest.,* 90 (3), 1138-1144, ISSN 0021-9738

Kunkel,E.J., Chomas,J.E., & Ley,K. (1998). Role of primary and secondary capture for leukocyte accumulation in vivo. *Circ. Res. 82*, 30-38, ISSN 0009-7330.

Kunkel,E.J. & Ley,K. (1996). Distinct phenotype of E-selectin-deficient mice. E-selectin is required for slow leukocyte rolling in vivo. *Circ. Res. 79*, 1196-1204, ISSN 0009-7330.

Lampugnani,M.G., Resnati,M., Raiteri,M., Pigott,R., Pisacane,A., Houen,G., Ruco,L.P., & Dejana,E. (1992). A novel endothelial-specific membrane protein is a marker of cell-cell contacts. *J. Cell Biol. 118*, 1511-1522, ISSN 0021-9525.

Lee,M., Calabresi,L., Chiesa,G., Franceschini,G., & Kovanen,P.T. (2002). Mast cell chymase degrades apoE and apoA-II in apoA-I-knockout mouse plasma and reduces its ability to promote cellular cholesterol efflux. *Arterioscler. Thromb. Vasc. Biol. 22*, 1475-1481, ISSN 1524-4636.

Lessner,S.M., Prado,H.L., Waller,E.K., & Galis,Z.S. (2002). Atherosclerotic lesions grow through recruitment and proliferation of circulating monocytes in a murine model. *Am. J. Pathol. 160*, 2145-2155, ISSN 0002-9440.

Leeuwenberg,J.F., Smeets,E.F., Neefjes,J.J., Shaffer,M.A., Cinek,T., Jeunhomme,T.M., Ahern,T.J., Buurman,W.A. (1992). E-selectin and intercellular adhesion molecule-1 are reslease by activated human endothelial cells in vitro. *Immunology. 77(4)*. 543-549. ISSN 0019-2805

Ley, K., Laudanna, C., Cybulsky, M., & Nourshargh,S. (2007). Getting to the site of inflammation: the leukocyte adhesion cascade updated. *Nat.Rev.Immunol.*, ISSN 1474-1741.

Ley,K. & Kansas,G.S. (2004). Selectins in T-cell recruitment to non-lymphoid tissues and sites of inflammation. *Nat. Rev. Immunol. 4*, 325-335, ISSN 1474-1733.

Lindstedt,K.A., Mayranpaa,M.I., & Kovanen,P.T. (2007). Mast cells in vulnerable atherosclerotic plaques--a view to a kill. *J. Cell Mol. Med. 11*, 739-758, ISSN 1582-1838.

Llodra,J., Angeli,V., Liu,J., Trogan,E., Fisher,E.A., & Randolph,G.J. (2004). Emigration of monocyte-derived cells from atherosclerotic lesions characterizes regressive, but not progressive, plaques. *Proc. Natl. Acad. Sci. U. S. A 101*, 11779-11784, ISSN 0027-8424.

Lotzer,K., Dopping,S., Connert,S., Grabner,R., Spanbroek,R., Lemser,B., Beer,M., Hildner,M., Hehlgans,T., van der,W.M., Mebius,R.E., Lovas,A., Randolph,G.J., Weih,F., & Habenicht,A.J. (2010). Mouse aorta smooth muscle cells differentiate into lymphoid tissue organizer-like cells on combined tumor necrosis factor receptor-1/lymphotoxin beta-receptor NF-kappaB signaling. *Arterioscler. Thromb. Vasc. Biol. 30*, 395-402, ISSN 1524-4636.

Luchtefeld,M., Grothusen,C., Gagalick,A., Jagavelu,K., Schuett,H., Tietge,U.J., Pabst,O., Grote,K., Drexler,H., Forster,R., & Schieffer,B. (2010). Chemokine receptor 7 knockout attenuates atherosclerotic plaque development. *Circulation 122*, 1621-1628, ISSN 1524-4539.

Luster,A.D., Alon,R., & von Andrian,U.H. (2005). Immune cell migration in inflammation: present and future therapeutic targets. *Nat. Immunol. 6*, 1182-1190, ISSN 1529-2908.

Mach,F., Sauty,A., Iarossi,A.S., Sukhova,G.K., Neote,K., Libby,P., & Luster,A.D. (1999). Differential expression of three T lymphocyte-activating CXC chemokines by human atheroma-associated cells. *J. Clin. Invest 104*, 1041-1050, ISSN 0021-9738.

Mallat,Z., Gojova,A., Brun,V., Esposito,B., Fournier,N., Cottrez,F., Tedgui,A., & Groux,H. (2003). Induction of a regulatory T cell type 1 response reduces the development of atherosclerosis in apolipoprotein E-knockout mice. *Circulation 108*, 1232-1237, ISSN 1524-4539.

Mandell,K.J. & Parkos,C.A. (2005). The JAM family of proteins. *Adv. Drug Deliv.* Rev. *57*, 857-867, ISSN 0169-409X.

Matloubian,M., David,A., Engel,S., Ryan,J.E., & Cyster,J.G. (2000). A transmembrane CXC chemokine is a ligand for HIV-coreceptor Bonzo. *Nat. Immunol. 1*, 298-304, ISSN 1529-2908.

Mayerl,C., Lukasser,M., Sedivy,R., Niederegger,H., Seiler,R., & Wick,G. (2006). Atherosclerosis research from past to present--on the track of two pathologists with opposing views, Carl von Rokitansky and Rudolf Virchow. Virchows Arch. *449*, 96-103, ISSN 0945-6317.

Mazzone,A., De,S.S., Ricevuti,G., Mazzucchelli,I., Fossati,G., Pasotti,D., Bramucci,E., Angoli,L., Marsico,F., & Specchia,G. (1993). Increased expression of neutrophil and monocyte adhesion molecules in unstable coronary artery disease. *Circulation 88*, 358-363, ISSN 0009-7322.

McEver,R.P. (2002). Selectins: lectins that initiate cell adhesion under flow. *Curr. Opin. Cell Biol. 14*, 581-586, ISSN 0955-0674.

Methe,H. & Weis,M. (2007). Atherogenesis and inflammation--was Virchow right? *Nephrol. Dial. Transplant. 22*, 1823-1827, ISSN 0931-0509.

Moos,M.P., John,N., Grabner,R., Nossmann,S., Gunther,B., Vollandt,R., Funk,C.D., Kaiser,B., & Habenicht,A.J. (2005). The lamina adventitia is the major site of immune cell accumulation in standard chow-fed apolipoprotein E-deficient mice. *Arterioscler. Thromb. Vasc. Biol. 25*, 2386-2391, ISSN 1524-4636.

Moreno,P.R., Purushothaman,K.R., Sirol,M., Levy,A.P., & Fuster,V. (2006). Neovascularization in human atherosclerosis. *Circulation 113*, 2245-2252, ISSN 1524-4539.

Mulligan-Kehoe,M.J. (2010). The vasa vasorum in diseased and nondiseased arteries. *Am. J. Physiol Heart Circ. Physiol 298*, H295-H305, ISSN 1522-1539.

Munro,J.M., van der Walt,J.D., Munro,C.S., Chalmers,J.A., & Cox,E.L. (1987). An immunohistochemical analysis of human aortic fatty streaks. *Hum. Pathol. 18*, 375-380, ISSN 0046-8177.

Murugesan,G., Sandhya Rani,M.R., Gerber,C.E., Mukhopadhyay,C., Ransohoff,R.M., Chisolm,G.M., Kottke-Marchant,K. (2003). Lysophosphatidylcholine regulates human microvascular endothelial cell expression of chemokines. *J. Mol. Cell. Cardiol. 35 (11)*, 1375-1384, ISSN 0022-2828.

Nageh,M.F., Sandberg,E.T., Marotti,K.R., Lin,A.H., Melchior,E.P., Bullard,D.C., & Beaudet,A.L. (1997). Deficiency of inflammatory cell adhesion molecules protects against atherosclerosis in mice. *Arterioscler. Thromb. Vasc. Biol. 17*, 1517-1520, ISSN 1079-5642.

Newman,P.J. (1997). The biology of PECAM-1. *J. Clin. Invest 99*, 3-8, ISSN 0021-9738.

Newman,W., Beall,L.D., Carson,C.W., Hunder,G.G., Graben,N., Randhawa,Z.I., Gopal,T.V., Wiener-Kronish,J., Matthay,M.A. (1993). Soluble E-selectin is found in supernatants of activated endothelial cells and is elevated in the serum of patients with septic shock. *J. Immunol. 150(2)*. 644-654. ISSN 0022-1767

Nicholls,S.J. & Hazen,S.L. (2009). Myeloperoxidase, modified lipoproteins, and atherogenesis. *J. Lipid Res. 50 Suppl*, S346-S351, ISSN 0022-2275.

Ostermann,G., Fraemohs,L., Baltus,T., Schober,A., Lietz,M., Zernecke,A., Liehn,E.A., & Weber,C. (2005). Involvement of JAM-A in mononuclear cell recruitment on inflamed or atherosclerotic endothelium: inhibition by soluble JAM-A. *Arterioscler. Thromb. Vasc. Biol. 25*, 729-735, ISSN 1524-4636.

Pan,J.H., Sukhova,G.K., Yang,J.T., Wang,B., Xie,T., Fu,H., Zhang,Y., Satoskar,A.R., David,J.R., Metz,C.N., Bucala,R., Fang,K., Simon,D.I., Chapman,H.A., Libby,P., & Shi,G.P. (2004). Macrophage migration inhibitory factor deficiency impairs atherosclerosis in low-density lipoprotein receptor-deficient mice. *Circulation 109*, 3149-3153, ISSN 1524-4539.

Parhami,F., Fang,Z.T., Fogelman,A.M., Andalibi,A., Territo,M.C., & Berliner,J.A. (1993). Minimally modified low density lipoprotein-induced inflammatory responses in endothelial cells are mediated by cyclic adenosine monophosphate. *J. Clin. Invest 92*, 471-478, ISSN 0021-9738.

Park,Y.M., Febbraio,M., & Silverstein,R.L. (2009). CD36 modulates migration of mouse and human macrophages in response to oxidized LDL and may contribute to macrophage trapping in the arterial intima. *J. Clin. Invest 119*, 136-145, ISSN 0021-9738.

Parums,D. & Mitchinson,M.J. (1981). Demonstration of immunoglobulin in the neighbourhood of advanced atherosclerotic plaques. *Atherosclerosis 38*, 211-216, ISSN 0021-9150.

Passlick,B., Flieger,D., & Ziegler-Heitbrock,H.W. (1989). Identification and characterization of a novel monocyte subpopulation in human peripheral blood. *Blood 74*, 2527-2534, ISSN 0006-4971.

Patel,S.S., Thiagarajan,R., Willerson,J.T., & Yeh,E.T. (1998). Inhibition of alpha4 integrin and ICAM-1 markedly attenuate macrophage homing to atherosclerotic plaques in ApoE-deficient mice. *Circulation 97*, 75-81, ISSN 0009-7322.

Pedersen,E.M., Oyre,S., Agerbaek,M., Kristensen,I.B., Ringgaard,S., Boesiger,P., & Paaske,W.P. (1999). Distribution of early atherosclerotic lesions in the human abdominal aorta correlates with wall shear stresses measured in vivo. *Eur. J. Vasc. Endovasc. Surg. 18*, 328-333, ISSN 1078-5884.

Piali,L., Weber,C., LaRosa,G., Mackay,C.R., Springer,T.A., Clark-Lewis,I., & Moser,B. (1998). The chemokine receptor CXCR3 mediates rapid and shear-resistant adhesion-induction of effector T lymphocytes by the chemokines IP10 and Mig. *Eur. J. Immunol. 28*, 961-972, ISSN 0014-2980 .

Pigot,R. Dillon,L.P., Hemingway,I.H., Gearing,A.J. (1992). Soluble forms of E-Selectin, ICAM-1 and VCAM-1 are present in the supernatants of cytokine activated cultured endothelial cells. *Biochem Biophys Res Commun. 187(2)*, 584-589. ISSN 0006-291X

Pillarisetti,S., Paka,L., Obunike,J.C., Berglund,L., & Goldberg,I.J. (1997). Subendothelial retention of lipoprotein (a). Evidence that reduced heparan sulfate promotes lipoprotein binding to subendothelial matrix. *J. Clin. Invest 100*, 867-874, ISSN 0021-9738.

Pober,J.S., Gimbrone,M.A., Jr., Cotran,R.S., Reiss,C.S., Burakoff,S.J., Fiers,W., & Ault,K.A. (1983). Ia expression by vascular endothelium is inducible by activated T cells and by human gamma interferon. *J. Exp. Med. 157*, 1339-1353, ISSN 0022-1007.

Potteaux,S., Gautier,E.L., Hutchison,S.B., van Rooijen N., Rader,D.J., Thomas,M.J., Sorci-Thomas,M.G., & Randolph,G.J. (2011). Suppressed monocyte recruitment drives macrophage removal from atherosclerotic plaques of Apoe-/- mice during disease regression. *J. Clin. Invest 121*, 2025-2036, ISSN 1558-8238.

Quinn,M.T., Parthasarathy,S., Fong,L.G., Steinberg,D. (1987). Oxidatively modified low density lipoproteins: a potential role in recruitment and retention of monocyte/macrophages during atherogenesis. *Proc. Natl. Acad. Sci. USA.*, 84(9), 2995-2998, ISSN 0027-8424

Quinn,M.T., Parthasarathy,S., Steinberg,D. (1988). Lysophosphatidylcholine: a chemotactic factor for human monocytes and its potential role in atherogenesis. *Proc. Natl. Acad. Sci. USA.*, 85(8), 2805-2809, ISSN 0027-8424

Ramos,C.L., Huo,Y., Jung,U., Ghosh,S., Manka,D.R., Sarembock,I.J., & Ley,K. (1999). Direct demonstration of P-selectin- and VCAM-1-dependent mononuclear cell rolling in early atherosclerotic lesions of apolipoprotein E-deficient mice. *Circ. Res. 84*, 1237-1244, ISSN 0009-7330.

Ranjbaran,H., Wang,Y., Manes,T.D., Yakimov,A.O., Akhtar,S., Kluger,M.S., Pober,J.S., & Tellides,G. (2006). Heparin displaces interferon-gamma-inducible chemokines (IP-10, I-TAC, and Mig) sequestered in the vasculature and inhibits the transendothelial migration and arterial recruitment of T cells. *Circulation 114*, 1293-1300, 1524-4539.

Reape,T.J., Rayner,K., Manning,C.D., Gee,A.N., Barnette,M.S., Burnand,K.G., & Groot,P.H. (1999). Expression and cellular localization of the CC chemokines PARC and ELC in human atherosclerotic plaques. *Am. J. Pathol. 154*, 365-374, ISSN 0002-9440 .

Ritman,E.L. & Lerman,A. (2007). The dynamic vasa vasorum. *Cardiovasc. Res. 75*, 649-658, ISSN 0008-6363.

Roldan,V., Marin,F., Lip,G.Y.H., Blann,A.D. (2003). Soluble E-selectin in cardiovascular disease and its risk factors. A review of the literature. *Throm. Haemost. 90(6)*, 1007-1020, ISSN 0340-6245

Rotzius,P., Thams,S., Soehnlein,O., Kenne,E., Tseng,C.N., Bjorkstrom,N.K., Malmberg,K.J., Lindbom,L., & Eriksson,E.E. (2010). Distinct infiltration of neutrophils in lesion shoulders in ApoE-/- mice. *Am. J. Pathol. 177*, 493-500, ISSN 1525-2191.

Sakaguchi,S., Yamaguchi,T., Nomura,T., & Ono,M. (2008). Regulatory T cells and immune tolerance. *Cell 133*, 775-787, ISSN 1879-0372 .

Serbina,N.V. & Pamer,E.G. (2006). Monocyte emigration from bone marrow during bacterial infection requires signals mediated by chemokine receptor CCR2. *Nat. Immunol. 7*, 311-317, ISSN 1529-2908.

Shagdarsuren,E., Djalali-Talab,Y., Aurrand-Lions,M., Bidzhekov,K., Liehn,E.A., Imhof,B.A., Weber,C., & Zernecke,A. (2009). Importance of junctional adhesion molecule-C for neointimal hyperplasia and monocyte recruitment in atherosclerosis-prone mice-brief report. *Arterioscler. Thromb. Vasc. Biol. 29*, 1161-1163, ISSN 1524-4636.

Shaw,S.K., Ma,S., Kim,M.B., Rao,R.M., Hartman,C.U., Froio,R.M., Yang,L., Jones,T., Liu,Y., Nusrat,A., Parkos,C.A., & Luscinskas,F.W. (2004). Coordinated redistribution of leukocyte LFA-1 and endothelial cell ICAM-1 accompany neutrophil transmigration. *J. Exp. Med. 200*, 1571-1580, ISSN 0022-1007.

Soehnlein,O., Lindbom,L., & Weber,C. (2009). Mechanisms underlying neutrophil-mediated monocyte recruitment. *Blood 114*, 4613-4623, ISSN 1528-0020.

Sprague, A.H., Khalil, R.A. (2009) Inflammatory cytokines in vascular dysfunction and vascular disease. *Biochem Pharmacol*, 78(6): 539-552, ISSN 1873-2968

Sun,J., Sukhova,G.K., Wolters,P.J., Yang,M., Kitamoto,S., Libby,P., MacFarlane,L.A., Mallen-St,C.J., & Shi,G.P. (2007). Mast cells promote atherosclerosis by releasing proinflammatory cytokines. *Nat. Med. 13*, 719-724, ISSN 1078-8956.

Sunderkotter,C., Nikolic,T., Dillon,M.J., van Rooijen N., Stehling,M., Drevets,D.A., & Leenen,P.J. (2004). Subpopulations of mouse blood monocytes differ in maturation stage and inflammatory response. *J. Immunol. 172*, 4410-4417, ISSN 0022-1767.

Swirski,F.K., Libby,P., Aikawa,E., Alcaide,P., Luscinskas,F.W., Weissleder,R., & Pittet,M.J. (2007). Ly-6Chi monocytes dominate hypercholesterolemia-associated monocytosis and give rise to macrophages in atheromata. *J. Clin. Invest 117*, 195-205, ISSN 0021-9738.

Swirski,F.K., Nahrendorf,M., Etzrodt,M., Wildgruber,M., Cortez-Retamozo,V., Panizzi,P., Figueiredo,J.L., Kohler,R.H., Chudnovskiy,A., Waterman,P., Aikawa,E., Mempel,T.R., Libby,P., Weissleder,R., & Pittet,M.J. (2009). Identification of splenic reservoir monocytes and their deployment to inflammatory sites. *Science 325*, 612-616, ISSN 1095-9203.

Swirski,F.K., Pittet,M.J., Kircher,M.F., Aikawa,E., Jaffer,F.A., Libby,P., & Weissleder,R. (2006). Monocyte accumulation in mouse atherogenesis is progressive and proportional to extent of disease. *Proc. Natl. Acad. Sci. U. S. A 103*, 10340-10345, ISSN 0027-8424.

Tacke,F., Alvarez,D., Kaplan,T.J., Jakubzick,C., Spanbroek,R., Llodra,J., Garin,A., Liu,J., Mack,M., van,R.N., Lira,S.A., Habenicht,A.J., & Randolph,G.J. (2007). Monocyte subsets differentially employ CCR2, CCR5, and CX3CR1 to accumulate within atherosclerotic plaques. *J. Clin. Invest 117*, 185-194, ISSN 0021-9738.

Tanaka,K., Nagata,D., Hirata,Y., Tabata,Y., Nagai,R., & Sata,M. (2011). Augmented angiogenesis in adventitia promotes growth of atherosclerotic plaque in apolipoprotein E-deficient mice. *Atherosclerosis 215*, 366-373, ISSN 1879-1484 .

Tedgui,A. & Mallat,Z. (2006). Cytokines in atherosclerosis: pathogenic and regulatory pathways. *Physiol Rev. 86*, 515-581, ISSN 0031-9333.

Trogan,E., Feig,J.E., Dogan,S., Rothblat,G.H., Angeli,V., Tacke,F., Randolph,G.J., & Fisher, E.A. (2006). Gene expression changes in foam cells and the role of chemokine receptor CCR7 during atherosclerosis regression in ApoE-deficient mice. *Proc. Natl. Acad. Sci. U. S. A 103*, 3781-3786, ISSN 0027-8424.

Tsou,C.L., Peters,W., Si,Y., Slaymaker,S., Aslanian,A.M., Weisberg,S.P., Mack,M., & Charo,I.F. (2007). Critical roles for CCR2 and MCP-3 in monocyte mobilization from bone marrow and recruitment to inflammatory sites. *J.Clin. Invest 117*, 902-909, ISSN 0021-9738.

Tsou,J.K., Gower,R.M., Ting,H.J., Schaff,U.Y., Insana,M.F., Passerini,A.G., & Simon,S.I. (2008). Spatial regulation of inflammation by human aortic endothelial cells in a linear gradient of shear stress. *Microcirculation. 15*, 311-323, ISSN 1073-9688.

Tu,L., Poe,J.C., Kadono,T., Venturi,G.M., Bullard,D.C., Tedder,T.F., Steeber,D.A. (2002). A functional role for circulating mouse L-selectin in regulating leukocyte/endothelial cell interactions in vivo. *J. Immunol. 169(4)*. 2034-2043. ISSN 0022-1767.

VanderLaan,P.A., Reardon,C.A., & Getz,G.S. (2004). Site specificity of atherosclerosis: site-selective responses to atherosclerotic modulators. Arterioscler. *Thromb. Vasc. Biol. 24*, 12-22, ISSN 1524-4636 .

Vestweber,D. (2007). Adhesion and signalling molecules controlling the transmigration of leukocytes through endothelium. *Immunol. Rev. 218*, 178-196, ISSN 0105-2896 .

von Hundelshausen, P., Koenen,R.R., Sack,M., Mause,S.F., Adriaens,W., Proudfoot,A.E., Hackeng,T.M., & Weber,C. (2005). Heterophilic interactions of platelet factor 4 and RANTES promote monocyte arrest on endothelium. *Blood 105*, 924-930, ISSN 0006-4971.

von Hundelshausen, P., Weber,K.S., Huo,Y., Proudfoot,A.E., Nelson,P.J., Ley,K., & Weber,C. (2001). RANTES deposition by platelets triggers monocyte arrest on inflamed and atherosclerotic endothelium. *Circulation 103*, 1772-1777, ISSN 1524-4539.

Weber,K.S., von Hundelshausen,P., Clark-Lewis,I., Weber,P.C., & Weber,C. (1999). Differential immobilization and hierarchical involvement of chemokines in monocyte arrest and transmigration on inflamed endothelium in shear flow. *Eur. J. Immunol. 29*, 700-712, ISSN 0014-2980.

Wick,G., Romen,M., Amberger,A., Metzler,B., Mayr,M., Falkensammer,G., & Xu,Q. (1997). Atherosclerosis, autoimmunity, and vascular-associated lymphoid tissue. *FASEB J. 11*, 1199-1207, ISSN 0892-6638.

Zarbock,A., Lowell,C.A., & Ley,K. (2007). Spleen tyrosine kinase Syk is necessary for E-selectin-induced alpha(L)beta(2) integrin-mediated rolling on intercellular adhesion molecule-1. *Immunity. 26*, 773-783, ISSN 1074-7613.

Zhang,J., Alcaide, P., Liu, L., Sun, J., He, A., Luscinskas, F.W., Shi, G.P. (2011). Regulation of endothelial cell adhesion molecule expression by mast cells, macrophages, and neutrophils. *PLoS One.* 14; 1-10, ISSN 1932-6203.

Zhou, X., & Hansson G.K. Detection of B cells and proinflammatory cytokines in atherosclerotic plaques of hypercholesterolaemic apolipoprotein E knockout mice. (1999). *Scand. J. Immunol.* 50, 25-30, ISSN 1365-3083.

Zernecke,A., Bot,I., Djalali-Talab,Y., Shagdarsuren,E., Bidzhekov,K., Meiler,S., Krohn,R., Schober,A., Sperandio,M., Soehnlein,O., Bornemann,J., Tacke,F., Biessen,E.A., & Weber,C. (2008). Protective role of CXC receptor 4/CXC ligand 12 unveils the importance of neutrophils in atherosclerosis. *Circ. Res. 102*, 209-217, ISSN 1524-4571.

Zernecke,A., Liehn,E.A., Fraemohs,L., von Hundelshausen, P., Koenen,R.R., Corada,M., Dejana,E., & Weber,C. (2006). Importance of junctional adhesion molecule-A for neointimal lesion formation and infiltration in atherosclerosis-prone mice. *Arterioscler. Thromb. Vasc. Biol. 26*, e10-e13, ISSN 1524-4636.

Zernecke, A & Weber, C., (2010). Chemokines in the vascular inflammatory response of atherosclerosis. *Cardiovasc. Research*. 86, 192-201, ISSN 1755-3245.

11

# (Auto)Phagocytosis in Atherosclerosis: Implications for Plaque Stability and Therapeutic Challenges

Dorien M. Schrijvers, Guido R.Y. De Meyer and Wim Martinet
*University of Antwerp, Laboratory of Pharmacology*
*Belgium*

## 1. Introduction

This chapter is intended to describe the interactions between cell death, phagocytosis and autophagic survival in atherosclerosis, and how these processes could be attractive therapeutic targets for atherosclerotic plaque stabilization.
Atherosclerosis is a long-term, progressive inflammatory disease characterized by the formation of atherosclerotic plaques in the intima of medium- and large-sized arteries. Progression of the disease is accelerated by well-known risk factors including gender, age, hypercholesterolemia, diabetes mellitus, hypertension, smoking, obesity and a sedentary life-style (Kannel et al., 2004). In the advanced stage, plaques can partially or totally occlude the blood vessel, known as arterial stenosis. However, not only the degree of stenosis, but also the composition and stability of the plaque determines the clinical outcome of the disease (Hansson, 2005). Indeed, plaques may become extremely unstable and prone to rupture through the presence of many inflammatory cells and mediators, a large necrotic core consisting of uncleared cell debris and lipids, a high degree of cell death leading to a scarce amount of smooth muscle cells, and the formation of leaky neovessels inside the plaque. Occlusive thrombi, as a result of plaque rupture, in turn cause acute (and often fatal) clinical manifestations, such as myocardial infarction and stroke. Current clinical therapy is focused on chirurgical interventions (stents, endarterectomy, bypass) and plasma cholesterol lowering drugs (e.g. statins). In addition, changes in diet and exercise have made significant inroads in preventing acute atherothrombotic events (Getz & Reardon, 2006). Although these aforementioned approaches have provided significant improvements, they are far from sufficient. Analysis of the cell death and phagocytosis machinery as well as survival strategies of cells in plaques could provide additional insights for development of new plaque stabilizing strategies.

## 2. Phagocytosis of apoptotic cells

Billions of cells in the human body die each day by the process of apoptosis (Henson et al., 2001). A critical process, called phagocytosis, is coupled with each of these cell death events. Macrophages and nonprofessional phagocytes remove apoptotic cells (AC) via phagocytosis in a rapid and efficient manner. This results in at least five critical protective effects: (1) it actively suppresses the secretion of inflammatory cytokines from the phagocyte, via autocrine/paracrine secretion of transforming growth factor beta (TGFβ), prostaglandin E2 (PGE2), and platelet-activating factor (PAF) (Fadok et al., 1998), (2) it prevents leakage of proinflammatory intracellular material from the dying cell, before membrane damage occurs, (3) it triggers a potent survival pathway in the phagocyte, involving Akt, NF-κB and cholesterol efflux (Reddy et al., 2002; Kiss et al., 2006), (4) it can promote cell growth and wound healing through the release of vascular endothelial growth factor (VEGF) and TGFβ, respectively (Golpon et al., 2004; Sindrilaru et al., 2009), and (5) it has a vital role in maintaining immunological tolerance against cell-associated antigens, as the TGFβ, produced by the dying cells or the engulfing cells induce the differentiation of inducible regulatory T cells, which inhibit immune responses (Green et al., 2009). The entire process of phagocytosis (recognition, tethering, binding, internalization) is tightly regulated and involves a wide array of molecules, including receptors on the phagocyte, ligands on the AC and soluble bridging molecules (Figure 1). The multiplicity of ways in which phagocytes recognize and engulf AC suggests that a hierarchy of engulfment mechanisms and back-up mechanisms exists. Indeed, upon blocking essential receptors phagocytosis of AC is decreased but this inhibition is never complete, suggesting cooperation between different mechanisms of phagocytosis (Pradhan et al., 1997).

Changes in composition and molecular topology of the plasma membrane of the AC involve the loss of "don't-eat-me" signals, also called self-associated molecular patterns (SAMPs), such as CD31 (Brown et al., 2002) and CD47 (Gardai et al., 2005) and the exposure of "eat-me" signals, also known as apoptotic cell-associated molecular patterns (ACAMPs). The most renowned ACAMP is the redistributed phosphatidylserine (PS) (Fadok et al., 1992;, 1999; Callahan et al., 2000; Hoffmann et al., 2001), which on viable cells is actively confined to the inner leaflet of the plasma membrane. Annexin-1 is a caspase-dependent engulfment ligand that is recruited from the cytosol and exported to the outer plasma membrane leaflet, colocalizes with PS, and is required for efficient clearance of ACs (Arur et al., 2003). Similar to PS, calreticulin acts as a facultative recognition ligand on AC (Martins et al., 2010). Phagocyte pattern recognition receptors such as CD14 (Devitt et al., 1998; Schlegel et al., 1999), scavenger receptors such as CD36, and integrins such as αvβ3 (Savill et al., 1992), together with PS receptors such as BAI-1 (D. Park et al., 2007), TIM-4 (Miyanishi et al., 2007) and stabilin-2 (S.Y. Park et al., 2008), or PS bridging molecules such as MFG-E8 (lactadherin) and Gas-6—which bind to PS on the AC and to integrins or MerTK on the phagocyte, respectively (Qingxian et al., 2010)—are well known phagocytic receptors. Upon engagement, strong tethering is achieved, the phagocytic synapse is set, and engulfment response pathways are activated. Other phagocyte receptors include an unidentified PS receptor (PSR), transglutaminase 2 (TG2) (Szondy et al., 2003), low density lipoprotein receptor-related protein 1 (LRP1) (Lillis et al., 2008), ATP binding cassette 7 (ABCA7), purinergic receptor P2Y2, CD91 (Martins et al., 2010) and fractalkine receptor 1 (CX3CR1).

Recognition signals and receptors are crucial for efficient phagocytosis. However, these signals can only be effective when the phagocyte and the AC are in close proximity. Soluble "come-get-me" signals are secreted by AC to attract phagocytes to sites of AC death (Grimsley & Ravichandran, 2003) (Table 1).

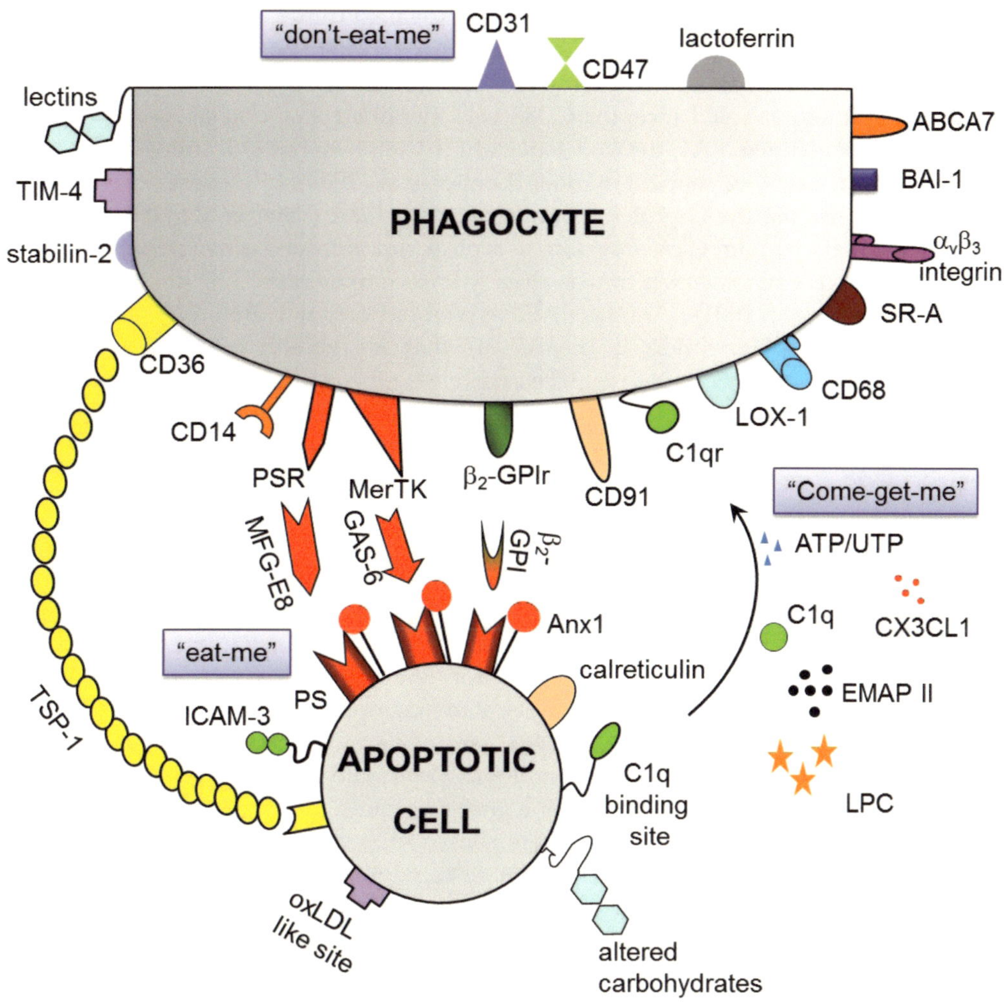


Fig. 1. Phagocyte recognition of apoptotic cells. Several receptors on the phagocyte membrane are involved and interact either directly with their ligands on the AC surface ("eat-me") or via bridging molecules. AC can send out chemoattractant signals to attract macrophages to the site of cell death ("come-get-me"). To prevent phagocytosis of healthy cells, the latter express molecules to identify themselves ("don't-eat-me"). ABCA7, ATP-binding cassette-7; CD14, lipopolysaccharide receptor; LOX-1, lectin-like oxidized low density lipoprotein receptor-1; CD36, thrombospondin receptor; CD68, macrosialin; SRA, scavenger receptor class A; FcR, Fc fragment of immunoglobulin G receptor; LRP, LDL receptor-related protein; CD91, α2-macroglobulin; GAS-6, growth arrest-specific gene 6; β2-GPI, beta 2-glycoprotein 2; TSP, thrombospondin; PS, phosphatidylserine; PSR, PS receptor; αvβ3, vitronectin receptor; MFG-E8, milk-fat globule epidermal growth factor 8; ICAM-3, intracellular adhesion molecule-1; C1q, complement complex 1q; Anx1, annexin 1; BAI-1, brain angiogenesis inhibitor-1; TIM-4, T-cell immunoglobulin and mucin domain-containing protein 4; MerTK, c-mer proto-oncogene tyrosine kinase; LPC, lysophosphatidylcholine; CX3CL1, fractalkine; EMAP II, endothelial monocyte-activating polypeptide II.

The first identified attraction signal of AC was the covalent dimer of ribosomal protein S19 (dRP S19) (Horino et al., 1998). It is an essential monocyte chemoattractant in the synovium of patients with rheumatoid arthritis (Nishiura et al., 1996). By using neutralizing antibodies, G-protein coupled receptor CD88 was identified as a crucial receptor for dRP S19. The most characterized AC-derived attractant is lysophosphatidylcholine (LPC), which is secreted in a caspase-3 dependent manner (Lauber et al., 2003). LPC exerts its chemotactic effect on monocytes via the G-protein coupled receptor G2A (Peter et al., 2008). Knockout mice that are deficient in G2A develop a typical autoimmune phenotype resembling systemic lupus erythematosus, which was already known to be caused by deficiencies in AC recognition (Le et al., 2001). Another AC-derived attraction signal is the endothelial monocyte-activating polypeptide II (EMAP II) that is proteolytically cleaved during apoptosis but not during necrosis to mature and release the active p23 protein (Knies et al., 1998). Processing of pro-EMAP II was observed to be a rather late event in the course of apoptosis, occurring several hours after poly (ADP-ribose) polymerase cleavage. Since AC are phagocytised at an early stage, it was suggested that mature EMAP II serves as a back-up signal at sites of excessive cell death (Behrensdorf et al., 2000). Importantly, *in vitro* experiments showed that human pro-EMAP II is not cleaved by caspases and mature EMAP II could not be found in AC, as opposed to murine EMAP II. Thus, it is not entirely clear whether mature EMAP II or its precursor is the real cytokine (Martinet et al., 2010). The only receptor that has been reported in the context of EMAP II is CX3CR1, but it remains to be elucidated whether this is the crucial sensor for EMAP II p23 (Hou et al., 2006). C1q facilitates the ingestion of apoptotic cells by human macrophages via binding to calreticulin (Ogden et al., 2001). Thrombospondin-1 (TSP1) modulates a number of processes, including migration, proliferation and angiogenesis and was also found to be actively secreted during apoptosis (Savill et al., 1992). It serves as a bridging molecule to physically connect the phagocyte to the AC, though the phagocyte sensor involved remains obscure. Recently, nucleotides such as ATP and UTP, which can be recognized by purinergic receptor P2Y2, were found to be released from AC and incite migration of monocytes and macrophages (Elliott et al., 2009). Membrane-bound fractalkine (CX3CL1) can be released from AC by a so far unknown protease, to induce recruitment of macrophages (Truman et al., 2008). The CX3CR1-fractalkine system seems to be particularly important in germinal centers, and is limited to certain cell types, such as B cells and neurons. Two less characterized AC-derived chemokines are sphingosine-1-phosphate (S1P) and the N-terminal fragment of tyrosyl tRNA synthetases (mini TyrRS) (Gude et al., 2008; Wakasugi & Schimmel, 1999). Both were identified in *in vitro* settings and might contribute to the anti-inflammatory character of AC clearance. While it is clear that apoptosis can be executed in the absence of blebbing and that phagocytic engulfment is not restricted to 'bite-sized' apoptotic bodies, it has been suggested that fragmentation of the AC may be important for chemotactic signaling to mononuclear phagocytes (Segundo et al., 1999; Hugel et al., 2005; Simons & Raposo, 2009). Yet, the range of action and the phagocyte sensors remain to be resolved.

Note that plasma membrane-damaged cells (i.e. late apoptotic and necrotic cells) can also release or expose endogenous and exogenous signals, known as alarmins or damage-associated molecular patterns (DAMPs), to alert the organism to tissue injury (Patel et al., 2006; Peter et al., 2010) (Table 1). One such protein is the high mobility group box 1 protein (HMGB-1), which is released from necrotic cells, but not during apoptosis, and actively stimulates the secretion of proinflammatory cytokines (Scaffidi et al., 2002; Andersson et al.,

2000). Toll like receptors (TLR)-2 and 4 have been described to be engaged in HMGB-1 signaling (Yu et al., 2006). Another necrotic cell-derived danger signal, that is closely related to HMGB-1 is the hepatoma-derived growth factor (HDGF) (Nakamura et al., 1994). It is mainly located in the nucleus and remains trapped there during apoptosis, but is passively released during necrosis. The family of the calgranulin proteins, also referred to as the S100 proteins, are potent chemoattractant proteins and play a significant role in the propagation of inflammation (Donato, 2003; Foell et al., 2008). Specifically, the S100A8-S100A9 complex and S100A12 proved to be useful diagnostic markers of inflammatory diseases, like arthritis and COPD, where they are found in high concentrations in the blood, sputum, stool and synovial fluid (Foell et al., 2004). Future studies need to clarify whether these proteins also represent therapeutic targets. Heat shock proteins (HSP) 70, 90 and 98 are released during heat-induced necrosis, probably via exosomes (Basu et al., 2000). Yet, knowledge about the secretion and exact functions is confusing and needs clarification. For example, apart from their TLR-mediated pro-inflammatory signaling, HSP also display anti-inflammatory effects (Wieten et al., 2007; Tang et al., 2007). Finally, concentrations of uric acid are increased during cell injury. Uric acid has the ability to prime T cells in the generation of helper and cytotoxic T cells (Shi et al., 2002; Ghaemi-Oskouie & Shi, 2011).

| "don't-eat-me" | "eat-me" | "come-get-me" | "alarmins" |
|---|---|---|---|
| CD31 | PS | LPC | HMGB-1 |
| CD47 | Anx1 | EMAP-II (p23) | HDGF |
| lactoferrin | calreticulin | ATP/UTP | S100 proteins |
| | | TSP1 | HSPs |
| | | CX3CL1 | uric acid |
| | | C1q | |
| | | dRP S19 | |
| | | mini TyrRS | |
| | | S1P | |
| | | microblebs | |

Table 1. Comprehensive list of signals that are presented and/or secreted by healthy cells ("don't-eat-me"), apoptotic cells (cell surface "eat-me" signals and soluble "come-get-me"signals) or necrotic cells ("alarmins"). Abbreviations: PS, phosphatidylserine; Anx1, annexin 1; LPC, lysophosphatidylcholine, EMAP-II (p23), endothelial monocyte-activating polypeptide II active protein; TSP1, thrombospondin 1; CX3CL1, fractalkine; C1q, complement complex 1q; dRP S19, dimer of ribosomal protein S19; mini TyrRS, N-terminal fraction tyrosyl tRNA synthetase; S1P, sphingosine-1-phosphate; HMGB-1, high mobility group box 1 protein; HDGF, hepatoma-derived growth factor; S100 proteins, calgranulin family of proteins; HSP, heat-shock protein.

Recognition of necrotic cells by phagocytes is less well understood than recognition of ACs, but an increasing number of recent studies are highlighting its importance. (Krysko et al., 2006). C1q, mannose-binding lectin (MBL) and pentraxin-3 (PTX3) were demonstrated exclusively on late ACs and necrotic cells (Gaipl et al., 2001; Nauta et al., 2003; Rovere et al., 2000). C-reactive protein (CRP), an acute phase protein binds to secondary necrotic neutrophils (Hart et al., 2005). However, CRP does not uniquely bind to necrotic cells. The same is true for TSP1. Future studies are needed to identify the differences and similarities between the macrophage interaction with AC and necrotic cells. A pitfall in this area is the lack of a good cell culture system to study this. Current cell culture models are still very variable, displaying a mixture of early and late ACs and necrosis. In addition, detailed information on mechanisms of binding and internalization of necrotic cells is sparse. Importantly, the trigger provoking necrotic death has an important impact on the kind of immunological response of phagocytes (Hirt & Leist, 2003). Phagocytic uptake of late apoptotic/necrotic cells by antigen-presenting cells, such as DCs, can lead to the presentation of autoantigens to autoreactive T cells in a proinflammatory context, thus facilitating the onset of an autoimmune response (Poon et al., 2010). However, there are several studies reporting non-inflammatory responses of phagocytes, including modulation of anti-tumor immunity and tissue repair via VEGF induction (M. Li et al., 2001).

For more comprehensive details of the molecular complexity of the clearance phases and engulfment signaling pathways, the reader is referred to recent reviews (Elliott & Ravichandran, 2010; Kinchen 2010; Poon et al., 2010; Devitt & Marshall, 2011).

### 2.1 Phagocytosis of apoptotic cells in atherosclerosis

In early human atherosclerotic plaques, phagocytic clearance of AC by macrophages is very efficient (Tabas, 2005) (Figure 2). Conversely, phagocytosis in advanced human atherosclerotic plaques is defective, resulting in secondary necrosis, expansion of the necrotic core and increased plaque vulnerability (Schrijvers et al., 2005; Thorp & Tabas, 2009; Thorp, 2010). Similar results have been found in mouse models of advanced atherosclerosis. The impact of defective clearance of AC on the plaque further exacerbated when essential effector molecules in phagocytosis were targeted. Examples of these effector molecules are MerTK (Thorp et al., 2008; Ait-Oufella et al., 2008), MFG-E8 (Ait-Oufella et al., 2007), C1q (Bhatia et al., 2007), LRP-1 (Yancey et al., 2010), TSP1 (Moura et al., 2008), TG2 (Boisvert et al., 2006) and ABCA7 (Jehle et al., 2006).

The mechanisms of defective phagocytosis in advanced atherosclerotic plaques are not entirely clear, although *in vitro* experiments have put forward several plausible explanations (Schrijvers et al., 2005). It is unlikely that overwhelming apoptosis is a major factor, since phagocytosis is very efficient in early plaques, where phagocytosis is not defective, when excessive apoptosis is induced through genetic manipulation (Tabas, 2010). In addition, AC in plaques are found in the vicinity of macrophages, which rules out a possible geographic problem. Moreover, atherosclerotic plaques are highly inflamed tissue and contain large areas of macrophage infiltration. Therefore, it is not the quantity of the phagocytes that is important for phagocytosis, but their functionality. Most likely, phagocytosis itself becomes ineffective in advanced plaques.

One of the first discovered mechanisms that contribute to defective clearance of AC in atherosclerosis is the competition of oxidized low density lipoproteins (oxLDL), but not acetylated LDL, with AC and oxidatively damaged cells for macrophage binding (Sambrano & Steinberg, 1995). AC, oxLDL as well as oxidized red blood cells share oxidatively modified moieties on their surfaces that serve as ligands for macrophage recognition, thereby profoundly inhibiting the phagocytosis of AC. Furthermore, secretion of MFG-E8 (lactadherin), a macrophage-derived molecule that facilitates phagocytosis of AC, is down-regulated upon free cholesterol-loading in macrophages (Su et al., 2005). Electron microscopy images from macrophage-derived foam cells in atherosclerotic plaques show that these cells are often crammed with large lipid droplets. It is therefore tempting to speculate that these macrophages are no longer able to engulf AC ("full is full"). Uptake of AC in macrophages treated *in vitro* with an excess of platelets or aggregated LDL is not inhibited, most likely because foam cells in culture rarely reach the same degree of foam cell formation as seen in human plaques, but phagocytosis of beads results in a nearly complete inhibition of phagocytosis of AC (Schrijvers et al., 2005). These findings confirm a study by Moller et al. (2002) showing that uptake of indigestible, rigid particles by macrophages induces cellular 'stiffening' so that changes in cellular shape, which are needed to form pseudopodia for phagocytosis, are inhibited. In addition to foam cell formation, increased oxidative stress is a hallmark of advanced atherosclerotic plaques. Although several reactive oxygen species (ROS) can be found in human plaques, peroxynitrite ($ONOO^-$) plays a central role in the pathophysiology of atherosclerosis as it induces protein nitrosylation and oxidative DNA damage. The peroxynitrite donor SIN1A concentration-dependently decreases phagocytosis of AC *in vitro* (Schrijvers et al., 2005), suggesting that PS or other factors present on macrophages or dying cells required for phagocytosis may be sensitive to oxidative conditions. Proteolytic cleavage of macrophage receptors exacerbates disease in cystic fibrosis and bronchiectasis (Vandivier et al., 2002). Potent proteases, such as matrix metalloproteinases and ADAM proteins (a disintegrin and metalloproteinase) are upregulated in advanced plaques. *In vitro* cleavage of MerTK leads to generation of soluble Mer, that binds to AC and prevents their uptake by macrophages (Sather et al., 2007). Interestingly, gene polymorphisms in CD31 ("don't eat me") and increasing levels of its soluble form have been associated with ischemic stroke, suggesting that extracellular CD31 could affect phagocyte interactions with AC (Wei et al., 2009). These, and other ideas, will require careful assessment in advanced atherosclerotic plaques.

The accumulation of AC has a number of consequences that promote plaque progression and destabilization (Figure 2). Firstly, impaired phagocytosis of AC results in enhanced secretion of proinflammatory cytokines including TNFα and IL-6 by the phagocyte, and a reduced release of anti-inflammatory proteins such as TGFβ and IL-10 (Fadok et al., 1998; Erwig & Henson, 2007). Deregulated expression of these cytokines may result in inflammatory autoimmune responses, as seen in systemic lupus erythematosus and rheumatoid arthritis, two non-atherosclerotic inflammatory disorders with a similar defect in phagocytosis of dying cells by macrophages. Secondly, tissue factor (TF) expression co-localizes with AC, especially around the lipid core of human atherosclerotic plaques, suggesting that uncleared AC are an important source of this molecule (Tedgui & Mallat, 2001). TF is a key element in the initiation of the coagulation cascade and mediates thrombus formation after rupture of an unstable plaque, when free AC are exposed to the blood stream. Thirdly, macrophages that have ingested cholesterol-loaded AC show a remarkable set of survival responses, some of which are not present during the loading of macrophages with lipoprotein-derived cholesterol (Cui et al., 2007). These responses include cholesterol esterification and massive cholesterol efflux, as well as the triggering of cell survival signal transduction pathways involving PI3-kinase/Akt and NF- κB. Consequently, impaired phagocytosis of AC renders the phagocyte more susceptible to cholesterol-induced death (Yvan-Charvet et al., 2010). Finally, expansion of the necrotic core is stimulated due to secondary necrosis of free AC. The interaction of macrophages with necrotic cells or compounds released from necrotic cells (alarmins) often results in an additional inflammatory response (Scaffidi et al., 2002). Necrotic cells also passively release matrix degrading proteases. In this way, post-apoptotic necrosis may contribute to plaque instability through enlargement of the necrotic core, matrix breakdown and stimulation of inflammation and neovascularization (Figure 2).

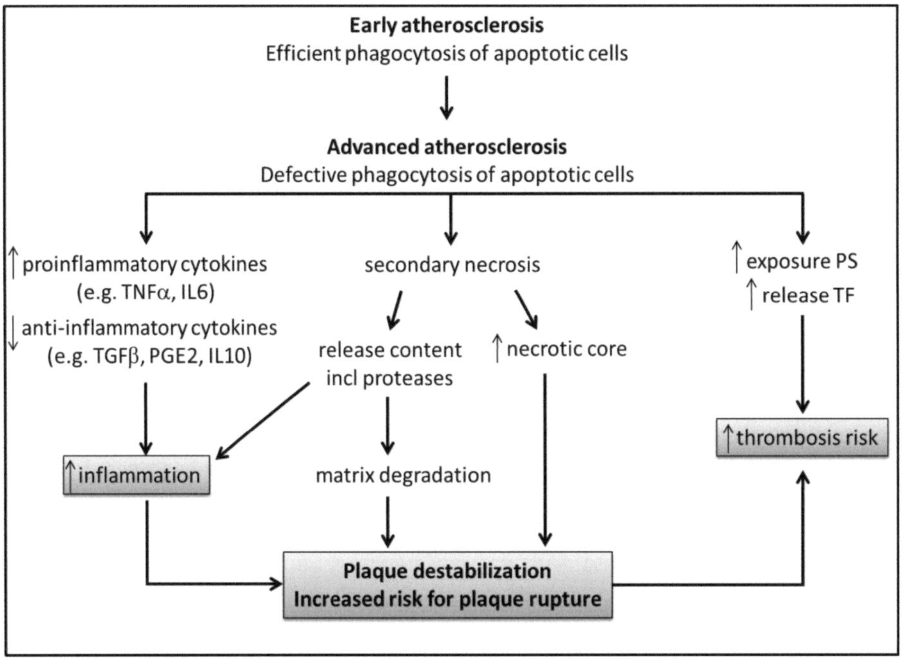


Fig. 2. Consequences of defective phagocytosis of apoptotic cells in atherosclerotic plaques. In early plaques, AC numbers are low and phagocytosis is very efficient, which stimulates active suppression of inflammatory pathways, prevents release of intracellular contents from the dying cells and promotes macrophage survival. In advanced plaques however, phagocytosis of ACs is severely impaired, leading to plaque progression and destabilization through various mechanisms. Unstable plaques are at risk for rupture, which results in the formation of an occlusive thrombus and subsequent, possible fatale, ischemic events. In addition, ACs expose phosphatidylserine (PS) and are a source of tissue factor (TF), both highly thrombogenic.

### 2.2 Therapeutic possibilities

Defective AC clearance can alter immune responses in ways that exacerbate human diseases, e.g. acceleration of SLE, COPD, cystic fibrosis and atherosclerosis. Therefore, a promising approach to stabilize atherosclerotic plaques would be to therapeutically enhance the phagocytic capacity of macrophages. Importantly, non-specific enhancement of phagocytosis is not desirable, because of the adverse effects associated with phagocytosis of lipoproteins, platelets or erythrocytes (Schrijvers et al., 2007).

Statins are an important class of drugs in the treatment of atherosclerosis. They were discovered as drugs that reduce cholesterol levels by inhibiting the 3-hydroxy-3-methylglutaryl coenzyme A (HMG-CoA), but they also have an anti-inflammatory action by virtue of their ability to block prenylation of signaling molecules, i.e. Rho GTPases. Interestingly, it has been shown that lovastatin increases phagocytosis of ACs by macrophages from COPD patients in an HMG-CoA reductase-dependent manner (Morimoto et al., 2006). In contrast, simvastatin impairs Fc-receptor mediated phagocytosis of bacteria (phagocytosis followed by oxidative burst and bacterial killing) and at the same time enhances the production of proinflammatory mediators (Benati et al., 2010). These data should be assessed to prevent potential side-effects in patients undergoing long-term treatment with this statin, who become exposed to an opportunistic pathogen such as *S. aureus*, that is commonly found on the skin and in the upper airways.

Because oxLDL or oxLDL antibodies interfere with phagocytosis of AC, it is tempting to speculate that antioxidants can improve clearance of dying cells. However, clinical trials in humans with antioxidants showed only limited success in preventing coronary artery disease. Possibly the antioxidants lose activity too quickly or do not penetrate the plaque deep enough to reach the phagocytes. This idea is supported by the fact that antioxidants do not prevent the oxidation of phagocytized lipoproteins in the lysosome of macrophages (Wen & Leake, 2007). It is possible that more encouraging results will be obtained in the future through the use of drugs that are targeted to specific oxidation reactions in atherosclerosis. It should also be noted that certain antioxidants may not promote but inhibit recognition of AC by phagocytes by inhibiting oxidation of externalized PS (Tyurina et al., 2004).

In obesity and type 2 diabetes, the defect in efferocytosis of macrophages seems to be related to increased concentrations of saturated fatty acids (FA) and/or decreased concentrations of the ω-3 FA eicosapentaenoic acid (EPA) and docosahexaenoic acid (DHA) (S. Li et al., 2009). This change in membrane lipid composition may lead to defective PI3K activation and failure to generate PIP3 in the macrophage phagocytic membrane. Interestingly, feeding ob/ob mice a fish oil diet increases ω-3 FA without appreciable changes in the content of saturated FA and leads to a reversal of the defect in efferocytosis and a reduction in plaque size (S. Li et al., 2009). These findings suggest that the level of ω-3 FA in the macrophage membrane is an important factor contributing to efficient efferocytosis.

Examples of other drugs that promote phagocytic clearance of AC are chemerin, an endogenous chemoattractant (Cash et al., 2010), the macrolide antibiotic azithromycin (Hodge et al., 2006), members of the lipoxin family (Godson et al., 2000), inflammation resolution mediators such as resolvins (Serhan et al., 2008), inhibitors of MerTK cleavage (Sather et al., 2007), PPARδ activators (Mukundan et al., 2009), LXR activators which increase expression of MerTK, as well as compounds that induce secretion of the efferocytosis effector apolipoprotein E and ABCA1/G1-mediated efflux of toxic sterols (A-Gonzalez et al., 2009; Yancey et al., 2010; Yvan-Charvet et al., 2010).

Phagocyte populations in atherosclerosis are heterogeneous (Waldo et al., 2008; Shimada, 2009) and express different express markers and phagocytic receptors, depending on their spatial location in the plaque and surrounding milieu. *In vitro*, alternatively activated macrophages (M2 phenotype) preferentially clear AC and secrete anti-inflammatory cytokines, including IL-10 and TGFβ (W. Xu et al., 2006). On the other hand, classically activated (M1) macrophages secrete proinflammatory cytokines, such as TNFα and IL-6, that can negatively affect phagocytosis. It would be interesting to elucidate whether communication between these subsets affects phagocytosis efficiency. Plaque phagocytes can polarize towards a spectrum of activation states, resulting in altered phagocytic capacities (Peng et al., 2009). Taking advantage of the fact that some subpopulations are more efficient phagocytes, might be a very attractive way to restore and enhance defective

AC clearance in atherosclerotic plaques. For example, activation of PPARγ stimulates macrophage polarization to the anti-inflammatory M2 phenotype (Bouhlel et al., 2007). Whether or not these aforementioned approaches will be effective at stabilizing atherosclerotic plaques through the amelioration of phagocytic clearance remains to be elucidated.

## 3. Autophagy

### 3.1 General principles

While phagocytosis reflects clearance of non-self particles, autophagy represents a process for cells to dispose of their own unwanted or damaged proteins and organelles (Klionsky, 2007). Autophagy or "self eating" refers to a conserved cellular process for the turnover of organelles and proteins that occurs in all eukaryotic cells (Yoshimori, 2004). It is activated as an adaptive response to environmental stress (e.g. nutrient deprivation, hypoxia, oxidative stress, exposure to xenobiotics) to promote cell survival through the recycling of precursors (amino acids, free fatty acids, nucleotides) derived from the degradation of endogenous cellular components. Typical of autophagy is the formation of double-membrane structures, called phagophores, that engulf intracellular material such as protein aggregates, lipid droplets and complete organelles for degradation (Figure 3). The phagophore expands and, on completion, forms an autophagosome, which then fuses with lysosomes, thereby generating an autophagolysosome (Shintani & Klionsky, 2004). Incorporation of the outer autophagosomal membrane in the lysosomal membrane allows the degradation of the remaining inner single membrane and the cytoplasmic content of the autophagosome by lysosomal hydrolases.

Autophagy generally acts as a housekeeping mechanism, and is crucially involved in the maintenance of normal cellular homeostasis. Hereby, turnover of damaged or dysfunctional organelles, such as mitochondria, peroxisomes and endoplasmic reticulum, is facilitated to maintain a healthy population of these organelles. When stimulated by cellular stress conditions, autophagy functions as a self-cannibalization pathway that promotes cell survival in an unfavorable environment. This pro-survival function of autophagy has been demonstrated at the cellular and tissue level in different contexts, such as nutrient and growth factor deprivation, endoplasmic reticulum stress, development, microbial infection, and diseases characterized by the accumulation of protein aggregates. Preclinical studies have demonstrated that autophagy is associated with cancer, neurodegenerative disorders (e.g. Alzheimer's, Parkinson's and Huntington's disease), embryogenesis, aging and immunity, but also with cardiovascular disease including ischemia-reperfusion injury of the heart, cardiomyopathy and atherosclerosis (Mathew et al., 2007; Levine & Kroemer, 2008; Mizushima et al., 2008; Martinet & De Meyer, 2008,2009a). Despite tremendous recent advances in this field, the functional significance of autophagy in human disease remains incompletely understood, and potentially involves both adaptive and maladaptive outcomes.

There are three main types of autophagy, namely macroautophagy, microautophagy or chaperone-mediated autophagy (Klionsky et al., 2007). Macroautophagy is the most extensively analysed and quantitatively more important type of autophagy in which entire portions of the cytosol are sequestered by a de novo-formed phagophore that seals into an autophagosome (Figure 3). In addition to this 'in bulk' degradation, selective sequestration of cellular structures into autophagosomes is a common mechanism for removal of organelles or particulate protein complexes (aggregates). This is then referred to as selective macroautophagy. The process of microautophagy is poorly characterized, at least in mammalian cells. Like in macroautophagy, entire cytosolic regions constitute the microautophagy cargo, but it is the lysosomal membrane itself that invaginates or protrudes to seclude the cytosolic components. Selective autophagy of soluble cytosolic proteins can occur via chaperone-mediated autophagy, the only type of autophagy that requires unfolding of the protein cargo before internalization into lysosomes (Dice, 2007). Selectivity is determined via the recognition of a pentapeptide in the amino acid sequence of the substrate proteins that are delivered to the surface of the lysosomes by a cytosolic chaperone (Hsc70). To reach the lysosomal lumen, these proteins interact with the lysosome-associated protein type 2A (LAMP-2A) receptor, and a complex of lysosomal chaperones at both sides of the lysosomal membrane.

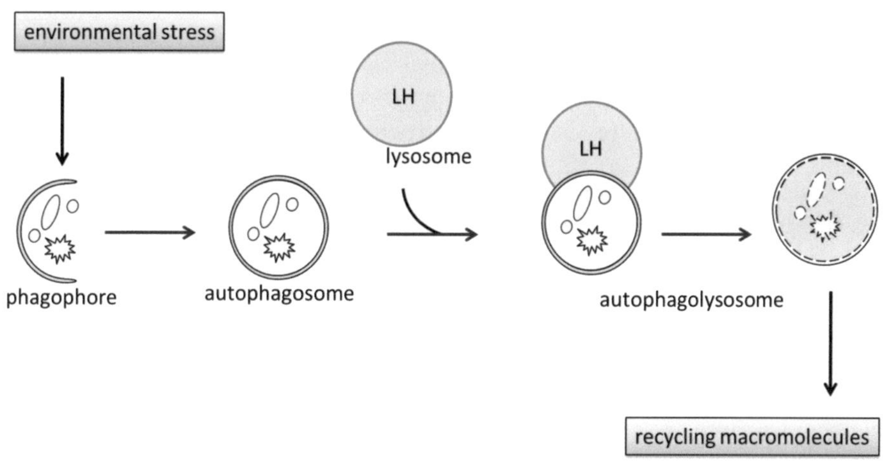


Fig. 3. Schematic depiction of the autophagy process. A phagophore is formed at the initiation of autophagy, in response to environmental stress (e.g. nutrient deprivation) to sequester cytoplasmic components for degradation. Upon completion, the phagophore forms a double-membraned vesicle called an autophagosome. After fusion with a lysosome, the content is degraded by lysosomal hydrolases (LH). Following breakdown, the resulting macromolecules (e.g. nucleic acids, amino acids, free fatty acids) are released back into the cytosol for reuse by the cell.

### 3.2 Molecular mechanisms of autophagy

The molecular machinery and signaling cascades that regulate autophagy are very complex (Ravikumar et al., 2010; Yang & Klionsky, 2010). Briefly, the key regulator of autophagy in human and murine cells is the mammalian target of rapamycin (mTOR) kinase, which suppresses autophagy in conditions of sufficient nutrients and growth factors, via class I phoshatidylinositol-3-kinases (PI3Ks) and Akt. Activation of the mTOR complex 1 (mTORC1) - and consequent repression of autophagy - can also be mediated by mitogen-activated protein kinases (MAPKs), by activation of the p90 ribosomal S6 kinase, as well as by the Wnt signaling pathway. Other prominent regulators of autophagy include (but are not limited to): AMP-activated protein kinase (AMPK), which inhibits mTOR in response to reduced ATP levels; eukaryotic translation initiation factor 2α (eIF2α), which responds to nutrient deprivation; c-Jun N-terminal kinase (JNK), which is involved in multiple signaling cascades activated by stressful conditions; members of the Bcl-2 protein family that contain a single Bcl-2 homology (BH) domain, the so-called BH3-only proteins, which displace (and hence derepress) the essential autophagy modulator Beclin 1 from inhibitory complexes with Bcl-2 or Bcl-XL; Sirtuin 1, which responds to high NAD+ levels, de facto acting as a sensor of nutrient availability; the oncosuppressor protein p53, which inhibits autophagy when present in the cytoplasm; the IκB kinase (IKK) complex, which is also essential for the activation of NF-κB by stress; the inositol 1,4,5-trisphosphate (IP3) receptor (IP3R) at the level of the ER and transglutaminase 2. Finally, autophagy is positively regulated by the transcription factor activity of E2F1, FoxO3a, NF-κB and p53 among others.

### 3.3 Autophagy in atherosclerosis

Autophagy in atherosclerotic plaques has not yet been analysed in full detail due to technical limitations, in particular the lack of adequate marker proteins. As a consequence, the role of autophagy in atherosclerosis is unclear and currently under intense investigation. However, transmission electron microscopy of smooth muscle cells (SMCs) in the fibrous cap of advanced plaques revealed ultrastructural features of autophagy such as vacuolization and formation of myelin figures (Martinet & De Meyer, 2009b). The latter structures, composed of phospholipids and membrane fragments, refer to autophagic degradation of membranous cellular components. Moreover, Western blot analysis of human carotid plaques showed processing of microtubule-associated protein 1 light chain 3 (LC3) into the autophagosome-specific isoform LC3-II, indicating activation of autophagy. Importantly, these kind of data have to be interpreted with great caution. Autophagy is a dynamic process: formation of autophagosomes, followed by their degradation after lysosomal fusion (Figure 3). Many groups, including our own, have measured increased autophagosome formation or LC3 processing, and labelled this as increased autophagic activity. However, these parameters can also reflect impaired degradation. Therefore, it is essential to measure autophagic flux (Gottlieb & Mentzer, 2010). In tissue, this can be very challenging. A very elegant method now widely accepted to measure flux is using a tandem fusion protein of LC3 with the red acid-insensitive mCherry (or RFP) and the green acid-sensitive GFP proteins to measure formation of autolysosomes and their degradation (Kimura et al., 2007). GFP fluorescence is quenched in the acidic environment of the lysosome, while mCherry (or RFP) fluorescence is stable at low pH. As a consequence, detection of yellow fluorescence (overlap of GFP and mCherry) reflects impaired flux, and the presence of red fluorescence reflects quenching of GFP and thus ongoing degradation in the lysosome (Mizushima et al., 2010). Besides LC3, levels of other autophagy substrates can be used for measuring autophagic flux, of which the best studied is p62, an adaptor protein that links ubiquitinated proteins to LC3. Accumulation of p62 reflects impaired degradation in the autophagolysosome, whereas low p62 levels indicate active degradation. Unfortunately, no data is available on p62 levels during atherosclerotic plaque formation and destabilization.

*In vitro* studies identified several potential triggers for autophagy that are present in atherosclerotic plaques, such as inflammation (Heymann, 2006; Jia et al., 2006), ROS production (Scherz-Shouval & Elazar, 2011), accumulation of oxidized lipoproteins (Muller et al., 2011; Nowicki et al., 2007) and endoplasmic reticulum stress (Qin et al., 2010). Also hypoxia is a common feature of advanced human atherosclerotic plaques (Sluimer et al.,

2008), caused by inadequate vascularization, nutrient and growth factor deprivation, a well-known condition leading to induction of autophagy (Azad et al., 2008).

### 3.3.1 Dual role of autophagy in atherosclerosis

Autophagy can protect plaque cells against oxidative stress by degrading damaged intracellular material, in particular polarized mitochondria (Kiffin et al., 2006). In this way, successful autophagy of the damaged components promotes cell survival by limiting the release of pro-apoptotic proteins such as cytochrome c into the cytosol (Gozuacik & Kimchi, 2004). The protective role of autophagy in atherosclerosis was illustrated by *in vitro* findings showing that death of smooth muscle cells (SMC) induced by low concentrations of statins is attenuated by the autophagy inducer 7-ketocholesterol (Martinet et al., 2008). Also excess free cholesterol or exposure of SMCs to lipid peroxidation products such as 4-hydroxynonenal activates autophagy, thereby prolonging SMC survival (K. Xu et al., 2010). Also, autophagy safeguards efficient phagocytosis of AC (Qu et al., 2007), which is beneficial for plaque stability (Figure 2). Altogether, induction of autophagy represents a vital component of a general stress response in vascular cells and could therefore be an important determinant of the stability of atherosclerotic plaques (Figure 4).

In contrast, excessive autophagy in SMCs or endothelial cells may cause autophagic cell death (Levine & Yuan, 2005). SMC death in turn results in plaque destabilization owing to the reduced synthesis of collagen and thinning of the fibrous cap. Also endothelial cell death may be detrimental for the structure of the plaque as endothelial injury and/or death represents a primary mechanism for acute clinical events by promoting lesional thrombosis. In view of plaque stability and regression, these observations might advise against excessive autophagy induction in plaques. Conversely, autophagic death of macrophages is considered a promising approach to stabilize advanced plaques (Martinet et al., 2007).

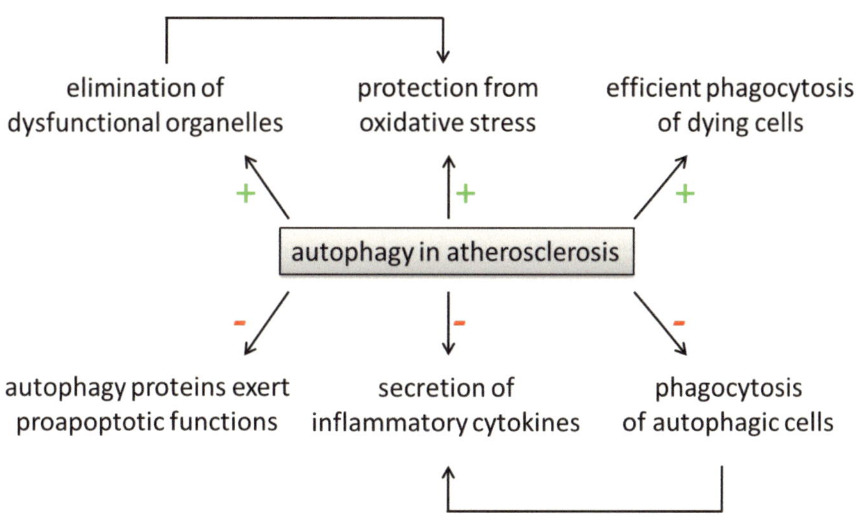


Fig. 4. Consequences of autophagy in atherosclerosis. While autophagy contributes beneficially to plaque stability by protecting cells from oxidative stress and ensuring efficient clearance of dead cells, it can also exert functions that are unfavorable in terms of plaque stability. Autophagy has a very potent inflammatory component and is very tightly linked to other forms of cell death, especially apoptosis.

However, recent evidence indicates that phagocytosis of cells dying through autophagy results in an inflammatory response through inflammasome activation, IL-1β release and subsequent IL-6 and TNFα induction in neighboring phagocytes (Petrovski et al., 2007) (Figure 4). Moreover, autophagy proteins themselves can exert proapoptotic functions. For example, Beclin-1 (Atg6), a key protein involved in autophagy, can interact with the anti-apoptotic proteins Bcl-2 or Bcl-xL. This interaction is pro-apoptotic and antiautophagic, at least under non-autophagic stimuli. However, during autophagic conditions, Beclin-1 binding to Bcl-xL is antiapoptotic (Pattingre et al., 2005; Wang, 2008). In addition, Atg5 (when cleaved by activated calpain) can bind to Bcl-xL and induce apoptosis (Yousefi et al., 2006; Yousefi & Simon, 2007). On the other hand, inactivation of autophagy genes (e.g. Atg5) also causes cell death (Komatsu et al., 2006), making matters even more complicated. These data demonstrate that the crosstalk between autophagy and apoptosis should not be neglected when designing interventions aimed at stabilizing atherosclerotic plaques via autophagy.

### 3.3.2 Is autophagy an interesting drug target for plaque stabilization?

Pharmacological modulation of autophagy can be achieved by targeting key players in the autophagy machinery (Rubinzstein et al., 2007). For example, rapamycin or its derivatives (e.g. everolimus) inhibit mTOR, thereby activating autophagy. Another way to modulate autophagy is to target the mTOR-independent route, mainly regulated by inositol-1,4,5-triphosphate (IP3) levels. This can be achieved with drugs such as lithium, sodium valproate and carbamezapine. The first line of evidence that demonstrates the beneficial effects of autophagy induction in atherosclerosis was obtained after stent-based delivery of the rapamycin derivative everolimus in plaques of cholesterol-fed rabbits (Verheye et al., 2007). This treatment resulted in a marked reduction of macrophages via autophagic cell death without affecting the SMCs. However, recent *in vitro* work in our laboratory has demonstrated that pharmacological induction of autophagy in macrophages triggers secretion of proinflammatory cytokines such as IL-6, MCP1 and TNFα (Martinet, De Meyer, unpublished data), suggesting that the autophagic process is not immunologically silent. This cocktail of cytokines has the potential to induce SMC death and exacerbate the inflammatory infiltration of leukocytes in the plaque. Combined treatment with anti-inflammatory agents such as glucocorticosteroids may help to prevent the adverse effects of drug-induced autophagy. On the other hand, induction of autophagy in free cholesterol-loaded SMCs by rapamycin inhibited AC death (K. Xu et al., 2010), possibly through the degradation of dysfunctional organelles such as mitochondria and endoplasmic reticulum. These findings provide a rationale for the use of rapamycin or analogs such as everolimus to stabilize advanced atherosclerotic plaques.

Several studies have shed light on the potential detrimental consequences of autophagy inhibition with regard to plaque stability. Firstly, autophagy is essential for efficient phagocytosis of dying cells (Qu et al., 2007). ACs derived from cells lacking essential autophagy genes (Atg5 or beclin-1) fail to present the "eat-me" signal PS and secrete lower levels of the "come-get-me" signal lysophosphatidylcholine (Qu et al., 2007). This will result in a marked decrease in the engulfment of apoptotic corpses, enhanced plaque necrosis and recruitment of inflammatory cells (Gautier et al., 2009). Thus, inhibition of autophagy may further destabilize advanced plaques, where phagocytosis of ACs is already compromised (Schrijvers et al., 2005). Additionally, inhibition of autophagy using 3-methyladenine in free cholesterol-treated SMCs enhances apoptosis and necrosis (K. Xu et al., 2010), indicating that a strong interaction exists between autophagy and other forms of cell death (Maiuri et al., 2007). Of note, altering autophagy using pharmacological agents can be problematic, as they can interfere with general processes, such as glucose metabolism (e.g. metformin, deoxyglucose) or mitochondrial respiration (e.g. oligomycin). Broad-spectrum PI3 kinase inhibitors wortmannin and 3-methyladenine, widely used in autophagy research, inhibit Akt activation. Thus, results using these agents must always be interpreted carefully.

## 4. Concluding remarks

(Auto)phagocytosis plays a key role in maintaining atherosclerotic plaque stability (Figure 5). Efficient phagocytosis of AC is required to prevent accumulation of dead cells, expansion of the necrotic core in plaques and inflammatory responses resulting from secondary necrosis of residual AC. These factors will undoubtedly promote plaque inflammation, destabilization and rupture, leading to possible fatal ischemic events (e.g. myocardial infarction and stroke). Autophagy may be viewed as a "cry for survival," and such survival is the result of an adaptive response to fight against cellular stress. If this stress—such as oxidative damage in atherosclerotic plaques—is mild, autophagy is activated in order to

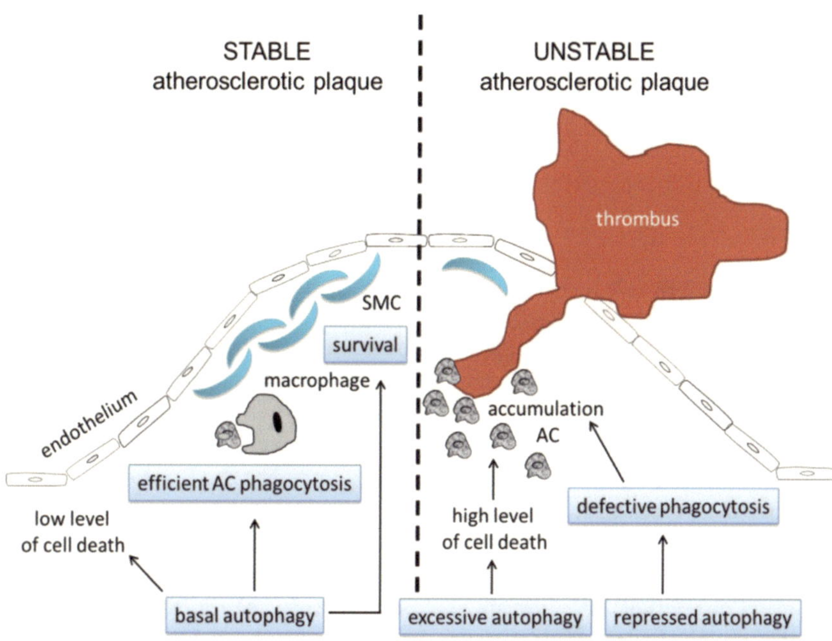


Fig. 5. Implications of dysfunctional phagocytosis and autophagy on the stability of atherosclerotic plaques. In stable plaques, AC numbers are low and phagocytosis is very efficient. Basal autophagy contributes to maintain efficient phagocytosis and promote cell survival. In unstable plaques, however, phagocytosis of AC is severely impaired, leading to accumulation of AC, expansion of the necrotic core, thereby increasing the risk for plaque rupture, which results in the formation of an occlusive thrombus. Decreased autophagy probably worsens phagocytosis efficiency, which is already compromised in advanced plaques, whereas excessive autophagy can result in cell death and inflammatory responses.

survive. On the other hand, if cellular stress is overwhelming or continuous, the adaptive response fails and cells undergo an autophagic type of death. Crossbreeding of mouse models for atherosclerosis (e.g. ApoE or LDL receptor knockout animals) with autophagy-deficient mice (e.g. conditional Atg5 or Atg7 knockout animals) will undoubtedly shed more light on the potential role of autophagy in atherosclerosis. Based on the literature and promising experiments in our lab and that of others, it is definite that cells need autophagy to be able to survive under stressful circumstances. Therefore, controlled (moderate) induction of autophagy, but not excessive induction or inhibition of autophagy, seems to be a promising strategy for stabilization of atherosclerotic plaques. The challenge for the future in the stabilization of atherosclerotic plaques will be to turn on the protective pro-survival effects of autophagy in a selective manner, without activating unwanted death pathways or proinflammatory signaling cascades. With progress being made in tissue-specific drug targeting using nanoparticles, one potential future approach to stabilize atherosclerotic plaques would be to develop macrophage-specific phagocytosis and/or autophagy inducers combined with anti-inflammatory drugs. However, stimulation of autophagy can only be beneficial if autophagic flux is not impaired, since this condition could lead to lysosomal leakage or ejection of autophagosomes as well as the induction of cell death. Altogether, (auto)phagocytosis is a crucial process involved in atherogenesis that significantly affects the stability of the atherosclerotic plaque.

## 5. Acknowledgements

This work was supported by the Fund for Scientific Research-Flanders and the University of Antwerp.

## 6. References

A-Gonzalez, N., Bensinger, S.J., Hong, C., Beceiro, S., Bradley, M.N., Zelcer, N., Deniz, J., Ramirez, C., Díaz, M., Gallardo, G., de Galarreta, C.R., Salazar, J., Lopez, F., Edwards, P., Parks, J., Andujar, M., Tontonoz, P. & Castrillo, A. (2009) Apoptotic cells promote their own clearance and immune tolerance through activation of the nuclear receptor LXR. *Immunity*,31,2,pp.245-58.

Ait-Oufella, H., Kinugawa, K., Zoll, J., Simon, T., Boddaert, J., Heeneman, S., Blanc-Brude, O., Barateau, V., Potteaux, S., Merval, R., Esposito, B., Teissier, E., Daemen, M.J., Lesèche, G., Boulanger, C., Tedgui, A. & Mallat, Z. (2007) Lactadherin deficiency leads to apoptotic cell accumulation and accelerated atherosclerosis in mice. *Circulation*,115,16,pp.2168-77.

Ait-Oufella, H., Pouresmail, V., Simon, T., Blanc-Brude, O., Kinugawa, K., Merval, R., Offenstadt, G., Lesèche, G., Cohen, P.L., Tedgui, A. & Mallat, Z. (2008) Defective mer receptor tyrosine kinase signaling in bone marrow cells promotes apoptotic cell accumulation and accelerates atherosclerosis. *Arterioscler Thromb Vasc Biol*,28,8, pp.1429-31.

Andersson, U., Wang, H., Palmblad, K., Aveberger, A.C., Bloom, O., Erlandsson-Harris, H., Janson, A., Kokkola, R., Zhang, M., Yang, H. & Tracey, K.J. (2000) High mobility group 1 protein (HMG-1) stimulates proinflammatory cytokine synthesis in human monocytes. *J Exp Med*,192,4,pp. 565-70.

Arur, S., Uche, U.E., Rezaul, K., Fong, M., Scranton, V., Cowan, A.E., Mohler, W. & Han, D.K. (2003) Annexin I is an endogenous ligand that mediates apoptotic cell engulfment. *Dev Cell*,4,4,pp.587-98.

Azad, M.B., Chen, Y., Henson, E.S., Cizeau, J., McMillan-Ward, E., Israels, S.J. & Gibson, S.B. (2008) Hypoxia induces autophagic cell death in apoptosis-competent cells through a mechanism involving BNIP3. *Autophagy*,4,2,pp.195-204.

Basu, S., Binder, R.J., Suto, R., Anderson, K.M. & Srivastava, P.K. (2000) Necrotic but not apoptotic cell death releases heat shock proteins, which deliver a partial maturation signal to dendritic cells and activate the NF-kappa B pathway. *Int Immunol*, 12,11,pp.1539-46.

Behrensdorf, H.A., van de Craen, M., Knies, U.E., Vandenabeele, P. & Clauss, M. (2000) The endothelial monocyte-activating polypeptide II (EMAP II) is a substrate for caspase-7. *FEBS Lett*,466,1,pp.143-7.

Benati, D., Ferro, M., Savino, M.T., Ulivieri, C., Schiavo, E., Nuccitelli, A., Pasini, F.L. & Baldari, C.T. (2010) Opposite effects of simvastatin on the bactericidal and inflammatory response of macrophages to opsonized S. aureus. *J Leukoc Biol*, 87,3,pp.433-42.

Bhatia, V.K., Yun, S., Leung,V., Grimsditch, D.C., Benson, G.M., Botto, M.B., Boyle, J.J. & Haskard, D.O. (2007) Complement C1q reduces early atherosclerosis in low-density lipoprotein receptor-deficient mice. *Am J Pathol*,170,1,pp. 416-23.

Boisvert, W.A., Rose, D.M., Boullier, A., Quehenberger, O., Sydlaske, A., Johnson, K.A., Curtiss, L.K. & Terkeltaub, R. (2006) Leukocyte transglutaminase 2 expression limits atherosclerotic lesion size. *Arterioscler Thromb Vasc Biol*,26,3,pp.563-9.

Bouhlel, M.A., Derudas, B., Rigamonti, E., Dièvart, R., Brozek, J., Haulon, S., Zawadzki, C., Jude, B., Torpier, G., Marx, N., Staels, B. & Chinetti-Gbaguidi, G. (2007) PPARgamma activation primes human monocytes into alternative M2 macrophages with anti-inflammatory properties. *Cell Metab*,6,2,pp.137-43.

Brown, S., Heinisch, I., Ross, E., Shaw, K., Buckley, C.D. & Savill, J. (2002) Apoptosis disables CD31-mediated cell detachment from phagocytes promoting binding and engulfment. *Nature*,418,6894,pp.200-3.

Callahan, M.K., Williamson, P. & Schlegel, R.A. (2000) Surface expression of phosphatidylserine on macrophages is required for phagocytosis of apoptotic thymocytes. *Cell Death Differ*,7,7,pp.645-53.

Cash, J.L., Christian, A.R. & Greaves, D.R. (2010) Chemerin peptides promote phagocytosis in a ChemR23- and Syk-dependent manner. *J Immunol*,184,9,pp.5315-24.

Cui, D., Thorp, E., Li, Y., Wang, N., Yvan-Charvet, L., Tall, A.R. & Tabas, I. (2007) Pivotal advance: macrophages become resistant to cholesterol-induced death after phagocytosis of apoptotic cells. *J Leukoc Biol*,82,5,pp.1040-50.

Devitt, A., Moffatt, O.D., Raykundalia, C., Capra, J.D., Simmons, D.L. & Gregory, C.D. (1998) Human CD14 mediates recognition and phagocytosis of apoptotic cells. *Nature*,392,6675,pp.505-9.

Devitt, A. & Marshall, L.J. (2011) The innate immune system and the clearance of apoptotic cells. *J Leukoc Biol*. May 11. [Epub ahead of print]

Dice, J.F. (2007) Chaperone-mediated autophagy. *Autophagy*,3,4,pp.295-9.

Donato, R. (2003) Intracellular and extracellular roles of S100 proteins. *Microsc Res Tech*, 60,6,pp.540-51.

Elliott, M.R., Chekeni, F.B., Trampont, P.C., Lazarowski, E.R., Kadl, A., Walk, S.F., Park, D., Woodson, R.I., Ostankovich, M., Sharma, P., Lysiak, J.J., Harden, T.K., Leitinger, N. & Ravichandran, K.S. (2009) Nucleotides released by apoptotic cells act as a find-me signal to promote phagocytic clearance. *Nature*,461,7261,pp.282-6.

Elliott, M.R. & Ravichandran K.S. (2010) Clearance of apoptotic cells: implications in health and disease. *J Cell Biol*,189,pp.1059–70.

Erwig, L.P.& Henson, P.M. (2007) Immunological consequences of apoptotic cell phagocytosis. *Am J Pathol*,171,1,pp.2-8.

Fadok, V.A., Voelker, D.R., Campbell, P.A., Cohen, J.J., Bratton, D.L. & Henson, P.M. (1992) Exposure of phosphatidylserine on the surface of apoptotic lymphocytes triggers specific recognition and removal by macrophages. *J Immunol*,148,7,pp.2207-16.

Fadok, V.A., Bratton, D.L., Konowal, A., Freed, P.W., Westcott, J.Y. & Henson, P.M. (1998) Macrophages that have ingested apoptotic cells in vitro inhibit proinflammatory cytokine production through autocrine/paracrine mechanisms involving TGF-beta, PGE2, and PAF. *J Clin Invest*,101,4,pp.890-8.

Foell, D., Frosch, M., Sorg, C. & Roth, J. (2004) Phagocyte-specific calcium-binding S100 proteins as clinical laboratory markers of inflammation. *Clin Chim Acta*,344,1,pp.37-51.

Foell, D., Wittkowski, H., Ren, Z., Turton, J., Pang, G., Daebritz, J., Ehrchen, J., Heidemann. J., Borody, T., Roth, J. & Clancy, R. (2008) Phagocyte-specific S100 proteins are released from affected mucosa and promote immune responses during inflammatory bowel disease. *J Pathol*,216,2,pp.183-92.

Gaipl, U.S., Kuenkele, S., Voll, R.E., Beyer, T.D., Kolowos, W., Heyder, P., Kalden, J.R. & Herrmann, M. (2001) Complement binding is an early feature of necrotic and a rather late event during apoptotic cell death. *Cell Death Differ*,8,4,pp.327-34.

Gardai, S.J., McPhillips, K.A., Frasch, S.C., Janssen, W.J., Starefeldt, A., Murphy-Ullrich, J.E., Bratton, D.L., Oldenborg, P.A., Michalak, M. & Henson, P.M. (2005) Cell-surface calreticulin initiates clearance of viable or apoptotic cells through trans-activation of LRP on the phagocyte. *Cell*,123,2,pp.321-34.

Gautier, E.L., Huby, T., Witztum, J.L., Ouzilleau, B., Miller, E.R., Saint-Charles, F., Aucouturier, P., Chapman, M.J. & Lesnik, P. (2009) Macrophage apoptosis exerts divergent effects on atherogenesis as a function of lesion stage. *Circulation*,119, pp.1795-1804.

Getz, G.S. & Reardon, C.A. (2006) Diet and murine atherosclerosis. *Arterioscler Thromb Vasc Biol*,26,2,pp.242-9.

Ghaemi-Oskouie, F. & Shi, Y. (2011) The role of uric acid as an endogenous danger signal in immunity and inflammation. *Curr Rheumatol Rep*,13,2,pp.160-6.

Godson, C., Mitchell, S., Harvey, K., Petasis, N.A., Hogg, N. & Brady, H.R. (2000) Cutting edge: lipoxins rapidly stimulate nonphlogistic phagocytosis of apoptotic neutrophils by monocyte-derived macrophages. *J Immunol*,164,4,pp.1663-7.

Golpon, H.A., Fadok, V.A., Taraseviciene-Stewart, L., Scerbavicius, R., Sauer, C., Welte, T., Henson, P.M. & Voelkel, N.F. (2004) Life after corpse engulfment: phagocytosis of apoptotic cells leads to VEGF secretion and cell growth. *FASEB J*,18,pp.1716–1718.

Gottlieb, R.A. & Mentzer, R.M. (2010) Autophagy during cardiac stress: joys and frustrations of autophagy. *Annu Rev Physiol*,72,pp.45-59.

Gozuacik, D. & Kimchi, A. (2004) Autophagy as a cell death and tumor suppressor mechanism. *Oncogene*,23,pp.2891–2906.

Green, D.R., Ferguson, T., Zitvogel, L. & Kroemer, G. (2009) Immunogenic and tolerogenic cell death. *Nat Rev Immunol*,9,pp.353–363.

Grimsley, C. & Ravichandran, K.S. (2003) Cues for apoptotic cell engulfment: eat-me, don't eat-me and come-get-me signals. *Trends Cell Biol*,13,pp.648–656.

Gude, D.R., Alvarez, S.E., Paugh, S.W., Mitra, P., Yu, J., Griffiths, R., Barbour, S.E., Milstien, S.& Spiegel, S. (2008) Apoptosis induces expression of sphingosine kinase 1 to release sphingosine-1-phosphate as a "come-and-get-me" signal. *FASEB J*, 22,8,pp.2629-38.

Hansson, G.K. (2005) Inflammation, atherosclerosis, and coronary artery disease. *N Engl J Med*,352,16,pp.1685-95.

Hart, S.P., Alexander, K.M., MacCall, S.M. & Dransfield, I. (2005) C-reactive protein does not opsonize early apoptotic human neutrophils, but binds only membrane-permeable late apoptotic cells and has no effect on their phagocytosis by macrophages. *J Inflamm (Lond)*,31,pp.2-5.

Henson, P.M., Bratton, D.L. & Fadok, V.A. (2001) Apoptotic cell removal. *Curr Biol*, 11,19,pp.R795-805.

Heymann, D. (2006) Autophagy: a protective mechanism in response to stress and inflammation. *Curr Opin Investig Drugs*,7,pp.443–450.

Hirt, U.A. & Leist, M. (2003) Rapid, noninflammatory and PS-dependent phagocytic clearance of necrotic cells. *Cell Death Differ*,10,10,pp.1156-64.

Hodge, S., Hodge, G., Brozyna, S., Jersmann, H., Holmes, M. & Reynolds, P.N. (2006) Azithromycin increases phagocytosis of apoptotic bronchial epithelial cells by alveolar macrophages. *Eur Respir J*,28,3,pp.486-95.

Hoffmann, P.R., deCathelineau, A.M., Ogden, C.A., Leverrier, Y., Bratton, D.L., Daleke, D.L., Ridley, A.J., Fadok, V.A. & Henson, P.M. (2001) Phosphatidylserine (PS) induces PS receptor-mediated macropinocytosis and promotes clearance of apoptotic cells. *J Cell Biol*,155,4,pp.649-59.

Horino, K., Nishiura, H., Ohsako, T., Shibuya, Y., Hiraoka, T., Kitamura, N. & Yamamoto, T. (1998) A monocyte chemotactic factor, S19 ribosomal protein dimer, in phagocytic clearance of apoptotic cells. *Lab Invest*,78,5,pp.603-17.

Hou, Y., Plett, P.A., Ingram, D.A., Rajashekhar, G., Orschell, C.M., Yoder, M.C., March, K.L. & Clauss, M. (2006) Endothelial-monocyte-activating polypeptide II induces migration of endothelial progenitor cells via the chemokine receptor CXCR3. *Exp Hematol*,34,8,pp.1125-32.

Hugel, B., Martínez, M.C., Kunzelmann, C. & Freyssinet, J.M. (2005) Membrane microparticles: two sides of the coin. *Physiology (Bethesda)*,20,pp.22-7.

Jehle, A.W., Gardai, S.J., Li, S., Linsel-Nitschke, P., Morimoto, K., Janssen, W.J., Vandivier, R.W., Wang, N., Greenberg, S., Dale, B.M., Qin, C., Henson, P.M. & Tall, A.R. (2006) ATP-binding cassette transporter A7 enhances phagocytosis of apoptotic cells and associated ERK signaling in macrophages. *J Cell Biol*,174,4,pp.547-56.

Jia, G., Cheng, G., Gangahar, D.M. & Agrawal, D.K. (2006) Insulin-like growth factor-1 and TNF-alpha regulate autophagy through c-jun N-terminal kinase and Akt pathways in human atherosclerotic vascular smooth cells. *Immunol Cell Biol*,84,pp.448–454.

Kannel,. W.B., D'Agostino, R.B., Sullivan, L. & Wilson, P.W. (2004) Concept and usefulness of cardiovascular risk profiles. *Am Heart J*,148,1,pp.16-26.

Kiffin, R., Bandyopadhyay, U. & Cuervo, A.M. (2006) Oxidative stress and autophagy. *Antioxid Redox Signal*,8,pp.152–62.

Kimura, S., Noda, T. & Yoshimori, T. (2007) Dissection of the autophagosome maturation process by a novel reporter protein, tandem fluorescent-tagged LC3. *Autophagy*, 3,pp.452-60.

Kinchen, J.M. (2010) A model to die for: signaling to apoptotic cell removal in worm, fly and mouse. *Apoptosis*,15,998–1006.

Kiss, R.S., Elliott, M.R., Ma, Z., Marcel, Y.L. & Ravichandran, K.S. (2006) Apoptotic cells induce a phosphatidylserine-dependent homeostatic response from phagocytes. *Curr Biol.* 16,22,pp.2252-8.

Klionsky, D.J. (2007) Autophagy: from phenomenology to molecular understanding in less than a decade. *Nat Rev Mol Cell Biol*,8,11,pp.931-7.

Klionsky, D.J., Cuervo, A.M., Dunn, W.A. Jr, Levine, B., van der Klei, I. & Seglen, P.O. (2007) How shall I eat thee? *Autophagy*,3,5,pp.413-6.

Knies, U.E., Behrensdorf, H.A., Mitchell, C.A., Deutsch, U., Risau, W., Drexler, H.C. & Clauss, M. (1998) Regulation of endothelial monocyte-activating polypeptide II release by apoptosis. *Proc Natl Acad Sci U S A*,95,21,pp.12322-7.

Komatsu, M., Waguri, S., Chiba, T., Murata, S., Iwata, J., Tanida, I., Ueno, T., Koike, M., Uchiyama, Y., Kominami, E. & Tanaka, K. (2006) Loss of autophagy in the central nervous system causes neurodegeneration in mice. *Nature*,441,pp.880–884.

Krysko, D.V., D'Herde, K. & Vandenabeele, P. (2006) Clearance of apoptotic and necrotic cells and its immunological consequences. *Apoptosis*,11,10,pp.1709-26.

Lauber, K., Bohn, E., Krober, S.M., Xiao, Y.J., Blumenthal, S.G., Lindemann, R.K., Marini, P., Wiedig, C., Zobywalski, A., Baksh, S., Xu, Y., Autenrieth, I.B., Schulze-Osthoff, K., Belka, C., Stuhler, G. & Wesselborg, S. (2003) Apoptotic cells induce migration of phagocytes via caspase-3-mediated release of a lipid attraction signal. *Cell*,113,6, pp.717–730.

Le, L.Q., Kabarowski, J.H., Weng, Z., Satterthwaite, A.B., Harvill, E.T., Jensen, E.R., Miller, J.F. & Witte, O.N. (2001) Mice lacking the orphan G protein-coupled receptor G2A develop a late-onset autoimmune syndrome. *Immunity*,14,5,pp.561-71.

Levine, B. & Yuan, J. (2005) Autophagy in cell death: an innocent convict? *J Clin Invest*, 115,pp.2679–88.

Levine, B. & Kroemer, G. (2008) Autophagy in the pathogenesis of disease. *Cell*,132,pp.27-42.

Li, M., Carpio, D.F., Zheng, Y., Bruzzo, P., Singh, V., Ouaaz, F., Medzhitov, R.M. & Beg, A.A. (2001) An essential role of the NF-kappa B/Toll-like receptor pathway in induction of inflammatory and tissue-repair gene expression by necrotic cells. *J Immunol*, 166,12,pp.7128-35.

Li, S., Sun, Y., Liang, C.P., Thorp, E.B., Han, S., Jehle, A.W., Saraswathi, V., Pridgen, B., Kanter, J.E., Li, R., Welch, C.L., Hasty, A.H., Bornfeldt, K.E., Breslow, J.L., Tabas, I. & Tall, AR. (2009) Defective phagocytosis of apoptotic cells by macrophages in atherosclerotic lesions of ob/ob mice and reversal by a fish oil diet. *Circ Res*,105,11,pp.1072-82.

Lillis, A.P., Van Duyn, L.B., Murphy-Ullrich, J.E. & Strickland, D.K. (2008) LDL receptor-related protein 1: unique tissue-specific functions revealed by selective gene knockout studies. *Physiol Rev*,88,3,pp.887-918.

Maiuri, M.C., Zalckvar, E., Kimchi, A. & Kroemer, G. (2007) Self-eating and self-killing: crosstalk between autophagy and apoptosis. *Nat Rev Mol Cell Biol*,8,pp.741–52.

Mathew, R., Karantza-Wadsworth, V. & White, E. (2007) Role of autophagy in cancer. *Nat Rev Cancer*,7,pp.961–7.

Martinet, W., Verheye, S. & De Meyer, G.R.Y. (2007) Selective depletion of macrophages in atherosclerotic plaques via macrophage-specific initiation of cell death. *Trends Cardiovasc Med*,17,pp.69-75.

Martinet, W. & De Meyer G.R.Y. (2008) Autophagy in atherosclerosis. *Curr Atheroscler Rep*,10,3,pp.216-23.

Martinet, W., Schrijvers D,M., Timmermans, J.P. & Bult, H. (2008) Interactions between cell death induced by statins and 7-ketocholesterol in rabbit aorta smooth muscle cells. *Br J Pharmacol*,154,pp.1236–46.

Martinet, W. & De Meyer, G.R.Y. (2009a) Autophagy in the cardiovascular system. *Biochim Biophys Acta*,1793,pp.1485-95.

Martinet, W. & De Meyer, G.R.Y. (2009b) Autophagy in atherosclerosis: a cell survival and death phenomenon with therapeutic potential. *Circ Res*,104,3,pp.304-17.

Martinet, W., De Meyer, I., Cools, N., Timmerman, V., Bult, H., Bosmans, J. & De Meyer G.R.Y. (2010) Cell death-mediated cleavage of the attraction signal p43 in human atherosclerosis: implications for plaque destabilization. *Arterioscler Thromb Vasc Biol*,30,7,pp.1415-22.

Martins, I., Kepp, O., Galluzzi, L., Senovilla, L., Schlemmer, F., Adjemian, S., Menger, L., Michaud, M., Zitvogel, L. & Kroemer, G. (2010) Surface-exposed calreticulin in the interaction between dying cells and phagocytes. *Ann N Y Acad Sci*,1209,pp.77-82.

Miyanishi, M., Tada, K., Koike, M., Uchiyama, Y., Kitamura, T. & Nagata, S. (2007) Identification of Tim4 as a phosphatidylserine receptor. *Nature*, 450,7168,pp.435-9.

Mizushima, N., Levine, B., Cuervo, A.M. & Klionsky, D.J. (2008) Autophagy fights disease through cellular self-digestion. *Nature*,45,pp.1069-75.

Mizushima, N., Yoshimori, T. & Levine, B. (2010) Methods in mammalian autophagy research. *Cell*,140,pp.313-26.

Möller, W., Hofer, T., Ziesenis, A., Karg, E. & Heyder, J. (2002) Ultrafine particles cause cytoskeletal dysfunctions in macrophages. *Toxicol Appl Pharmacol*,182,3,pp.197-207.

Morimoto, K., Janssen, W.J., Fessler, M.B., McPhillips, K.A., Borges, V.M., Bowler, R.P., Xiao, Y.Q., Kench, J.A., Henson, P.M. & Vandivier, R.W. (2006) Lovastatin enhances clearance of apoptotic cells (efferocytosis) with implications for chronic obstructive pulmonary disease. *J Immunol*,176,12,pp.7657-65.

Moura, R., Tjwa, M., Vandervoort, P., Van Kerckhoven, S., Holvoet, P. & Hoylaerts, M.F. (2008) Thrombospondin-1 deficiency accelerates atherosclerotic plaque maturation in ApoE-/- mice. *Circ Res*,103,10,pp.1181-9.

Mukundan, L., Odegaard, J.I., Morel, C.R., Heredia, J.E., Mwangi, J.W., Ricardo-Gonzalez, R.R., Goh, Y.P., Eagle, A.R., Dunn, S.E., Awakuni, J.U., Nguyen, K.D., Steinman, L., Michie, S.A. & Chawla, A. (2009) PPAR-delta senses and orchestrates clearance of apoptotic cells to promote tolerance. *Nat Med*,15,11,pp.1266-72.

Muller, M., Salvayre, R., Negre-Salvayre, A. & Vindis, C. (2011) Oxidized LDLs trigger endoplasmic reticulum stress and autophagy: Prevention by HDLs. *Autophagy*, 7,pp.541-543.

Nakamura, H., Izumoto, Y., Kambe, H., Kuroda, T., Mori, T., Kawamura, K., Yamamoto, H. & Kishimoto, T. (1994) Molecular cloning of complementary DNA for a novel human hepatoma-derived growth factor. Its homology with high mobility group-1 protein. *J Biol Chem*,269,40,pp.25143-9.

Nauta, A.J., Raaschou-Jensen, N., Roos, A., Daha, M.R., Madsen, H.O., Borrias-Essers, M.C., Ryder, L.P., Koch, C. & Garred, P. (2003) Mannose-binding lectin engagement with late apoptotic and necrotic cells. *Eur J Immunol*,33,10,pp.2853-63.

Nishiura, H., Shibuya, Y., Matsubara, S., Tanase, S., Kambara, T. & Yamamoto, T. (1996) Monocyte chemotactic factor in rheumatoid arthritis synovial tissue. Probably a cross-linked derivative of S19 ribosomal protein. *J Biol Chem*,271,2,pp.878-82.

Nowicki, M., Zabirnyk, O., Duerrschmidt, N., Borlak, J. & Spanel-Borowski, K. (2007) No upregulation of lectin-like oxidized low-density lipoprotein receptor-1 in serum-deprived EA.hy926 endothelial cells under oxLDL exposure, but increase in autophagy. *Eur J Cell Biol*,86,pp.605–16.

Ogden, C.A., deCathelineau, A., Hoffmann, P.R., Bratton, D., Ghebrehiwet, B., Fadok, V.A. & Henson, P.M. (2001) C1q and mannose binding lectin engagement of cell surface calreticulin and CD91 initiates macropinocytosis and uptake of apoptotic cells. *J Exp Med*,194,6,pp.781-95.

Park, D., Tosello-Trampont, A.C., Elliott, M.R., Lu, M., Haney, L.B., Ma, Z., Klibanov, A.L., Mandell, J.W. & Ravichandran, K.S. (2007) BAI1 is an engulfment receptor for apoptotic cells upstream of the ELMO/Dock180/Rac module. *Nature*, 450,7168,pp.430-4.

Park, S.Y., Jung, M.Y., Kim, H.J., Lee, S.J., Kim, S.Y., Lee, B.H., Kwon, T.H., Park, R.W. & Kim, I.S. (2008) Rapid cell corpse clearance by stabilin-2, a membrane phosphatidylserine receptor. *Cell Death Differ*,15,1,pp.192-201.

Patel, V.A., Longacre, A., Hsiao, K., Fan, H., Meng, F., Mitchell, J.E., Rauch, J., Ucker, D.S. & Levine, J.S. (2006) Apoptotic cells, at all stages of the death process, trigger characteristic signaling events that are divergent from and dominant over those triggered by necrotic cells: Implications for the delayed clearance model of autoimmunity. *J Biol Chem*,281,8,pp.4663-70.

Pattingre, S., Tassa, A., Qu, X., Garuti, R., Liang, X.H., Mizushima, N., Packer, M., Schneider, M.D. & Levine, B. (2005) Bcl-2 antiapoptotic proteins inhibit Beclin 1-dependent autophagy. *Cell*,122,pp.927–39.

Peng, Y., Latchman, Y. & Elkon, KB. (2009) Ly6C(low) monocytes differentiate into dendritic cells and cross-tolerize T cells through PDL-1. *J Immunol*,182,5,pp.2777-85.

Peter, C., Waibe, M., Radu, C.G., Yang, L.V., Witte, O.N., Schulze-Osthoff, K., Wesselborg, S. & Lauber, K. (2008) Migration to apoptotic "find-me" signals is mediated via the phagocyte receptor G2A. *J Biol Chem*,283,9,pp.5296-305.

Peter, C., Wesselborg, S., Herrmann, M. & Lauber, K. (2010) Dangerous attraction: phagocyte recruitment and danger signals of apoptotic and necrotic cells. *Apoptosis*, 15,9,pp.1007-28.

Petrovski, G., Zahuczky, G., Májai, G. & Fésüs, L. (2007) Phagocytosis of cells dying through autophagy evokes a proinflammatory response in macrophages. *Autophagy*, 3,5,pp.509-11.

Poon, I.K., Hulett, M.D. & Parish, C.R. (2010) Molecular mechanisms of late apoptotic/necrotic cell clearance. *Cell Death Differ*,17,3,pp.381-97.

Pradhan, D., Krahling, S., Williamson, P. & Schlegel, R.A. (1997) Multiple systems for recognition of apoptotic lymphocytes by macrophages. *Mol Biol Cell*,8,5,pp.767-78.

Qin, L., Wang, Z., Tao, L. & Wang, Y. (2010) ER stress negatively regulates AKT/TSC/mTOR pathway to enhance autophagy. *Autophagy*,6,pp.239-247.

Qingxian L, Qiutang L, Qingjun L. (2010) Regulation of phagocytosis by TAM receptors and their ligands. *Front Biol*,5,3,pp.227-37.

Qu, X., Zou, Z., Sun, Q., Luby-Phelps, K., Cheng, P., Hogan, R.N., Gilpin, C. & Levine, B. (2007) Autophagy gene-dependent clearance of apoptotic cells during embryonic development. *Cell*,128,pp.931-46.

Ravikumar, B., Sarkar, S., Davies, J.E., Futter, M., Garcia-Arencibia, M., Green-Thompson, Z.W., Jimenez-Sanchez, M., Korolchuk, V.I., Lichtenberg, M., Luo, S., Massey, D.C., Menzies, F.M., Moreau, K., Narayanan, U., Renna, M., Siddiqi, F.H., Underwood, B.R., Winslow, A.R. & Rubinsztein, D.C. (2010) Regulation of mammalian autophagy in physiology and pathophysiology. *Physiol Rev*,90,pp.1383-435.

Reddy, S.M., Hsiao, K.H., Abernethy, V.E., Fan, H., Longacre, A., Lieberthal, W., Rauch, J., Koh, J.S. & Levine, J.S. (2002) Phagocytosis of apoptotic cells by macrophages induces novel signaling events leading to cytokine-independent survival and inhibition of proliferation: activation of Akt and inhibition of extracellular signal-regulated kinases 1 and 2. *J Immunol*,169,2,pp.702-13.

Rovere, P., Peri, G., Fazzini, F., Bottazzi, B., Doni, A., Bondanza, A., Zimmermann, V.S., Garlanda, C., Fascio, U., Sabbadini, M.G., Rugarli, C., Mantovani, A. & Manfredi, A.A. (2000) The long pentraxin PTX3 binds to apoptotic cells and regulates their clearance by antigen-presenting dendritic cells. *Blood*,96,13,pp.4300-6.

Rubinsztein, D.C., Gestwicki, J.E., Murphy, L.O. & Klionsky, D.J. (2007) Potential therapeutic applications of autophagy. *Nat Rev Drug Discov*,6,pp.304-12.

Sambrano, G.R. & Steinberg, D. (1995) Recognition of oxidatively damaged and apoptotic cells by an oxidized low density lipoprotein receptor on mouse peritoneal macrophages: role of membrane phosphatidylserine. *Proc Natl Acad Sci U S A*, 92,pp.1396–400.

Sather, S., Kenyon, K.D., Lefkowitz, J.B., Liang, X., Varnum, B.C., Henson, P.M. & Graham, D.K. (2007) A soluble form of the Mer receptor tyrosine kinase inhibits macrophage clearance of apoptotic cells and platelet aggregation. *Blood*,109,3,pp.1026-33.

Savill, J., Hogg, N., Ren, Y. & Haslett, C. (1992) Thrombospondin cooperates with CD36 and the vitronectin receptor in macrophage recognition of neutrophils undergoing apoptosis. *J Clin Invest*,90,4,pp.1513-22.

Scaffidi, P., Misteli, T. & Bianchi, M.E. (2002) Release of chromatin protein HMGB1 by necrotic cells triggers inflammation. *Nature*,418,6894,pp.191-5.

Scannell, M., Flanagan, M.B., deStefani, A., Wynne, K.J., Cagney, G., Godson, C. & Maderna, P. (2007) Annexin-1 and peptide derivatives are released by apoptotic cells and stimulate phagocytosis of apoptotic neutrophils by macrophages. *J Immunol*,178,7, pp.4595-605.

Scherz-Shouval, R. & Elazar, Z. (2011) Regulation of autophagy by ROS: physiology and pathology. *Trends Biochem Sci*,36,pp.30-38.

Schlegel, R.A., Krahling, S., Callahan, M.K. & Williamson, P. (1999) CD14 is a component of multiple recognition systems used by macrophages to phagocytose apoptotic lymphocytes. *Cell Death Differ*,6,6,pp.583-92.

Schrijvers, D.M., De Meyer, G.R., Kockx, M.M., Herman, A.G. & Martinet, W. (2005) Phagocytosis of apoptotic cells by macrophages is impaired in atherosclerosis. *Arterioscl Thromb Vasc Biol*,25,6,pp.1256-61.

Schrijvers, D.M., De Meyer, G.R.Y., Herman, A.G. & Martinet, W. (2007) Phagocytosis in atherosclerosis: Molecular mechanisms and implications for plaque progression and stability. *Cardiovasc Res*,73,3,pp.470-80.

Segundo, C., Medina, F., Rodríguez, C., Martínez-Palencia, R., Leyva-Cobián, F.& Brieva, J.A. (1999) Surface molecule loss and bleb formation by human germinal center B cells undergoing apoptosis: role of apoptotic blebs in monocyte chemotaxis. *Blood*, 94,3,pp.1012-20.

Serhan, C.N., Chiang, N. & Van Dyke, T.E. (2008) Resolving inflammation: dual anti-inflammatory and pro-resolution lipid mediators. *Nat Rev Immunol*,8,5,pp.349-61.

Shi, Y., Evans, J.E. & Rock, K.L. (2003) Molecular identification of a danger signal that alerts the immune system to dying cells. *Nature*,425,6957,pp.516-21.

Shimada, K. (2009) Immune system and atherosclerotic disease: heterogeneity of leukocyte subsets participating in the pathogenesis of atherosclerosis. *Circ J*,73,6,pp.994-1001.

Shintani, T. & Klionsky, D.J. (2004) Autophagy in health and disease: a double-edged sword. *Science*,306,pp.990-5.

Simons, M. & Raposo, G. (2009) Exosomes—vesicular carriers for intercellular communication. *Curr Opin Cell Biol*,21,pp.575–81.

Sindrilaru, A., Peters, T., Schymeinsky, J., Oreshkova, T., Wang, H., Gompf, A., Mannella, F., Wlaschek, M., Sunderkötter, C., Rudolph, K.L., Walzog, B., Bustelo, X.R., Fischer, K.D. & Scharffetter-Kochanek, K. (2009) Wound healing defect of Vav3-/- mice due to impaired {beta}2-integrin-dependent macrophage phagocytosis of apoptotic neutrophils. *Blood*,113,21,pp.5266-76.

Sluimer, J.C., Gasc, J.M., van Wanroij, J.L., Kisters, N., Groeneweg, M., Sollewijn, G., Cleutjens, J.P., van den Akker, L.H., Corvol, P., Wouters, B.G., Daemen, M.J. & Bijnens, A.P. (2008) Hypoxia, hypoxia-inducible transcription factor, and macrophages in human atherosclerotic plaques are correlated with intraplaque angiogenesis. *J Am Coll Cardiol*,51,pp.1258–65.

Su, Y.R., Dove, D.E., Major, A.S., Hasty, A.H., Boone, B., Linton, M.F. & Fazio, S. (2005) Reduced ABCA1-mediated cholesterol efflux and accelerated atherosclerosis in apolipoprotein E-deficient mice lacking macrophage-derived ACAT1. *Circulation*, 111,18,pp.2373-81.

Szondy, Z., Sarang, Z., Molnar, P., Nemeth, T., Piacentini, M., Mastroberardino, P.G., Falasca, L., Aeschlimann, D., Kovacs, J., Kiss, I., Szegezdi, E., Lakos, G., Rajnavolgyi, E., Birckbichler, P.J., Melino, G. & Fesus, L. (2003) Transglutaminase 2 -/- mice reveal a phagocytosis-associated crosstalk between macrophages and apoptotic cells. *Proc Natl Acad Sci U S A*,100,13,pp.7812-7.

Tabas, I. (2005) Consequences and therapeutic implications of macrophage apoptosis in atherosclerosis: the importance of lesion stage and phagocytic efficiency. *Arterioscler Thromb Vasc Biol*,25,11,pp.2255-64.

Tabas, I. (2010) Macrophage death and defective inflammation resolution in atherosclerosis. *Nat Rev Immunol*,10,1,pp.36-46.

Tang, D., Kang, R., Xiao, W., Wang, H., Calderwood, S.K. & Xiao, X. (2007) The anti-inflammatory effects of heat shock protein 72 involve inhibition of high-mobility-group box 1 release and proinflammatory function in macrophages. *J Immunol*, 179,2,pp.1236-44.

Tedgui, A. & Mallat, Z. (2001) Apoptosis as a determinant of atherothrombosis. *Thromb Haemost*, 86,1,pp.420-6.

Thorp, E., Cui, D., Schrijvers, D.M., Kuriakose, G. & Tabas, I. (2008) Mertk receptor mutation reduces efferocytosis efficiency and promotes apoptotic cell accumulation and plaque necrosis in atherosclerotic lesions of apoe-/- mice. *Arterioscler Thromb Vasc Biol*,28,8,pp.1421-8.

Thorp, E. & Tabas, I. (2009) Mechanisms and consequences of efferocytosis in advanced atherosclerosis. *J Leukoc Biol*,86,5,pp.1089-95.

Thorp, E.B. (2010) Mechanisms of failed apoptotic cell clearance by phagocyte subsets in cardiovascular disease. *Apoptosis*,15,pp.1124-36.

Truman, L.A., Ford, C.A., Pasikowska, M., Pound, J.D., Wilkinson, S.J., Dumitriu, I.E., Melville, L., Melrose, L.A., Ogden, C.A., Nibbs, R., Graham, G., Combadiere, C. & Gregory, C.D. (2008) CX3CL1/fractalkine is released from apoptotic lymphocytes to stimulate macrophage chemotaxis. *Blood*,112,13,pp.5026-36.

Tyurina, Y.Y., Serinkan, F.B., Tyurin, V.A., Kini, V., Yalowich, J.C., Schroit, A.J., Fadeel, B. & Kagan, V.E. (2004) Lipid antioxidant, etoposide, inhibits phosphatidylserine externalization and macrophage clearance of apoptotic cells by preventing phosphatidylserine oxidation. *J Biol Chem*,279,7,pp.6056-64.

Vandivier, R.W., Fadok, V.A., Hoffmann, P.R., Bratton, D.L., Penvari, C., Brown, K.K., Brain, J.D., Accurso, F.J. & Henson, P.M. (2002) Elastase-mediated phosphatidylserine receptor cleavage impairs apoptotic cell clearance in cystic fibrosis and bronchiectasis. *J Clin Invest*,109,5,pp.661-70.

Verheye, S., Martinet, W., Kockx, M.M., Knaapen, M.W.M., Salu, K., Timmermans, J.P., Ellis, J.T., Kilpatrick, D.L. & De Meyer, G.R.Y. (2007) Selective clearance of macrophages in atherosclerotic plaques by autophagy. *J Am Coll Cardiol*,49,pp.706-15.

Wakasugi, K. & Schimmel, P. (1999) Two distinct cytokines released from a human aminoacyl-tRNA synthetase. *Science*,284,5411,pp.147-51.

Waldo, S.W., Li, Y., Buono, C., Zhao, B., Billings, E.M., Chang, J. & Kruth, H.S. (2008) Heterogeneity of human macrophages in culture and in atherosclerotic plaques. *Am J Pathol*,172,4,pp.1112-26.

Wang, J. (2008) Beclin-1 bridges autophagy, apoptosis and differentiation. *Autophagy*, 4,pp.947-8.

Wei, Y.S., Lan, Y., Liu, Y.G., Meng, L.Q., Xu, Q.Q. & Xie, H.Y. (2009) Platelet-endothelial cell adhesion molecule-1 gene polymorphism and its soluble level are associated with ischemic stroke. *DNA Cell Biol*,28,3,pp.151-8.

Wen, Y. & Leake, D.S. (2007) Low density lipoprotein undergoes oxidation within lysosomes in cells. *Circ Res*,100,9,pp.1337-43.

Wieten, L., Broere, F., van der Zee, R., Koerkamp, E.K., Wagenaar, J. & van Eden, W. (2007) Cell stress induced HSP are targets of regulatory T cells: a role for HSP inducing compounds as anti-inflammatory immuno-modulators? *FEBS Lett*,581,pp.3716-22.

Xu, W., Roos, A., Schlagwein, N., Woltman, A.M., Daha, M.R., van Kooten, C. (2006) IL-10-producing macrophages preferentially clear early apoptotic cells. *Blood*, 107,12,pp.4930-7.

Xu, K., Yang, Y., Yan, M., Zhan, J., Fu, X. & Zheng, X. (2010) Autophagy plays a protective role in free cholesterol overload-induced death of smooth muscle cells. *J Lipid Res*, 51,pp.2581-90.

Yancey, P.G., Blakemore, J., Ding, L., Fan, D., Overton, C.D., Zhang, Y., Linton, M.F. & Fazio, S. (2010) Macrophage LRP-1 controls plaque cellularity by regulating efferocytosis and Akt activation. *Arterioscler Thromb Vasc Biol*,30,4,pp.787-95.

Yang, Z. & Klionsky, D.J. (2010) Mammalian autophagy: core molecular machinery and signaling regulation. *Curr Opin Cell Biol*,22,pp.124-31.

Yoshimori, T. (2004) Autophagy: a regulated bulk degradation process inside cells. *Biochem Biophys Res Commun*,313,pp.453-458.

Yousefi, S., Perozzo, R., Schmid, I., Ziemiecki, A., Schaffner, T., Scapozza, L., Brunner, T. & Simon, H.U. (2006) Calpain-mediated cleavage of Atg5 switches autophagy to apoptosis. *Nat Cell Biol*,8,pp.1124–32.

Yousefi, S. & Simon, H.U. (2007) Apoptosis regulation by autophagy gene 5. *Crit Rev Oncol Hematol*,63,pp.241-4.

Yu, M., Wang, H., Ding, A., Golenbock, D.T., Latz, E., Czura, C.J., Fenton, M.J., Tracey, K.J. & Yang, H. (2006) HMGB1 signals through toll-like receptor (TLR) 4 and TLR2. *Shock*,26,2,pp.174-9.

Yvan-Charvet, L., Pagler, T.A., Seimon, T.A., Thorp, E., Welch, C.L., Witztum, J.L., Tabas, I. & Tall, A.R. (2010) ABCA1 and ABCG1 protect against oxidative stress-induced macrophage apoptosis during efferocytosis. *Circ Res*,106,12,pp.1861-9

# 12

# Innate Immune Receptors in Atherosclerosis

Jennifer E. Cole, Anusha N. Seneviratne and Claudia Monaco
*Kennedy Institute of Rheumatology, Imperial College London*
*United Kingdom*

## 1. Introduction

The inflammatory response is an important process, aiming to restore tissue homeostasis following tissue injury or infection. Acute inflammation is a tightly controlled process. If an inflammatory stimulus persists or if normal immune function is perturbed, inflammation may become chronic. Atherosclerosis is a chronic inflammatory disorder involving components of both the innate and adaptive immune systems (Ross, 1999). The innate immune system provides the first line of defence against invading pathogens. Innate immune detection of pathogens relies on a set of pattern recognition receptors (PRRs) that recognise and respond to conserved pathogen-associated molecular patterns (PAMPs). Growing evidence supports roles for PRRs in the initiation and progression of atherosclerosis. In this chapter, the agonists, signalling pathways, expression and functions of PRRs, in particular in reference to atherosclerosis, will be discussed. The potential therapeutic benefit of targeting PRRs for treatment of atherosclerosis will also be explored.

## 2. Pattern recognition receptors

PAMPs are recognised by an expanding number of PRRs, which currently includes at least 50 members. PRRs can be categorised into one of three families: Toll-like receptors (TLRs), Retinoic acid inducible gene I (RIG-I)-like receptors (RLRs), and Nucleotide-binding oligomerization domain (NOD)-like receptors (NLRs). Both extracellular and intracellular compartments are patrolled by PRRs with each family of receptors specialising in surveying a given location. TLRs are transmembrane PRRs either located in the cellular membrane (interacting with the extracellular space) or within intracellular vesicles such as endosomes or lysosomes. Cytosolic PRRs include RLRs and NLRs that detect intracellular PAMPs. While cytosolic PRRs are universally expressed in the majority of cells in the body (Takeuchi & Akira, 2010), TLR expression is more restricted. TLR, NLR and RLR ligation by an agonist stimulates downstream signalling cascades activating 2 major types of transcription factor: the nuclear factor kB (NFκB), and interferon response factors (IRFs).

### 2.1 Toll-like receptors (TLRs)

The TLR family contains at least 13 different members in mammals. Following ligand binding, TLRs dimerise, with most receptors (with the exception of TLR2 and TLR4) forming homodimers. Components of the bacterial cell wall including bacterial lipoproteins, endotoxin and flagellin are sensed by TLR2, TLR4 and TLR5 respectively. TLR3, TLR7, TLR8 and TLR9 are not located on the cell surface and are instead located on the membranes of endoplasmic reticulum (ER), endosomes and lysosomes, where they detect nucleic acids derived from bacteria or viruses. The TLR family share their cytoplasmic Toll/Interleukin-1 Receptor (TIR) domain – essential for signal transduction - with their larger parent family which includes interleukin-1-receptor (IL-1Rs). The extracellular regions of TLRs contain tandemly arranged leucine rich repeats (LRR) creating a horseshoe-shaped solenoid structure (Liu et al., 2008a). TLRs are connected to their downstream signalling cascades via five TLR adaptor molecules that are recruited to and homophilically interact with the TIR domain: myeloid differentiation protein 88 (MyD88), Toll–interleukin-1 receptor domain-containing adaptor inducing interferon-β (TRIF), TIR domain-containing adaptor protein (TIRAP)/MyD88-adaptor-like (MAL), TRIF related adaptor molecule (TRAM) and sterile alpha and HEAT/Armadillo motif (SARM).

### 2.2 RIG-I-like receptors (RLRs)

Double stranded RNA (dsRNA) in the cytoplasm can be sensed in both immune and non-immune cells via RLRs. The RLR family includes retinoic acid inducible gene I (RIG-I), melanoma differentiation associated gene 5 (MDA5) and laboratory of genetics and physiology 2 (LGP2). RLRs possess a central RNA helicase domain with the ATPase binding motif DExD/H. The C-terminal regulatory domain is responsible for binding to dsRNAs. RIG-I and MDA5 have two N-terminal caspase activation and recruitment domains (CARDs), which allows homophilic interactions between activated RIG-I or MDA5 and the adaptor protein mitochondrial antiviral signaling (MAVS, also known as IPS-1, VISA, and Cardif), which is found in the outer mitochondrial membrane (Takeuchi & Akira, 2010).

### 2.3 NOD-like receptors (NLRs)

NLRs belong to a large family of soluble proteins that are present in the cytoplasm and detect intracellular ligands. There are 23 NLR genes in humans and 34 in mice. Three distinct subfamilies of NLRs exist: NODs, NLRPs (or NALPs) and IL-1β-converting enzyme (ICE)-protease activating factor (IPAF). NLRs are composed of the following domains: a C-terminal ligand-sensing leucine-rich repeat (LRR) domain, a central nucleotide-binding and oligomerization (NACHT) domain (responsible for oligomerization), and an N-terminal effector pyrin domain (PYD), caspase recruitment domain family (CARD) or baculoviral IAP repeat (BIR) mediating homophilic interactions in downstream signalling. The physiological function of most NLRs is still not understood.

## 3. PRR agonists in atherosclerosis

A vast and diverse array of ligands including viruses, lipids and extracellular matrix components are collectively recognised by PRRs (Lundberg & Hansson, 2010). Each individual PRR exhibits specificity in the repertoire of ligands that it recognises and responds to. In a process known as 'sterile inflammation', activation of PRRs can occur in the absence of exogenous stimuli (Rifkin et al., 2005). The PRR agonists in this context are generated as a result of tissue damage and inflammation and are known as 'damage-associated molecular patterns' (DAMPs). Thus, PRR ligands encompass both exogenous PAMPs and endogenous DAMPs. Increasing evidence suggests that different co-receptors and accessory molecules and thus different mechanisms of action are used by TLRs in response to ligation by PAMPs and DAMPs (reviewed in (Piccinini & Midwood, 2010)). Exogenous PRR ligands, such as viruses and bacteria, and endogenous PRR ligands, including extracellular matrix components, modified lipids and heat shock proteins are PRR ligands that may be relevant in the context of atherosclerosis.

### 3.1 Exogenous PRR agonists

Exogenous agonists are the best defined PRR ligands and include components of bacteria and viruses. TLR2 recognises a diverse array of PAMPs using heterodimerisation with TLR1 or TLR6. TLR2 is key in the recognition of Gram-positive bacteria (Underhill et al., 1999a; Underhill et al., 1999b). Lipoteichoic acid, is a ligand of TLR2/TLR6 heterodimers as are peptidoglycan and zymosan (Gantner et al., 2003; Ozinsky et al., 2000; Schroder et al., 2003). Using CD36 as a co-receptor, TLR2/TLR6 heterodimers also recognise mycoplasma diacylated lipoproteins peptide (Brightbill et al., 1999; Hoebe et al., 2005; Takeuchi et al., 2001). Triacylated lipoproteins are ligands for TLR1/TLR2 heterodimers (Jin et al., 2007; Takeuchi et al., 2002). Endotoxin (lipopolysaccharide), a component of the outer membrane of Gram-negative bacteria, is an agonist for the TLR4 signalling complex (Shimazu et al., 1999; Wright et al., 1990). Compared to TLR2 and TLR4, other TLRs have a relatively limited repertoire of TLR ligands. TLR3 senses viral double-stranded RNA and some small interfering RNAs. A synthetic dsRNA analogue Poly(I:C) is commonly used as a TLR3 activator (Takeuchi & Akira, 2010). Bacterial flagellin is recognised by TLR5 and TLR9 detects unmethylated CpG DNA, typically of bacterial origin (O'Neill & Bowie, 2007). TLR7 is the main sensor of ssRNA derived from RNA viruses including human immunodeficiency virus and influenza A. More recently, TLR7 on myeloid dendritic cells has also been shown to be capable of sensing bacterial RNA (Mancuso et al., 2009).

Genomic RNA of dsRNA viruses and dsRNA generated as the replication intermediate of ssRNA viruses in the cytosol are ligands for RLRs. Short dsRNAs with 5′ triphosphate ends are sensed by RIG-I whereas MDA5 recognises longer dsRNAs (Kato et al., 2006). NOD1 and NOD2 sense peptidoglycan. NOD1 recognises a peptidoglycan motif: dipeptide γ-d-glutamyl-meso-dia-minopimelic acid (iE-DAP) and NOD2 recognises muramyl dipeptide (Chamaillard et al., 2003; Girardin et al., 2003a; Girardin et al., 2003b; Inohara et al., 2003). Whole pathogens including bacteria with pore-forming toxins and viruses including influenza virus are activators of the NLRP3 inflammasome (reviewed in (Schroder & Tschopp, 2010)).

Numerous exogenous PAMPS may be ligands for PRRs in atherosclerosis. *Chlamydia pneumonia, porphyromonas gingivalis* and cytomegalovirus are exogenous PRR ligands found in atherosclerotic plaques (Chiu et al., 1997; Kuo et al., 1993). These bacterial and viral infectious agents have been associated with an increased risk of atherosclerosis development (Kalayoglu et al., 2002; Kiechl et al., 2001; Scannapieco et al., 2003) and are recognised by TLR2 and TLR4 (Burns et al., 2006; Compton et al., 2003; Naiki et al., 2008). The failure to detect active viral replication within atherosclerotic plaques (Kol et al., 1995; Zhou et al., 1999) suggests PRR activation by infectious agents and not viral replication itself is the link between infectious disease and cardiovascular risk. Exogenous heat shock proteins (HSPs), nucleic acids (Lehtiniemi et al., 2005; Ott et al., 2006) and peptidoglycan

(Laman et al., 2002) are also present in atherosclerotic lesions and thus may activate PRRs in atherogenesis.

### 3.2 Endogenous PRR agonists

Many endogenous PRR ligands are present in atherosclerotic lesions and thus PRR activation in atherosclerosis could result from a combination of exogenous and endogenous ligand sensing. Indeed, work by Curtiss and colleagues supports a role for endogenous TLR ligands in atherogenesis (Mullick et al., 2005). Extracellular matrix (ECM) is degraded during tissue injury and remodelling leading to the generation of ECM components, which can function as PRR ligands. Fibrinogen can activate TLR4 signalling as can the fibronectin alternatively spliced exon encoding type III extra domain A (EDA) and tenascin C (Midwood & Orend, 2009; Okamura et al., 2001; Smiley et al., 2001). Hyaluronan, a large glycosaminoglycan component of the ECM, and biglycan activate TLR2 and TLR4 signalling (Schaefer et al., 2005; Scheibner et al., 2006; Taylor et al., 2004). Hyaluronan can induce IL-1 release by macrophages in a NLRP3-dependent manner (Yamasaki et al., 2009) while biglycan also activates the NLRP3 inflammasome (Babelova et al., 2009). The large ECM proteoglycan versican is a TLR2/6 ligand associated with cytokine production in tumor-infiltrating macrophages (Kim et al., 2009). These ECM components may be generated during injury and remodeling of the vessel wall and thus may activate PRRs in atherosclerosis.

Lipids, key components of atherosclerotic plaques, are TLR ligands. Minimally modified low-density lipoproteins induce cytokine and reactive oxygen species generation via TLR4 signalling complexes (Miller et al., 2003). In association with CD36, TLR4/TLR6 hetero-dimers sense oxidized LDL leading to increased chemokine expression (Stewart et al., 2010). Saturated fatty acids elicit TLR4 activation whereas polyunsaturated fatty acids inhibit TLR4 activation (Lee et al., 2003). However, the ability of saturated fatty acids to directly induce TLR signaling has been questioned (Erridge & Samani, 2009). TLR2 can also sense ApoCIII, a component of very-low-density lipoprotein (VLDL) (Kawakami et al., 2008).

HSPs are present in murine atherosclerotic lesions and are ligands for TLR2 and TLR4 (Asea et al., 2002; Kanwar et al., 2001). However, some studies using low-endotoxin preparations have disputed the role of HSPs as ligands for TLRs (Bausinger et al., 2002). The nuclear protein high-mobility group box-1 (HMGB-1) is expressed in human atherosclerotic smooth muscle cells (Porto et al., 2006). HMGB1 binds DNA and is a ligand for TLR2, TLR4, TLR9 and other nucleic acid sensors (Park et al., 2004; Yanai et al., 2009). mRNA from necrotic cells, which may be present in atherosclerotic plaques, is a TLR3 agonist (Kariko et al., 2004).

The NLRP3 inflammasome can be activated by many factors including extracellular ATP, potassium efflux and reactive oxygen species. In addition, intracellular crystals such as monosodium urate crystals and cholesterol crystals can activate the NLRP3 inflammasome (Duewell et al., 2010; Martinon et al., 2006).

## 4. Signalling of pattern recognition receptors

### 4.1 Toll-like receptor signalling

TLR signalling is composed of two distinct signalling pathways depending on whether the adaptor molecule MyD88 is used following ligation and activation (Figure 1).

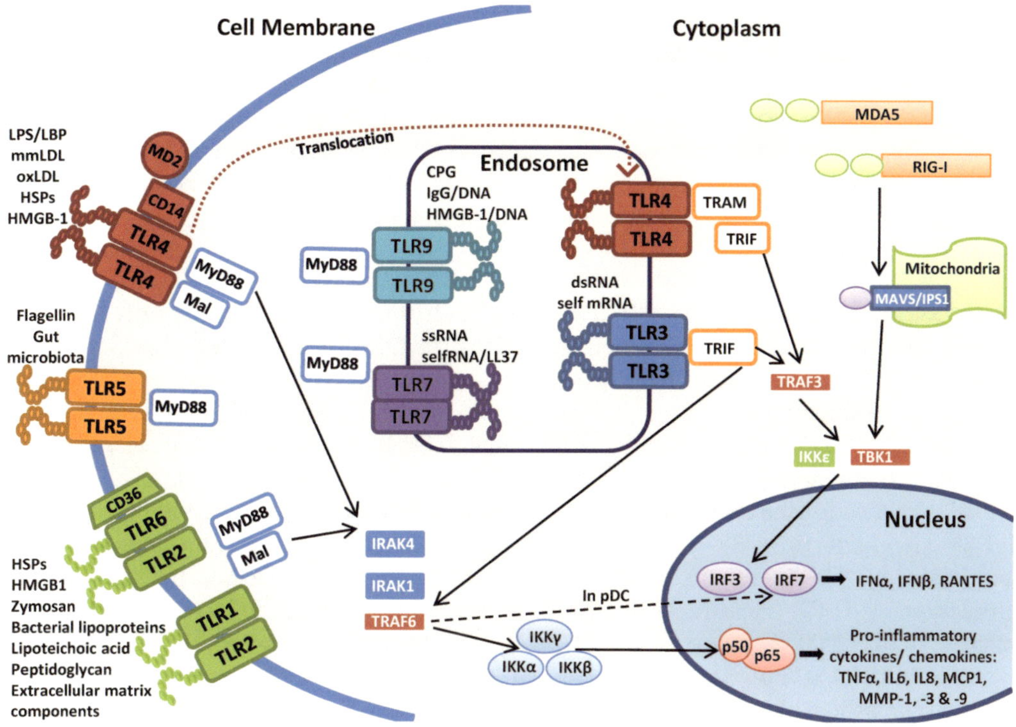


Fig. 1. **Toll-like receptor & RIG-I-like receptor signalling. MyD88-dependent signalling:** All TLRs, except TLR3, recruit the adaptor protein MyD88. MyD88 recruits IRAK1 and IRAK4 to its death domain, which then recruit TRAF6. IRAK1 with TRAF6 subsequently activate a complex consisting of TAK1, which activates the canonical IκB kinase (IKK) complex and the mitogen-activated protein kinase pathway (not shown). NFκB (p50/p65) is then activated to transcribe multiple proinflammatory cytokine genes. The production of type I IFNs by TLR7 and TLR9 depends on MyD88 in plasmacytoid dendritic cells (pDCs). **TRIF-dependent signalling:** TLR3 and endosomal TLR4 (via TRAM), utilise TRIF to interact with the non-canonical IKKs, TBK-1 and IKKε via TRAF3, which phosphorylate IRF3 to induce expression of IFNs. **RIG-I-like receptor signalling:** RIG-I and MDA5 interact with IPS-1 to activate TBK1 enabling the phosphorylation of IRF3 and IRF7. These transcription factors then homo- or heterodimerize, translocate into the nucleus and activate the transcription of type I IFN genes.

#### 4.1.1 MyD88-dependent signalling pathway

All TLRs with the exception of TLR3 use MyD88 to initiate downstream signalling. TLR2 and TLR4 require TIRAP/MAL as a bridge between the TLR and MyD88 (Kagan & Medzhitov, 2006; Yamamoto et al., 2002). Following PAMP recognition by TLRs, MyD88 recruits members of the IL-1 receptor-associated kinase (IRAK) family, including IRAK4, IRAK1, IRAK2 and IRAKM. IRAK4 is activated first, followed by IRAK1 and IRAK2, with all being essential for robust activation of NFκB and MAPK (Kawagoe et al., 2008). The IRAKs then dissociate from MyD88 and associate with TRAF6, an E3 ubiquitin ligase, leading to the activation of a complex consisting of transforming growth factor-β-activated kinase 1 (TAK1), TAK1 binding protein (TAB)1, TAB2 and TAB3. This complex translocates into the cytosol where TAK1 phosphorylates IKKβ. Subsequently, the IKK complex, consisting of IKKα, IKKβ and NFκB essential modulator (NEMO), phosphorylates IκBα, an NFκB inhibitory protein. Phosphorylated IκBα is degraded by the ubiquitin proteosome system, freeing NFκB to translocate to the nucleus and mediate transcription of inflammatory genes. TAK1 also phosphorylates MAPK6 activating the MAP kinases Erk1, Erk2, p38 and Jnk. Activation of the MAPK pathway triggers the formation of activated protein (AP)-1, a transcription factor complex controlling genes encoding many cytokines (Johnson & Lapadat, 2002).

TLR7 and TLR9 induce the production of type 1 IFNs and NFκB-dependent cytokines via the MyD88 dependent pathway. Plasmacytoid dendritic cells (pDCs) constitutively express Interferon Regulatory Factor (IRF)7 which binds to MyD88 forming a complex with IRAK1, IRAK4, TRAF3, TRAF6 and IKKα (Kawai & Akira, 2008). Phosphorylated IRF7 then translocates to the nucleus and facilitates the production of type 1 IFNs (Kawai & Akira, 2010). In contrast, conventional dendritic cells (cDCs) mediate the activation of IRF1 resulting in IFN-β gene expression (Negishi et al., 2006; Schmitz et al., 2007).

MyD88 is critical for the downstream inflammatory effects following ligation of many TLRs. MyD88 knockout ($MyD88^{-/-}$) mice do not respond to peptidoglycan and lipoprotein stimulation of TLR2 (Takeuchi et al., 2002; Takeuchi et al., 2000), Imidazoquinoline stimulation of TLR7 (Hemmi et al., 2002) or stimulation of TLR9 by CpG DNA motifs (Häcker et al., 2000; Schnare et al., 2000). Similarly, $MyD88^{-/-}$ mice have an abolished response to TLR4 stimulation by LPS (Kawai et al., 1999) or TLR5 stimulation by bacterial flagellin (Hayashi et al., 2001).

### 4.1.2 TRIF-dependent signalling pathway

TLR3 utilises signalling via TRIF to elicit responses (Alexopoulou et al., 2001). TRIF associates with TRAF3 and TRAF6 via its N-terminal TRAF binding-motifs (Takeuchi & Akira, 2010). TRAF3 activates 2 noncanonical IKK-related kinases, TBK1 and IKKε which phosphorylate IRF3 enabling its nuclear translocation (Häcker & Karin, 2006; Oganesyan et al., 2006). IRF3 mediates the production of proinflammatory cytokines, type 1 IFNs and increased expression of IFN-induced genes including Adar1, Ifit3 and IRF7 (Tenoever et al., 2007). TRIF also interacts with RIP1 and RIP3 (Takeuchi & Akira, 2010). The TNFR-associated death domain protein (TRADD) is involved in TRIF dependent signalling (Ermolaeva et al., 2008). A complex is formed consisting of TRADD, FADD and RIP1. TRADD triggers the ubiquitination of RIP1 activating NF-κB. Following stimulation by Poly(I:C), a synthetic dsRNA analogue, FADD activates caspase-8 and caspase-10 (Takahashi et al., 2006). These cleaved caspases activate NFκB (Takahashi et al., 2006). In addition, TRIF associates with TRAF6 to activate TAK1. This is thought to occur in an ubiquitination-dependent mechanism similar to the MyD88-dependent pathway resulting in phosphorylation of the inhibitory molecule IκBα by IKKα and IKKβ (Alexopoulou et al., 2001). SARM is a an inhibitor of TRIF-mediated signalling in humans (Carty et al., 2006).

TLR4 is unique in that it can utilise both the MyD88 and TRIF dependent pathways with the sequential activation of 4 adaptor molecules. It appears that the receptor's cellular localisation determines which pathway is triggered (Kagan et al., 2008; Tanimura et al., 2008). Upon ligand binding, membrane bound TLR4 recruits MyD88 which binds to MAL to activate NFκB and MAPK (Kagan & Medzhitov, 2006). Secondly, TLR4 translocates to the endosome via dynamin-dependent endocytosis. There TLR4 associates with TRAM to trigger the TRIF-dependent pathway resulting in IRF3 activation and late phase activation of NFκB and MAPK (Kagan et al., 2008; Rowe et al., 2006; Tanimura et al., 2008).

### 4.2 RIG-I-like receptor (RLR) signalling

RLR signalling activates NFκB, MAPK, and IRFs to induce type I IFNs. LGP2 may regulate the functions of RIG-I and MDA5 as LGP2-deficient mice have elevated levels of type I IFNs. Overexpression of IPS-1 (also called MAVS) activates the promoters of NFκB and type I IFNs inhibiting viral replication. The induction of IFNβ by IPS-1 requires TBK1 and IKKi (Kawai et al., 2005). IPS-1 has a C-terminal transmembrane domain required for mitochondrial targeting (Seth et al., 2005), and deleting this region of IPS-1 prevents IRF3 and NF-κB activation. TRAF3 directly binds both IPS-1 and TBK1/IKKi enabling type I IFN induction in response to ssRNA viral infection. TBK1 is broadly expressed in many tissues while IKKi expression is stimulated upon pro-inflammatory signals such as TNF-α and IFN-γ. It has been suggested that TBK1 aids the initiation of signalling following viral infection while IKKi regulates the immune response in the later stages of viral infection (Kawai & Akira, 2007). IKKi can phosphorylate STAT1 and IRF3 to regulate antiviral gene expression. IPS-1 also interacts with RIP-1 and FADD (Kawai et al., 2005) forming a complex with caspase-10 and caspase-8. The detection of poly I:C triggers the cleavage of these caspases (Takahashi et al., 2006) activating their death effector domain to activate NF-κB.

### 4.3 NOD-like receptor (NLR) signalling

NODs activate MAPKs and NFκB via the serine–threonine kinase RICK and consequently activate TAK1 kinase. NLRs activate the release of the IL-1 family of inflammatory cytokines through the formation of large cytoplasmic complexes known as 'inflammasomes', which include caspase-1. Inflammasomes are characterised into three main complexes —the NLRP3/NALP3 inflammasome, the NLRP1/NALP1 inflammasome and the IPAF/NLRC4 inflammasome. The NLRP3 inflammasome is currently the most studied and consists of the NLRP3 scaffold, the apoptosis-associated speck-like protein-containing CARD (ASC) adaptor, and caspase-1. ASC links the NLR and caspase; normally caspase 1 and 11 (Wang et al., 1998). Upon activation, caspase-1 cleaves the precursor cytokines into their bioactive form, most notably activating IL-1β and IL-18.

### 4.4 Integration of pattern recognition signalling

The pattern recognition system involves numerous interactions between components of different pathways. NOD stimulation, TLR activation and proinflammatory cytokine stimulation can act as priming signals leading to NFκB activation, pro-IL1β synthesis, and the activation of inflammasomal components such as caspase-11 and NLRP3 (Mariathasan & Monack, 2007). A second signal then activates caspase-1 in the inflammasome complex. Such second signals include activation by ATP of the P2X7 purinergic receptor with potassium efflux, PAMPs and DAMPs such as oxidative stress, large particles and ultraviolet light (Wang et al., 1998).

The interaction of IPS-1 with NLR proteins can modulate the activation of NFκB and IRF3 signalling. NLRX1/NOD5 may interact with IPS-1 and inhibit its binding to RIG-I and the production of type I IFNs and pro-inflammatory cytokines. RIG-I can also directly activate the inflammasome. Finally, NOD2 can translocate into mitochondria, and signal via IPS-1, inducing type I IFN secretion via IRF3 during viral infection (reviewed in (Ting et al.,2010)).

## 5. Expression of PRRs in health and atherosclerotic disease

TLRs are expressed by both leukocyte subsets and resident tissue cells (reviewed in (Cole et al., 2010)). In contrast to veins, which are relatively atherosclerosis-resistant, the arterial system is more predisposed to atherosclerotic lesion formation. This is mirrored by the sensitivity of venous and arterial cells to TLR agonists with arterial cells responding to a broader range of TLR agonists than venous cells (Erridge et al., 2008). Different arterial beds exhibit heterogeneity in their TLR mRNA expression. Carotid arteries and the aorta share a similar pattern of TLR expression with high expression of TLRs 1 through 6 and minimal to no expression of TLRs 7, 8 and 9. Iliac arteries display the broadest expression of TLRs expressing all but TLR3 whereas mesenteric and subclavian arteries express a narrower range of TLRs. TLR2 and TLR4 are the only TLR described to be ubiquitously expressed in normal human arteries (Pryshchep et al., 2008). During human atherogenesis, TLR expression (in particular expression of TLR1, TLR2 and TLR4) is increased in diseased vessels compared to healthy vessels (Edfeldt et al., 2002). Increased expression of TLR2 and TLR4 are found both in macrophages and in resident cells including adventitial fibroblasts, endothelial cells and smooth muscle cells from human atherosclerotic vessels (Edfeldt et al., 2002; Otsui et al., 2007; Vink et al., 2002; Xu et al., 2001). Similar to human atherosclerotic tissue, expression of TLR2 and TLR4 is increased in murine models of the disease (Mullick et al., 2008; Xu et al., 2001).

In early atherosclerotic lesions, endothelial cells are the first cells to display TLR expression. In LDLR-/- mice endothelial cells at atherosclerosis-prone regions of the vasculature, such as the inner curve of the aortic arch, display increased TLR2 expression, which is also associated with areas of monocyte recruitment (Mullick et al., 2008). Whether endothelial TLR2 expression is a cause or effect of monocyte recruitment is unknown. Smooth muscle cells (SMC) also respond to PAMPs and express TLRs. TLR-1, -3, -4 and -6 are constitutively expressed at the mRNA level by cultured human vascular smooth muscle cells and TLR2, TLR3 and TLR4 stimulation induces SMC production of cytokines and chemokines such as IL6 and MCP1 (Stoll et al., 2004; Yang et al., 2005a; Yang et al., 2005b; Yang et al., 2006). Recently, atheroma-derived SMC have been shown to exhibit a specific increase in TLR3 expression and TLR3-dependent functional responses compared to control aortic SMC (Cole et al., 2011).

Although all leukocyte populations express TLRs, TLR expression on monocytes/ macrophages and dendritic cells is the best characterised. Monocytes, which constitute 5-10% of circulating blood leukocytes in both mouse and man, are key players at all stages of atherogenesis. Constant recruitment of monocytes into atherosclerotic plaques occurs and their recruitment is proportional to plaque size (Swirski et al., 2006). Human blood monocytes highly express TLR2 and TLR4 mRNA and respond to stimulation with their respective TLR ligands by secreting pro-inflammatory cytokines including TNFα and IL6 (Kadowaki et al., 2001; Visintin et al., 2001). TLR4 expression on peripheral blood monocytes appears to correlate with disease activity with monocytes from patients with acute coronary syndromes expressing more TLR4 than monocytes from patients with stable angina (Methe et al., 2005; Shiraki et al., 2006). Similarly, TLR2 expression is also increased on circulating blood monocytes from patients with atherosclerotic disease (Kuwahata et al., 2009; Mizoguchi et al., 2007). Circulating monocytes in ApoE-/- mice with advanced atherosclerosis also exhibit increased expression of TLR2 and TLR4 (Schoneveld et al., 2008). Subsets of monocytes and macrophages with differing characteristics have been described.

The balance of these subsets in disease may determine the outcome for the patient. In both humans and mice, two major subsets of monocytes; 'inflammatory' and 'resident', have been described (Gordon & Taylor, 2005), which can be distinguished on the basis of size, granularity and expression pattern of adhesion molecules and chemokine receptors. Macrophages can also be divided into subsets and can be broadly defined as M1 'classically activated' or M2 'alternatively activated' (Gordon & Taylor, 2005). In terms of TLR responses, differing levels of LPS responsiveness has been described in two subsets of CD14+ peripheral blood monocytes (Moreno-Altamirano et al., 2007), type I interferon production following TLR2 stimulation has been shown to occur specifically in murine inflammatory monocytes from bone marrow and spleen (Barbalat et al., 2009) and M2 macrophages have been shown to exhibit 12-fold higher expression of TLR5 than M1 macrophages (Martinez et al., 2006). Despite these few studies, as yet, the differential expression of TLRs on monocyte and macrophage subsets has not been examined in detail.

The role of dendritic cells (DC) in atherosclerosis is unknown however in normal arteries dendritic cells form networks in the intima, which is described as being part of a 'vascular-associated lymphoid tissue' (Bobryshev & Lord, 1995; Millonig et al., 2001; Wick et al., 1997). Their location in the healthy vessel wall, particularly in regions prone to atherosclerotic lesion development such as branch-points, suggests a role in atherosclerosis development (Lord & Bobryshev, 1999; Millonig et al., 2001). DCs can be broadly classified as either myeloid (mDC) or plasmacytoid (pDC) with both subsets being present in atherosclerotic plaques (Erbel et al., 2007; Niessner et al., 2006). mDCs express TLRs 2-8 at the mRNA level and secrete cytokines and upregulate costimulatory molecule expression in response to TLR-2, -3 and -4 activation (Jarrossay et al., 2001; Matsumoto et al., 2003). On the other hand, pDCs strongly express TLR7 and TLR9 mRNA and are activated, mature and secrete cytokines following exposure to the TLR9 ligand CpG (Hornung et al., 2002; Jarrossay et al., 2001; Kadowaki et al., 2001; Matsumoto et al., 2003). Both mDCs and pDCs express and respond to TLR7 ligation with R848 albeit with different functional outcomes: mDCs express IL12 while pDCs express IFNα (Ito et al., 2002).

Although less is known regarding the expression of RLR and NLRs in atherosclerosis, increasing evidence supports a similar trend to that seen for TLRs. Intimal macrophages in aortic atherosclerotic lesions highly express RIG-I (Imaizumi et al., 2007). In healthy human coronary artery ring cultures, IFNγ treatment augmented the expression of the RNA sensors TLR3, MDA5 and RIG-I (Ahmad et al., 2010).

## 6. Functional consequences of PRR activation in atherosclerosis

### 6.1 The role of the IL1/TLR superfamily in atherosclerotic lesion development

The use of mice deficient in IL1/TLR superfamily molecules has revealed key roles for these signalling pathways in atherosclerotic lesion development. Deletion of MyD88 in ApoE-/- mice inhibits atherosclerotic lesion formation by 60% and also results in a 75% reduction in macrophage recruitment (Bjorkbacka et al., 2004; Michelsen et al., 2004). In addition, following carotid ligation, an 89% reduction in lesion formation is observed in ApoE-/- mice bred with an IRAK4 kinase-inactive knock-in mouse (Rekhter et al., 2008). MyD88 and IRAK4 are part of both the TLR and interleukin receptor (IL1R and IL18R) signalling pathways. ApoE-/-IL18-/- double knockout mice exhibit smaller lesions with a more stable phenotype compared to ApoE-/- (Elhage et al., 2003). Similarly, IL1β deficiency in ApoE-/- mice leads to a 30% reduction in lesion size and a reduction in pro-inflammatory mediators such as VCAM-1 and MCP-1 (Kirii et al., 2003). Overexpression of the endogenous IL1 inhibitor, IL1 receptor antagonist (IL1RA), attenuates lesion production (Merhi-Soussi et al., 2005) whereas IL1RA deletion in ApoE-/- augments lesion development at early timepoints (Isoda et al., 2004).

TLR2 and TLR4 have been the most extensively studied in animal models of atherosclerosis. A missense mutation in the TLR4 gene causing resistance to endotoxin has been identified in C3H/HeJ mice (Poltorak et al., 1998; Qureshi et al., 1999). These mice are resistant to diet-induced atherosclerosis (Nishina et al., 1993). However, no effect on lesion development was observed when bone marrow from C3H/HeJ mice was transplanted into ApoE-/- mice (Shi et al., 2000) suggesting resident vascular cell TLR4 signalling may be more important than TLR4 on hematopoietic cells. Interestingly, a similar observation has been made for TLR2, with TLR2-/- bone marrow transfer into LDLR-/- mice having no effect on lesion development. However, a role for hematopoietic cells in recognition of exogenous TLR2 ligands was revealed when LDLR-/- mice were transplanted with TLR2-/- bone marrow prior to stimulation with a synthetic TLR2 ligand as this led to reduced lesion development (Mullick et al., 2005). In vascular injury models, deficiency of TLR2 or TLR4 leads to reduced neointima formation and activation of TLR2 and TLR4 with agonists augments neointima formation (Schoneveld et al., 2005; Vink et al., 2002). Furthermore, genetic deletion of either TLR2 or TLR4 in atherosclerosis-prone mice confers marked protection from atherosclerotic lesion development attenuating plaque formation by 30-69% (TLR2-deletion) and 55% (TLR4-deletion) (Liu et al., 2008b; Michelsen et al., 2004; Mullick et al., 2005). Lesional macrophage content is also significantly reduced in these TLR deficient animals (Liu et al., 2008b; Michelsen et al., 2004). Administration of a TLR2 agonist to LDLR-/- mice promotes lesion development (Mullick et al., 2005). A rabbit hypercholesterolemia model has revealed that the expression of TLR2 and TLR4 may have a synergistic effect on lesion development (Shinohara et al., 2007).

A protective role for TLR3 in arterial injury and early atherosclerosis has been described, challenging the prevailing view that TLRs are purely detrimental in atherogenesis. TLR3 activation using the synthetic ligand Poly(I:C) led to attenuated neointima formation in C57BL/6 but not TLR3-/- mice following carotid injury (Cole et al., 2011). Furthermore, TLR3 was shown to mediate protection against medial damage even in the absence of exogenous TLR3 stimulation suggesting that following injury an endogenous TLR3 ligand is released which maintains the integrity of the vessel wall. In addition, ApoE-/-TLR3-/- mice exhibited increased lesion formation compared to ApoE-/- at an early but not later timepoint (Cole et al., 2011). The mechanisms of the protective effects of TLR3 remain to be explored as does the identification of endogenous TLR3 ligands in atherosclerosis. mRNA from necrotic cells and stathmin, a microtubule regulatory protein have both been identified as potential endogenous TLR3 ligands (Bsibsi et al., 2010; Kariko et al., 2004). A recent study showed that intravenous administration of poly(I:C) induces endothelial dysfunction and increased atherosclerotic lesion development (Zimmer et al., 2011). Together the studies of Cole *et al.,* and Zimmer and colleagues suggest a complex role for dsRNA sensing in atherosclerosis.

Evidence from human polymorphism and atheroma-cell culture studies also support roles for TLRs in atherosclerosis. Asp299Gly and Thr399Ile are two single-nucleotide TLR4 polymorphisms that are associated with reduced responses to inhaled LPS (Arbour et al., 2000). Despite individuals who carry these polymorphisms having lower circulating levels of proinflammatory cytokines and adhesion molecules (Cook et al., 2004), no definitive effect of these polymorphisms on cardiovascular disease has been identified (reviewed in (Frantz et al., 2007)). The TLR2 polymorphism Arg753Gln has been found, in a relatively small study, to be associated with restenosis and an increased risk of developing mycobacterial disease (Hamann et al., 2005). In human atherosclerosis, TLR2 and MyD88 have been shown to play a predominant role in NFκB activation, the production of proinflammatory cytokines including MCP-1 and IL6 and the generation of the matrix degrading enzymes MMP-1, -2, -3 and -9 (Monaco et al., 2009). This finding suggests that TLR2 signalling may promote plaque vulnerability and rupture. The same study found that TLR4 and its adaptor protein TRAM were not rate-limiting for cytokine production in human atherosclerosis but may have a role in MMP-1 and -3 production (Monaco et al., 2009).

### 6.2 Involvement of TLRs in lipid-associated signalling

Foam cells are a hallmark feature of atherosclerotic lesions. TLR2, TLR4 and TLR9 ligation on macrophages promotes lipid uptake and foam cell formation (Funk et al., 1993; Kim et al., 2009; Lee et al., 2008; Oiknine & Aviram, 1992). Whilst TLR4-dependent fluid phase uptake (macropinocytosis) of lipids occurs in differentiated macrophages (Choi et al., 2009), TLRs also promote macrophage lipid uptake indirectly. In response to TLR3, TLR4 and TLR9 activation, macrophage expression of the scavenger receptors SRA, macrophage receptor with collagenous structure (MARCO) and lectin-like oxidised low-density lipoprotein receptor-1 (LOX-1) is increased (Doyle et al., 2004; Lee et al., 2008). Similarly TLR2, TLR3 and TLR4 ligation induces expression of fatty acid binding proteins such as aP2 and Mal1 in murine but not human macrophages (Feingold et al., 2010; Kazemi et al., 2005). Lipid-X receptors (LXRs) regulate expression of genes including ATP-binding cassette transporter A1 (ABCA1) and G1 (ABCG1), which are involved in cholesterol efflux. Activation of TLR3 and TLR4, via signalling pathways involving IRF3, leads to attenuated expression of ABCA1 and ABCG1 through inhibition of LXR transcriptional activity (Castrillo et al., 2003). Furthermore, in a recent study, low-grade endotoxemia *in vivo* inhibited reverse cholesterol transport in mice and also impaired cholesterol efflux in *ex vivo* cultured human macrophages (McGillicuddy et al., 2009). Thus TLR signalling can both promote lipid uptake and disrupt cholesterol efflux therefore promoting foam cell formation and atherosclerotic lesion development.

### 6.3 The role of NLR and RIG-I in atherosclerosis

The role of NLR in the development of atherosclerosis is emerging. The NLRP3 inflammasome, is the best characterised NLR thus far in atherosclerosis. Neointima formation is reduced in ASC-/- mice compared to control mice following wire-injury of the femoral artery (Yajima et al., 2008). In addition, neointima in ASC-/- mice exhibited attenuated IL1β and IL18 expression. BMT experiments revealed hematopoietic cell ASC expression is important for neointima formation in this model (Yajima et al., 2008). Cholesterol crystals, previously thought to be present only in advanced atherosclerotic lesions have been shown to be present in lesions of ApoE-/- mice as soon as 2 weeks after the initiation of high-fat feeding (Duewell et al., 2010). Cholesterol crystals can activate the NLRP3 inflammasome in human and murine macrophages leading to caspase-1 cleavage and IL1β release suggesting that these crystals may be endogenous danger signals in atherosclerosis (Duewell et al., 2010; Rajamaki et al., 2010). Bone marrow transfer of hematopoietic cells from mice lacking NLRP3, ASC or IL1α/β into LDLR-/- mice leads to attenuated lesion formation and reduced serum IL18 levels compared to mice receiving bone marrow cells from wild-type mice (Duewell et al., 2010). However more recently, Menu *et al* have crossed ApoE-/- mice with NLRP3-/-, ASC-/- and caspase1-/- mice to create double knockout mice (Menu et al., 2011). Suprisingly, deletion of these 3 key components of the NLRP3 inflammasome in ApoE-/- mice did not greatly affect atherosclerotic lesion development, macrophage recruitment nor lesion stability suggesting that these molecules do not affect atherosclerosis (Menu et al., 2011). The use of different murine models may explain the differences between these findings and those of Duewell and colleagues. The role of other NLRs and RIG-I in atherosclerosis remains to be examined.

## 7. The therapeutic potential of PRRs in treating atherosclerosis

Atherosclerosis, the leading cause of coronary artery and cerebrovascular disease, which together comprise the leading causes of death worldwide (Lopez et al., 2006), are a significant social and economic burden. Thus, there is a pressing need to identify new molecular targets and develop novel therapeutics for the treatment of atherosclerosis. Since PRRs are key players at all stages of atherosclerotic lesion development, targeting PRRs is an exciting prospect for the treatment of cardiovascular disease.

TLR2 and TLR4 are the best-characterised PRRs in atherosclerosis. Both receptors have been ascribed pro-atherogenic roles and thus inhibition of these receptors is currently the most appealing prospect for generation of PRR therapeutics. Reduction of protein expression of TLR2 and TLR4 in murine and human cells has been achieved using angiotensin II blockade, statin and insulin treatment (Ahn et al., 2007; Foldes et al., 2008; Ghanim et al., 2008). Whether such reductions translate to inhibition of functional responses and whether this inhibition is achievable in patients with cardiovascular disease remains to be determined. TLR2 blockade can inhibit cytokine, chemokine and MMP production in human atherosclerosis, while disruption of TLR4 signalling had little effect on the same outcomes (Monaco et al., 2009). Blockade of TLR2 is also beneficial in a murine model of myocardial ischemia/reperfusion injury (Arslan et al., 2010). TLR4 antagonists such as Eritoran are in development for immune disorders (reviewed in (Hennessy et al., 2010)) and may be beneficial in the treatment of cardiovascular disease. However, caution is needed when extrapolating murine data into human targets and therapeutics. Deletion of IL-1, TLR-2 and TLR-4 is equally effective in murine models of atherosclerosis, however only TLR-2 has a predominant role in human disease (Monaco et al., 2009). In addition to developing antagonists of pro-atherogenic PRRs, it is important to consider generating PRR agonists to target athero-protective PRRs such as TLR3.

Before the most effective PRR therapeutics can be generated, it will be important to discern the precise pattern of PRR expression and the consequence of PRR signalling on all cell types in the vessel wall in both health and disease. As lesions develop, the composition of atherosclerotic plaques change and thus different PRRs and cell types may need to be targeted at different time-points during disease progression.

## 8. Concluding remarks

Evidence supporting a key role for PRRs in the initiation and development of atherosclerosis is growing and yet the full contribution of PRR activation and signalling to atherogenesis is only just emerging. Prominent pro-atherogenic roles have been assigned to TLR2 and TLR4 as these receptors have been shown to promote foam cell formation, macrophage recruitment and cytokine/MMP production - all key components of atherosclerotic plaque development. However, recent data has shown TLR3 to be atheroprotective. Furthermore, the roles and functions of the other PRRs including NODs and RIG-I remain to be explored. Given the complex consequences of TLR activation, further studies are required to fully elucidate the expression patterns, ligands (both endogenous and exogenous), signalling pathways and functions of PRRs in both health and at all stages of disease development. With increased knowledge, it may then be possible to design novel therapeutics targeting PRRs for the treatment of cardiovascular disease.

## 9. References

Ahmad, U., Ali, R., Lebastchi, A.H., Qin, L., Lo, S.F., Yakimov, A.O., Khan, S.F., Choy, J.C., Geirsson, A., Pober, J.S., & Tellides, G. (2010). IFN-gamma primes intact human coronary arteries and cultured coronary smooth muscle cells to double-stranded RNA- and self-RNA-induced inflammatory responses by upregulating TLR3 and melanoma differentiation-associated gene 5. *J Immunol*, Vol. 185, No. 2, pp. 1283-1294

Ahn, K.O., Lim, S.W., Li, C., Yang, H.J., Ghee, J.Y., Kim, J.Y., Kim, S.H., Kim, J., & Yang, C.W. (2007). Influence of angiotensin II on expression of toll-like receptor 2 and maturation of dendritic cells in chronic cyclosporine nephropathy. *Transplantation*, Vol. 83, No. 7, pp. 938-947

Alexopoulou, L., Holt, A., Medzhitov, R., & Flavell, R. (2001). Recognition of double-stranded RNA and activation of NF-κB by Toll-like receptor 3. *Nature*, Vol. 413, pp. 732-738

Arbour, N.C., Lorenz, E., Schutte, B.C., Zabner, J., Kline, J.N., Jones, M., Frees, K., Watt, J.L., & Schwartz, D.A. (2000). TLR4 mutations are associated with endotoxin hyporesponsiveness in humans. *Nat Genet*, Vol. 25, No. 2, pp. 187-191

Arslan, F., Smeets, M., O'Neill, L., Keogh, B., McGuirk, P., Timmers, L., Tersteeg, C., Hoefer, I., Doevendans, P., Pasterkamp, G., & de Kleijn, D. (2010). Myocardial ischemia/reperfusion injury is mediated by leukocytic toll-like receptor-2 and reduced by systemic administration of a novel anti-toll-like receptor-2 antibody. *Circulation*, Vol. 121, No. 1, pp. 80-90

Asea, A., Rehli, M., Kabingu, E., Boch, J.A., Bare, O., Auron, P.E., Stevenson, M.A., & Calderwood, S.K. (2002). Novel signal transduction pathway utilized by extracellular HSP70: role of toll-like receptor (TLR) 2 and TLR4. *J Biol Chem*, Vol. 277, No. 17, pp. 15028-15034

Babelova, A., Moreth, K., Tsalastra-Greul, W., Zeng-Brouwers, J., Eickelberg, O., Young, M.F., Bruckner, P., Pfeilschifter, J., Schaefer, R.M., Grone, H.J., & Schaefer, L. (2009). Biglycan, a danger signal that activates the NLRP3 inflammasome via toll-like and P2X receptors. *J Biol Chem*, Vol. 284, No. 36, pp. 24035-24048

Barbalat, R., Lau, L., Locksley, R., & Barton, G. (2009). Toll-like receptor 2 on inflammatory monocytes induces type I interferon in response to viral but not bacterial ligands. *Nat Immunol*, Vol. 10, No. 11, pp. 1200-1207

Bausinger, H., Lipsker, D., Ziylan, U., Manie, S., Briand, J.P., Cazenave, J.P., Muller, S., Haeuw, J.F., Ravanat, C., de la Salle, H., & Hanau, D. (2002). Endotoxin-free heat-shock protein 70 fails to induce APC activation. *Eur J Immunol*, Vol. 32, No. 12, pp. 3708-3713

Bjorkbacka, H., Kunjathoor, V.V., Moore, K.J., Koehn, S., Ordija, C.M., Lee, M.A., Means, T., Halmen, K., Luster, A.D., Golenbock, D.T., & Freeman, M.W. (2004). Reduced atherosclerosis in MyD88-null mice links elevated serum cholesterol levels to activation of innate immunity signaling pathways. *Nat Med*, Vol. 10, No. 4, pp. 416-421

Bobryshev, Y.V., & Lord, R.S. (1995). Ultrastructural recognition of cells with dendritic cell morphology in human aortic intima. Contacting interactions of Vascular Dendritic Cells in athero-resistant and athero-prone areas of the normal aorta. *Arch Histol Cytol*, Vol. 58, No. 3, pp. 307-322

Brightbill, H.D., Libraty, D.H., Krutzik, S.R., Yang, R.B., Belisle, J.T., Bleharski, J.R., Maitland, M., Norgard, M.V., Plevy, S.E., Smale, S.T., Brennan, P.J., Bloom, B.R., Godowski, P.J., & Modlin, R.L. (1999). Host defense mechanisms triggered by microbial lipoproteins through toll-like receptors. *Science*, Vol. 285, No. 5428, pp. 732-736

Bsibsi, M., Bajramovic, J.J., Vogt, M.H., van Duijvenvoorden, E., Baghat, A., Persoon-Deen, C., Tielen, F., Verbeek, R., Huitinga, I., Ryffel, B., Kros, A., Gerritsen, W.H., Amor, S., & van Noort, J.M. (2010). The microtubule regulator stathmin is an endogenous protein agonist for TLR3. *J Immunol*, Vol. 184, No. 12, pp. 6929-6937

Burns, E., Bachrach, G., Shapira, L., & Nussbaum, G. (2006). Cutting Edge: TLR2 is required for the innate response to Porphyromonas gingivalis: activation leads to bacterial persistence and TLR2 deficiency attenuates induced alveolar bone resorption. *J Immunol*, Vol. 177, No. 12, pp. 8296-8300

Carty, M., Goodbody, R., Schroder, M., Stack, J., Moynagh, P.N., & Bowie, A.G. (2006). The human adaptor SARM negatively regulates adaptor protein TRIF-dependent Toll-like receptor signaling. *Nat Immunol*, Vol. 7, pp. 1074-1081

Castrillo, A., Joseph, S., Vaidya, S., Haberland, M., Fogelman, A., Cheng, G., & Tontonoz, P. (2003). Crosstalk between LXR and toll-like receptor signaling mediates bacterial and viral antagonism of cholesterol metabolism. *Mol Cell*, Vol. 12, No. 4, pp. 805-816

Chamaillard, M., Hashimoto, M., Horie, Y., Masumoto, J., Qiu, S., Saab, L., Ogura, Y., Kawasaki, A., Fukase, K., Kusumoto, S., Valvano, M.A., Foster, S.J., Mak, T.W., Nunez, G., & Inohara, N. (2003). An essential role for NOD1 in host recognition of bacterial peptidoglycan containing diaminopimelic acid. *Nat Immunol*, Vol. 4, No. 7, pp. 702-707

Chiu, B., Viira, E., Tucker, W., & Fong, I.W. (1997). Chlamydia pneumoniae, cytomegalovirus, and herpes simplex virus in atherosclerosis of the carotid artery. *Circulation*, Vol. 96, No. 7, pp. 2144-2148

Choi, S., Harkewicz, R., Lee, J., Boullier, A., Almazan, F., Li, A., Witztum, J., Bae, Y., & Miller, Y. (2009). Lipoprotein accumulation in macrophages via toll-like receptor-4-dependent fluid phase uptake. *Circ Res*, Vol. 104, No. 12, pp. 1355-1363

Cole, J.E., Georgiou, E., & Monaco, C. (2010). The expression and functions of toll-like receptors in atherosclerosis. *Mediators Inflamm*, Vol. 2010, p. 393946

Cole, J.E., Navin, T.J., Cross, A.J., Goddard, M.E., Alexopoulou, L., Mitra, A.T., Davies, A.H., Flavell, R.A., Feldmann, M., & Monaco, C. (2011). From the Cover: Unexpected protective role for Toll-like receptor 3 in the arterial wall. *Proc Natl Acad Sci U S A*, Vol. 108, No. 6, pp. 2372-2377

Compton, T., Kurt-Jones, E.A., Boehme, K.W., Belko, J., Latz, E., Golenbock, D.T., & Finberg, R.W. (2003). Human cytomegalovirus activates inflammatory cytokine responses via CD14 and Toll-like receptor 2. *J Virol*, Vol. 77, No. 8, pp. 4588-4596

Conforti, R., Ma, Y., Morel, Y., Paturel, C., Terme, M., Viaud, S., Ryffel, B., Ferrantini, M., Uppaluri, R., Schreiber, R., Combadière, C., Chaput, N., André, F., Kroemer, G., & Zitvogel, L. (2010). Opposing effects of toll-like receptor (TLR3) signaling in tumors can be therapeutically uncoupled to optimize the anticancer efficacy of TLR3 ligands. *Cancer Res*, Vol. 70, No. 2, pp. 490-500

Cook, D.N., Pisetsky, D.S., & Schwartz, D.A. (2004). Toll-like receptors in the pathogenesis of human disease. *Nat Immunol*, Vol. 5, No. 10, pp. 975-979

Doyle, S., O'Connell, R., Miranda, G., Vaidya, S., Chow, E., Liu, P., Suzuki, S., Suzuki, N., Modlin, R., Yeh, W., Lane, T., & Cheng, G. (2004). Toll-like receptors induce a phagocytic gene program through p38. *J Exp Med*, Vol. 199, No. 1, pp. 81-90

Duewell, P., Kono, H., Rayner, K.J., Sirois, C.M., Vladimer, G., Bauernfeind, F.G., Abela, G.S., Franchi, L., Nuñez, G., Schnurr, M., Espevik, T., Lien, E., Fitzgerald, K.A., Rock, K.L., Moore, K.J., Wright, S.D., Hornung, V., & Latz, E. (2010). NLRP3 inflammasomes are required for atherogenesis and activated by cholesterol crystals. *Nature*, Vol. 464, No. 7293, pp. 1357-1361

Edfeldt, K., Swedenborg, J., Hansson, G., & Yan, Z. (2002). Expression of toll-like receptors in human atherosclerotic lesions: a possible pathway for plaque activation. *Circulation*, Vol. 105, No. 10, pp. 1158-1161

Elhage, R., Jawien, J., Rudling, M., Ljunggren, H.G., Takeda, K., Akira, S., Bayard, F., & Hansson, G.K. (2003). Reduced atherosclerosis in interleukin-18 deficient apolipoprotein E-knockout mice. *Cardiovasc Res*, Vol. 59, No. 1, pp. 234-240

Erbel, C., Sato, K., Meyer, F., Kopecky, S., Frye, R., Goronzy, J., & Weyand, C. (2007). Functional profile of activated dendritic cells in unstable atherosclerotic plaque. *Basic Res Cardiol*, Vol. 102, No. 2, pp. 123-132

Ermolaeva, M.A., Michallet, M.-C., Papadopoulou, N., Utermöhlen, O., Kranidioti, K., Kollias, G., Tschopp, J., & Pasparakis, M. (2008). Function of TRADD in tumor necrosis factor receptor 1 signaling and in TRIF-dependent inflammatory responses. *Nature immunology*, Vol. 9, pp. 1037-1046

Erridge, C., Burdess, A., Jackson, A.J., Murray, C., Riggio, M., Lappin, D., Milligan, S., Spickett, C.M., & Webb, D.J. (2008). Vascular cell responsiveness to Toll-like receptor ligands in carotid atheroma. *Eur J Clin Invest*, Vol. 38, No. 10, pp. 713-720

Erridge, C., & Samani, N.J. (2009). Saturated fatty acids do not directly stimulate Toll-like receptor signaling. *Arterioscler Thromb Vasc Biol*, Vol. 29, No. 11, pp. 1944-1949

Feingold, K.R., Kazemi, M.R., Magra, A.L., McDonald, C.M., Chui, L.G., Shigenaga, J.K., Patzek, S.M., Chan, Z.W., Londos, C., & Grunfeld, C. (2010). ADRP/ADFP and Mal1 expression are increased in macrophages treated with TLR agonists. *Atherosclerosis*, Vol. 209, No. 1, pp. 81-88

Foldes, G., von Haehling, S., Okonko, D.O., Jankowska, E.A., Poole-Wilson, P.A., & Anker, S.D. (2008). Fluvastatin reduces increased blood monocyte Toll-like receptor 4 expression in whole blood from patients with chronic heart failure. *Int J Cardiol*, Vol. 124, No. 1, pp. 80-85

Frantz, S., Ertl, G., & Bauersachs, J. (2007). Mechanisms of disease: Toll-like receptors in cardiovascular disease. *Nat Clin Pract Cardiovasc Med*, Vol. 4, No. 8, pp. 444-454

Funk, J., Feingold, K., Moser, A., & Grunfeld, C. (1993). Lipopolysaccharide stimulation of RAW 264.7 macrophages induces lipid accumulation and foam cell formation. *Atherosclerosis*, Vol. 98, No. 1, pp. 67-82

Gantner, B.N., Simmons, R.M., Canavera, S.J., Akira, S., & Underhill, D.M. (2003). Collaborative induction of inflammatory responses by dectin-1 and Toll-like receptor 2. *J Exp Med*, Vol. 197, No. 9, pp. 1107-1117

Ghanim, H., Mohanty, P., Deopurkar, R., Sia, C.L., Korzeniewski, K., Abuaysheh, S., Chaudhuri, A., & Dandona, P. (2008). Acute modulation of toll-like receptors by insulin. *Diabetes Care*, Vol. 31, No. 9, pp. 1827-1831

Girardin, S.E., Boneca, I.G., Carneiro, L.A., Antignac, A., Jehanno, M., Viala, J., Tedin, K., Taha, M.K., Labigne, A., Zahringer, U., Coyle, A.J., DiStefano, P.S., Bertin, J., Sansonetti, P.J., & Philpott, D.J. (2003a). Nod1 detects a unique muropeptide from gram-negative bacterial peptidoglycan. *Science*, Vol. 300, No. 5625, pp. 1584-1587

Girardin, S.E., Boneca, I.G., Viala, J., Chamaillard, M., Labigne, A., Thomas, G., Philpott, D.J., & Sansonetti, P.J. (2003b). Nod2 is a general sensor of peptidoglycan through muramyl dipeptide (MDP) detection. *J Biol Chem*, Vol. 278, No. 11, pp. 8869-8872

Gordon, S., & Taylor, P. (2005). Monocyte and macrophage heterogeneity. *Nat Rev Immunol*, Vol. 5, No. 12, pp. 953-964

Häcker, H., Vabulas, R.M., Takeuchi, O., Hoshino, K., Akira, S., & Wagner, H. (2000). Immune cell activation by bacterial CpG-DNA through myeloid differentiation marker 88 and tumor necrosis factor receptor-associated factor (TRAF)6. *The Journal of experimental medicine*, Vol. 192, pp. 595-600

Häcker, H., & Karin, M. (2006). Regulation and function of IKK and IKK-related kinases. *Science's STKE : signal transduction knowledge environment*, Vol. 2006, p. re13

Hamann, L., Gomma, A., Schroder, N.W., Stamme, C., Glaeser, C., Schulz, S., Gross, M., Anker, S.D., Fox, K., & Schumann, R.R. (2005). A frequent toll-like receptor (TLR)-2 polymorphism is a risk factor for coronary restenosis. *J Mol Med*, Vol. 83, No. 6, pp. 478-485

Hayashi, F., Smith, K.D., Ozinsky, A., Hawn, T.R., Yi, E.C., Goodlett, D.R., Eng, J.K., Akira, S., Underhill, D.M., & Aderem, A. (2001). The innate immune response to bacterial flagellin is mediated by Toll-like receptor 5. *Nature*, Vol. 410, pp. 1099-1103

Hemmi, H., Kaisho, T., Takeuchi, O., Sato, S., Sanjo, H., Hoshino, K., Horiuchi, T., Tomizawa, H., Takeda, K., & Akira, S. (2002). Small anti-viral compounds activate immune cells via the TLR7 MyD88-dependent signaling pathway. *Nature immunology*, Vol. 3, pp. 196-200

Hennessy, E.J., Parker, A.E., & O'Neill, L.A. (2010). Targeting Toll-like receptors: emerging therapeutics? *Nat Rev Drug Discov*, Vol. 9, No. 4, pp. 293-307

Hoebe, K., Georgel, P., Rutschmann, S., Du, X., Mudd, S., Crozat, K., Sovath, S., Shamel, L., Hartung, T., Zähringer, U., & Beutler, B. (2005). CD36 is a sensor of diacylglycerides. *Nature*, Vol. 433, pp. 523-527

Hornung, V., Rothenfusser, S., Britsch, S., Krug, A., Jahrsdorfer, B., Giese, T., Endres, S., & Hartmann, G. (2002). Quantitative expression of toll-like receptor 1-10 mRNA in cellular subsets of human peripheral blood mononuclear cells and sensitivity to CpG oligodeoxynucleotides. *J Immunol*, Vol. 168, No. 9, pp. 4531-4537

Imaizumi, T., Yagihashi, N., Kubota, K., Yoshida, H., Sakaki, H., Yagihashi, S., Kimura, H., & Satoh, K. (2007). Expression of retinoic acid-inducible gene-I (RIG-I) in macrophages: possible involvement of RIG-I in atherosclerosis. *J Atheroscler Thromb*, Vol. 14, No. 2, pp. 51-55

Inohara, N., Ogura, Y., Fontalba, A., Gutierrez, O., Pons, F., Crespo, J., Fukase, K., Inamura, S., Kusumoto, S., Hashimoto, M., Foster, S.J., Moran, A.P., Fernandez-Luna, J.L., & Nunez, G. (2003). Host recognition of bacterial muramyl dipeptide mediated through NOD2. Implications for Crohn's disease. *J Biol Chem*, Vol. 278, No. 8, pp. 5509-5512

Isoda, K., Sawada, S., Ishigami, N., Matsuki, T., Miyazaki, K., Kusuhara, M., Iwakura, Y., & Ohsuzu, F. (2004). Lack of interleukin-1 receptor antagonist modulates plaque composition in apolipoprotein E-deficient mice. *Arterioscler Thromb Vasc Biol*, Vol. 24, No. 6, pp. 1068-1073

Ito, T., Amakawa, R., Kaisho, T., Hemmi, H., Tajima, K., Uehira, K., Ozaki, Y., Tomizawa, H., Akira, S., & Fukuhara, S. (2002). Interferon-alpha and interleukin-12 are induced differentially by Toll-like receptor 7 ligands in human blood dendritic cell subsets. *J Exp Med*, Vol. 195, No. 11, pp. 1507-1512

Jarrossay, D., Napolitani, G., Colonna, M., Sallusto, F., & Lanzavecchia, A. (2001). Specialization and complementarity in microbial molecule recognition by human myeloid and plasmacytoid dendritic cells. *Eur J Immunol*, Vol. 31, No. 11, pp. 3388-3393

Jin, M.S., Kim, S.E., Heo, J.Y., Lee, M.E., Kim, H.M., Paik, S.G., Lee, H., & Lee, J.O. (2007). Crystal structure of the TLR1-TLR2 heterodimer induced by binding of a tri-acylated lipopeptide. *Cell*, Vol. 130, No. 6, pp. 1071-1082

Johnson, G.L., & Lapadat, R. (2002). Mitogen-activated protein kinase pathways mediated by ERK, JNK, and p38 protein kinases. *Science (New York, NY)*, Vol. 298, pp. 1911-1912

Kadowaki, N., Ho, S., Antonenko, S., Malefyt, R.W., Kastelein, R.A., Bazan, F., & Liu, Y.J. (2001). Subsets of human dendritic cell precursors express different toll-like receptors and respond to different microbial antigens. *J Exp Med*, Vol. 194, No. 6, pp. 863-869

Kagan, J.C., & Medzhitov, R. (2006). Phosphoinositide-mediated adaptor recruitment controls Toll-like receptor signaling. *Cell*, Vol. 125, pp. 943-955

Kagan, J.C., Su, T., Horng, T., Chow, A., Akira, S., & Medzhitov, R. (2008). TRAM couples endocytosis of Toll-like receptor 4 to the induction of interferon-beta. *Nat Immunol*, Vol. 9, pp. 361-368

Kalayoglu, M.V., Libby, P., & Byrne, G.I. (2002). Chlamydia pneumoniae as an emerging risk factor in cardiovascular disease. *JAMA*, Vol. 288, No. 21, pp. 2724-2731

Kanwar, R., Kanwar, J., Wang, D., Ormrod, D., & Krissansen, G. (2001). Temporal expression of heat shock proteins 60 and 70 at lesion-prone sites during atherogenesis in ApoE-deficient mice. *Arterioscler Thromb Vasc Biol*, Vol. 21, No. 12, pp. 1991-1997

Kariko, K., Ni, H., Capodici, J., Lamphier, M., & Weissman, D. (2004). mRNA is an endogenous ligand for Toll-like receptor 3. *J Biol Chem*, Vol. 279, No. 13, pp. 12542-12550

Kato, H., Takeuchi, O., Sato, S., Yoneyama, M., Yamamoto, M., Matsui, K., Uematsu, S., Jung, A., Kawai, T., Ishii, K.J., Yamaguchi, O., Otsu, K., Tsujimura, T., Koh, C.S., Reis e Sousa, C., Matsuura, Y., Fujita, T., & Akira, S. (2006). Differential roles of MDA5 and RIG-I helicases in the recognition of RNA viruses. *Nature*, Vol. 441, No. 7089, pp. 101-105

Kawagoe, T., Sato, S., Matsushita, K., Kato, H., Matsui, K., Kumagai, Y., Saitoh, T., Kawai, T., Takeuchi, O., & Akira, S. (2008). Sequential control of Toll-like receptor-dependent responses by IRAK1 and IRAK2. *Nat Immunol*, Vol. 9, No. 6, pp. 684-691

Kawai, T., Adachi, O., Ogawa, T., Takeda, K., & Akira, S. (1999). Unresponsiveness of MyD88-deficient mice to endotoxin. *Immunity*, Vol. 11, pp. 115-122

Kawai, T., Takahashi, K., Sato, S., Coban, C., Kumar, H., Kato, H., Ishii, K.J., Takeuchi, O., & Akira, S. (2005). IPS-1, an adaptor triggering RIG-I- and Mda5-mediated type I interferon induction. *Nature immunology*, Vol. 6, pp. 981-988

Kawai, T., & Akira, S. (2007). Signaling to NF-kappaB by Toll-like receptors. *Trends in molecular medicine*, Vol. 13, pp. 460-469

Kawai, T., & Akira, S. (2008). Toll-like receptor and RIG-I-like receptor signaling. *Ann N Y Acad Sci*, Vol. 1143, pp. 1-20

Kawai, T., & Akira, S. (2010). The role of pattern-recognition receptors in innate immunity: update on Toll-like receptors. *Nat Immunol*, Vol. 11, pp. 373-384

Kawakami, A., Osaka, M., Aikawa, M., Uematsu, S., Akira, S., Libby, P., Shimokado, K., Sacks, F.M., & Yoshida, M. (2008). Toll-Like Receptor 2 Mediates Apolipoprotein CIII-Induced Monocyte Activation. *Circulation Research*, Vol. 103, No. 12, pp. 1402-1409

Kazemi, M., McDonald, C., Shigenaga, J., Grunfeld, C., & Feingold, K. (2005). Adipocyte fatty acid-binding protein expression and lipid accumulation are increased during activation of murine macrophages by toll-like receptor agonists. *Arterioscler Thromb Vasc Biol*, Vol. 25, No. 6, pp. 1220-1224

Kiechl, S., Egger, G., Mayr, M., Wiedermann, C.J., Bonora, E., Oberhollenzer, F., Muggeo, M., Xu, Q., Wick, G., Poewe, W., & Willeit, J. (2001). Chronic infections and the risk of carotid atherosclerosis: prospective results from a large population study. *Circulation*, Vol. 103, No. 8, pp. 1064-1070

Kim, S., Takahashi, H., Lin, W.W., Descargues, P., Grivennikov, S., Kim, Y., Luo, J.L., & Karin, M. (2009). Carcinoma-produced factors activate myeloid cells through TLR2 to stimulate metastasis. *Nature*, Vol. 457, No. 7225, pp. 102-106

Kirii, H., Niwa, T., Yamada, Y., Wada, H., Saito, K., Iwakura, Y., Asano, M., Moriwaki, H., & Seishima, M. (2003). Lack of interleukin-1beta decreases the severity of atherosclerosis in ApoE-deficient mice. *Arterioscler Thromb Vasc Biol*, Vol. 23, No. 4, pp. 656-660

Kol, A., Sperti, G., Shani, J., Schulhoff, N., van de Greef, W., Landini, M.P., La Placa, M., Maseri, A., & Crea, F. (1995). Cytomegalovirus replication is not a cause of instability in unstable angina. *Circulation*, Vol. 91, No. 7, pp. 1910-1913

Kuo, C., Gown, A., Benditt, E., & Grayston, J. (1993). Detection of Chlamydia pneumoniae in aortic lesions of atherosclerosis by immunocytochemical stain. *Arterioscler Thromb*, Vol. 13, No. 10, pp. 1501-1504

Kuwahata, S., Fujita, S., Orihara, K., Hamasaki, S., Oba, R., Hirai, H., Nagata, K., Ishida, S., Kataoka, T., Oketani, N., Ichiki, H., Iriki, Y., Saihara, K., Okui, H., Ninomiya, Y., &

Tei, C. (2009). High expression level of Toll-like receptor 2 on monocytes is an important risk factor for arteriosclerotic disease. *Atherosclerosis*, Vol. 209, No. 1, pp. 248-254

Laman, J.D., Schoneveld, A.H., Moll, F.L., van Meurs, M., & Pasterkamp, G. (2002). Significance of peptidoglycan, a proinflammatory bacterial antigen in atherosclerotic arteries and its association with vulnerable plaques. *Am J Cardiol*, Vol. 90, No. 2, pp. 119-123

Lee, J., Ye, J., Gao, Z., Youn, H., Lee, W., Zhao, L., Sizemore, N., & Hwang, D. (2003). Reciprocal modulation of Toll-like receptor-4 signaling pathways involving MyD88 and phosphatidylinositol 3-kinase/AKT by saturated and polyunsaturated fatty acids. *J Biol Chem*, Vol. 278, No. 39, pp. 37041-37051

Lee, J., Lim, E., Park, D., Lee, S., Kim, J., & Baek, S. (2008). A combination of Lox-1 and Nox1 regulates TLR9-mediated foam cell formation. *Cell Signal*, Vol. 20, No. 12, pp. 2266-2275

Lehtiniemi, J., Karhunen, P.J., Goebeler, S., Nikkari, S., & Nikkari, S.T. (2005). Identification of different bacterial DNAs in human coronary arteries. *Eur J Clin Invest*, Vol. 35, No. 1, pp. 13-16

Liu, L., Botos, I., Wang, Y., Leonard, J.N., Shiloach, J., Segal, D.M., & Davies, D.R. (2008a). Structural basis of toll-like receptor 3 signaling with double-stranded RNA. *Science*, Vol. 320, pp. 379-381

Liu, X., Ukai, T., Yumoto, H., Davey, M., Goswami, S., Gibson, F.C., & Genco, C.A. (2008b). Toll-like receptor 2 plays a critical role in the progression of atherosclerosis that is independent of dietary lipids. *Atherosclerosis*, Vol. 196, No. 1, pp. 146-154

Lopez, A.D., Mathers, C.D., Ezzati, M., Jamison, D.T., & Murray, C.J. (2006). Global and regional burden of disease and risk factors, 2001: systematic analysis of population health data. *Lancet*, Vol. 367, No. 9524, pp. 1747-1757

Lord, R.S., & Bobryshev, Y.V. (1999). Clustering of dendritic cells in athero-prone areas of the aorta. *Atherosclerosis*, Vol. 146, No. 1, pp. 197-198

Lundberg, A.M., & Hansson, G.K. (2010). Innate immune signals in atherosclerosis. *Clin Immunol*, Vol. 134, No. 1, pp. 5-24

Mancuso, G., Gambuzza, M., Midiri, A., Biondo, C., Papasergi, S., Akira, S., Teti, G., & Beninati, C. (2009). Bacterial recognition by TLR7 in the lysosomes of conventional dendritic cells. *Nat Immunol*, Vol. 10, No. 6, pp. 587-594

Mariathasan, S., & Monack, D.M. (2007). Inflammasome adaptors and sensors: intracellular regulators of infection and inflammation. *Nat Rev Immunol*, Vol. 7, pp. 31-40

Martinez, F.O., Gordon, S., Locati, M., & Mantovani, A. (2006). Transcriptional profiling of the human monocyte-to-macrophage differentiation and polarization: new molecules and patterns of gene expression. *J Immunol*, Vol. 177, No. 10, pp. 7303-7311

Martinon, F., Pétrilli, V., Mayor, A., Tardivel, A., & Tschopp, J. (2006). Gout-associated uric acid crystals activate the NALP3 inflammasome. *Nature*, Vol. 440, No. 7081, pp. 237-241

Matsumoto, M., Funami, K., Tanabe, M., Oshiumi, H., Shingai, M., Seto, Y., Yamamoto, A., & Seya, T. (2003). Subcellular localization of Toll-like receptor 3 in human dendritic cells. *J Immunol*, Vol. 171, No. 6, pp. 3154-3162

McGillicuddy, F.C., de la Llera Moya, M., Hinkle, C.C., Joshi, M.R., Chiquoine, E.H., Billheimer, J.T., Rothblat, G.H., & Reilly, M.P. (2009). Inflammation impairs reverse cholesterol transport in vivo. *Circulation*, Vol. 119, No. 8, pp. 1135-1145

Menu, P., Pellegrin, M., Aubert, J.F., Bouzourene, K., Tardivel, A., Mazzolai, L., & Tschopp, J. (2011). Atherosclerosis in ApoE-deficient mice progresses independently of the NLRP3 inflammasome. *Cell Death Dis*, Vol. 2, p. e137

Merhi-Soussi, F., Kwak, B.R., Magne, D., Chadjichristos, C., Berti, M., Pelli, G., James, R.W., Mach, F., & Gabay, C. (2005). Interleukin-1 plays a major role in vascular inflammation and atherosclerosis in male apolipoprotein E-knockout mice. *Cardiovasc Res*, Vol. 66, No. 3, pp. 583-593

Methe, H., Kim, J., Kofler, S., Weis, M., Nabauer, M., & Koglin, J. (2005). Expansion of circulating Toll-like receptor 4-positive monocytes in patients with acute coronary syndrome. *Circulation*, Vol. 111, No. 20, pp. 2654-2661

Michelsen, K.S., Wong, M.H., Shah, P.K., Zhang, W., Yano, J., Doherty, T.M., Akira, S., Rajavashisth, T.B., & Arditi, M. (2004). Lack of Toll-like receptor 4 or myeloid differentiation factor 88 reduces atherosclerosis and alters plaque phenotype in mice deficient in apolipoprotein E. *Proc Natl Acad Sci USA*, Vol. 101, No. 29, pp. 10679-10684

Midwood, K.S., & Orend, G. (2009). The role of tenascin-C in tissue injury and tumorigenesis. *J Cell Commun Signal*, Vol. 3, No. 3-4, pp. 287-310

Miller, Y.I., Viriyakosol, S., Binder, C.J., Feramisco, J.R., Kirkland, T.N., & Witztum, J.L. (2003). Minimally modified LDL binds to CD14, induces macrophage spreading via TLR4/MD-2, and inhibits phagocytosis of apoptotic cells. *J Biol Chem*, Vol. 278, No. 3, pp. 1561-1568

Millonig, G., Niederegger, H., Rabl, W., Hochleitner, B., Hoefer, D., Romani, N., & Wick, G. (2001). Network of vascular-associated dendritic cells in intima of healthy young individuals. *Arterioscler Thromb Vasc Biol*, Vol. 21, No. 4, pp. 503-508

Mizoguchi, E., Orihara, K., Hamasaki, S., Ishida, S., Kataoka, T., Ogawa, M., Saihara, K., Okui, H., Fukudome, T., Shinsato, T., Shirasawa, T., Ichiki, H., Kubozono, T., Ninomiya, Y., Otsuji, Y., & Tei, C. (2007). Association between Toll-like receptors and the extent and severity of coronary artery disease in patients with stable angina. *Coron Artery Dis*, Vol. 18, No. 1, pp. 31-38

Monaco, C., Gregan, S.M., Navin, T.J., Foxwell, B.M., Davies, A.H., & Feldmann, M. (2009). Toll-like receptor-2 mediates inflammation and matrix degradation in human atherosclerosis. *Circulation*, Vol. 120, No. 24, pp. 2462-2469

Moreno-Altamirano, M.M., Aguilar-Carmona, I., & Sanchez-Garcia, F.J. (2007). Expression of GM1, a marker of lipid rafts, defines two subsets of human monocytes with differential endocytic capacity and lipopolysaccharide responsiveness. *Immunology*, Vol. 120, No. 4, pp. 536-543

Mullick, A., Tobias, P., & Curtiss, L. (2005). Modulation of atherosclerosis in mice by Toll-like receptor 2. *J Clin Invest*, Vol. 115, No. 11, pp. 3149-3156

Mullick, A.E., Soldau, K., Kiosses, W.B., Bell, T.A., 3rd, Tobias, P.S., & Curtiss, L.K. (2008). Increased endothelial expression of Toll-like receptor 2 at sites of disturbed blood flow exacerbates early atherogenic events. *J Exp Med*, Vol. 205, No. 2, pp. 373-383

Naiki, Y., Sorrentino, R., Wong, M.H., Michelsen, K.S., Shimada, K., Chen, S., Yilmaz, A., Slepenkin, A., Schröder, N.W.J., Crother, T.R., Bulut, Y., Doherty, T.M., Bradley, M.,

Shaposhnik, Z., Peterson, E.M., Tontonoz, P., Shah, P.K., & Arditi, M. (2008). TLR/MyD88 and liver X receptor alpha signaling pathways reciprocally control Chlamydia pneumoniae-induced acceleration of atherosclerosis. *J Immunol*, Vol. 181, No. 10, pp. 7176-7185

Negishi, H., Fujita, Y., Yanai, H., Sakaguchi, S., Ouyang, X., Shinohara, M., Takayanagi, H., Ohba, Y., Taniguchi, T., & Honda, K. (2006). Evidence for licensing of IFN-gamma-induced IFN regulatory factor 1 transcription factor by MyD88 in Toll-like receptor-dependent gene induction program. *Proceedings of the National Academy of Sciences of the United States of America*, Vol. 103, pp. 15136-15141

Niessner, A., Sato, K., Chaikof, E., Colmegna, I., Goronzy, J., & Weyand, C. (2006). Pathogen-sensing plasmacytoid dendritic cells stimulate cytotoxic T-cell function in the atherosclerotic plaque through interferon-alpha. *Circulation*, Vol. 114, No. 23, pp. 2482-2489

Nishina, P., Wang, J., Toyofuku, W., Kuypers, F., Ishida, B., & Paigen, B. (1993). Atherosclerosis and plasma and liver lipids in nine inbred strains of mice. *Lipids*, Vol. 28, No. 7, pp. 599-605

O'Neill, L.A., & Bowie, A.G. (2007). The family of five: TIR-domain-containing adaptors in Toll-like receptor signalling. *Nat Rev Immunol*, Vol. 7, pp. 353-364

Oganesyan, G., Saha, S.K., Guo, B., He, J.Q., Shahangian, A., Zarnegar, B., Perry, A., & Cheng, G. (2006). Critical role of TRAF3 in the Toll-like receptor-dependent and -independent antiviral response. *Nature*, Vol. 439, pp. 208-211

Oiknine, J., & Aviram, M. (1992). Increased susceptibility to activation and increased uptake of low density lipoprotein by cholesterol-loaded macrophages. *Arterioscler Thromb*, Vol. 12, No. 6, pp. 745-753

Okamura, Y., Watari, M., Jerud, E.S., Young, D.W., Ishizaka, S.T., Rose, J., Chow, J.C., & Strauss, J.F., 3rd (2001). The extra domain A of fibronectin activates Toll-like receptor 4. *J Biol Chem*, Vol. 276, No. 13, pp. 10229-10233

Otsui, K., Inoue, N., Kobayashi, S., Shiraki, R., Honjo, T., Takahashi, M., Hirata, K., Kawashima, S., & Yokoyama, M. (2007). Enhanced expression of TLR4 in smooth muscle cells in human atherosclerotic coronary arteries. *Heart Vessels*, Vol. 22, No. 6, pp. 416-422

Ott, S., El Mokhtari, N., Musfeldt, M., Hellmig, S., Freitag, S., Rehman, A., Kuhbacher, T., Nikolaus, S., Namsolleck, P., Blaut, M., Hampe, J., Sahly, H., Reinecke, A., Haake, N., Gunther, R., Kruger, D., Lins, M., Herrmann, G., Folsch, U., Simon, R., & Schreiber, S. (2006). Detection of diverse bacterial signatures in atherosclerotic lesions of patients with coronary heart disease. *Circulation*, Vol. 113, No. 7, pp. 929-937

Ozinsky, A., Underhill, D.M., Fontenot, J.D., Hajjar, A.M., Smith, K.D., Wilson, C.B., Schroeder, L., & Aderem, A. (2000). The repertoire for pattern recognition of pathogens by the innate immune system is defined by cooperation between toll-like receptors. *Proc Natl Acad Sci U S A*, Vol. 97, No. 25, pp. 13766-13771

Park, J., Svetkauskaite, D., He, Q., Kim, J., Strassheim, D., Ishizaka, A., & Abraham, E. (2004). Involvement of toll-like receptors 2 and 4 in cellular activation by high mobility group box 1 protein. *J Biol Chem*, Vol. 279, No. 9, pp. 7370-7377

Piccinini, A.M., & Midwood, K.S. (2010). DAMPening inflammation by modulating TLR signalling. *Mediators Inflamm*, Vol. In press,

Poltorak, A., He, X., Smirnova, I., Liu, M., Van Huffel, C., Du, X., Birdwell, D., Alejos, E., Silva, M., Galanos, C., Freudenberg, M., Ricciardi-Castagnoli, P., Layton, B., & Beutler, B. (1998). Defective LPS signaling in C3H/HeJ and C57BL/10ScCr mice: mutations in Tlr4 gene. *Science*, Vol. 282, No. 5396, pp. 2085-2088

Porto, A., Palumbo, R., Pieroni, M., Aprigliano, G., Chiesa, R., Sanvito, F., Maseri, A., & Bianchi, M.E. (2006). Smooth muscle cells in human atherosclerotic plaques secrete and proliferate in response to high mobility group box 1 protein. *FASEB J*, Vol. 20, No. 14, pp. 2565-2566

Pryshchep, O., Ma-Krupa, W., Younge, B., Goronzy, J., & Weyand, C. (2008). Vessel-specific Toll-like receptor profiles in human medium and large arteries. *Circulation*, Vol. 118, No. 12, pp. 1276-1284

Qureshi, S.T., Lariviere, L., Leveque, G., Clermont, S., Moore, K.J., Gros, P., & Malo, D. (1999). Endotoxin-tolerant mice have mutations in Toll-like receptor 4 (Tlr4). *J Exp Med*, Vol. 189, No. 4, pp. 615-625

Rajamaki, K., Lappalainen, J., Oorni, K., Valimaki, E., Matikainen, S., Kovanen, P.T., & Eklund, K.K. (2010). Cholesterol crystals activate the NLRP3 inflammasome in human macrophages: a novel link between cholesterol metabolism and inflammation. *PLoS ONE*, Vol. 5, No. 7, p. e11765

Rekhter, M., Staschke, K., Estridge, T., Rutherford, P., Jackson, N., Gifford-Moore, D., Foxworthy, P., Reidy, C., Huang, X.D., Kalbfleisch, M., Hui, K., Kuo, M.S., Gilmour, R., & Vlahos, C.J. (2008). Genetic ablation of IRAK4 kinase activity inhibits vascular lesion formation. *Biochem Biophys Res Commun*, Vol. 367, No. 3, pp. 642-648

Rifkin, I., Leadbetter, E., Busconi, L., Viglianti, G., & Marshak-Rothstein, A. (2005). Toll-like receptors, endogenous ligands, and systemic autoimmune disease. *Immunol Rev*, Vol. 204, pp. 27-42

Ross, R. (1999). Atherosclerosis--an inflammatory disease. *N Engl J Med*, Vol. 340, No. 2, pp. 115-126

Rowe, D.C., McGettrick, A.F., Latz, E., Monks, B.G., Gay, N.J., Yamamoto, M., Akira, S., O'Neill, L.A., Fitzgerald, K.A., & Golenbock, D.T. (2006). The myristoylation of TRIF-related adaptor molecule is essential for Toll-like receptor 4 signal transduction. *Proceedings of the National Academy of Sciences of the United States of America*, Vol. 103, pp. 6299-6304

Scannapieco, F.A., Bush, R.B., & Paju, S. (2003). Associations between periodontal disease and risk for atherosclerosis, cardiovascular disease, and stroke. A systematic review. *Ann Periodontol*, Vol. 8, No. 1, pp. 38-53

Schaefer, L., Babelova, A., Kiss, E., Hausser, H.J., Baliova, M., Krzyzankova, M., Marsche, G., Young, M.F., Mihalik, D., Gotte, M., Malle, E., Schaefer, R.M., & Grone, H.J. (2005). The matrix component biglycan is proinflammatory and signals through Toll-like receptors 4 and 2 in macrophages. *J Clin Invest*, Vol. 115, No. 8, pp. 2223-2233

Scheibner, K.A., Lutz, M.A., Boodoo, S., Fenton, M.J., Powell, J.D., & Horton, M.R. (2006). Hyaluronan fragments act as an endogenous danger signal by engaging TLR2. *J Immunol*, Vol. 177, No. 2, pp. 1272-1281

Schmitz, F., Heit, A., Guggemoos, S., Krug, A., Mages, J., Schiemann, M., Adler, H., Drexler, I., Haas, T., Lang, R., & Wagner, H. (2007). Interferon-regulatory-factor 1 controls Toll-like receptor 9-mediated IFN-beta production in myeloid dendritic cells. *European journal of immunology*, Vol. 37, pp. 315-327

Schnare, M., Holt, A.C., Takeda, K., Akira, S., & Medzhitov, R. (2000). Recognition of CpG DNA is mediated by signaling pathways dependent on the adaptor protein MyD88. *Current biology : CB*, Vol. 10, pp. 1139-1142

Schoneveld, A., Hoefer, I., Sluijter, J., Laman, J., de Kleijn, D., & Pasterkamp, G. (2008). Atherosclerotic lesion development and Toll like receptor 2 and 4 responsiveness. *Atherosclerosis*, Vol. 197, No. 1, pp. 95-104

Schoneveld, A.H., Oude Nijhuis, M.M., van Middelaar, B., Laman, J.D., de Kleijn, D.P., & Pasterkamp, G. (2005). Toll-like receptor 2 stimulation induces intimal hyperplasia and atherosclerotic lesion development. *Cardiovasc Res*, Vol. 66, No. 1, pp. 162-169

Schroder, K., & Tschopp, J. (2010). The inflammasomes. *Cell*, Vol. 140, No. 6, pp. 821-832

Schroder, N.W., Morath, S., Alexander, C., Hamann, L., Hartung, T., Zahringer, U., Gobel, U.B., Weber, J.R., & Schumann, R.R. (2003). Lipoteichoic acid (LTA) of Streptococcus pneumoniae and Staphylococcus aureus activates immune cells via Toll-like receptor (TLR)-2, lipopolysaccharide-binding protein (LBP), and CD14, whereas TLR-4 and MD-2 are not involved. *J Biol Chem*, Vol. 278, No. 18, pp. 15587-15594

Seth, R.B., Sun, L., Ea, C.K., & Chen, Z.J. (2005). Identification and characterization of MAVS, a mitochondrial antiviral signaling protein that activates NF-kappaB and IRF 3. *Cell*, Vol. 122, pp. 669-682

Shi, W., Wang, N.J., Shih, D.M., Sun, V.Z., Wang, X., & Lusis, A.J. (2000). Determinants of atherosclerosis susceptibility in the C3H and C57BL/6 mouse model: evidence for involvement of endothelial cells but not blood cells or cholesterol metabolism. *Circ Res*, Vol. 86, No. 10, pp. 1078-1084

Shimazu, R., Akashi, S., Ogata, H., Nagai, Y., Fukudome, K., Miyake, K., & Kimoto, M. (1999). MD-2, a molecule that confers lipopolysaccharide responsiveness on Toll-like receptor 4. *J Exp Med*, Vol. 189, No. 11, pp. 1777-1782

Shinohara, M., Hirata, K., Yamashita, T., Takaya, T., Sasaki, N., Shiraki, R., Ueyama, T., Emoto, N., Inoue, N., Yokoyama, M., & Kawashima, S. (2007). Local overexpression of toll-like receptors at the vessel wall induces atherosclerotic lesion formation: synergism of TLR2 and TLR4. *Arterioscler Thromb Vasc Biol*, Vol. 27, No. 11, pp. 2384-2391

Shiraki, R., Inoue, N., Kobayashi, S., Ejiri, J., Otsui, K., Honjo, T., Takahashi, M., Hirata, K., Yokoyama, M., & Kawashima, S. (2006). Toll-like receptor 4 expressions on peripheral blood monocytes were enhanced in coronary artery disease even in patients with low C-reactive protein. *Life Sci*, Vol. 80, No. 1, pp. 59-66

Smiley, S.T., King, J.A., & Hancock, W.W. (2001). Fibrinogen stimulates macrophage chemokine secretion through toll-like receptor 4. *J Immunol*, Vol. 167, No. 5, pp. 2887-2894

Stewart, C.R., Stuart, L.M., Wilkinson, K., van Gils, J.M., Deng, J., Halle, A., Rayner, K.J., Boyer, L., Zhong, R., Frazier, W.A., Lacy-Hulbert, A., Khoury, J.E., Golenbock, D.T., & Moore, K.J. (2010). CD36 ligands promote sterile inflammation through assembly of a Toll-like receptor 4 and 6 heterodimer. *Nat Immunol*, Vol. 11, No. 2, pp. 155-161

Stoll, L., Denning, G., Li, W., Rice, J., Harrelson, A., Romig, S., Gunnlaugsson, S., Miller, F., & Weintraub, N. (2004). Regulation of endotoxin-induced proinflammatory activation in human coronary artery cells: expression of functional membrane-bound CD14 by human coronary artery smooth muscle cells. *J Immunol*, Vol. 173, No. 2, pp. 1336-1343

Swirski, F., Pittet, M., Kircher, M., Aikawa, E., Jaffer, F., Libby, P., & Weissleder, R. (2006). Monocyte accumulation in mouse atherogenesis is progressive and proportional to extent of disease. *Proc Natl Acad Sci U S A*, Vol. 103, No. 27, pp. 10340-10345

Takahashi, K., Kawai, T., Kumar, H., Sato, S., Yonehara, S., & Akira, S. (2006). Roles of caspase-8 and caspase-10 in innate immune responses to double-stranded RNA. *Journal of immunology (Baltimore, Md : 1950)*, Vol. 176, pp. 4520-4524

Takeuchi, O., Takeda, K., Hoshino, K., Adachi, O., Ogawa, T., & Akira, S. (2000). Cellular responses to bacterial cell wall components are mediated through MyD88-dependent signaling cascades. *International immunology*, Vol. 12, pp. 113-117

Takeuchi, O., Kawai, T., Muhlradt, P., Morr, M., Radolf, J., Zychlinsky, A., Takeda, K., & Akira, S. (2001). Discrimination of bacterial lipoproteins by Toll-like receptor 6. *Int Immunol*, Vol. 13, No. 7, pp. 933-940

Takeuchi, O., Sato, S., Horiuchi, T., Hoshino, K., Takeda, K., Dong, Z., Modlin, R., & Akira, S. (2002). Cutting edge: role of Toll-like receptor 1 in mediating immune response to microbial lipoproteins. *J Immunol*, Vol. 169, No. 1, pp. 10-14

Takeuchi, O., & Akira, S. (2010). Pattern recognition receptors and inflammation. *Cell*, Vol. 140, pp. 805-820

Tanimura, N., Saitoh, S., Matsumoto, F., Akashi-Takamura, S., & Miyake, K. (2008). Roles for LPS-dependent interaction and relocation of TLR4 and TRAM in TRIF-signaling. *Biochemical and biophysical research communications*, Vol. 368, pp. 94-99

Taylor, K.R., Trowbridge, J.M., Rudisill, J.A., Termeer, C.C., Simon, J.C., & Gallo, R.L. (2004). Hyaluronan fragments stimulate endothelial recognition of injury through TLR4. *J Biol Chem*, Vol. 279, No. 17, pp. 17079-17084

Tenoever, B.R., Ng, S.-L., Chua, M.A., McWhirter, S.M., García-Sastre, A., & Maniatis, T. (2007). Multiple functions of the IKK-related kinase IKKepsilon in interferon-mediated antiviral immunity. *Science (New York, NY)*, Vol. 315, pp. 1274-1278

Ting, J.P.Y., Duncan, J.A., & Lei, Y. (2010). How the noninflammasome NLRs function in the innate immune system. *Science*, Vol. 327, pp. 286-290

Underhill, D.M., Ozinsky, A., Hajjar, A.M., Stevens, A., Wilson, C.B., Bassetti, M., & Aderem, A. (1999a). The Toll-like receptor 2 is recruited to macrophage phagosomes and discriminates between pathogens. *Nature*, Vol. 401, pp. 811-815

Underhill, D.M., Ozinsky, A., Smith, K.D., & Aderem, A. (1999b). Toll-like receptor-2 mediates mycobacteria-induced proinflammatory signaling in macrophages. *Proc Natl Acad Sci U S A*, Vol. 96, No. 25, pp. 14459-14463

Vink, A., Schoneveld, A.H., van der Meer, J.J., van Middelaar, B.J., Sluijter, J.P., Smeets, M.B., Quax, P.H., Lim, S.K., Borst, C., Pasterkamp, G., & de Kleijn, D.P. (2002). In vivo evidence for a role of toll-like receptor 4 in the development of intimal lesions. *Circulation*, Vol. 106, No. 15, pp. 1985-1990

Visintin, A., Mazzoni, A., Spitzer, J., Wyllie, D., Dower, S., & Segal, D. (2001). Regulation of Toll-like receptors in human monocytes and dendritic cells. *J Immunol*, Vol. 166, No. 1, pp. 249-255

Wang, S., Miura, M., Jung, Y.K., Zhu, H., Li, E., & Yuan, J. (1998). Murine caspase-11, an ICE-interacting protease, is essential for the activation of ICE. *Cell*, Vol. 92, pp. 501-509

Wick, G., Romen, M., Amberger, A., Metzler, B., Mayr, M., Falkensammer, G., & Xu, Q. (1997). Atherosclerosis, autoimmunity, and vascular-associated lymphoid tissue. *FASEB J*, Vol. 11, No. 13, pp. 1199-1207

Wright, S.D., Ramos, R.A., Tobias, P.S., Ulevitch, R.J., & Mathison, J.C. (1990). CD14, a receptor for complexes of lipopolysaccharide (LPS) and LPS binding protein. *Science*, Vol. 249, No. 4975, pp. 1431-1433

Xu, X.H., Shah, P.K., Faure, E., Equils, O., Thomas, L., Fishbein, M.C., Luthringer, D., Xu, X.P., Rajavashisth, T.B., Yano, J., Kaul, S., & Arditi, M. (2001). Toll-like receptor-4 is expressed by macrophages in murine and human lipid-rich atherosclerotic plaques and upregulated by oxidized LDL. *Circulation*, Vol. 104, No. 25, pp. 3103-3108

Yajima, N., Takahashi, M., Morimoto, H., Shiba, Y., Takahashi, Y., Masumoto, J., Ise, H., Sagara, J., Nakayama, J., Taniguchi, S.i., & Ikeda, U. (2008). Critical role of bone marrow apoptosis-associated speck-like protein, an inflammasome adaptor molecule, in neointimal formation after vascular injury in mice. *Circulation*, Vol. 117, No. 24, pp. 3079-3087

Yamamoto, M., Sato, S., Hemmi, H., Sanjo, H., Uematsu, S., Kaisho, T., Hoshino, K., Takeuchi, O., Kobayashi, M., Fujita, T., Takeda, K., & Akira, S. (2002). Essential role for TIRAP in activation of the signalling cascade shared by TLR2 and TLR4. *Nature*, Vol. 420, pp. 324-329

Yamasaki, K., Muto, J., Taylor, K.R., Cogen, A.L., Audish, D., Bertin, J., Grant, E.P., Coyle, A.J., Misaghi, A., Hoffman, H.M., & Gallo, R.L. (2009). NLRP3/cryopyrin is necessary for interleukin-1beta (IL-1beta) release in response to hyaluronan, an endogenous trigger of inflammation in response to injury. *J Biol Chem*, Vol. 284, No. 19, pp. 12762-12771

Yanai, H., Ban, T., Wang, Z., Choi, M.K., Kawamura, T., Negishi, H., Nakasato, M., Lu, Y., Hangai, S., Koshiba, R., Savitsky, D., Ronfani, L., Akira, S., Bianchi, M.E., Honda, K., Tamura, T., Kodama, T., & Taniguchi, T. (2009). HMGB proteins function as universal sentinels for nucleic-acid-mediated innate immune responses. *Nature*, Vol. 462, No. 7269, pp. 99-103

Yang, X., Coriolan, D., Murthy, V., Schultz, K., Golenbock, D.T., & Beasley, D. (2005a). Proinflammatory phenotype of vascular smooth muscle cells: role of efficient Toll-like receptor 4 signaling. *Am J Physiol Heart Circ Physiol*, Vol. 289, No. 3, pp. H1069-1076

Yang, X., Coriolan, D., Schultz, K., Golenbock, D., & Beasley, D. (2005b). Toll-like receptor 2 mediates persistent chemokine release by Chlamydia pneumoniae-infected vascular smooth muscle cells. *Arterioscler Thromb Vasc Biol*, Vol. 25, No. 11, pp. 2308-2314

Yang, X., Murthy, V., Schultz, K., Tatro, J., Fitzgerald, K., & Beasley, D. (2006). Toll-like receptor 3 signaling evokes a proinflammatory and proliferative phenotype in human vascular smooth muscle cells. *Am J Physiol Heart Circ Physiol*, Vol. 291, No. 5, pp. H2334-2343

Zhou, Y.F., Shou, M., Guetta, E., Guzman, R., Unger, E.F., Yu, Z.X., Zhang, J., Finkel, T., & Epstein, S.E. (1999). Cytomegalovirus infection of rats increases the neointimal response to vascular injury without consistent evidence of direct infection of the vascular wall. *Circulation*, Vol. 100, No. 14, pp. 1569-1575

Zimmer, S., Steinmetz, M., Asdonk, T., Motz, I., Coch, C., Hartmann, E., Barchet, W., Wassmann, S., Hartmann, G., & Nickenig, G. (2011). Activation of endothelial toll-like receptor 3 impairs endothelial function. *Circ Res*, Vol. 108, No. 11, pp. 1358-1366

# 13

# Cholesterol and Inflammation at the Crossroads of Non-Alcoholic Fatty Liver Disease (NAFLD) and Atherogenesis

Gregor Lorbek and Damjana Rozman
*Center for Functional Genomics and Bio-Chips, Institute of Biochemistry, Faculty of Medicine, University of Ljubljana*
*Slovenia*

## 1. Introduction

Non-alcoholic fatty liver disease (NAFLD) encompasses a variety of diseases ranging from simple steatosis or fatty liver through non-alcoholic steatohepatisis (NASH) to fibrosis that can eventually lead to irreversible cirrhosis. NASH was first described by Ludwig et al. (Ludwig et al., 1980) in a number of patients who reported no "significant" alcohol intake but whose liver histology resembled that of alcoholic liver disease. Today the term NAFLD is used either when referring to a full spectrum of liver disease or when the aetiology of the disease is unknown, excluding secondary causative factors such as excessive alcohol intake, hepatotoxic drugs, metabolic/genetic and other liver diseases (for instance autoimmune or viral hepatitis) (Treeprasertsuk et al., 2011).

The occurrence of NAFLD has been persistently increasing in parallel with the concerning worldwide epidemic of obesity and diabetes and is expected to rise in the future (Portincasa et al., 2005). In the Western countries NAFLD is already becoming the most common cause of liver disease with the estimates of prevalence being between 17 and 33 % in the general population (McCullough, 2005) and rising as high as 90 % in morbidly obese individuals (Machado et al., 2006). NASH, the most severe and clinically significant form of NAFLD, is less common and is expected to be present between 5.7 and 17 % of the population (McCullough, 2005), again the numbers increase in the morbidly obese (up to 37 %) (Machado et al., 2006). Although NAFLD can occur in lean patients, the majority of the patients are overweight or obese (McCullough, 2005). Of particular concern, especially in the view of the future disease burden, is the presence of NAFLD in children and adolescents. For instance, the prevalence of obesity among US children has tripled in just one decade, rising from 5 % in 1980 to 15 % in 1990 and is currently around 17 %(Centers for Disease Control and Prevention CDC, 2011). The estimates of NAFLD prevalence in childhood have risen accordingly and are already between 2.6 and 9.6 % among the general pediatric population (Pacifico et al., 2010), reaching 68 % in obese children (Fu et al., 2011). Most cases of NAFLD arise in the detrimental environment of various metabolic disorders commonly known as the metabolic syndrome. The disease is strongly associated with insulin resistance, hypertension, glucose intolerance, central obesity and dyslipidemia and is thus recognized as the hepatic manifestation of the metabolic syndrome (Marchesini et al., 2005). Simple steatosis is largely benign and has a good prognosis. Nevertheless, a significant proportion of steatotic patients will develop steatohepatitis, which is characterized by hepatocyte injury and inflammation with 20-25 % possibility of progression to advanced fibrosis and cirrhosis (Farrell et al., 2005). In patients with cirrhosis liver failure is the most common cause of death warranting a liver transplantation (Grattagliano et al., 2011). NAFLD is also significantly associated with cardiovascular disease (CVD) independently of metabolic syndrome components and the classical risk factors (Nakao & Yoneda, 2009; Targher & Arcaro, 2007). In fact, one of the leading causes of death in NAFLD patients is coronary artery disease (Adams et al., 2005; Matteoni et al., 1999). Recent evidence thus suggests that NAFLD might play an important role in the development of atherosclerosis (see Chapter 4). NASH has also been found to be associated with increased risk of hepatocellular carcinoma (Marrero et al., 2002).

NAFLD is clinically silent. The symptoms usually described by the patients, such as fatigue and vague discomfort over the liver, are quite non-specific (Farrell et al., 2005). The presence of the disease is often suspected upon abnormal results of routinely performed liver tests in the presence of metabolic syndrome risk factors and exclusion of secondary causes. It should be noted, however, that elevated liver enzymes have poor sensitivity since serum transaminases can be normal in up to 80 % of patients with steatosis (Browning et al., 2004). Hepatic imaging, which can be ordered as a part of investigations into abdominal pain or elevated liver enzymes, usually provides the first clues of the presence of steatosis. Hepatic ultrasound, where steatosis is seen as increased echogenicity or "bright liver", has a quite high sensitivity, especially when more than 33 % of hepatocytes are fatty. The same sensitivity has been found with the use of computerized tomography and magnetic resonance imaging, but unfortunately all three methods are unable to detect features of fibrosis and cirrhosis, which present the greatest risk of liver failure (Saadeh et al., 2002). Today liver biopsy is the gold standard for diagnosing NASH, since only histological evaluation of the liver tissue is able to discern simple steatosis from steatosis with inflammation, which represents the hallmark of NASH. It is of vital clinical importance to distinguish advanced liver disease from the more benign states because of its poor outcome. Guidelines on when to perform the liver biopsy are still a matter of discussion since the procedure is costly, invasive, prone to complications such as pain or even death (0.01 % procedural mortality) and inclined to sampling variability (Guha et al., 2006; Poynard et al., 2006). Indication for liver biopsy is currently based upon risk assessment for fibrosis, which takes into consideration obesity, diabetes, age over 45 and aspartate transaminase (AST) to alanine transaminase (ALT) ratio over 1 (Angulo & Lindor, 2002).

Despite an ever increasing knowledge about the mechanisms of NAFLD pathogenesis (see Chapter 3), an efficient therapy remains elusive. Several key pieces of information for targeted treatment are still missing, such as why only a certain proportion of patients with simple steatosis progress to steatohepatitis and a better understanding of causal relationships of NAFLD and metabolic syndrome components. In fact, the use of term NAFLD itself suggests an unknown aetiology of the disease. Because of this and because of strong association of NAFLD to metabolic syndrome, the therapy is primarily directed towards lifestyle modifications. Patients are encouraged to lose weight through physical exercise improving body mass index (BMI), insulin resistance and diabetic control (Musso et al., 2010). It was shown that the benefits of relatively consistent weight loss are removal of fat from hepatocytes, which can even lead to improved necroinflammation and decreased fibrosis (Hickman et al., 2002; Palmer & Schaffner, 1990; Ueno et al., 1997). It is estimated that a change in nutritional habits in which we would reduce caloric intake by as little as 100 kilocalories per day would prevent epidemic of both obesity and NAFLD (Hill et al., 2003). Pharmacological interventions are indicated for patients with a risk of developing advanced liver disease. Because insulin resistance is the single most prevalent predisposing factor for NAFLD (Bugianesi et al., 2005b), treatment is mainly aimed to improve insulin sensitivity. Insulin sensitizers metformin and thiazolidinediones are gaining acknowledgement as drugs with beneficial effects on NAFLD (Ahmed & Byrne, 2009). Other therapy strategies are directed towards improving dyslipidemia and oxidative stress, which are commonly associated with NAFLD, and drugs such as statins, polyunsaturated fatty acids, vitamins C and E and ursodeoxycholic acid are currently being evaluated in clinical trials (Musso et al., 2010).

At present, NAFLD can best be described as a multi-factorial disorder with no specific diagnostic tests and no approved treatment regimen. Increasing interest in the research of this complex disease is implicating more and more factors that contribute to the pathogenesis of NAFLD. In this chapter we will first describe pathology and pathogenesis of NALFD and move on to establish a link between NAFLD and atherosclerosis. Subsequently we will depict the interplay of cholesterol metabolism and inflammation and their relation to atherosclerosis through NAFLD.

## 2. Pathology of NAFLD

NAFLD covers a wide range of pathological states and it is often difficult to draw the line where one condition ends and the other begins. First efforts were put into defining histopathological criteria for the diagnosis of NASH. In order to avoid the early confusions, it was proposed that liver biopsies of NASH should closely resemble those of alcoholic steatohepatitis (Lee, 1995). However, many of the more subtle forms of steatosis with inflammation were thus unjustifiably excluded from being designated as NASH. To overcome the diagnostic inconsistencies, Matteoni et al. (Matteoni et al., 1999) divided NAFLD into four categories (Table 1).

| Category of NAFLD | Pathology | Clinical correlation |
|---|---|---|
| **Type 1** | Simple fatty liver (steatosis) | Not progressive with a good prognosis |
| **Type 2** | Steatosis and lobular inflammation (steatohepatitis) | Probably benign, does not resemble alcoholic steatohepatitis, not diagnosed as NASH |
| **Type 3** | Steatosis, lobular inflammation and ballooning degeneration (steatonecrosis) | NASH without fibrosis - may progress to cirrhosis |
| **Type 4** | Steatosis, ballooning degeneration and Mallory bodies, and/or fibrosis | NASH with fibrosis - may progress to cirrhosis and liver failure |

Table 1. Categories of non-alcoholic fatty liver disease (NAFLD) and their clinical correlation (Farrell et al., 2005; Matteoni et al., 1999).

Steatosis (or fatty liver) is the hallmark of NAFLD and is characterized by the accumulation of fat droplets in hepatocytes. To diagnose steatosis at least 5 % of fatty hepatocytes need to be present (Kleiner et al., 2005), while less liver fat accumulation can be physiological and is transient in nature. At the histological level, fat is seen as a single macrovesicular droplet that displaces the nucleus to the periphery of the cell although a smaller amount of fat accumulation can be microvesicular (smaller vacuoles around the rim of the cell) (Hall & Kirsch, 2005). Steatosis, which is entirely microvesicular, is prompting other aetiology such as excessive alcohol intake or drugs (Hall & Kirsch, 2005). Other types of lipid accumulation that can be present in steatosis are lipogranulomas and fat cysts (Brunt, 2011).

Steatosis with lobular inflammation is considered a type 2 NAFLD. The inflammation infiltrate comprises of neutrophils, lymphocytes, plasma cells and macrophages. It is usually present as scattered clusters of cells across the lobule, but it can also be seen in portal tracts (Yerian, 2011). It is rather difficult to delineate simple steatosis from steatosis with lobular inflammation, because truly simple steatosis is very uncommon. One large study that evaluated 933 adult and pediatric liver biopsies found out that only four were completely void of inflammatory infiltration (Brunt et al., 2009). On the other hand, just one or two focal collections of mononuclear cells in the parenchyma are not enough to diagnose a type 2 NAFLD. Minimum criteria to define any type of hepatitis in fatty liver are yet to be defined (Hall & Kirsch, 2005).

The third prerequisite to diagnose NASH, besides the fatty hepatocytes and inflammatory infiltrate, is the hepatocyte injury present either as reversible hepatic ballooning degeneration or irreversible hepatic necrosis or apoptosis. Ballooned hepatocytes are large in size and have a pale, "cobweb-like" cytoplasm that is a consequence of fluid retention (Yerian, 2011). They are quite difficult to distinguish from fatty hepatocytes with small fat droplets that resemble mildly hidropic cells. It is possible to discern fat from fluid with certain histochemical stainings of liver tissue but these are not routinely performed (Brunt & Tiniakos, 2010). Mallory bodies are often seen in ballooned hepatocytes and they appear as irregularly shaped eosinophilic masses in the cytoplasm. They are composed of cytokeratin polypeptides and can be stained with antibody to ubiquitin (French, 2000). Mallory bodies are not required for the diagnosis of NASH. Apoptotic hepatocytes are observed as deeply eosinophilic cytoplasmic aggregates that may or may not be surrounded by Kupffer cells (liver macrophages), however, apoptosis of hepatocytes in NAFLD is never so prominent as in viral hepatitis (Hall & Kirsch, 2005).

In the progressive forms of liver disease fibrosis and cirrhosis may occur. The former is characterized as aberrant deposition of extracellular matrix (collagen) by activated hepatic stellate cells as part of the injury healing process. Fibrosis is characteristically pericellular in distribution and is first observed in the centrilobular region of the liver. With progression it extends towards portal areas (Brunt, 2011). Cirrhosis or liver scarring is defined as a complete loss of the normal lobular architecture and replacement of liver tissue by fibrosis, scar tissue and regenerative nodules of hepatocytes (Grattagliano et al., 2011). It eventually leads to the loss of liver function.

## 3. Pathogenesis of NAFLD

### 3.1 Insulin resistance as a predominant factor for NAFLD

NAFLD is strongly associated with components of the metabolic syndrome and the majority of cases of NAFLD occur in patients with obesity (60–95 %), type 2 diabetes mellitus (28–55

%) and hyperlipidemia (27–92 %) (Marchesini & Bugianesi, 2005). Insulin resistance (IR), being the cardinal feature of the metabolic syndrome, is almost uniformly found in patients with NAFLD (Bugianesi et al., 2005a; Comert et al., 2001; Marchesini et al., 1999; Sanyal et al., 2001). The causes of IR are as of yet unknown and are being researched extensively. IR can be classified as either peripheral IR in which we have reduced insulin-mediated uptake of glucose by skeletal muscle and adypocites or hepatic IR where insulin is unable to suppress glucose production in the liver. There is mounting evidence that the main pathological event leading to peripheral IR is ectopic accumulation of fat (fatty acid metabolites) in skeletal muscle, which causes a defect either in glucose transport or phosphorylation of insulin receptors (Samuel & Shulman, 2005). The same mechanism is believed to cause hepatic IR (Kim et al., 2001). In the presence of peripheral IR, insulin is unable to efficiently exert its antilipolytic effects on adipose tissue resulting in increased free fatty acid (FFA) flux into the bloodstream. Hyperlipidemia thus arising exacerbates IR in the muscle and adipose tissue and causes fat deposition in the liver affecting its function and inducing hepatic IR. It was found out that not only in obese, but also in lean NAFLD patients with normal glucose tolerance and lipid levels lipolysis and lipid oxidation at the basal level were increased and inefficiently inhibited after insulin administration (Marchesini & Bugianesi, 2005). The source of increased FFA flux in NAFLD patients is not clear but it seems that visceral adiposity may play an important role since it is more insulin resistant than subcutaneous adipose tissue (Lefebvre et al., 1998). This notion is supported by the fact that the aforementioned lean NAFLD patients had enlarged waist girth, which is in good correlation with central (visceral) adiposity.

NAFLD could thus possibly stem from a defect in insulin sensitivity causing derangements in glucose metabolism (which explains its link with other metabolic disorders) and in lipid metabolism that predisposes to hepatic steatosis, which is the first step in the pathogenesis of advanced liver disease.

### 3.2 The two-hit hypothesis and beyond

According to the initial "two-hit" hypothesis NASH develops in two subsequent steps (Day & James, 1998). The "first hit" leads to hepatic accumulation of triglycerides (steatosis) that makes liver susceptible to hepatocyte injury mediated by "second hits" such as inflammatory cytokines, oxidative stress and mitochondrial dysfunction, which in turn promote inflammatory infiltration and fibrosis.

#### 3.2.1 Steatosis

Lipids that accumulate in the liver are mainly triglycerides formed from esterification of glycerol and FFA within the hepatocyte (Figure 1). Three distinct sources of FFA are: lipolysis in the adipose tissue, *de novo* lipogenesis in the liver and dietary sources. Mechanisms for FFA utilization in the liver are: use as energy source in the process of β-oxidation, storage in the form of triglyceride droplets or export in the form of very low-density lipoproteins (VLDL). Hepatic fat accumulation can therefore be a consequence of a malfunction of any of these three mechanisms of FFA utilization or because of an increased fat delivery. In the case of NAFLD the increased influx of FFA from adipose tissue as a consequence of IR and obesity plays the dominant role since 60 % of liver triglycerides derive from FFA overflow from adipose tissue, 25 % from *de novo* lipogenesis and 15 % from the diet (Donnelly et al., 2005). IR also has a more direct effect on the liver.

Hyperinsulinemia, which accompanies IR, inhibits β-oxidation of FFA (Postic & Girard, 2008) and at the same time increases expression of lipogenic genes through up-regulation of transcription factor, sterol regulatory element binding protein-1c (SREBP-1c) (Kohjima et al., 2008). As a consequence, synthesis of lipids is intensified, which further promotes hepatic steatosis. As an answer to the increased synthesis of triglycerides, the production of VLDL is also increased whereas insufficient to adequately remove fat from the liver (Zoltowska et al., 2001).

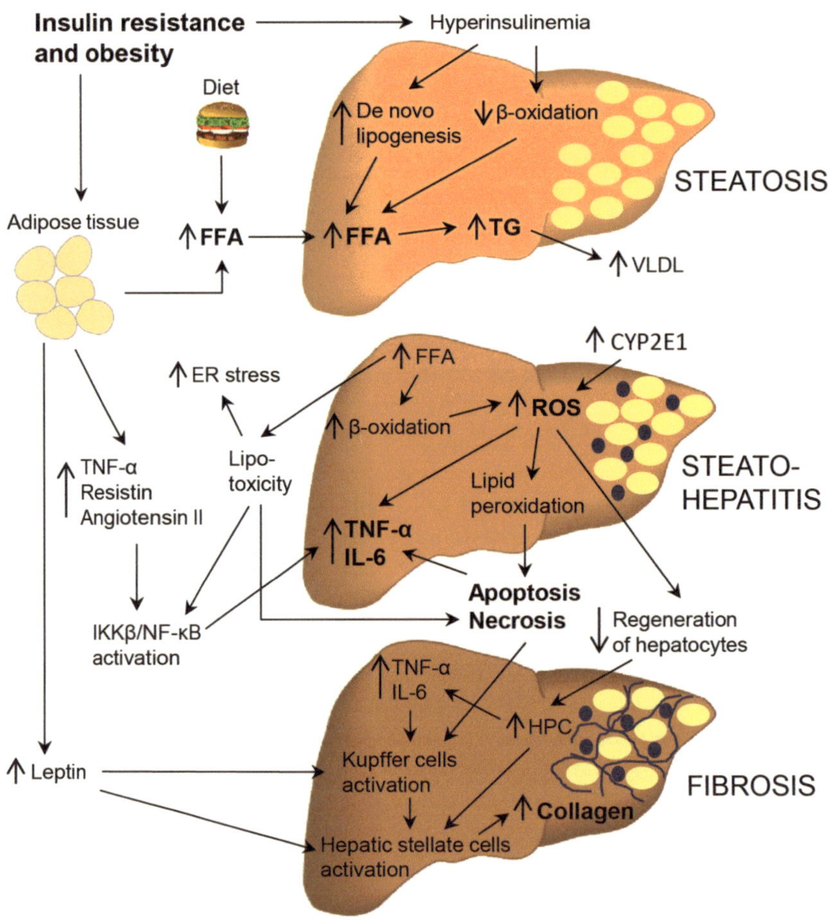


Fig. 1. Pathogenesis of NAFLD. Prominent feature of liver steatosis is the accumulation of excess FFA from the adipose tissue in the form of triglycerides. Gradual increase of FFA β-oxidation due to increased hepatic insulin resistance generates ROS, which activate inflammatory pathways and initiate lipid peroxidation. As a result, apoptosis and necrosis of hepatocytes, which are further aggravated by FFA lipotoxicity, activate Kupffer cells, which in turn stimulate hepatic stellate cells to produce excess amounts of collagen. CYP2E1: cytochrome P450 2E1; ER: endoplasmic reticulum; FFA: free fatty acids; HPC: hepatic progenitor cells; IKKβ/NF-κB: inhibitor kappa kinase beta/nuclear factor kappa B; IL-6: interleukin-6; TG: triglycerides; ROS: reactive oxygen species; TNF-α: tumor necrosis factor α; VLDL: very low-density lipoproteins.

### 3.2.2 Steatohepatitis and fibrosis

As was already stated, steatosis is tightly associated with hepatic inflammation. Again, visceral adipose tissue (insulin resistant) plays an important role in the transition from simple steatotic to inflamed liver, since it is not solely a site of energy storage, but also actively secreting endocrine organ. Most adipocyte-derived adipokines, such as tumor necrosis factor-α (TNF-α), resistin and angiotensin II, induce both IR and low-grade inflammation through activation of c-Jun NH2-terminal kinase-1 (JNK-1) and inhibitor kappa kinase beta (IKKβ)/nuclear factor kappa B (NF-κB) pathway in the liver. Induction of the latter pathway leads to feed forward loop of increased expression of pro-inflammatory cytokines like interleukin-6 (IL-6), interleukin 1-beta (IL-1β), TNF-α and activation of Kupffer cells (Cai et al., 2005; Wieckowska et al., 2008). Patients with NAFLD have elevated serum and hepatic levels of TNF-α (Haukeland et al., 2006; Hui et al., 2004) as well as IL-6 (Wieckowska et al., 2008). Concentrations of both correlate well with histological severity of NAFLD (Crespo et al., 2001; van der Poorten et al., 2008). Two additional well studied adipokines that have been implicated in NAFLD development are leptin and adiponectin. Leptin has an important role in the regulation of energy intake (Mantzoros, 1999) but also in the immune system (Lord, 2002) and in the promotion of fibrogenesis (Saxena et al., 2002). Together with TNF-α and IL-6 it activates hepatic stellate cells to deposit excessive amounts of collagen either directly (with binding to the receptors) or through stimulating secretion of transforming growth factor-β (TGF- β) by Kuppfer cells (Nieto, 2006; Shoelson et al., 2007). The obese and patients with NAFLD have higher levels of leptin and are considered to be leptin resistant (Uygun et al., 2000). In contrast to other adipokines, adiponectin protects the liver from inflammation and fibrogenesis. It antagonizes actions of TNF-α, inhibits lipogenesis (it down-regulates SREBP-1c) and increases insulin sensitivity (Polyzos et al., 2010; Whitehead et al., 2006). Circulatory levels of adiponection were found to be reduced in NAFLD patients (Bugianesi et al., 2005c) and it was shown that administration of recombinant adiponectin can substantially improve NASH in *ob/ob* mice, one of the animal models of NAFLD (Musso et al., 2010).

Oxidative stress and mitochondrial dysfunction are closely related and are both contributing to the liver injury. Mitochondria are the major site of free radical formation in the hepatocytes. Reactive oxygen species (ROS) are physiological by-products of energy production from glucose breakdown and FFA β-oxidation and are more or less successfully controlled by endogenous radical scavenging system. However, in the IR (NAFLD) state there is an increase of FFA delivery to the hepatocytes and gradual loss of suppression of fatty acid oxidation by insulin, generating levels of ROS that are beyond control of endogenous antioxidants (Sanyal et al., 2001). Mitochondria are the first to be exposed to the effects of ROS, which cause uncoupling of oxidation and phosphorylation process of forming adenosine triphosphate, and positive feedback loop of ROS production is thus created. ROS then activate inflammatory pathways through stimulated production of TNF-α and initiate lipid peroxidation, which is detrimental to mitochondria and which causes cell death either by signaling apoptosis or promoting necrosis (Mylonas & Kouretas, 1999; Tang et al., 2002). Hepatocyte apoptosis caused by peroxidation of excess triglycerides seems to be the critical step in progression from simple steatosis to NASH and cirrhosis (Syn et al., 2009). Apoptotic hepatocytes are phagocytized by adjacent Kupffer cells, leading to hepatic stellate cell activation and fibrogenesis. The role of apoptosis in the progression of liver injury was confirmed in a recent study on animal model of NASH where hepatic fibrosis was significantly improved upon inhibition of caspase signaling (Witek et al., 2009). Another potent source of ROS in NAFLD patients is overexpression of cytochrome P450 2E1 (CYP2E1), a microsomal fatty acid oxidizing enzyme (Weltman et al., 1998).

### 3.2.3 FFA lipotoxicity

Recently, new evidence has come into light that urge the "two-hit" hypothesis to be revised and modified. There is an increasing appreciation about a more direct role of FFA in promoting liver injury. It has been shown that accumulation of triglycerides in hepatocytes can actually be beneficial in preventing development of NAFLD. Inhibition of triglyceride synthesis in obese mice with NASH has improved steatosis, but worsened liver injury, inflammation and fibrosis (Yamaguchi et al., 2007). In the same mouse model the pathology of NAFLD has worsened in parallel with the FFA burden. It seems that hepatic triglyceride accumulation acts as a buffering system disabling FFA to exert their toxic effects on the liver. FFA directly induces lipotoxicity in the liver in the following manners:

1. Detergent effects at high concentrations, inhibition of ion pumps, ion channels and calcium ionophor activity (Bass & Merriman, 2005; Nguyen et al., 2000; Schonfeld et al., 2000).
2. Mediation of hepatocyte apoptosis through JNK-1 pathway. Saturated fatty acids seem to be more toxic than unsaturated fatty acids in this respect (Malhi et al., 2006).
3. Saturated fatty acids promote endoplasmic reticulum stress that is initially aimed at compensating for cell damage but can trigger hepatocyte apoptosis when dysregulated or activated for longer time like in the case of NAFLD (Wang et al., 2006). Endoplasmic reticulum stress can also be triggered by other biological stresses such as hyperinsulinemia and hyperlipidemia (Ron, 2002).
4. Adipokine-independent hepatocyte IKKβ/NF-κB pathway activation that leads to increased expression of pro-inflammatory cytokines (Boden, 2005).

### 3.2.4 The third hit

Recently, a "third-hit" was proposed to be involved in pathogenesis of NAFLD (Dowman et al., 2010; Syn et al., 2009). In the healthy liver, ability of mature hepatocytes to replicate in order to replace dead tissue is a core feature of liver's remarkable capability to regenerate itself after various injuries. Oxidative stress, especially excessive and prolonged production of $H_2O_2$ by mitochondria, results in impaired replication of mature hepatocytes, which in turn leads to expansion of the hepatic progenitor cells (HPCs). These cells reside in the Canal of Hering near the portal veins (periportal area) of the liver and upon activation first proliferate to intermediate hepatocyte-like cells that finally evolve into either cholangiocytes (epithelial cells of the bile duct) or mature hepatocytes, both contributing to liver repair. It seems that this type of response is an important factor in the development of late stage liver disease since numbers of HPCs and intermediate hepatocytes strongly correlate with the fibrosis stage (Roskams et al., 2003). Possible mechanisms for stimulating a progressive periportal fibrosis that is seen in advanced types of NAFLD include secretion of profibrogenic cytokines (IL-6, IL-8, TGF-β) by HPCs and intermediate hepatocytes (Svegliati-Baroni et al., 2008), as well as a possible transition of cholangiocytes to myofibroblasts (Xia et al., 2006). On the other hand, evidence exists that fibrosis preceds expansion of HPCs, suggesting a more complex interaction between both phenomena (Van Hul et al., 2009).

Why only a small portion of patients with simple steatosis progress to NASH and end-stage liver disease is still poorly explained. There is a rationale that genetic factors in concert with environmental factors might represent the missing link. A number of genes involved in oxidative stress, lipid metabolism and fibrosis are differentially up- or down-regulated in patients with NASH compared to patients with simple steatosis (Younossi et al., 2005). Several candidate genes are currently being investigated for their roles in the development of NAFLD (Day & Daly, 2005).

In respect to the overwhelming new knowledge about pathogenesis of NAFLD, it is perhaps reasonable to gradually abandon the notion of "two hits" acting one after the other in favor of multiple interactive pathogenic networks that centrally converge towards factors promoting liver fat accumulation in a fashion capable of causing liver injury. The underlying origin of these changes is probably a combination of genetic and environmental factors (Farrell & Larter, 2006).

## 4. NAFLD and atherogenesis

### 4.1 Associations of NAFLD and atherogenesis

A link between cardiovascular disease (CVD) and metabolic syndrome components has already been established (Dekker et al., 2005). Given the recent recognition of NAFLD as being a hepatic manifestation of the metabolic syndrome, patients with NAFLD would be expected to have an increased risk of CVD development and events. Moreover, NAFLD has actually been established as an independent risk factor of CVD regardless of other confounding metabolic disorders. Last but not least, a possibility exists that NAFLD is not solely a risk marker, but an early mediator of CVD development as well (Targher & Arcaro, 2007).

NAFLD has been shown to be associated with circulatory endothelial dysfunction, one of the early atherosclerosis markers. NAFLD patients in comparison with non-steatotic controls had a significant decrease in the brachial artery flow-mediated vasodilation that was related to the histological severity of NAFLD. In addition, these patients had an increased 10-year probability of CVD events (Villanova et al., 2005). Another reliable marker of subclinical atherosclerosis is an increase in the carotid artery intima-media thickness (IMT) (O'Leary & Polak, 2002). Again, NAFLD histology predicted the carotid IMT independently of age, sex, BMI and other traditional risk factors such as IR and features of the metabolic syndrome (Targher et al., 2006a). IMT has also been found to strongly correlate with elevated liver enzymes alanine aminotransferase and gamma-glutamyl transpeptidase, surrogate markers of NAFLD (Sookoian & Pirola, 2008).

Notably, there have been numerous reports about associations of NAFLD and increased CVD prevalence. In a study with a large sample of middle-aged male workers they found that people with NAFLD were more likely to have CVD than those without it, even more, the association was independent of obesity and other prognostic factors (Lin et al., 2005). Another study showed that the occurrence of NAFLD was significantly higher in subjects with acute myocardial infarction and also, that the severity of coronary artery disease was greater in these individuals independent of age, sex and BMI (Kessler et al., 2005).

Mortality rate among NAFLD patients is increased in comparison to the general population (Adams & Angulo, 2005). In one study, 132 patients with NAFLD were followed for approximately 18 years and it was reported that CVD was the second most common cause of death, right after cancer and in the same numbers as liver-related mortality (Matteoni et al., 1999). Another study with greater number of patients (420), but with mean follow-up of only 7.6 years, also found CVD and malignancy to have the highest rates of mortality that was overall higher in comparison to the people without NAFLD (Adams et al., 2005). It is questionable whether findings of these studies are applicable to the broader population since the number of patients was relatively low and the data originated from non-NAFLD oriented institutions (Targher & Arcaro, 2007). However, as in the case of subclinical atherosclerosis, elevated liver enzymes have been found to have a strong correlation not just with CVD risk, but also with increased CVD-related deaths in studies with a much higher number of participants (Lee et al., 2007; Schindhelm et al., 2007; Wannamethee et al., 1995). Practically in all of these studies NAFLD has been shown to be a risk factor of CVD independently of traditional risk factors or components of metabolic syndrome.

It has recently been suggested that childhood NAFLD could be an early contributing factor for development of atherosclerosis (Schwimmer et al., 2005). The authors of the study proposed that the process of atherosclerosis could already start in childhood and progress to symptomatic CVD in adulthood. Namely, in a sample of 817 children, atherosclerosis was twice as prevalent in children with fatty liver as in those without fatty liver. It is therefore reasonable to assume that steatosis is a potential early mediator of atherosclerosis, and this notion predicts an even greater epidemic of CVD in the future in parallel with increasing prevalence of NAFLD in pediatric population.

It seems that NAFLD brings with it an increased risk of developing atherosclerosis independently of other predictive factors. Whether this is true will need to be confirmed in subsequent studies with a larger number of patients and well defined and uniform diagnostic criteria for NAFLD. Nevertheless, a body of evidence clearly points in the direction that NAFLD is not just an innocent by-stander, but a pathological state that is actively contributing to atherosclerosis. From the clinician point of view these findings suggest that when NAFLD is detected either by ultrasound imaging or routinely performed liver enzyme tests, attention should be directed towards establishing whether other underlying CVD risk factors are also present. Similar if not greater efforts than for the treatment of NAFLD should then be considered to prevent development of atherosclerosis, since many NAFLD patients will die because of a major CVD event before the end-stage liver disease actually develops (Targher, 2007).

### 4.2 Mechanisms linking NAFLD and atherogenesis

Many studies clearly established a strong association of NAFLD and CVD, however, the mechanistic links between both diseases are still inadequately understood. One of the main problems in inferring causal relationships between NAFLD and accelerated atherosclerosis is their almost uniform coexistence with IR and other components of the metabolic syndrome. In this respect we will need to harness the aid of different NAFLD animal models that provide unique and to a certain extent controllable (patho)physiological conditions, which enable us to study these intertwined mechanisms separately from one another or in various combinations (Larter & Yeh, 2008). What are the possible routes of interaction between fatty liver disease and atherosclerosis?

#### 4.2.1 Inflammation

One of the principal features of NAFLD, especially NASH, is increased oxidative stress and chronic, subclinical inflammation. The key pro-inflammatory cytokine that plays a vital role in mediating inflammation is believed to be TNF-α (Figure 2). Expanded and insulin resistant abdominal adipose tissue is secreting increased amounts of TNF-α into the bloodstream that activates hepatic production of TNF-α through activation of IKKβ/NF-κB pathway. Activation of Kupffer cells by cytokines or hepatocyte damage further increases expression of TNF-α and IL-6 elevating both liver and systemic levels of pro-inflammatory cytokines. These enhance the inflammation and IR of the adipose tissue as well as the liver, and the vicious circle is closed. Another reinforcing route for inflammation starts with the inability of the insulin to suppress lipolysis in the adipose tissue that causes excess FFA flux to the liver where FFA are subjected to increased hepatic β-oxidation. Elevated levels of ROS cause oxidative damage that further intensifies the activation of inflammatory pathways in the liver (see Chapter 3). TNF-α promotes expression of IL-6 and IL-6 is the main hepatic stimulus for the production of C-reactive protein (CRP) (Heinrich et al., 1990). It has been known for a long time that inflammatory processes mediate the initiation and development of atherosclerotic lesions (Ross, 1999). Levels of TNF-α and IL-6 have been commonly associated with increased risk of coronary events (Ridker et al., 2000; Ridker et al., 2000). Until recently, CRP was thought to be an inactive downstream marker of the inflammation process. However, it has been shown that it can actively contribute to the development of atherosclerosis. CRP causes expression of cell adhesion molecules, activation of complement as well as mediating low-density lipoprotein (LDL) uptake by macrophages (Blake & Ridker, 2002). In NAFLD patients the levels of CRP were expectedly found to be increased compared to controls (Brea et al., 2005).

On the other side of the inflammation spectrum adiponectin acts as an anti-inflammatory mediator, mainly by antagonizing effects of TNF-α (Whitehead et al., 2006). Adiponectin has also been found to have antithrombotic effects, inhibiting thrombus formation and platelet aggregation (Kato et al., 2006). In NAFLD patients adiponectin levels are decreased (Hui et al., 2004; Targher et al., 2006b), thus lacking its protective effects against vascular diseases (Dekker et al., 2008).

In addition to direct predisposition of cytokines to atherosclerosis, the reinforcing inflammatory response through liver-adipose tissue axis exerts its effect indirectly as well. It has been shown that TNF-α interferes with intracellular insulin signaling cascade in the liver, adding to both hepatic and peripheral IR (Pandey et al., 2009). One of the dominant features of IR is atherogenic dyslipidemia, which will be discussed in the next subchapter. In corroboration of the effects of inflammatory cytokines on lipid status it has been shown that administration of recombinant TNF-α to treat cancer patients resulted in increased concentrations of VLDL and triglycerides and decreased high-density lipoprotein (HDL) particles (Sherman et al., 1988).

### 4.2.2 Dyslipidemia and aberrant cholesterol metabolism

Patients with metabolic syndrome usually have a state of dyslipidemia characterized by high triglycerides, low HDL-cholesterol, increased small dense LDL particles and increased apolipoprotein B100 concentration (Targher et al., 2008), which have all been recognized as atherogenic with strong associations to increased CVD risk (Heine & Dekker, 2002). In healthy people insulin suppresses hepatic production of VLDL in order to maintain normal hepatic lipid homeostasis (Sparks & Sparks, 1990). However, in the state of hepatic IR that has been further aggravated by steatosis, the secretion of VLDL is increased in conjunction with excessive triglyceride production (Adiels et al., 2006). After VLDL enters the blood, triglycerides are gradually removed by the action of lipoprotein lipase resulting in small, dense LDL (the most atherogenic subclass of LDL) (Fon Tacer & Rozman, 2011). Concentrations of triglycerides, VLDL and small dense LDL particles have been increased in patients with fatty liver (Adiels et al., 2006; Cali et al., 2007; Sugino et al., 2011). Additionally, it has been shown that hepatic steatosis is a better predictor of the composition and severity of dyslipidemia than hyperglycemia or IR in type-2 diabetic patients (Toledo et al., 2006). In patients with NAFLD, HDL or "the good cholesterol" has been found to be decreased as a secondary abnormality due to increased VLDL and LDL (Cali et al., 2007). Contrary to the simple fatty liver, VLDL synthesis and secretion are impaired in the state of steatohepatitis, contributing further to the accumulation of triglycerides in the liver and thus promoting lipid oxidative damage (Fujita et al., 2009).

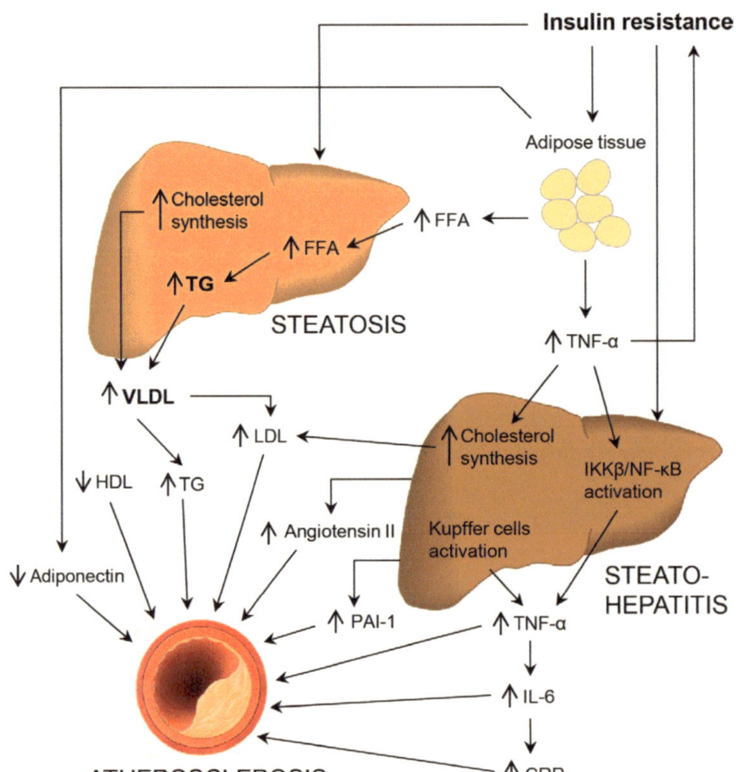


Fig. 2. Mechanisms linking NAFLD and atherosclerosis. Two principal atherogenic features of NAFLD are dyslipidemia and chronic subclinical inflammation. Increased cholesterol and triglyceride synthesis are the driving forces of increased secretion of VLDL and consequentially increased concentrations of LDL and TG. As a secondary abnormality HDL is decreased. Inflammed liver are producing excessive amounts of TNF-α, IL-6, CRP, PA-1, angiotensin II and cholesterol, which all stimulate the process of atherosclerosis. CRP: C-reactive protein; HDL: high-density lipoprotein FFA: free fatty acids; IKKβ/NF-κB: inhibitor kappa kinase beta/nuclear factor kappa B; IL-6: interleukin-6; LDL: low-density lipoprotein; PAI-1: plasminogen activator inhibitor -1; TG: triglycerides; TNF-α: tumor necrosis factor α; VLDL: very low-density lipoproteins.

Alongside aberrant lipoprotein metabolism driven mainly by IR, disturbances of cholesterol metabolism have also been found in patients with NAFLD. Detrimental effects of hypercholesterolemia on the progression of atherosclerosis have long been established. Cholesterol is capable of accumulating within the vascular wall, causing alterations in vascular structure and interfering with endothelial function leading to lesions, plaques, occlusions and emboli. Excess cholesterol concentration has also been associated with endothelial cell dysfunction, elevated oxidative stress and strong pro-inflammatory state in microcirculation (Stapleton et al., 2010). In humans cholesterol originates either from *de novo* synthesis or from the diet and is excreted mainly in the form of bile acids. Elevated concentrations of cholesterol have been found in the fatty liver of obese hyperlipidemic individuals compared to those without fatty liver (Reunanen et al., 1969). Obesity, metabolic syndrome, type 2-diabetes and IR have all been associated with increased cholesterol synthesis and lowered absorption of dietary cholesterol (Gylling et al., 2007; Miettinen & Gylling, 2000; Pihlajamaki et al., 2004; Simonen et al., 2002). Recent study has shown that the same happens in NAFLD patients (Simonen et al., 2011), where an increase in expression of cholesterogenic genes has been observed (Nakamuta et al., 2009). It seems that excess cholesterol synthesis, along with increased synthesis of triglycerides, presents one of the driving factors for increased production of VLDL particles in hepatic steatosis (Fon Tacer & Rozman, 2011).

Emerging evidence has started to place cholesterol in the "second hit" group that mediates the transition from simple steatosis to steatohepatitis. It has been shown that mitochondrial loading of free cholesterol, rather than FFA or triglycerides, sensitizes the liver to TNF-α induced steatohepatitis (Mari et al., 2006). In hyperlipidemic mouse models of NASH, dietary cholesterol, and not steatosis, predisposed to hepatic inflammation (Wouters et al., 2008). TNF-α also has a direct influence on lipid homeostasis since it activates cholesterol synthesis and inhibits formation of bile acids, thus increasing LDL-cholesterol and decreasing HDL-cholesterol (Fon Tacer et al., 2007; Fon Tacer et al., 2010). In contrast to its role in atherosclerosis, cholesterols implication in NAFLD has been poorly investigated. Nevertheless, limited research in this area is indicating an important role of cholesterol in pathogenesis of NAFLD as well as a novel link between disrupted cholesterol metabolism in NAFLD and atherosclerosis.

### 4.2.3 Other factors connecting fatty liver and the process of atherosclerosis

Apart from many positive feedback loops between fatty liver and IR, visceral adipose tissue, hyperglycemia and dyslipidemia, several other factors are mediating a cross-talk between atherosclerosis and NAFLD. Many coagulation factors are synthesized by hepatocytes. In NAFLD patients several are overproduced, and of particular concern is plasminogen activator inhibitor-1, which has direct atherogenic effects (Bansilal et al., 2007). Hepatocytes also produce angiotensinogen, a precursor of angiotensin II, and hepatic stellate cells are even capable of synthesizing and secreting mature form of angiotensin II upon activation by hepatocyte damage (Bataller et al., 2003). Angiotensin II is a pro-atherogenic vasoconstrictive peptide that predisposes to elevated blood pressure (Bataller et al., 2003; Massiera et al., 2001) and possibly also to CVD (Silventoinen et al., 2008).

Many other factors that contribute to both NAFLD and increased risk of atherosclerosis, like disturbances in endocrine system, hypoxia and ectopic fat deposition, are reviewed elsewhere (Loria et al., 2008).

## 5. Conclusion – The intertwined roles of cholesterol and inflammation in NAFLD and atherogenesis

In affluent economies NAFLD is already the most common cause of liver-related diseases and a major cause of morbidity and mortality. Sedentary life style and increased caloric intake, a hallmark of modern societies, are of particular concern in this respect, since NAFLD is found exclusively in obese individuals with insulin resistance. One of the emerging problems is also the increasing prevalence of fatty liver in children and adolescents, forecasting an even bigger social and economic impact of the disease in the future. Even though simple steatosis is benign, if not averted, it could predispose to more severe forms of liver disease with poor outcome. Despite the fact that the first description of NAFLD was made as many as 30 years ago, the decisive factor tipping the scales towards NASH is largely unknown. Genetic factors might play an important role here. Because of poorly understood mechanisms linking different stages of NAFLD, therapy is directed mainly towards improving the metabolic disorders without liver-specific drugs yet available. Surprisingly, cardiovascular events are among the leading causes of death in NAFLD patients, and recent research has enthroned NAFLD as an independent risk factor for CVD. Many direct as well as indirect links between fatty liver and atherosclerotic vessels have been established in the recent years. Inflammation and dyslipidemia are the most important factors contributing to both diseases with disrupted cholesterol metabolism gaining recognition, especially in the pathogenesis of NAFLD. Unfortunately, information about the role of cholesterol in NAFLD is limited, and hopefully new and emerging animal models (Horvat et al., 2011; Keber et al., 2011) of disturbed cholesterol metabolism will provide the missing insights. Better understanding of these mechanisms is important since inhibition of cholesterol synthesis by statins has proven beneficial in NAFLD patients (Ekstedt et al., 2007). However, the use of statins presents a risk of developing adverse drug reactions such as elevation of liver enzymes or hepatotoxicity due to drug interactions (Rozman & Monostory, 2010).

## 6. Acknowledgements

This work was supported by Slovenian Research Agency Programme grant P1-0104. Gregor Lorbek is funded as young researcher by the Slovenian Research Agency.

## 7. References

Adams, L.A. & Angulo, P. (2005). Recent concepts in non-alcoholic fatty liver disease. *Diabetic medicine : a journal of the British Diabetic Association,* Vol.22, No.9, pp. 1129-33, ISSN 0742-3071.

Adams, L.A.; Lymp, J.F.; St Sauver, J.; Sanderson, S.O.; Lindor, K.D.; Feldstein, A. & Angulo, P. (2005). The natural history of nonalcoholic fatty liver disease: a population-based cohort study. *Gastroenterology,* Vol.129, No.1, pp. 113-21, ISSN 0016-5085.

Adiels, M.; Taskinen, M.R.; Packard, C.; Caslake, M.J.; Soro-Paavonen, A.; Westerbacka, J.; Vehkavaara, S.; Hakkinen, A.; Olofsson, S.O.; Yki-Jarvinen, H. & Boren, J. (2006). Overproduction of large VLDL particles is driven by increased liver fat content in man. *Diabetologia,* Vol.49, No.4, pp. 755-65, ISSN 0012-186X.

Ahmed, M.H. & Byrne, C.D. (2009). Current treatment of non-alcoholic fatty liver disease. *Diabetes, obesity & metabolism,* Vol.11, No.3, pp. 188-95, ISSN 1463-1326.

Angulo, P. & Lindor, K.D. (2002). Non-alcoholic fatty liver disease. *Journal of gastroenterology and hepatology,* Vol.17 Suppl, S186-90, ISSN 0815-9319.

Bansilal, S.; Farkouh, M.E. & Fuster, V. (2007). Role of insulin resistance and hyperglycemia in the development of atherosclerosis. *The American journal of cardiology,* Vol.99, No.4A, pp. 6B-14B, ISSN 0002-9149.

Bass, M.N. & Merriman, R.B. (2005). Fatty acid metabolism and lipotoxicity in the pathogenesis of NAFLD/NASH, In: *Fatty Liver Disease: NASH and Related Disorders,* G. C. Farrell, J. George, P. M. Hall and A. J. McCullough, pp. 109-122, Blackwell Publishing, ISBN 1-4051-1292-1, USA.

Bataller, R.; Sancho-Bru, P.; Gines, P.; Lora, J.M.; Al-Garawi, A.; Sole, M.; Colmenero, J.; Nicolas, J.M.; Jimenez, W.; Weich, N.; Gutierrez-Ramos, J.C.; Arroyo, V. & Rodes, J. (2003). Activated human hepatic stellate cells express the renin-angiotensin system and synthesize angiotensin II. *Gastroenterology,* Vol.125, No.1, pp. 117-25, ISSN 0016-5085.

Blake, G.J. & Ridker, P.M. (2002). Inflammatory bio-markers and cardiovascular risk prediction. *Journal of internal medicine,* Vol.252, No.4, pp. 283-94, ISSN 0954-6820.

Boden, G. (2005). Free fatty acids and insulin secretion in humans. *Current diabetes reports,* Vol.5, No.3, pp. 167-70, ISSN 1534-4827.

Brea, A.; Mosquera, D.; Martin, E.; Arizti, A.; Cordero, J.L. & Ros, E. (2005). Nonalcoholic fatty liver disease is associated with carotid atherosclerosis: a case-control study. *Arteriosclerosis, thrombosis, and vascular biology,* Vol.25, No.5, pp. 1045-50, ISSN 1524-4636.

Browning, J.D.; Szczepaniak, L.S.; Dobbins, R.; Nuremberg, P.; Horton, J.D.; Cohen, J.C.; Grundy, S.M. & Hobbs, H.H. (2004). Prevalence of hepatic steatosis in an urban population in the United States: impact of ethnicity. *Hepatology,* Vol.40, No.6, pp. 1387-95, ISSN 0270-9139.

Brunt, E.M. (2011). Non-alcoholic fatty liver disease: what's new under the microscope? *Gut,* ISSN 1468-3288.

Brunt, E.M.; Kleiner, D.E.; Wilson, L.A.; Unalp, A.; Behling, C.E.; Lavine, J.E. & Neuschwander-Tetri, B.A. (2009). Portal chronic inflammation in nonalcoholic fatty liver disease (NAFLD): a histologic marker of advanced NAFLD-Clinicopathologic correlations from the nonalcoholic steatohepatitis clinical research network. *Hepatology,* Vol.49, No.3, pp. 809-20, ISSN 1527-3350.

Brunt, E.M. & Tiniakos, D.G. (2010). Histopathology of nonalcoholic fatty liver disease. *World journal of gastroenterology : WJG,* Vol.16, No.42, pp. 5286-96, ISSN 1007-9327.

Bugianesi, E.; Gastaldelli, A.; Vanni, E.; Gambino, R.; Cassader, M.; Baldi, S.; Ponti, V.; Pagano, G.; Ferrannini, E. & Rizzetto, M. (2005). Insulin resistance in non-diabetic patients with non-alcoholic fatty liver disease: sites and mechanisms. *Diabetologia,* Vol.48, No.4, pp. 634-42, ISSN 0012-186X.

Bugianesi, E.; McCullough, A.J. & Marchesini, G. (2005). Insulin resistance: a metabolic pathway to chronic liver disease. *Hepatology,* Vol.42, No.5, pp. 987-1000, ISSN 0270-9139.

Bugianesi, E.; Pagotto, U.; Manini, R.; Vanni, E.; Gastaldelli, A.; de Iasio, R.; Gentilcore, E.; Natale, S.; Cassader, M.; Rizzetto, M.; Pasquali, R. & Marchesini, G. (2005). Plasma adiponectin in nonalcoholic fatty liver is related to hepatic insulin resistance and hepatic fat content, not to liver disease severity. *The Journal of clinical endocrinology and metabolism,* Vol.90, No.6, pp. 3498-504, ISSN 0021-972X.

Cai, D.; Yuan, M.; Frantz, D.F.; Melendez, P.A.; Hansen, L.; Lee, J. & Shoelson, S.E. (2005). Local and systemic insulin resistance resulting from hepatic activation of IKK-beta and NF-kappaB. *Nature medicine,* Vol.11, No.2, pp. 183-90, ISSN 1078-8956.

Cali, A.M.; Zern, T.L.; Taksali, S.E.; de Oliveira, A.M.; Dufour, S.; Otvos, J.D. & Caprio, S. (2007). Intrahepatic fat accumulation and alterations in lipoprotein composition in obese adolescents: a perfect proatherogenic state. *Diabetes care,* Vol.30, No.12, pp. 3093-8, ISSN 1935-5548.

Centers for Disease Control and Prevention [CDC] (2011). CDC grand rounds: childhood obesity in the United States. *MMWR. Morbidity and mortality weekly report,* Vol.60, No.2, pp. 42-6, ISSN 1545-861X.

Comert, B.; Mas, M.R.; Erdem, H.; Dinc, A.; Saglamkaya, U.; Cigerim, M.; Kuzhan, O.; Unal, T. & Kocabalkan, F. (2001). Insulin resistance in non-alcoholic steatohepatitis. *Digestive and liver disease : official journal of the Italian Society of Gastroenterology and the Italian Association for the Study of the Liver,* Vol.33, No.4, pp. 353-8, ISSN 1590-8658.

Crespo, J.; Cayon, A.; Fernandez-Gil, P.; Hernandez-Guerra, M.; Mayorga, M.; Dominguez-Diez, A.; Fernandez-Escalante, J.C. & Pons-Romero, F. (2001). Gene expression of tumor necrosis factor alpha and TNF-receptors, p55 and p75, in nonalcoholic steatohepatitis patients. *Hepatology,* Vol.34, No.6, pp. 1158-63, ISSN 0270-9139.

Day, C.P. & Daly, A.K. (2005). NASH is a genetically determined disease, In: *Fatty Liver Disease: NASH and Related Disorders*, G. C. Farrell, J. George, P. M. Hall and A. J. McCullough, pp. 66-75, Blackwell Publishing, ISBN 1-4051-1292-1, USA.

Day, C.P. & James, O.F. (1998). Steatohepatitis: a tale of two "hits"? *Gastroenterology,* Vol.114, No.4, pp. 842-5, ISSN 0016-5085.

Dekker, J.M.; Funahashi, T.; Nijpels, G.; Pilz, S.; Stehouwer, C.D.; Snijder, M.B.; Bouter, L.M.; Matsuzawa, Y.; Shimomura, I. & Heine, R.J. (2008). Prognostic value of adiponectin for cardiovascular disease and mortality. *The Journal of clinical endocrinology and metabolism,* Vol.93, No.4, pp. 1489-96, ISSN 0021-972X.

Dekker, J.M.; Girman, C.; Rhodes, T.; Nijpels, G.; Stehouwer, C.D.; Bouter, L.M. & Heine, R.J. (2005). Metabolic syndrome and 10-year cardiovascular disease risk in the Hoorn Study. *Circulation,* Vol.112, No.5, pp. 666-73, ISSN 1524-4539.

Donnelly, K.L.; Smith, C.I.; Schwarzenberg, S.J.; Jessurun, J.; Boldt, M.D. & Parks, E.J. (2005). Sources of fatty acids stored in liver and secreted via lipoproteins in patients with nonalcoholic fatty liver disease. *The Journal of clinical investigation,* Vol.115, No.5, pp. 1343-51, ISSN 0021-9738.

Dowman, J.K.; Tomlinson, J.W. & Newsome, P.N. (2010). Pathogenesis of non-alcoholic fatty liver disease. *QJM : monthly journal of the Association of Physicians,* Vol.103, No.2, pp. 71-83, ISSN 1460-2393.

Ekstedt, M.; Franzen, L.E.; Mathiesen, U.L.; Holmqvist, M.; Bodemar, G. & Kechagias, S. (2007). Statins in non-alcoholic fatty liver disease and chronically elevated liver enzymes: a histopathological follow-up study. *Journal of hepatology,* Vol.47, No.1, pp. 135-41, ISSN 0168-8278.

Farrell, G.C.; George, J.; Hall, P.M. & McCullough, A.J. (2005). Overview: an introduction to NASH and related disorders, In: *Fatty Liver Disease: NASH and Related Disorders*, G.

C. Farrell, J. George, P. M. Hall and A. J. McCullough, pp. 1-12, Blackwell Publishing, ISBN 1-4051-1292-1, USA.

Farrell, G.C. & Larter, C.Z. (2006). Nonalcoholic fatty liver disease: from steatosis to cirrhosis. *Hepatology,* Vol.43, No.2 Suppl 1, pp. S99-S112, ISSN 0270-9139.

Fon Tacer, K.; Kuzman, D.; Seliskar, M.; Pompon, D. & Rozman, D. (2007). TNF-alpha interferes with lipid homeostasis and activates acute and proatherogenic processes. *Physiological genomics,* Vol.31, No.2, pp. 216-27, ISSN 1531-2267.

Fon Tacer, K.; Pompon, D. & Rozman, D. (2010). Adaptation of cholesterol synthesis to fasting and TNF-alpha: profiling cholesterol intermediates in the liver, brain, and testis. *The Journal of steroid biochemistry and molecular biology,* Vol.121, No.3-5, pp. 619-25, ISSN 1879-1220.

Fon Tacer, K. & Rozman, D. (2011). Nonalcoholic Fatty liver disease: focus on lipoprotein and lipid deregulation. *Journal of lipids,* ISSN 2090-3049.

French, S.W. (2000). Mechanisms of alcoholic liver injury. *Canadian journal of gastroenterology = Journal canadien de gastroenterologie,* Vol.14, No.4, pp. 327-32, ISSN 0835-7900.

Fu, J.F.; Shi, H.B.; Liu, L.R.; Jiang, P.; Liang, L.; Wang, C.L. & Liu, X.Y. (2011). Non-alcoholic fatty liver disease: An early mediator predicting metabolic syndrome in obese children? *World journal of gastroenterology : WJG,* Vol.17, No.6, pp. 735-42, ISSN 1007-9327.

Fujita, K.; Nozaki, Y.; Wada, K.; Yoneda, M.; Fujimoto, Y.; Fujitake, M.; Endo, H.; Takahashi, H.; Inamori, M.; Kobayashi, N.; Kirikoshi, H.; Kubota, K.; Saito, S. & Nakajima, A. (2009). Dysfunctional very-low-density lipoprotein synthesis and release is a key factor in nonalcoholic steatohepatitis pathogenesis. *Hepatology,* Vol.50, No.3, pp. 772-80, ISSN 1527-3350.

Grattagliano, I.; Ubaldi, E.; Bonfrate, L. & Portincasa, P. (2011). Management of liver cirrhosis between primary care and specialists. *World journal of gastroenterology : WJG,* Vol.17, No.18, pp. 2273-82, ISSN 1007-9327.

Guha, I.N.; Parkes, J.; Roderick, P.R.; Harris, S. & Rosenberg, W.M. (2006). Non-invasive markers associated with liver fibrosis in non-alcoholic fatty liver disease. *Gut,* Vol.55, No.11, pp. 1650-60, ISSN 0017-5749.

Gylling, H.; Hallikainen, M.; Kolehmainen, M.; Toppinen, L.; Pihlajamaki, J.; Mykkanen, H.; Agren, J.J.; Rauramaa, R.; Laakso, M. & Miettinen, T.A. (2007). Cholesterol synthesis prevails over absorption in metabolic syndrome. *Translational research : the journal of laboratory and clinical medicine,* Vol.149, No.6, pp. 310-6, ISSN 1931-5244.

Hall, P.M. & Kirsch, R. (2005). Pathology of hepatic steatosis, NASH and related conditions, In: *Fatty Liver Disease: NASH and Related Disorders,* G. C. Farrell, J. George, P. M. Hall and A. J. McCullough, pp. 13-22, Blackwell Publishing, ISBN 1-4051-1292-1, USA.

Haukeland, J.W.; Damas, J.K.; Konopski, Z.; Loberg, E.M.; Haaland, T.; Goverud, I.; Torjesen, P.A.; Birkeland, K.; Bjoro, K. & Aukrust, P. (2006). Systemic inflammation in nonalcoholic fatty liver disease is characterized by elevated levels of CCL2. *Journal of hepatology,* Vol.44, No.6, pp. 1167-74, ISSN 0168-8278.

Heine, R.J. & Dekker, J.M. (2002). Beyond postprandial hyperglycaemia: metabolic factors associated with cardiovascular disease. *Diabetologia,* Vol.45, No.4, pp. 461-75, ISSN 0012-186X.

Heinrich, P.C.; Castell, J.V. & Andus, T. (1990). Interleukin-6 and the acute phase response. *The Biochemical journal,* Vol.265, No.3, pp. 621-36, ISSN 0264-6021.

Hickman, I.J.; Clouston, A.D.; Macdonald, G.A.; Purdie, D.M.; Prins, J.B.; Ash, S.; Jonsson, J.R. & Powell, E.E. (2002). Effect of weight reduction on liver histology and biochemistry in patients with chronic hepatitis C. *Gut,* Vol.51, No.1, pp. 89-94, ISSN 0017-5749.

Hill, J.O.; Wyatt, H.R.; Reed, G.W. & Peters, J.C. (2003). Obesity and the environment: where do we go from here? *Science,* Vol.299, No.5608, pp. 853-5, ISSN 1095-9203.

Horvat, S.; McWhir, J. & Rozman, D. (2011). Defects in cholesterol synthesis genes in mouse and in humans: lessons for drug development and safer treatments. *Drug metabolism reviews,* Vol.43, No.1, pp. 69-90, ISSN 1097-9883.

Hui, J.M.; Hodge, A.; Farrell, G.C.; Kench, J.G.; Kriketos, A. & George, J. (2004). Beyond insulin resistance in NASH: TNF-alpha or adiponectin? *Hepatology,* Vol.40, No.1, pp. 46-54, ISSN 0270-9139.

Kato, H.; Kashiwagi, H.; Shiraga, M.; Tadokoro, S.; Kamae, T.; Ujiie, H.; Honda, S.; Miyata, S.; Ijiri, Y.; Yamamoto, J.; Maeda, N.; Funahashi, T.; Kurata, Y.; Shimomura, I.; Tomiyama, Y. & Kanakura, Y. (2006). Adiponectin acts as an endogenous antithrombotic factor. *Arteriosclerosis, thrombosis, and vascular biology,* Vol.26, No.1, pp. 224-30, ISSN 1524-4636.

Keber, R.; Motaln, H.; Wagner, K.D.; Debeljak, N.; Rassoulzadegan, M.; Acimovic, J.; Rozman, D. & Horvat, S. (2011). Mouse knockout of the cholesterogenic cytochrome P450 lanosterol 14{alpha}-Demethylase (CYP51) resembles Antley-Bixler syndrome. *The Journal of biological chemistry,* ISSN 0021-9258

Kessler, A.; Levy, Y.; Roth, A.; Zelber-Sagi, S.; Leshno, M.; Blendis, L.; Halpern, Z. & Oren, R. (2005). Increased prevalence of NAFLD in patients with acute myocardial infarction independent of BMI. *Hepatology,* Vol.42, No.4, pp. 623a, ISSN 0270-9139.

Kim, J.K.; Fillmore, J.J.; Chen, Y.; Yu, C.; Moore, I.K.; Pypaert, M.; Lutz, E.P.; Kako, Y.; Velez-Carrasco, W.; Goldberg, I.J.; Breslow, J.L. & Shulman, G.I. (2001). Tissue-specific overexpression of lipoprotein lipase causes tissue-specific insulin resistance. *Proceedings of the National Academy of Sciences of the United States of America,* Vol.98, No.13, pp. 7522-7, ISSN 0027-8424.

Kleiner, D.E.; Brunt, E.M.; Van Natta, M.; Behling, C.; Contos, M.J.; Cummings, O.W.; Ferrell, L.D.; Liu, Y.C.; Torbenson, M.S.; Unalp-Arida, A.; Yeh, M.; McCullough, A.J. & Sanyal, A.J. (2005). Design and validation of a histological scoring system for nonalcoholic fatty liver disease. *Hepatology,* Vol.41, No.6, pp. 1313-21, ISSN 0270-9139.

Kohjima, M.; Higuchi, N.; Kato, M.; Kotoh, K.; Yoshimoto, T.; Fujino, T.; Yada, M.; Yada, R.; Harada, N.; Enjoji, M.; Takayanagi, R. & Nakamuta, M. (2008). SREBP-1c, regulated by the insulin and AMPK signaling pathways, plays a role in nonalcoholic fatty liver disease. *International journal of molecular medicine,* Vol.21, No.4, pp. 507-11, ISSN 1107-3756.

Larter, C.Z. & Yeh, M.M. (2008). Animal models of NASH: getting both pathology and metabolic context right. *Journal of gastroenterology and hepatology,* Vol.23, No.11, pp. 1635-48, ISSN 1440-1746.

Lee, D.S.; Evans, J.C.; Robins, S.J.; Wilson, P.W.; Albano, I.; Fox, C.S.; Wang, T.J.; Benjamin, E.J.; D'Agostino, R.B. & Vasan, R.S. (2007). Gamma glutamyl transferase and metabolic syndrome, cardiovascular disease, and mortality risk: the Framingham Heart Study. *Arteriosclerosis, thrombosis, and vascular biology,* Vol.27, No.1, pp. 127-33, ISSN 1524-4636.

Lee, R.G. (1995). Nonalcoholic Steatohepatitis - Tightening the Morphological Screws on a Hepatic Rambler. *Hepatology,* Vol.21, No.6, pp. 1742-1743, ISSN 0270-9139.

Lefebvre, A.M.; Laville, M.; Vega, N.; Riou, J.P.; van Gaal, L.; Auwerx, J. & Vidal, H. (1998). Depot-specific differences in adipose tissue gene expression in lean and obese subjects. *Diabetes,* Vol.47, No.1, pp. 98-103, ISSN 0012-1797.

Lin, Y.C.; Lo, H.M. & Chen, J.D. (2005). Sonographic fatty liver, overweight and ischemic heart disease. *World journal of gastroenterology : WJG,* Vol.11, No.31, pp. 4838-42, ISSN 1007-9327.

Lord, G. (2002). Role of leptin in immunology. *Nutrition reviews,* Vol.60, No.10 Pt 2, pp. S35-8; discussion S68-84, 85-7, ISSN 0029-6643.

Loria, P.; Lonardo, A. & Targher, G. (2008). Is liver fat detrimental to vessels?: intersections in the pathogenesis of NAFLD and atherosclerosis. *Clinical science,* Vol.115, No.1, pp. 1-12, ISSN 1470-8736.

Ludwig, J.; Viggiano, T.R.; McGill, D.B. & Oh, B.J. (1980). Nonalcoholic steatohepatitis: Mayo Clinic experiences with a hitherto unnamed disease. *Mayo Clinic proceedings. Mayo Clinic,* Vol.55, No.7, pp. 434-8, ISSN 0025-6196.

Machado, M.; Marques-Vidal, P. & Cortez-Pinto, H. (2006). Hepatic histology in obese patients undergoing bariatric surgery. *Journal of hepatology,* Vol.45, No.4, pp. 600-6, ISSN 0168-8278.

Malhi, H.; Bronk, S.F.; Werneburg, N.W. & Gores, G.J. (2006). Free fatty acids induce JNK-dependent hepatocyte lipoapoptosis. *The Journal of biological chemistry,* Vol.281, No.17, pp. 12093-101, ISSN 0021-9258.

Mantzoros, C.S. (1999). The role of leptin in human obesity and disease: a review of current evidence. *Annals of internal medicine,* Vol.130, No.8, pp. 671-80, ISSN 0003-4819.

Marchesini, G.; Brizi, M.; Morselli-Labate, A.M.; Bianchi, G.; Bugianesi, E.; McCullough, A.J.; Forlani, G. & Melchionda, N. (1999). Association of nonalcoholic fatty liver disease with insulin resistance. *The American journal of medicine,* Vol.107, No.5, pp. 450-5, ISSN 0002-9343.

Marchesini, G. & Bugianesi, E. (2005). NASH as part of the metabolic (insulin resistance) syndrome, In: *Fatty Liver Disease: NASH and Related Disorders*, G. C. Farrell, J. George, P. M. Hall and A. J. McCullough, pp. 55-65, Blackwell Publishing, ISBN 1-4051-1292-1, USA.

Marchesini, G.; Marzocchi, R.; Agostini, F. & Bugianesi, E. (2005). Nonalcoholic fatty liver disease and the metabolic syndrome. *Current opinion in lipidology,* Vol.16, No.4, pp. 421-7, ISSN 0957-9672.

Mari, M.; Caballero, F.; Colell, A.; Morales, A.; Caballeria, J.; Fernandez, A.; Enrich, C.; Fernandez-Checa, J.C. & Garcia-Ruiz, C. (2006). Mitochondrial free cholesterol loading sensitizes to TNF- and Fas-mediated steatohepatitis. *Cell metabolism,* Vol.4, No.3, pp. 185-98, ISSN 1550-4131.

Marrero, J.A.; Fontana, R.J.; Su, G.L.; Conjeevaram, H.S.; Emick, D.M. & Lok, A.S. (2002). NAFLD may be a common underlying liver disease in patients with hepatocellular carcinoma in the United States. *Hepatology,* Vol.36, No.6, pp. 1349-54, ISSN 0270-9139.

Massiera, F.; Bloch-Faure, M.; Ceiler, D.; Murakami, K.; Fukamizu, A.; Gasc, J.M.; Quignard-Boulange, A.; Negrel, R.; Ailhaud, G.; Seydoux, J.; Meneton, P. & Teboul, M. (2001). Adipose angiotensinogen is involved in adipose tissue growth and blood pressure regulation. *The FASEB journal : official publication of the Federation of American Societies for Experimental Biology,* Vol.15, No.14, pp. 2727-9, ISSN 1530-6860.

Matteoni, C.A.; Younossi, Z.M.; Gramlich, T.; Boparai, N.; Liu, Y.C. & McCullough, A.J. (1999). Nonalcoholic fatty liver disease: a spectrum of clinical and pathological severity. *Gastroenterology,* Vol.116, No.6, pp. 1413-9, ISSN 0016-5085.

McCullough, A.J. (2005). The epidemiology and risk factors of NASH, In: *Fatty Liver Disease: NASH and Related Disorders,* G. C. Farrell, J. George, P. M. Hall and A. J. McCullough, pp. 23-37, Blackwell Publishing, ISBN 1-4051-1292-1, USA.

Miettinen, T.A. & Gylling, H. (2000). Cholesterol absorption efficiency and sterol metabolism in obesity. *Atherosclerosis,* Vol.153, No.1, pp. 241-8, ISSN 0021-9150.

Musso, G.; Gambino, R. & Cassader, M. (2010). Non-alcoholic fatty liver disease from pathogenesis to management: an update. *Obesity reviews : an official journal of the International Association for the Study of Obesity,* Vol.11, No.6, pp. 430-45, ISSN 1467-789X.

Mylonas, C. & Kouretas, D. (1999). Lipid peroxidation and tissue damage. *In vivo,* Vol.13, No.3, pp. 295-309, ISSN 0258-851X.

Nakamuta, M.; Fujino, T.; Yada, R.; Yada, M.; Yasutake, K.; Yoshimoto, T.; Harada, N.; Higuchi, N.; Kato, M.; Kohjima, M.; Taketomi, A.; Maehara, Y.; Nakashima, M.; Kotoh, K. & Enjoji, M. (2009). Impact of cholesterol metabolism and the LXRalpha-SREBP-1c pathway on nonalcoholic fatty liver disease. *International journal of molecular medicine,* Vol.23, No.5, pp. 603-8, ISSN 1107-3756.

Nakao, H. & Yoneda, M. (2009). The intertwisted correlations among non-alcoholic fatty liver disease, atherosclerosis, and metabolic syndrome. *Journal of gastroenterology,* Vol.44, No.11, pp. 1162-4, ISSN 1435-5922.

Nguyen, N.; Glanz, D. & Glaesser, D. (2000). Fatty acid cytotoxicity to bovine lens epithelial cells: investigations on cell viability, ecto-ATPase, Na(+), K(+)-ATPase and intracellular sodium concentrations. *Experimental eye research,* Vol.71, No.4, pp. 405-13, ISSN 0014-4835.

Nieto, N. (2006). Oxidative-stress and IL-6 mediate the fibrogenic effects of [corrected] Kupffer cells on stellate cells. *Hepatology,* Vol.44, No.6, pp. 1487-501, ISSN 0270-9139.

O'Leary, D.H. & Polak, J.F. (2002). Intima-media thickness: a tool for atherosclerosis imaging and event prediction. *The American journal of cardiology,* Vol.90, No.10C, pp. 18L-21L, ISSN 0002-9149.

Pacifico, L.; Poggiogalle, E.; Cantisani, V.; Menichini, G.; Ricci, P.; Ferraro, F. & Chiesa, C. (2010). Pediatric nonalcoholic fatty liver disease: A clinical and laboratory challenge. *World journal of hepatology,* Vol.2, No.7, pp. 275-88, ISSN 1948-5182.

Palmer, M. & Schaffner, F. (1990). Effect of weight reduction on hepatic abnormalities in overweight patients. *Gastroenterology,* Vol.99, No.5, pp. 1408-13, ISSN 0016-5085.

Pandey, A.K.; Bhardwaj, V. & Datta, M. (2009). Tumour necrosis factor-alpha attenuates insulin action on phosphoenolpyruvate carboxykinase gene expression and gluconeogenesis by altering the cellular localization of Foxa2 in HepG2 cells. *The FEBS journal,* Vol.276, No.14, pp. 3757-69, ISSN 1742-4658.

Pihlajamaki, J.; Gylling, H.; Miettinen, T.A. & Laakso, M. (2004). Insulin resistance is associated with increased cholesterol synthesis and decreased cholesterol absorption in normoglycemic men. *Journal of Lipid Research,* Vol.45, No.3, pp. 507-12, ISSN 0022-2275.

Polyzos, S.A.; Kountouras, J.; Zavos, C. & Tsiaousi, E. (2010). The role of adiponectin in the pathogenesis and treatment of non-alcoholic fatty liver disease. *Diabetes, obesity & metabolism,* Vol.12, No.5, pp. 365-83, ISSN 1463-1326.

Portincasa, P.; Grattagliano, I.; Palmieri, V.O. & Palasciano, G. (2005). The emerging problem of nonalcoholic steatohepatitis (NASH). *Romanian journal of gastroenterology,* Vol.14, No.1, pp. 43-51, ISSN 1221-4167.

Postic, C. & Girard, J. (2008). The role of the lipogenic pathway in the development of hepatic steatosis. *Diabetes & metabolism,* Vol.34, No.6 Pt 2, pp. 643-8, ISSN 1262-3636.

Poynard, T.; Ratziu, V.; Charlotte, F.; Messous, D.; Munteanu, M.; Imbert-Bismut, F.; Massard, J.; Bonyhay, L.; Tahiri, M.; Thabut, D.; Cadranel, J.F.; Le Bail, B. & de Ledinghen, V. (2006). Diagnostic value of biochemical markers (NashTest) for the prediction of non alcoholo steato hepatitis in patients with non-alcoholic fatty liver disease. *BMC gastroenterology,* Vol.6, 34, ISSN 1471-230X.

Reunanen, A.; Miettinen, T.A. & Nikkila, E.A. (1969). Quantitative lipid analysis of human liver needle biopsy specimens. *Acta medica Scandinavica,* Vol.186, No.3, pp. 149-50, ISSN 0001-6101.

Ridker, P.M.; Rifai, N.; Pfeffer, M.; Sacks, F.; Lepage, S. & Braunwald, E. (2000). Elevation of tumor necrosis factor-alpha and increased risk of recurrent coronary events after myocardial infarction. *Circulation,* Vol.101, No.18, pp. 2149-53, ISSN 1524-4539.

Ridker, P.M.; Rifai, N.; Stampfer, M.J. & Hennekens, C.H. (2000). Plasma concentration of interleukin-6 and the risk of future myocardial infarction among apparently healthy men. *Circulation,* Vol.101, No.15, pp. 1767-72, ISSN 1524-4539.

Ron, D. (2002). Translational control in the endoplasmic reticulum stress response. *The Journal of clinical investigation,* Vol.110, No.10, pp. 1383-8, ISSN 0021-9738.

Roskams, T.; Yang, S.Q.; Koteish, A.; Durnez, A.; DeVos, R.; Huang, X.; Achten, R.; Verslype, C. & Diehl, A.M. (2003). Oxidative stress and oval cell accumulation in mice and humans with alcoholic and nonalcoholic fatty liver disease. *The American journal of pathology,* Vol.163, No.4, pp. 1301-11, ISSN 0002-9440.

Ross, R. (1999). Atherosclerosis--an inflammatory disease. *The New England journal of medicine,* Vol.340, No.2, pp. 115-26, ISSN 0028-4793.

Rozman, D. & Monostory, K. (2010). Perspectives of the non-statin hypolipidemic agents. *Pharmacology & therapeutics,* Vol.127, No.1, pp. 19-40, ISSN 1879-016X.

Saadeh, S.; Younossi, Z.M.; Remer, E.M.; Gramlich, T.; Ong, J.P.; Hurley, M.; Mullen, K.D.; Cooper, J.N. & Sheridan, M.J. (2002). The utility of radiological imaging in nonalcoholic fatty liver disease. *Gastroenterology,* Vol.123, No.3, pp. 745-50, ISSN 0016-5085.

Samuel, V.T. & Shulman, G.I. (2005). Insulin resistance in NAFLD: potential mechanisms and therapies, In: *Fatty Liver Disease: NASH and Related Disorders,* G. C. Farrell, J. George, P. M. Hall and A. J. McCullough, pp. 38-54, Blackwell Publishing, ISBN 1-4051-1292-1, USA.

Sanyal, A.J.; Campbell-Sargent, C.; Mirshahi, F.; Rizzo, W.B.; Contos, M.J.; Sterling, R.K.; Luketic, V.A.; Shiffman, M.L. & Clore, J.N. (2001). Nonalcoholic steatohepatitis: association of insulin resistance and mitochondrial abnormalities. *Gastroenterology,* Vol.120, No.5, pp. 1183-92, ISSN 0016-5085.

Saxena, N.K.; Ikeda, K.; Rockey, D.C.; Friedman, S.L. & Anania, F.A. (2002). Leptin in hepatic fibrosis: evidence for increased collagen production in stellate cells and lean littermates of ob/ob mice. *Hepatology,* Vol.35, No.4, pp. 762-71, ISSN 0270-9139.

Schindhelm, R.K.; Dekker, J.M.; Nijpels, G.; Bouter, L.M.; Stehouwer, C.D.; Heine, R.J. & Diamant, M. (2007). Alanine aminotransferase predicts coronary heart disease events: a 10-year follow-up of the Hoorn Study. *Atherosclerosis*, Vol.191, No.2, pp. 391-6, ISSN 0021-9150.

Schonfeld, P.; Wieckowski, M.R. & Wojtczak, L. (2000). Long-chain fatty acid-promoted swelling of mitochondria: further evidence for the protonophoric effect of fatty acids in the inner mitochondrial membrane. *FEBS letters*, Vol.471, No.1, pp. 108-12, ISSN 0014-5793.

Schwimmer, J.B.; Deutsch, R.; Behling, C. & Lavine, J.E. (2005). Fatty liver as a determinant of atherosclerosis. *Hepatology*, Vol.42, No.4, pp. 610a, ISSN 0270-9139.

Sherman, M.L.; Spriggs, D.R.; Arthur, K.A.; Imamura, K.; Frei, E., 3rd & Kufe, D.W. (1988). Recombinant human tumor necrosis factor administered as a five-day continuous infusion in cancer patients: phase I toxicity and effects on lipid metabolism. *Journal of clinical oncology : official journal of the American Society of Clinical Oncology*, Vol.6, No.2, pp. 344-50, ISSN 0732-183X.

Shoelson, S.E.; Herrero, L. & Naaz, A. (2007). Obesity, inflammation, and insulin resistance. *Gastroenterology*, Vol.132, No.6, pp. 2169-80, ISSN 0016-5085.

Silventoinen, K.; Magnusson, P.K.; Neovius, M.; Sundstrom, J.; Batty, G.D.; Tynelius, P. & Rasmussen, F. (2008). Does obesity modify the effect of blood pressure on the risk of cardiovascular disease? A population-based cohort study of more than one million Swedish men. *Circulation*, Vol.118, No.16, pp. 1637-42, ISSN 1524-4539.

Simonen, P.; Kotronen, A.; Hallikainen, M.; Sevastianova, K.; Makkonen, J.; Hakkarainen, A.; Lundbom, N.; Miettinen, T.A.; Gylling, H. & Yki-Jarvinen, H. (2011). Cholesterol synthesis is increased and absorption decreased in non-alcoholic fatty liver disease independent of obesity. *Journal of hepatology*, Vol.54, No.1, pp. 153-9, ISSN 0168-8278.

Simonen, P.P.; Gylling, H.K. & Miettinen, T.A. (2002). Diabetes contributes to cholesterol metabolism regardless of obesity. *Diabetes care*, Vol.25, No.9, pp. 1511-5, ISSN 0149-5992.

Sookoian, S. & Pirola, C.J. (2008). Non-alcoholic fatty liver disease is strongly associated with carotid atherosclerosis: a systematic review. *Journal of hepatology*, Vol.49, No.4, pp. 600-7, ISSN 0168-8278.

Sparks, J.D. & Sparks, C.E. (1990). Insulin modulation of hepatic synthesis and secretion of apolipoprotein B by rat hepatocytes. *The Journal of biological chemistry*, Vol.265, No.15, pp. 8854-62, ISSN 0021-9258.

Stapleton, P.A.; Goodwill, A.G.; James, M.E.; Brock, R.W. & Frisbee, J.C. (2010). Hypercholesterolemia and microvascular dysfunction: interventional strategies. *Journal of inflammation*, Vol.7, 54, ISSN 1476-9255.

Sugino, I.; Kuboki, K.; Matsumoto, T.; Murakami, E.; Nishimura, C. & Yoshino, G. (2011). Influence of fatty liver on plasma small, dense LDL- cholesterol in subjects with and without metabolic syndrome. *Journal of atherosclerosis and thrombosis*, Vol.18, No.1, pp. 1-7, ISSN 1880-3873.

Svegliati-Baroni, G.; De Minicis, S. & Marzioni, M. (2008). Hepatic fibrogenesis in response to chronic liver injury: novel insights on the role of cell-to-cell interaction and transition. *Liver international : official journal of the International Association for the Study of the Liver*, Vol.28, No.8, pp. 1052-64, ISSN 1478-3231.

Syn, W.K.; Choi, S.S. & Diehl, A.M. (2009). Apoptosis and cytokines in non-alcoholic steatohepatitis. *Clinics in liver disease*, Vol.13, No.4, pp. 565-80, ISSN 1557-8224.

Tang, D.G.; La, E.; Kern, J. & Kehrer, J.P. (2002). Fatty acid oxidation and signaling in apoptosis. *Biological chemistry*, Vol.383, No.3-4, pp. 425-42, ISSN 1431-6730.

Targher, G. (2007). Non-alcoholic fatty liver disease, the metabolic syndrome and the risk of cardiovascular disease: the plot thickens. *Diabetic Medicine*, Vol.24, No.1, pp. 1-6, ISSN 0742-3071.

Targher, G. & Arcaro, G. (2007). Non-alcoholic fatty liver disease and increased risk of cardiovascular disease. *Atherosclerosis*, Vol.191, No.2, pp. 235-40, ISSN 0021-9150.

Targher, G.; Bertolini, L.; Padovani, R.; Rodella, S.; Zoppini, G.; Zenari, L.; Cigolini, M.; Falezza, G. & Arcaro, G. (2006). Relations between carotid artery wall thickness and liver histology in subjects with nonalcoholic fatty liver disease. *Diabetes care*, Vol.29, No.6, pp. 1325-30, ISSN 0149-5992.

Targher, G.; Bertolini, L.; Rodella, S.; Zoppini, G.; Scala, L.; Zenari, L. & Falezza, G. (2006). Associations between plasma adiponectin concentrations and liver histology in patients with nonalcoholic fatty liver disease. *Clinical endocrinology*, Vol.64, No.6, pp. 679-83, ISSN 0300-0664.

Targher, G.; Marra, F. & Marchesini, G. (2008). Increased risk of cardiovascular disease in non-alcoholic fatty liver disease: causal effect or epiphenomenon? *Diabetologia*, Vol.51, No.11, pp. 1947-53, ISSN 0012-186X.

Toledo, F.G.; Sniderman, A.D. & Kelley, D.E. (2006). Influence of hepatic steatosis (fatty liver) on severity and composition of dyslipidemia in type 2 diabetes. *Diabetes care*, Vol.29, No.8, pp. 1845-50, ISSN 0149-5992.

Treeprasertsuk, S.; Lopez-Jimenez, F. & Lindor, K.D. (2011). Nonalcoholic fatty liver disease and the coronary artery disease. *Digestive diseases and sciences*, Vol.56, No.1, pp. 35-45, ISSN 1573-2568.

Ueno, T.; Sugawara, H.; Sujaku, K.; Hashimoto, O.; Tsuji, R.; Tamaki, S.; Torimura, T.; Inuzuka, S.; Sata, M. & Tanikawa, K. (1997). Therapeutic effects of restricted diet and exercise in obese patients with fatty liver. *Journal of hepatology*, Vol.27, No.1, pp. 103-7, ISSN 0168-8278.

Uygun, A.; Kadayifci, A.; Yesilova, Z.; Erdil, A.; Yaman, H.; Saka, M.; Deveci, M.S.; Bagci, S.; Gulsen, M.; Karaeren, N. & Dagalp, K. (2000). Serum leptin levels in patients with nonalcoholic steatohepatitis. *The American journal of gastroenterology*, Vol.95, No.12, pp. 3584-9, ISSN 0002-9270.

van der Poorten, D.; Milner, K.L.; Hui, J.; Hodge, A.; Trenell, M.I.; Kench, J.G.; London, R.; Peduto, T.; Chisholm, D.J. & George, J. (2008). Visceral fat: a key mediator of steatohepatitis in metabolic liver disease. *Hepatology*, Vol.48, No.2, pp. 449-57, ISSN 1527-3350.

Van Hul, N.K.; Abarca-Quinones, J.; Sempoux, C.; Horsmans, Y. & Leclercq, I.A. (2009). Relation between liver progenitor cell expansion and extracellular matrix deposition in a CDE-induced murine model of chronic liver injury. *Hepatology*, Vol.49, No.5, pp. 1625-35, ISSN 1527-3350.

Villanova, N.; Moscatiello, S.; Ramilli, S.; Bugianesi, E.; Magalotti, D.; Vanni, E.; Zoli, M. & Marchesini, G. (2005). Endothelial dysfunction and cardiovascular risk profile in nonalcoholic fatty liver disease. *Hepatology*, Vol.42, No.2, pp. 473-80, ISSN 0270-9139.

Wang, D.; Wei, Y. & Pagliassotti, M.J. (2006). Saturated fatty acids promote endoplasmic reticulum stress and liver injury in rats with hepatic steatosis. *Endocrinology*, Vol.147, No.2, pp. 943-51, ISSN 0013-7227.

Wannamethee, G.; Ebrahim, S. & Shaper, A.G. (1995). Gamma-glutamyltransferase: determinants and association with mortality from ischemic heart disease and all causes. *American journal of epidemiology*, Vol.142, No.7, pp. 699-708, ISSN 0002-9262.

Weltman, M.D.; Farrell, G.C.; Hall, P.; Ingelman-Sundberg, M. & Liddle, C. (1998). Hepatic cytochrome P450 2E1 is increased in patients with nonalcoholic steatohepatitis. *Hepatology*, Vol.27, No.1, pp. 128-33, ISSN 0270-9139.

Whitehead, J.P.; Richards, A.A.; Hickman, I.J.; Macdonald, G.A. & Prins, J.B. (2006). Adiponectin--a key adipokine in the metabolic syndrome. *Diabetes, obesity & metabolism*, Vol.8, No.3, pp. 264-80, ISSN 1462-8902.

Wieckowska, A.; Papouchado, B.G.; Li, Z.; Lopez, R.; Zein, N.N. & Feldstein, A.E. (2008). Increased hepatic and circulating interleukin-6 levels in human nonalcoholic steatohepatitis. *The American journal of gastroenterology*, Vol.103, No.6, pp. 1372-9, ISSN 1572-0241.

Witek, R.P.; Stone, W.C.; Karaca, F.G.; Syn, W.K.; Pereira, T.A.; Agboola, K.M.; Omenetti, A.; Jung, Y.; Teaberry, V.; Choi, S.S.; Guy, C.D.; Pollard, J.; Charlton, P. & Diehl, A.M. (2009). Pan-caspase inhibitor VX-166 reduces fibrosis in an animal model of nonalcoholic steatohepatitis. *Hepatology*, Vol.50, No.5, pp. 1421-30, ISSN 1527-3350.

Wouters, K.; van Gorp, P.J.; Bieghs, V.; Gijbels, M.J.; Duimel, H.; Lutjohann, D.; Kerksiek, A.; van Kruchten, R.; Maeda, N.; Staels, B.; van Bilsen, M.; Shiri-Sverdlov, R. & Hofker, M.H. (2008). Dietary cholesterol, rather than liver steatosis, leads to hepatic inflammation in hyperlipidemic mouse models of nonalcoholic steatohepatitis. *Hepatology*, Vol.48, No.2, pp. 474-86, ISSN 1527-3350.

Xia, J.L.; Dai, C.; Michalopoulos, G.K. & Liu, Y. (2006). Hepatocyte growth factor attenuates liver fibrosis induced by bile duct ligation. *The American journal of pathology*, Vol.168, No.5, pp. 1500-12, ISSN 0002-9440.

Yamaguchi, K.; Yang, L.; McCall, S.; Huang, J.; Yu, X.X.; Pandey, S.K.; Bhanot, S.; Monia, B.P.; Li, Y.X. & Diehl, A.M. (2007). Inhibiting triglyceride synthesis improves hepatic steatosis but exacerbates liver damage and fibrosis in obese mice with nonalcoholic steatohepatitis. *Hepatology*, Vol.45, No.6, pp. 1366-74, ISSN 0270-9139.

Yerian, L. (2011). Histopathological evaluation of fatty and alcoholic liver diseases. *Journal of digestive diseases*, Vol.12, No.1, pp. 17-24, ISSN 1751-2980.

Younossi, Z.M.; Baranova, A.; Ziegler, K.; Del Giacco, L.; Schlauch, K.; Born, T.L.; Elariny, H.; Gorreta, F.; VanMeter, A.; Younoszai, A.; Ong, J.P.; Goodman, Z. & Chandhoke, V. (2005). A genomic and proteomic study of the spectrum of nonalcoholic fatty liver disease. *Hepatology*, Vol.42, No.3, pp. 665-74, ISSN 0270-9139.

Zoltowska, M.; Ziv, E.; Delvin, E.; Stan, S.; Bar-On, H.; Kalman, R. & Levy, E. (2001). Circulating lipoproteins and hepatic sterol metabolism in Psammomys obesus prone to obesity, hyperglycemia and hyperinsulinemia. *Atherosclerosis*, Vol.157, No.1, pp. 85-96, ISSN 0021-9150.

14

# Macrophage Cholesterol Homeostasis and Atherogenesis: Critical Role of Intracellular Cholesteryl Ester Hydrolysis

Shobha Ghosh
*Virginia Commonwealth University Medical Center*
*USA*

## 1. Introduction

Coronary artery disease (CAD) is the leading cause of death in United States and contributes to significant mortality around the world. According to the Heart Disease and Stroke 2011 update, released by the American Heart Association, 82,600,000 American adults (>1 in 3) have 1 or more type of cardiovascular disease and >2200 Americans die of CAD every day which is an average of 1 in every 39 seconds. These are alarming statistics and underscore the importance of continued understanding of the processes involved in the development of CAD. Atherosclerosis, characterized by increased lipid accumulation in the artery wall, is the major underlying cause of CAD.

Atherosclerosis is a chronic disease that often starts during early teens and progresses silently without any overt clinical symptoms till about age 40 when it manifests as heart attack or even stroke. While it is well established that accumulation of lipid-laden macrophage foam cells in the artery wall is the hall mark of atherosclerosis, two different theories are proposed to describe the events leading to infiltration of macrophages and subsequent development of foam cells within the artery wall. According to "response to injury" hypothesis, the initiating event is injury to the endothelial lining of the artery wall leading to the subsequent migration of monocytes and circulating lipoproteins mainly the low density lipoprotein (LDL) into the intimal space. This is followed by the unregulated uptake of modified LDL (mLDL) by monocyte derived macrophages leading to the formation of foam cells (Ross et al, 1977, Ross, 1993). "Response to retention" hypothesis, on the other hand, proposes that LDL migrates into the intimal space and is retained by association with the proteoglycans and is modified. Subsequent uptake by infiltrating macrophages results in development of foam cells (Williams and Tabas, 1995). Regardless of the sequence of events, the end result is accumulation of foam cells in the intimal space of the artery wall. This initiates the formation of fatty streaks which develops into an atherosclerotic plaque with continued accretion of foam cells. Figure 1 below summarizes these major events that lead to the formation of atherosclerotic plaque.

Continuous accumulation of lipid laden foam cells in an atherosclerotic plaque not only contributes to its volume but also enhances plaque associated inflammation and thus determines its vulnerability to rupture (Davies and Thomas, 1985). Therefore, reduction in the lipid core of the plaque is an obvious strategy to target reduction in plaque volume as well as enhance plaque stability. However, no therapies are currently available to reduce the lipid burden of atherosclerotic plaque. The presently used therapies for CAD include cholesterol lowering drugs such as statins that reduce plasma cholesterol by inhibiting the endogenous cholesterol synthesis. As a consequence, there is reduction in plasma LDL cholesterol levels which limits further foam cell formation and progression of atherosclerotic plaque. Nonetheless, these cholesterol lowering drugs do not increase removal of lipid from existing plaques and, therefore, cannot achieve plaque regression. Cleveland Clinic study by Nissen et al (Nissen et al, 2003) provided the first direct evidence of the clinical benefit of enhancing removal of cholesterol from macrophage foam cells. A detailed understanding of the cellular mechanisms that regulate lipid accumulation within macrophage foam cells and processes that are critical for mobilization of stored lipid is central to future development of targeted strategies to reduce atherosclerotic plaque burden with the aim to reduce CAD.

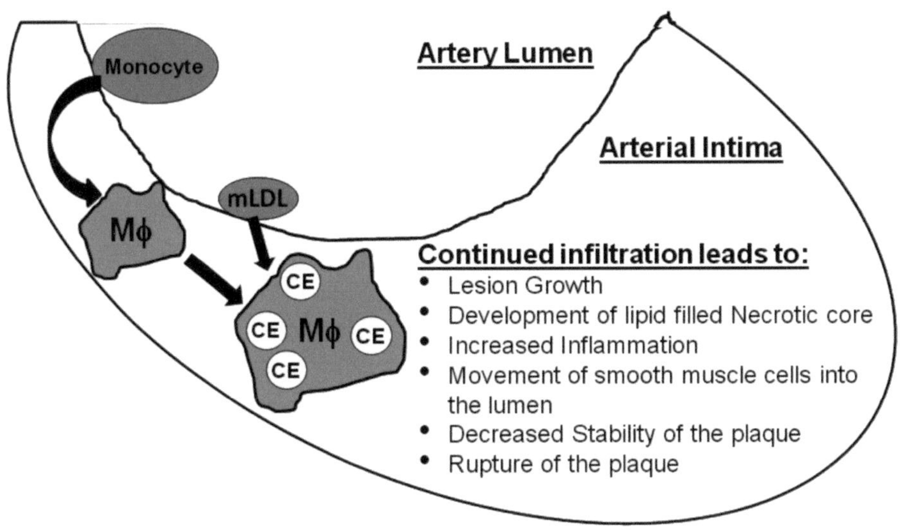


CE: Cholesteryl esters; Mϕ: macrophage; mLDL: modified LDL

Fig. 1. Schematic showing the events in the artery wall that lead to the formation of atherosclerotic plaque

## 2. Macrophage cholesterol homeostasis

Cholesterol homeostasis in macrophages and other peripheral cells is maintained by a balance between the influx and efflux processes. Cholesterol influx occurs by receptor and non-receptor mediated uptake of both normal and modified lipoproteins. The uptake of native LDL via the LDL receptor is regulated by the feedback inhibition of LDL receptor expression by cellular cholesterol levels and most peripheral cells limit their cholesterol uptake by this mechanism. Excess LDL returns to the liver where it is, once again, taken up via LDL receptor. Under conditions of increased dietary intake or increased endogenous synthesis of cholesterol, circulating LDL that cannot be taken by peripheral tissues or liver due to the inhibition of the expression of LDL receptor, becomes modified and is no longer a ligand for LDL receptor. Macrophages play a critical role in the removal of this modified

LDL. Macrophages express scavenger receptors, namely, scavenger receptor A (SR-A) and CD-36, that facilitate the uptake of modified LDL. Scavenger-receptor mediated uptake of modified LDL is largely unregulated and should be regarded as a mechanism that evolved to effectively clear modified lipoproteins from circulation and thus preventing the associated toxicity. Non-receptor mediated uptake pathways have recently been identified such as phagocytosis of aggregated LDL and macropinocytosis of native LDL that can also potentially contribute to lipid accumulation in macrophage foam cells. Cholesteryl esters (CE) associated with LDL are hydrolyzed in late endosomes/ lysosomes to free cholesterol (FC) which then traffics to and integrates into the plasma membrane. Excess membrane cholesterol and also a fraction of LDL-derived FC is transported to endoplasmic reticulum where it is re-esterified by acyl CoA:cholesterol acyltransferase-1 (ACAT1) and stored in cytoplasmic lipid droplets. While this re-esterification of cholesterol is initially beneficial to the cells in preventing the FC-associated cell toxicity, under conditions of unregulated or increased uptake of modified LDL, it leads to excessive accumulation of CE present as cytoplasmic lipid droplets giving the cells their characteristic "foamy" appearance. Cellular CE undergo constant cycle of hydrolysis and re-esterification (cholesteryl ester cycle) with a half life of 24h. Brown et al demonstrated for the first time that hydrolysis of stored CE is extra lysosomal and defined the "need" for a neutral cholesteryl ester hydrolase (CEH) (Brown et al, 1980) that can release FC from the lipid droplet associated CE which can either be re-esterified again by ACAT-1 or removed from the cells by extracellular acceptor-mediated cholesterol efflux. This acceptor mediated FC efflux is the major mechanism for the removal of cellular cholesterol. Efflux of FC occurs either by aqueous diffusion or via several transporters namely ATP binding cassette transporter A1 (ABCA1) and ABCG1. Bidirectional flux of FC also occurs through scavenger receptor BI (SR-BI). Since FC is extremely hydrophobic, its efflux from the cells is coupled to its association with specific extracellular acceptors. Macrophages secrete apolipoprotein E (ApoE) and it is believed that ApoE serves as the extracellular acceptor for FC that is effluxed via aqueous diffusion pathway. Serum albumin, present in the interstitial fluid, also serves as an important acceptor for FC effluxed via non-transporter mediated pathways. Apolipoprotein A1 that is synthesized in the liver and secreted as minimally lipidated particle containing small amount of phospholipids is the acceptor for FC effluxed via ABCA1. After acquiring some amount of FC, ApoA1 can no longer accept FC from ABCA1. Bulk of FC efflux occurs via ABCG1 and ApoA1 with some FC or high density lipoprotein (HDL) serve as the extracellular acceptor for this process. A small amount of FC is also converted into 27-hydroxycholesterol which can readily diffuse out of the cell and contribution of this pathway towards total FC removal from macrophages remains undefined. Figure 2 summarizes the various influx and efflux pathways involved in macrophage cholesterol homeostasis. Under normal physiological conditions a balance between these influx and efflux pathways maintains the levels of cellular cholesterol in macrophages and prevents foam cell formation. However, an imbalance between influx and efflux, occurring by either increased influx (under conditions with high levels of circulating LDL such as hypercholesterolemia) or decreased efflux (under conditions of aberrant cellular processes reducing FC availability for efflux or decreased levels of extracellular FC acceptors), cellular accumulation of CE containing lipid droplets increases resulting in the formation of foam cells and initiating atherogenesis. Improved understanding of these processes is, therefore, critical to developing new strategies to not only prevent foam cell formation but also to reduce CE burden of existing foam cells that may be associated with atherosclerotic lesions.

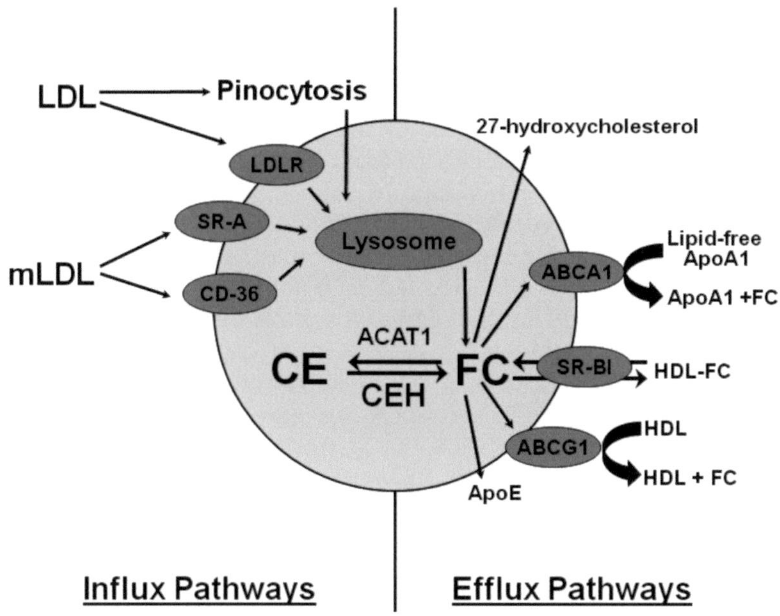


ABC: ATP binding cassette transporter; ACAT: Acyl-CoA cholesterol acyltransferase; ACEH: Acid cholesteryl ester hydrolase; ApoE: Apolipoprtoein E; CE: Cholesteryl ester; CEH: Cholesteryl ester hydrolase; FC: Free cholesterol; LDLR: LDL receptor; mLDL: Modified LDL; PL: Phospholipids; SR-A: Scavenger receptor type A; SR-BI: Scavenger receptor class B type I.

Fig. 2. Macrophage Cholesterol Homeostasis: Influx and Efflux Pathways

### 2.1 Cholesteryl ester accumulation

Cellular CEs exist in dynamic equilibrium with FC in a futile cholesteryl ester cycle with a half life of 24h. The two enzymes involved in this cycle are Acyl-CoA cholesterol acyltransferase (ACAT) and cholesteryl ester hydrolase (CEH). Two distinct genes have been identified for ACAT; ACAT1 is ubiquitously expressed in all cell types including macrophages and ACAT2 expression is restricted to liver and intestine. Since foam cells are characterized by accumulation of CE and ACAT1 is responsible for formation of CE, pharmacological inhibition of ACAT was initially pursued as a means to prevent or attenuate foam cell formation (Matsuda, 1994, Matsuo et al, 1995, Nicolosi et al, 1998, Sliskovic and White, 1991). However, increased plaque formation by preferential pharmacological inhibition of ACAT-1 was noted in mouse and rabbit models of atherosclerosis (Perrey et al, 2001). Ablation of ACAT1 gene resulted in marked systemic abnormalities in lipid homeostasis in hyper-cholesterolemic Apo-E deficient and LDL-receptor deficient mice, leading to extensive deposition of free cholesterol in skin and brain (Accad et al, 2000, Yagu et al, 2000). Further, ACAT1-deficient mice also displayed an increase in lesion area and the systemic lipid abnormalities. Inhibition or deficiency of ACAT1 also results in increased intracellular FC since it cannot be esterified to CE which is its inert and storage form. A rise in FC above its physiological concentration is associated with cellular toxicity (Glass and Witztum, 2001). Enrichment of the endoplasmic reticulum (ER) with FC induces ER stress leading to apoptosis. Therefore, although intuitively a logical strategy to limit cellular CE accumulation, inhibition or deficiency of ACAT1 has detrimental effects.

Alternatively, reduction in CEs stored in macrophage foam cells can also be achieved by enhancing mobilization. The first and the rate limiting step in cellular CE mobilization is CEH-mediated hydrolysis. Consistently, macrophages with high neutral CEH activity accumulate less cholesterol esters in the presence of atherogenic β-migrating very low-density lipoproteins (β-VLDL) in comparison to macrophages with low CEH activity (Ishii et al, 1992). Further, animal models of atherosclerosis, such as the hypercholesterolemic rabbit and the white Carneau pigeon, appear to possess macrophages in which stored cholesterol esters are resistant to hydrolysis and subsequent mobilization (Mathur et al, 1985, Yancey and St. Clair, 1994). While increased hydrolysis of CE will also lead to increase in FC but there is a fundamental difference between CEH activation and ACAT1 inhibition. Under conditions of ACAT1 inhibition, cellular FC has only one fate, namely, efflux to extracellular acceptors. However, FC generated as a result of CEH activation can either be re-esterified by ACAT1 or be effluxed to extracellular acceptor (two fates). Thus, CEH activation or over-expression does not result in an increase in cellular FC and is not associated with toxicity seen with ACAT1 inhibition indicating that CEH-mediated increase in cellular CE mobilization is a valid approach to target attenuation of foam cell formation (Ghosh et al, 2009).

### 2.2 Cholesteryl ester hydrolysis and cellular CE mobilization

Unregulated uptake of modified lipoproteins by macrophages can be regarded as a defence mechanism by which removal of these potentially toxic particles is facilitated. As discussed above, efflux of FC from macrophage foam cells is the major mechanism by which this CE accumulation can be reversed underscoring the importance of intracellular CE hydrolysis. Since the first description for the "need" of an extra lysosomal neutral CEH, several candidate enzymes have been identified as potential CE hydrolases in macrophages. Based on the observations that cAMP enhances FC efflux from macrophages and hormone sensitive lipase (HSL), an enzyme initially characterized from adipose tissue, requires protein kinase A and cAMP dependent activation, HSL was thought to be the likely candidate for macrophage CE hydrolysis (Goldberg and Khoo, 1990, Small et al, 1989). HSL is expressed in murine macrophages (Khoo et al, 1993) but its expression in human macrophages remains controversial (Johnson et al, 2000, Li and Hui, 1997, Reue et al 1997). Over-expression of HSL by transient transfection in murine macrophages led to increased mobilization of CE in the presence of an ACAT inhibitor (Escary et al 1998) but macrophage-specific transgenic expression of HSL led to a paradoxical increase in atherosclerosis and macrophages isolated from these mice stored 2-3 fold higher CE when incubated with AcLDL in vitro (Escary et al 1999). In addition, macrophages from HSL deficient mice did not have reduced CE mobilization suggestive of a limited, if any, role of HSL in macrophage CE mobilization. Since the effects of HSL deficiency on atherosclerosis have not been studied, it remains to be seen whether HSL plays a role in atherogenesis.

The second candidate enzyme speculated to play a role in macrophage CE mobilization was carboxyl ester lipase or CEL. CEL was first characterized from pancreas as a bile salt dependent cholesteryl esterase (Gallo, 1981, Kissel et al, 1989) that was also present in other tissues and was secreted in milk to facilitate digestion of CE in infants and newborns (Hui and Kissel, 1990). Li and Hui demonstrated the presence of CEL in human monocyte/macrophage cell line THP1 as well as primary blood derived monocyte macrophages and reported the absence of HSL in these cells (Li and Hui, 1997). However, since CEL is a secretory enzyme and it was thought to play a limited role in intracellular CE metabolism.

Pursuing the characterization of neutral CEH, we purified and cloned rat liver neutral cytosolic CEH which belonged to the carboxylesterase family and was distinctly different from HSL and CEL although it shared the same catalytic triad (Ghosh and Grogan, 1991, Ghosh et al, 1995). Using the strategy of homology cloning, we subsequently identified human macrophage CEH (Official gene symbol *CES1, Accession number NG_012057*) and demonstrated its expression in the THP1 human monocyte/macrophage cell line, as well as in human peripheral blood monocyte/macrophages (Ghosh, 2000). This enzyme associated with the surface of lipid droplets in lipid-laden cells (its physiological substrate) and hydrolyzed CE present in lipid droplets (Zhao et al, 2005). Over-expression of this enzyme resulted in mobilization of cellular CE (Ghosh et al, 2003) demonstrating its role in regulating cellular CE accumulation. Stable over-expression of this CEH in human monocyte/macrophage cell line, THP1, resulted in significantly higher FC efflux to ApoAI, HDL and serum demonstrating that FC released by CEH-mediated hydrolysis of intracellular CE is available for efflux by all known pathways (Zhao et al, 2007). Taken together, these data support the role of this enzyme in regulating macrophage CE content and FC efflux.

Stating the inability to measure CE hydrolytic activity associated with human CEH and its murine orthologue triglyceride lipase (TGL), Okazaki et al used a proteomics approach to identify another enzyme containing lipase consensus motifs and $\alpha/\beta$-hydrolase folds and reported the characterization of murine orthologue of AADACL1 (a deacetylase) also known as KIAA1363 (Okazaki et al, 2008). While its deficiency significantly reduced the deacetylase activity it did not affect CE hydrolase activity (Buchebner et al, 2010). These authors also found no difference in lipid droplet formation and cellular CE and FC content of HSL-deficient macrophages. Based on the data obtained with HSL and AADACL1 or KIAA1363 deficient macrophages, it can be concluded that macrophage CE hydrolysis is likely a multi-enzyme process. Considering the importance of CE hydrolysis in cellular CE mobilization, natural redundancy in enzymes capable of catalyzing this reaction is probably a protective mechanism evolved to prevent pathological consequences of lipid accumulation.

### 2.3 CEH and atherogenesis

Despite the apparent uncertainty surrounding the identity of macrophage CE hydrolase, the importance of this step in mobilization of CE and thereby attenuating atherosclerosis cannot be over-emphasized. The hypothesis that enhancing CE hydrolysis will reduce foam cell formation and consequently attenuate atherogenesis, was initially tested by development of HSL transgenic mice (Escary et al, 1999). Paradoxically, these mice had increased atherosclerosis and it was thought to be due to limiting levels of extra cellular acceptors. Subsequently, Choy et al developed ApoA IV and HSL double transgenics in C57BL/6 background and demonstrated a decrease in diet-induced atherosclerosis compared to HSL transgenics (Choy et al, 2003). HSL deficiency, however, did not have any effect on macrophage CE hydrolytic activity (Osuga et al, 2000) precluding its role in macrophage cholesterol homeostasis (Contreras, 2002) and no studies have been performed to date to directly assess the development of atherosclerosis in HSL deficient mice.

Since CEL expression was demonstrated in human macrophages, Kodvawala et al developed macrophage-specific CEL transgenic mice to evaluate the role of this CE hydrolase in the development of atherosclerosis (Kodvawala et al, 2005). In athero-susceptible ApoE-/- background, CEL transgenic mice displayed an approximate 4-fold higher atherosclerotic lesion area than ApoE(-/-) mice without the CEL transgene. It was speculated that perhaps its extracellular location or its hydrolysis of ceramide and lysophosphatidylcholine leads to increased cholesterol esterification and decreased cholesterol efflux resulting in increased atherosclerosis. Regardless of the underlying mechanisms, these studies demonstrate a minimal role for CEL in macrophage CE mobilization and thereby in atherogenesis.

To evaluate the role of CEH in foam cell formation and atherogenesis, we developed macrophage-specific CEH transgenic mice and crossed them into an atherosusceptible LDLR-/- background. High-fat high-cholesterol diet induced atherosclerosis was evaluated and we reported almost a 50% reduction in lesion area in LDLR-/-CEH transgenic mice compared to LDLR-/- mice (Zhao et al, 2007). In addition, CEH-mediated increase in CE mobilization also reduced total cholesterol and CE content of the lesions resulting in significantly reduced lesion necrosis. Consistent with our *in vitro* studies, macrophages from CEH transgenic mice showed higher FC efflux and decreased cellular CE levels upon loading with modified LDL. Over-expression of CEH in macrophages alone increased the process of reverse cholesterol transport and there was increased elimination of cholesterol in the feces of CEH transgenic mice (Zhao et al, 2007). The success in attenuating atherosclerosis and lesion necrosis by transgenic expression of CEH underscores the importance of the role of CE hydrolysis in atherogenesis. Transgenic mice over-expressing the newly identified CE hydrolase (AADACL1 or KIAA1363) have not yet been developed and the role of this enzyme in affecting atherogenesis remains to be evaluated.

### 2.4 CEH and elimination of cholesterol from the body

While hydrolysis of CE stored in macrophage represents the first step towards removal of FC from lesion associated foam cells, final removal of FC occurs from the liver either via direct secretion into bile or by conversion into bile acids, both of which are excreted in the feces. Figure 3 below summarizes the different steps involved in the movement of FC from macrophages to liver for final elimination, a process called Reverse Cholesterol Transport. FC effluxed from macrophages becomes associated with extracellular cholesterol acceptors and apolipoprotein A1 (ApoA1) is the major acceptor. Lipid free ApoA1 accepts FC transported via ABCA1 and this partially lipidated ApoA1 or nascent HDL (High density lipoprotein) then becomes the acceptor of FC transported via ABCG1. Bulk of FC efflux to HDL occurs via ABCG1 although bidirectional flux of FC also occurs through SR-BI. In the plasma compartment, FC in HDL particle is esterified by plasma Lecithin cholesterol acyltransferase (LCAT) and CE constitutes greater than 80% of total cholesterol carried by the HDL particle. In the liver, HDL binds to its receptor SR-BI and delivers its lipid "cargo", and lipid poor HDL is presumed to return into circulation to further serve as the extracellular cholesterol acceptor and facilitate removal of cholesterol from peripheral tissues including artery wall associated macrophage foam cells. This function of HDL is responsible for its alias "Good cholesterol" in contrast to LDL or "Bad cholesterol" that delivers cholesterol to the peripheral tissues and is responsible for CE accumulation in macrophages.

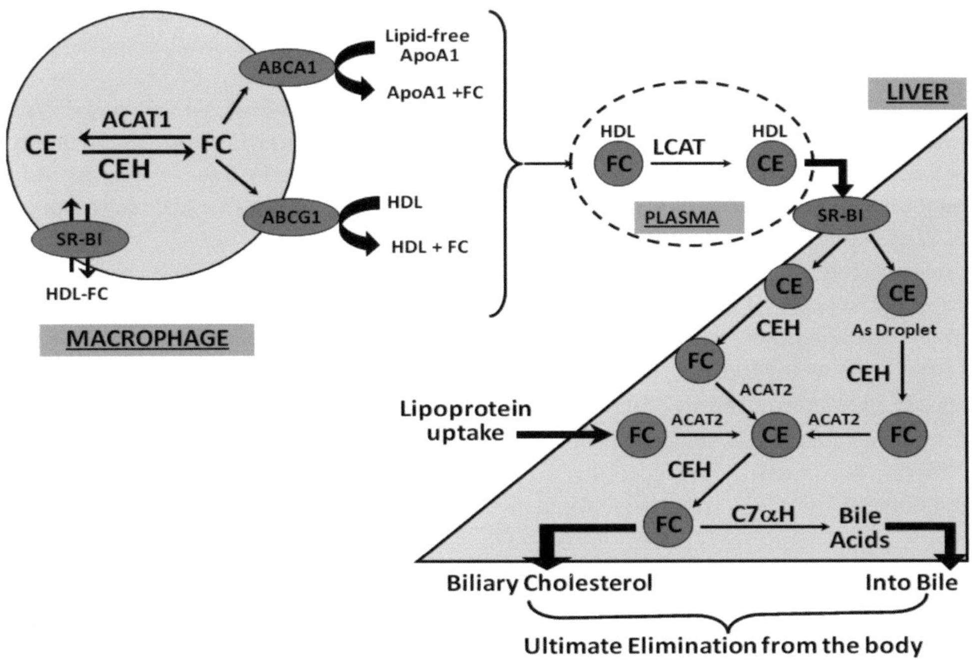


Fig. 3. Reverse Cholesterol Transport

FC delivered to the liver via SR-BI is believed to be directly secreted into bile (Kozarsky et al, 1997). On the other hand, for generation of FC, the HDL-delivered CE, once again, needs to be hydrolyzed underscoring the importance of CEH in hepatic CE metabolism. FC enters the hepatic metabolic pool where it is either re-esterified by ACAT2 (distinct from ACAT1 present in macrophages) or secreted into bile or converted into bile acids where the rate-limiting step is catalyzed by cholesterol 7α hydroxylase (C7αH). It should be emphasized that although humans and other mammals can synthesize cholesterol starting from acetate, they lack the enzymes required to degrade the steroid nucleus. Extremely hydrophobic cholesterol requires several modifications to increase its water solubility and to facilitate its excretion. Conversion of cholesterol to water soluble bile acids is one such mechanism which along with direct secretion of cholesterol in bile represents the major route of cholesterol elimination from the body.

### 2.4.1 Hepatic CE hydrolysis

Based on immunological cross reactivity and observed variations in CE hydrolytic activities in rat liver, Harrison speculated that hepatic CE hydrolytic activity is due to the uptake of pancreatic cholesterol esterase and that liver does not synthesize a similar enzyme (Harrison, 1988). This concept gained further support by the observed similarity between pancreatic and liver enzymes (Camulli, 1989, Chen 1997). However, we purified and characterized a rat hepatic CEH that was immunologically distinct from pancreatic CEH (Ghosh 1991). Molecular cloning of this rat liver CEH identified it as a member of the carboxylesterase family of enzymes (Ghosh et al., 1995). Biochemical, physiological and developmental characterization of this enzyme confirmed its role in regulating hepatic cholesterol homeostasis (Natarajan et al, 1996, 1998, Ghosh et al 1998). Homology cloning, based on this rat liver CEH, was used to identify the human macrophage CEH described above (Ghosh 2000). We also cloned CEH from human liver and demonstrated that, unlike ACAT, hepatic and macrophage CEH are products of the same gene *Ces1* (Zhao et al., 2005). To evaluate the role of hepatic CEH in regulating hepatic cholesterol metabolism, we over expressed CEH in mouse liver using adenovirus. Our data demonstrated a significant increase in bile acid secretion following adenovirus-mediated over-expression suggesting that CEH plays an important role in regulating this last step of RCT and enhances the elimination of cholesterol from the body (Zhao et al, 2008). To address the question whether enhancing CEH mediated CE hydrolysis in liver can increase in vivo RCT, we utilized "macrophage-to-feces" in vivo RCT model described by Zhang et al (Zhang et al, 2003). Adenovirus mediated over-expression of CEH led to a significant increase in the flux of cholesterol from macrophages to feces, predominantly in fecal bile acids (Zhao et al, 2008). These data demonstrate that increase in hepatic CEH alone can increase the flux of cholesterol from peripheral tissues such as macrophages to liver and ultimate elimination from the body into feces. Such enhanced elimination of cholesterol from the body should be potentially anti-atherogenic and to test the hypothesis that increase in hepatic CEH alone can reduce atherosclerosis, we have developed liver-specific CEH transgenic mice and studies are in progress to evaluate the effects on diet-induced atherosclerosis in these transgenic mice in an LDLR-/- background.

Initially HSL was thought be not expressed in liver (Holm et al, 1987), but re-evaluation of HSL-/- mice has provided some evidence that suggests that HSL might be expressed in liver and may contribute to CE hydrolysis in hepatocytes (Sekiya et al 2008, Fernandez et al 2008). However, to date, there are no reports of direct evaluation of HSL in regulating bile acid synthesis precluding the determination of its role in RCT and cholesterol elimination from the body. Expression of AADLAC1 or KIAA1363 is negligible in human and mouse liver and it is unlikely to play a significant role in either hepatic cholesterol homeostasis or in regulating the terminal step of RCT, namely hydrolysis of HDL-delivered CE.

### 2.5 Metabolic consequence of CE accumulation in macrophages

Intracellular accumulation of CE or cholesterol is considered to enhance the expression of pro-inflammatory mediators. Fazio and Linton proposed a feedback loop linking macrophage cholesterol balance and inflammatory mediators and suggested that a primary defect in cellular cholesterol balance may induce changes in the inflammatory status of the macrophage (Fazio and Linton 2001). Close relationship between macrophage cholesterol efflux and inflammation is also exemplified by attenuation of in vitro efflux and in vivo RCT by endotoxins (McGillicuddy et al 2009). In addition, pro-inflammatory cytokines such as IL-1$\beta$ and TNF$\alpha$ enhance lipid accumulation and foam cell formation by reducing lipid catabolism (Persson et al 2008). Consistently, under conditions of enhanced cholesterol accumulation, for example by deficiency of cholesterol transporter ABCA1, there was a marked increase in TNF-$\alpha$ secretion from macrophages (Koseki et al 2007) and increased inflammation with resulting loss in pancreatic beta cell function (Tang and Oram, 2009). It is also noteworthy that macrophages from ldlr-/-Abca1-/- mice with 80-fold increase in cellular CE content display an exaggerated inflammatory response (Francone et al, 2005). Thus, accumulation of CE in macrophages is likely to be central to the development of multiple metabolic disorders including atherogenesis, diabetes and hepatic steatosis (Figure 4).

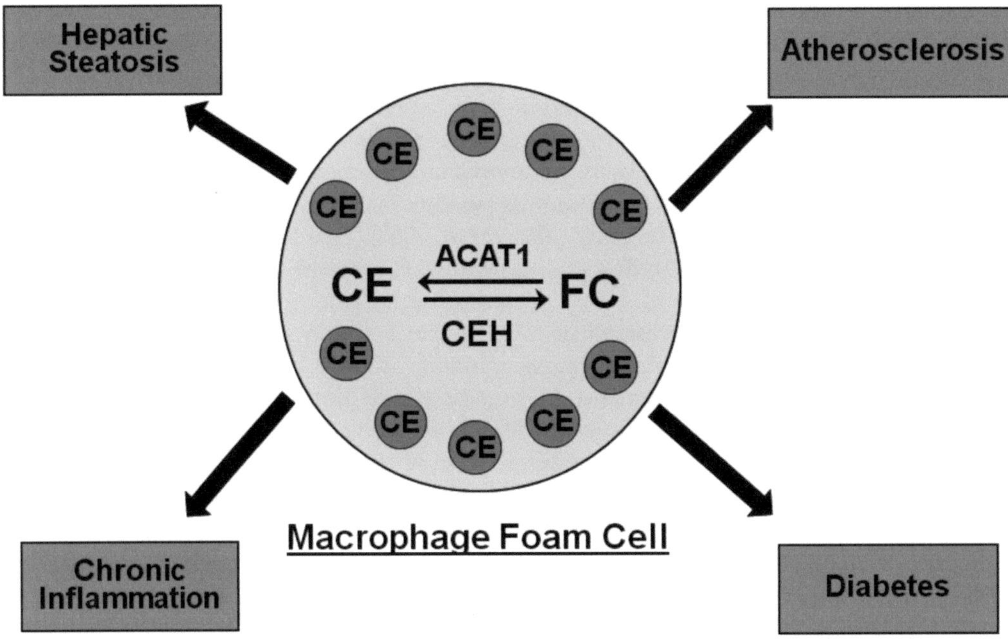


Fig. 4. Role of macrophage foam cell in regulating multiple metabolic disorders

### 2.5.1 CEH-mediated CE mobilization and inflammation

In contrast to CE accumulation, over-expression of ApoA1 that enhances CE removal and decreases cellular cholesterol levels results in attenuated response to pro-inflammatory insult by LPS (Levine et al 1993). Further, a recent clinical study demonstrated beneficial effects of re-constituted HDL infusions that enhance cholesterol efflux from cells on suppression of inflammation (Patel et al 2009) underscoring the importance of cholesterol removal in modulating inflammatory processes.

The observed decrease in lesion necrosis in CEH transgenic mice (Zhao et al 2007) was the first indication that CEH-mediated increase in macrophage CE mobilization is likely to be anti-inflammatory. We, therefore, directly examined the effects of CEH mediated hydrolysis of intracellular CE on reducing inflammation and inflammation-linked pathologies. Macrophage-specific transgenic expression of CEH significantly improved glucose tolerance and insulin sensitivity in LDLR-/- mice (Bie et al, 2010) demonstrating a critical role for CE mobilization in the development of insulin resistance and Type-2 diabetes mellitus (T2DM). Chronic low grade inflammation is increasingly being recognized as a key step in the pathogenesis of obesity-induced insulin resistance and T2DM and expanding adipose tissue was initially recognized as the site of production of pro-inflammatory mediators (Trayhurn and Wood 2004, Weiss 2004) responsible for this low grade inflammation. However, recent studies have demonstrated that majority of adipose tissue derived cytokines (TNF$\alpha$, IL-6 and IL-1$\beta$) actually originate in non-fat cells and among them, infiltrated macrophages play the most prominent role. This low-grade inflammation is mediated by the activation and recruitment of macrophages into the expanding adipose tissue (Bouloumié et al 2005). The level of macrophages within a tissue represents a balance between recruitment, survival/expansion and emigration which is facilitated by several chemokines and growth factors produced by adipocytes as well as infiltrated resident macrophages. These include monocyte chemoattracttant protein 1 (MCP-1) (Kanda et al, 2006), macrophage colony stimulating factor (M-CSF) and granulocyte-macrophage colony stimulating factor (GM-CSF) (Kim et al, 2008) that recruit and assist in expansion or colonization of macrophages, respectively. Whether accumulation of cholesterol in macrophages can affect macrophage recruitment into the adipose tissue due to increased production of these pro-inflammatory mediators has not been explored. Subramanian et al have recently reported that addition of relatively small amount (0.15%) of dietary cholesterol resulted in marked increase in accumulation of macrophages in adipose tissue (Subramanian et al, 2008). Although this study provides the first evidence that cholesterol plays an important role in macrophage infiltration into the adipose tissue, the role of macrophage cholesterol balance in regulating this process remains undefined. We demonstrated that CEH-mediated increase in CE mobilization in macrophages decreased activation of pro-inflammatory transcription factor NF-κB resulting in decreased expression of pro-inflammatory chemokines (e.g., MCP-1) and cytokines (e.g., IL-1β and IL-6) resulting in significant reduction in circulating cytokines. Macrophage infiltration into expanding adipose tissue was also significantly reduced in CEH transgenic mice. Further, insulin signaling in adipocytes was not dramatically perturbed by CEH over-expressing macrophages (Bie et al, 2010). Collectively, these data led us to propose the following model (Figure 5) whereby CEH-mediated reduction in macrophage CE levels regulate infiltration of macrophages into the expanding adipose tissue. Reduction in the number of macrophages limits the deleterious effects of macrophage-adipocyte interactions that are central to the development of insulin resistance.

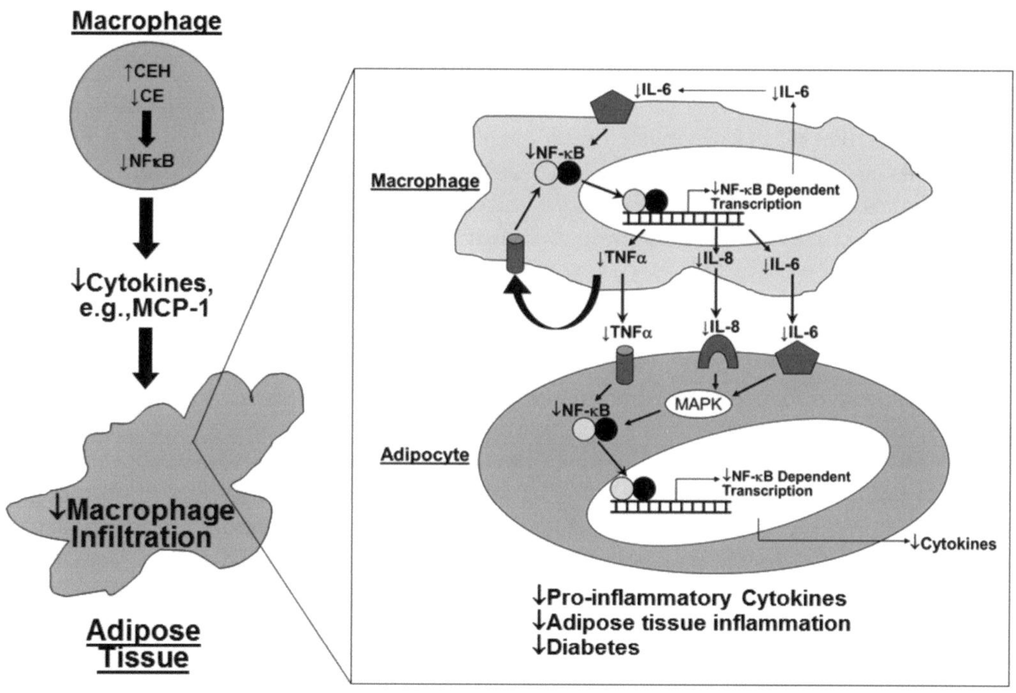


Fig. 5. Proposed model for Improved Insulin Sensitivity by CEH-mediated macrophage CE mobilization

Besides hypercholesterolemia, chronic low grade inflammation, obesity and T2DM are additional risk factors for development of atherosclerosis and CAD. Our data showing CEH-mediated attenuation of insulin resistance and systemic as well as adipose tissue inflammation establishes macrophage CE mobilization as an important therapeutic target that can simultaneously affect multiple and linked metabolic disease processes.

### 2.5.2 CEH-mediated CE mobilization and hepatic steatosis

In addition to the development of obesity and insulin resistance, both of which are risk factors for atherosclerosis, excessive intake of high calorie or high fat food also leads to the ectopic deposition of excess fat in tissues other than the physiological fat depots such as adipose tissue. Increased accumulation of lipids in liver results in hepatic steatosis that is central to the development of non-alcoholic fatty liver disease and which progresses into non-alcoholic steatohepatitis. The etiology of this disease is distinct from a similar liver pathology seen with alcoholism and hence the name.

Upon excessive lipid storage liver overproduces multiple cardiovascular risk factors such as glucose, very low density lipoproteins, plasminogen activator inhibitor-1 (PAI-1) coagulation factors and C-reactive protein (CRP). In addition, liver fat content is closely related to fasting insulin concentrations and direct measures of hepatic insulin sensitivity and increase in hepatic lipid contents predicts T2DM (Yki-Jarvinen, 2005). The mechanism(s) responsible for increased intra-hepatic triglyceride accumulation are not completely understood. It has been suggested that dysfunctional adipose tissue, characterized by adipocyte hypertrophy, macrophage infiltration, impaired insulin signaling, and insulin resistance, releases a host of inflammatory adipokines and excessive amounts of free fatty acids (FFA) that promote ectopic fat deposition in liver (Cusi, 2010). Alterations in FFA uptake regulated at the level of fatty acid transporter, CD36 expression is thought to be involved in increased triglyceride accumulation and hepatic CD36 expression is directly correlated with liver fat in human subjects (Greco et al, 2008).

Kupffer cells are resident macrophages present in the liver and, therefore, changes in macrophage metabolism and/or phenotype will also affect kupffer cells. However, the role of hepatocyte microenvironment namely the effect of Kupffer cells in regulating triglyceride accumulation in hepatocytes is not completely defined. Pro-inflammatory cytokines (namely, IL-1β, IL-6 or TNFα) secreted by Kupffer cells activate hepatocytes (Scott et al, 2005), affect gluconeogenesis (Yerkovich et al, 2004), increase the expression of acute phase proteins (Knolle et al, 1995) and enzymes involved in xenobiotic metabolism (Milosevic et al, 1999). On the other hand, anti-inflammatory cytokine IL-10 secreted by Kupffer cells is essential for hepatocyte homeostasis and its loss under conditions of Kupffer cell depletion is associated with increased STAT3-dependent signalling and steatosis leading to decreased insulin signalling (Clementi et al, 2009). These studies underscore the importance of understanding the mechanisms involved in regulating the inflammatory status of Kupffer cells. To directly evaluate the role of kupffer cells, we examined hepatocyte triglyceride (TG) accumulation in livers of leptin-deficient obese (ob/ob) mice that were crossed with macrophage-specific CEH transgenic mice. Leptin deficiency in these ob/ob mice leads to increased obesity resulting in significant ectopic lipid accumulation in the liver and, thus, providing an ideal model to test the effects of decreased CE accumulation in kupffer cells as a result of transgenic expression of CEH on hepatocyte TG metabolism. Accumulated lipids are stored as cytoplsamic lipid droplets that continue to occupy greater cellular area and total area occupied by lipid was used as a measure of total lipid accumulation and percent area occupied by lipid was significantly reduced by transgenic expression of CEH (Table 1). These data were confirmed by direct quantification of TG in total hepatic lipids where a significant decrease in hepatic TG content was observed in ob/ob-CEH transgenic mice. It is important to note that expression of CEH transgene in this model is macrophages-specific and, therefore, the observed effects are due to the changes in kupffer cell CE metabolism.

| Gentotype | Percent area occupied by lipid | Total TG (μg/mg tissue) |
|---|---|---|
| ob/ob | 45.4 ± 5.3 | 32.3 ± 4.3 |
| ob/ob-CEH Transgenic | 39.5 ± 3.1** | 23.1 ± 4.2** |

Table 1. Macrophage-specific transgenic expression of significantly decreases hepatic lipid accumulation **P<0.05

Consistent with a reduction in hepatic lipid content, ob/ob-CEH transgenic mice showed improved glucose tolerance and insulin sensitivity.

Macrophage polarization plays a pivotal role in the development of insulin resistance and it is promoted by a transition from an alternative M2 activation state maintained by STAT6 and PPARs to a classical M1 activation state driven by NF-κB, AP1, and other signal-dependent transcription factors that play crucial roles in innate immunity (Olefsky and Glass, 2010). While IL-1β, IL-6 and TNFα are the predominant cytokines secreted by M1 macrophages, M2 macrophages secrete anti-inflammatory cytokines IL-10 and IL-13. M1 activation by LPS via Toll-like receptor 4 (TLR4) or by free fatty acids as identified recently, triggers inflammatory responses (Bilan et al, 2009). Intracellular lipid content, specifically the cholesterol content, is increasingly being recognized as another major factor that contributes to macrophage activation. While cholesterol loading of macrophages activated TLR4 (Sun et al, 2009), HDL or ApoA1-mimetic stimulated removal of cellular cholesterol abolished LPS-induced mRNA expression of pro-inflammatory mediators such as MCP-1, MIP-1, RANTES, IL-6, and TNF-alpha but significantly up-regulated LPS-induced anti-inflammatory IL-10 expression (Smythies et al, 2010). Interaction of ApoA1 with cholesterol transporter ABCA1, suppressed the ability of LPS to induce pro-inflammatory cytokine expression suggesting that cholesterol removal from macrophages is an anti-inflammatory event (Tang et al, 2009). CEH-mediated increase in CE mobilization and subsequent decrease in cellular cholesterol content is, therefore, likely to polarize the macrophages to an M2 or anti-inflammatory phenotype. This is consistent with our earlier data demonstrating a decrease in expression of pro-inflammatory cytokines via reduced activation of NF-κB and AP-1 in CEH transgenic macrophages (Bie et al, 2010) that leads to a decrease in the levels of pro-inflammatory cytokines (e.g., IL-6) in circulation and reduction in systemic inflammation. Based on these data, we propose the following model (Figure 6) to integrate the cellular events and interactions that lead to the increased accumulation of TG in the liver and how CEH-mediated reduction in cellular CE content resulting in M2 polarization of Kupffer cells as well as decrease in circulating cytokines such as IL-6 can attenuate this process.

The studies described above and the recent developments linking cellular CE content to macrophage phenotype and inflammation underscore the importance of macrophage cholesterol homeostasis in regulating multiple metabolic disorders.

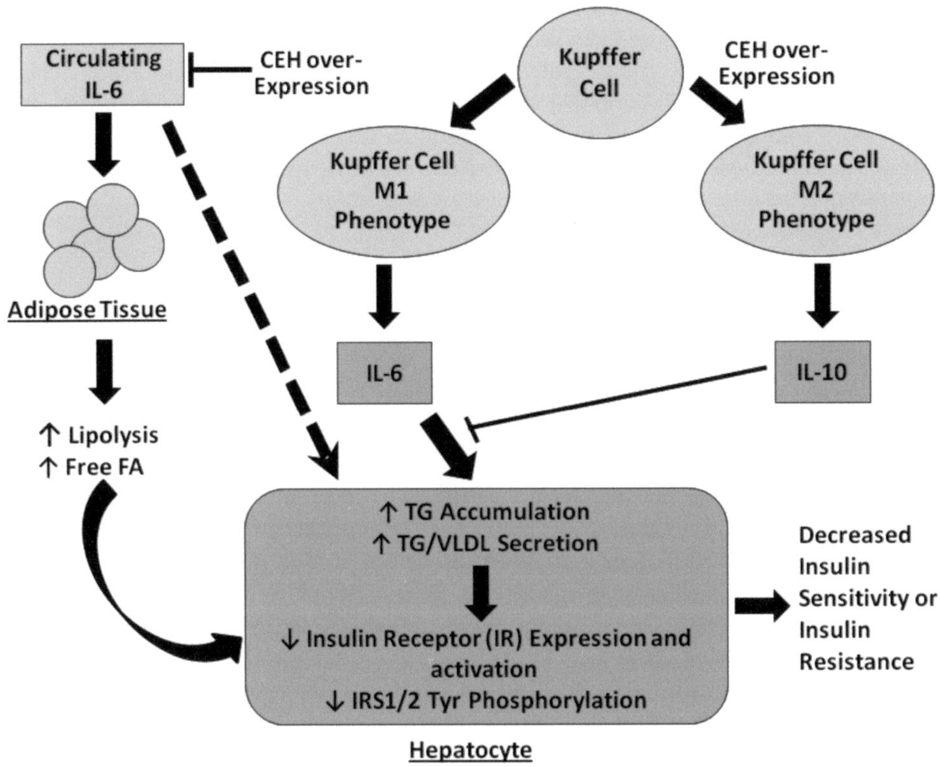


Fig. 6. Proposed model by which CEH-mediated macrophage CE mobilization attenuates hepatic TG accumulation and improves insulin sensitivity.

### 2.5.3 CEH-mediated CE mobilization and atherosclerotic plaque stability

In recent years, there has been a shift in the paradigm of arterial re-modelling during progression of atherosclerosis and improved understanding of the mechanism underlying acute coronary syndromes or sudden heart attacks. The earlier notion of gradual narrowing of the arterial lumen that eventually occludes the coronary artery resulting in heart attacks is being replaced by the concept of a developing plaque in the arterial wall (that may or may not affect the lumen) that becomes unstable and prone to rupture. Thrombotic events resulting from the sudden release of lipid contents of the plaque into circulation is now considered as the primary cause of acute coronary events. Large necrotic cores as well as increased inflammation associated with plaques are the two main factors that determine plaque stability.

Macrophage content of plaque is variable during the development of plaques (from fatty streaks to complex plaques) and is determined by processes involved in macrophage recruitment, apoptosis and egress. A balance between these processes limits plaque progression and is also likely to maintain favourable plaque characteristics. With increased lipid accumulation, plaque-associated foam cells undergo apoptosis and functional macrophages are required for efficient clearance of apoptotic cells (or efferocytosis). Inability to effectively clear the apoptotic cells results in accumulation of released lipids and other inflammatory mediators that lead to secondary necrosis. Growth of acellular necrotic core not only destabilizes the plaque by altering its physical characteristics, but it also limits smooth muscle cell proliferation required to maintain the integrity of the fibrous cap of the plaque. Our earlier studies have demonstrated a decrease in lesion necrosis in macrophage-specific CEH transgenic mice. These lesions also contained increased number of macrophages and significantly less number of apoptotic cells (Zhao et al, 2007). Collectively, these characteristics are suggestive of a more stable plaque.

Khallou-Laschet et al evaluated the phenotype of macrophages associated with progression of atherosclerosis in mice and demonstrated that early lesions were infiltrated with alternatively activated and anti-inflammatory M2 macrophages which favoured smooth cell proliferation and deposition of extra-cellular matrix (tissue repair phenotype). However, a phenotypic switch of existing macrophages within the plaques from M2 to M1 (classically activated macrophages with pro-inflammatory properties) occurred during plaque progression resulting in increased inflammation (Khallou-Laschet et al, 2010). M1 macrophages, identified by high expression of Ly6C surface antigen ($Ly6C^{Hi}$), increase with hypercholesterolemia, actively adhere to endothelium, become lesional macrophages and represent a newly recognized component of the inflammatory response in atherosclerosis (Swirski et al, 2007). We examined the phenotype of diet-induced lesion associated macrophages isolated from LDLR-/- and LDLR-/-CEH transgenic mice. Consistent with our earlier results described above, increased polarization towards M2 phenotype was noted in lesional macrophages from CEH transgenic mice. Studies are in progress to determine the effects of CEH-mediated shift in macrophage polarization on lesion-associated inflammation.

Increase in inflammation with increasing cellular cholesterol content has been known for a long time. Recent studies have also shown that deficiency of cholesterol transporter ABCA1 in LDLR-/- mice that results in massive CE accumulation, leads to an exacerbated response to lipopolysaccharide and increased inflammation (Francone et al, 2005). Increased inflammatory gene expression was also noted in macrophages from ABCG1 deficient macrophages (Balden et al, 2008). However, cellular mechanisms that directly link changes in cellular cholesterol homeostasis to inflammatory pathways remain undefined. In cells with increased CE accumulation, we demonstrated that CEH-mediated CE mobilization directly attenuated NF-κB and AP1-driven gene expression suggesting that pro-inflammatory transcription factor-driven gene expression is directly affected by cellular CE content (Bie et al 2010). However, the intracellular processes that are involved in "sensing" and "linking" of cellular CE content to inflammatory gene expression still remain to be elucidated.

## 3. Conclusions

Maintaining macrophage cholesterol homeostasis is central to atherogenesis. While unregulated uptake of modified LDL results in increased cellular CE content and foam cell formation, CEH-mediated mobilization of CE represent an important mechanism by which macrophages reduce the lipid burden. Given the importance of this step, intracellular CE hydrolysis is a multi-enzyme process and several enzymes catalyze this reaction. It is extremely important that the future focus is maintained on intracellular CE hydrolysis and not on establishing the "major" CE hydrolase in either human or mouse macrophages. Current strategies of single gene ablation are likely to be inconclusive not only due to the presence of multiple enzymes but also due to as yet unrecognized compensatory mechanisms that may become operative under conditions of single gene deficiency leading to erroneous dismissal of the candidate CE hydrolase as unimportant .

Removal of cholesterol from arterial wall associated macrophage foam cells represents the first step in prevention of atherosclerotic plaque formation or regression of existing plaques. Our results with CEH over-expression conclusively demonstrate the anti-atherogenic role of this enzyme in mobilizing stored CE from macrophages and attenuating atherogenesis. Cholesterol removed from the periphery including artery wall associated macrophages is returned to the liver via HDL and liver is the only organ that facilitates final elimination of cholesterol from the body. Since 80% of the total cholesterol delivered by HDL is CE, hepatic hydrolysis of CE is crucial to further metabolism of cholesterol. Consistently, increase in hepatic CE hydrolysis enhances elimination of cholesterol as bile acids in faeces. More importantly, increasing CE hydrolysis in liver alone stimulates movement of cholesterol from macrophages to faeces. Thus, hydrolysis of CE is an extremely important step in removal of cholesterol from the body and intracellular CE hydrolysis represents an important anti-atherogenic step that should be targeted for therapeutic benefit.

Although macrophage cholesterol homeostasis is intuitively linked to atherogenesis as the primary disease process, continuing characterization of macrophage-specific CEH transgenic mice has revealed novel roles of CEH in regulating several disease processes and has established the central role of macrophage cholesterol homeostasis. By modulating infiltration of macrophages into adipose tissue and thus affecting adipose tissue as well as systemic inflammation, mobilization of CE from macrophages improves glucose tolerance and insulin sensitivity. Similarly, by altering the polarization towards a more anti-inflammatory phenotype, increased CE mobilization from kupffer cells attenuates hepatic steatosis. Altered polarization towards M2 phenotype in atherosclerotic lesions also leads to decreased lesion necrosis and increased macrophage survival. Collectively, these studies clearly establish CEH as an important therapeutic target with a potential to simultaneously affect multiple disease processes. Ongoing studies will establish the direct link(s) between cellular CE content and inflammatory pathways and identify the intracellular pathways involved.

From a clinical and translational perspective, future studies are necessary to delineate endogenous mechanisms that regulate these CE hydrolases such that these can be specifically targeted (e.g., by pharmacological means) to increase the activity in vivo.

## 4. Acknowledgments

The research in my laboratory is supported by funding from NIH-NHLBI (HL069946 and HL097346) and American Diabetes Association. I would like to also acknowledge the following people in my laboratory who contributed to the research described here - Post-doctoral fellows, Drs. Bin Zhao and Jinghua Bie and the Technicians Ms. Jingmei Song, Jing Wang and Barbara Szomju. The contribution of Ms Kathryn Marqueen is also acknowledged.

## 5. References

Accad, M., Smith, S., Newland, D., Sanan, D., King, J.L., Linton, M., Fazio, S. & Farese, J.R. (2000). Massive xanthomatosis and altered composition of atherosclerotic lesions in hyperlipidemic mice lacking acyl CoA:cholesterol acyltransferase-1. *J. Clin. Invest.*, 105, 711-719.

Baldán, A., Gomes, A.V., Ping, P. & Edwards, P.A. (2008). Loss of ABCG1 results in chronic pulmonary inflammation. *J Immunol.* , 180, 3560-3568.

Bie, J., Zhao, B., Song, J., & Ghosh, S. (2010). Improved insulin sensitivity in high fat- and high cholesterol-fed Ldlr-/- mice with macrophage-specific transgenic expression of cholesteryl ester hydrolase: role of macrophage inflammation and infiltration into adipose tissue. *J Biol Chem.*, 285:13630-13637.

Bilan, P.J., Samokhvalov, V., Koshkina, A., Schertzer, J.D., Samaan, M.C. & Klip, A. (2009). Direct and macrophage-mediated actions of fatty acids causing insulin resistance in muscle cells. *Arch Physiol Biochem.*, 115, 176-190.

Bouloumié, A., Curat, C.A., Sengenès, C., Lolmède, K., Miranville, A. & Busse, R. (2005). Role of macrophage tissue infiltration in metabolic diseases. *Curr Opin Clin Nutr Metab Care.*, 8, 347-354.

Brown, M.S., Ho, Y.K. and Goldstein, J.L. (1980). The cholesteryl ester cycle in macrophage foam cells. Continual hydrolysis and re-esterification of cytoplasmic cholesteryl esters. *J Biol Chem.*, 255, 9344-9352.

Buchebner, M., Pfeifer, T., Rathke, N., Chandak, P.G., Lass, A., Schreiber, R., Kratzer, A., Zimmermann, R., Sattler, W., Koefeler, H., Fröhlich, E., Kostner, G.M., Birner-Gruenberger, R., Chiang, K.P., Haemmerle, G., Zechner, R., Levak-Frank, S., Cravatt, B. & Kratky, D. (2010). Cholesteryl ester hydrolase activity is abolished in HSL-/- macrophages but unchanged in macrophages lacking KIAA1363. *J Lipid Res.*, 51:2896-2908.

Camulli, E.D., Linke, M.J., Brockman, H.L. & Hui, D.Y. (1989). Identity of a cytosolic neutral cholesterol esterase in rat liver with the bile salt stimulated cholesterol esterase in pancreas. *Biochim Biophys Acta.*, 1005, 177-182.

Chen, X., Harrison, E.H. & Fisher, E.A. (1997). Molecular cloning of the cDNA for rat hepatic, bile salt-dependent cholesteryl ester/retinyl ester hydrolase demonstrates identity with pancreatic carboxylester lipase. *Proc Soc Exp Biol Med.*, 215, 186-191.

Choy, H.A., Wang, X.P. & Schotz, M.C. (2003). Reduced atherosclerosis in hormone-sensitive lipase transgenic mice overexpressing cholesterol acceptors. *Biochim Biophys Acta.*, 1634, 76-85.

Clementi, A.H., Gaudy, A.M., van Rooijen, N., Pierce, R.H. & Mooney RA. (2009). Loss of Kupffer cells in diet-induced obesity is associated with increased hepatic steatosis, STAT3 signaling, and further decreases in insulin signaling. *Biochim Biophys Acta.*, 1792, 1062-1072.

Contreras, J.A. (2002). Hormone sensitive lipase is not required for cholesteryl ester hydrolysis in macrophages. *Biochem. Biophys. Res. Comm.*, 292, 900-903.

Cusi K. (2010). The role of adipose tissue and lipotoxicity in the pathogenesis of type 2 diabetes. *Curr Diab Rep.*, 10: 306-315.

Davies, M.J. & Thomas, A.C. (1985). Plaque fissuring the cause of acute myocardical infarction, sudden ischaemic death and crescendo angina. *Br Heart J.*, 53, 363-373.

Escary, J., Choy, H.A., Reue, K., Wang, X., Castellani, L.W., Glass, C.K., Lusis, A.J. & Schotz, M.C. (1999). Paradoxical effect on atherosclerosis of hormone-sensitive lipase overexpression in macrophages. *J Lipid Res.*, 40, 397-404.

Escary, J.L., Choy, H.A., Reue, K. & Schotz, M.C. (1998). Hormone-sensitive lipase overexpression increases cholesteryl ester hydrolysis in macrophage foam cells. *Arterioscler Thromb Vasc Biol.*, 18, 991-998.

Fazio, S. & Linton, M.F. (2001). The inflamed plaque: cytokine production and cellular cholesterol balance in the vessel wall. *Am J Cardiol.*, 88, 12E-15E.

Fernandez, C., Lindholm, M. & Krogh M. (2008). Disturbed cholesterol homeostasis in hormone-sensitive lipase-null mice. *Am J Physiol Endocrinol Metab.*, 295, E820-831 (2008).

Francone, O. L., Royer, L., Boucher, G., Haghpassand, M., Freeman, A., Brees, D., Aiello, R. J. (2005). Increased cholesterol deposition, expression of scavenger receptors, and response to chemotactic factors in Abca1-deficient macrophages. *Arterioscler. Thromb. Vasc. Biol.*, 25, 1198–1205.

Francone, O.L., Royer, L., Boucher, G., Haghpassand, M., Freeman, A., Brees, D. & Aiello, R.J. (2005). Increased cholesterol deposition, expression of scavenger receptors, and response to chemotactic factors in Abca1-deficient macrophages. *Arterioscler Thromb Vasc Biol.*, 25, 1198-1205.

Gallo, L.L. (1981). Sterol ester hydrolase from rat pancreas. *Methods Enzymol.*, 71, 664-74.

Ghosh, S. & Grogan, W.M. (1991). Rapid three-step purification of a hepatic neutral cholesteryl ester hydrolase which is not the pancreatic enzyme. *Lipids.*, 10, 793-798.

Ghosh, S. & Grogan, W.M. (1991). Rapid three-step purification of a hepatic neutral cholesteryl ester hydrolase which is not the pancreatic enzyme. *Lipids*, 26, 793-798.

Ghosh, S. (2000). Cholesteryl ester hydrolase in human monocyte/macrophage: cloning, sequencing and expression of full-length cDNA. *Physiol. Genomics*, 2, 1-8.

Ghosh, S., Mallonee, D.H., Hylemon, P.B. & Grogan, W.M. (1995). Molecular cloning and expression of rat hepatic neutral cholesteryl ester hydrolase. *Biochim Biophys Acta.*, 1259, 305-312.

Ghosh, S., Natarajan, R., Pandak, W.M., Hylemon, P.B. & Grogan, W.M. (1998). Regulation of hepatic neutral cholesteryl ester hydrolase by hormones and changes in cholesterol flux. *Am J Physiol. 274 (4 Pt 1)*, G662-668).

Ghosh, S., St Clair, R.W. & Rudel, L.L. (2003). Mobilization of cytoplasmic CE droplets by over-expression of human macrophage cholesteryl ester hydrolase. *J Lipid Res.*, 44, 1833-1840.

Ghosh, S., Zhao, B., Bie, J. & Song, J. 2010. Macrophage Cholesteryl Ester Mobilization and Atherosclerosis. *Vascul Pharmacol.* 52, 1-10.

Glass, C.K. & Witztum, J.L. (2001). Atherosclerosis: The road ahead. *Cell*, 104, 503-516.

Goldberg, D.I. and Khoo, J.C. (1990). Stimulation of neutral cholesteryl ester hydrolase by cAMP in P388D1 macrophages. *Biochim. Biophys. Acta*, 1042, 132-137.

Greco, D., Kotronen, A., Westerbacka, J., Puig, O., Arkkila, P., Kiviluoto, T., Laitinen, S., Kolak, M., Fisher, R.M., Hamsten, A., Auvinen, P. & Yki-Järvinen H (2998). Gene expression in human NAFLD. *Am J Physiol Gastrointest Liver Physiol.*, 294, G1281-G1287.

Harrison, E.H. (1988). Bile salt-dependent, neutral cholesteryl ester hydrolase of rat liver: possible relationship with pancreatic cholesteryl ester hydrolase. *Biochim Biophys Acta*. 963, 28-34.

Holm, C., Belfrage, P. & Fredrikson, G. (1987). Immunological evidence for the presence of hormone-sensitive lipase in rat tissues other than adipose tissue. *Biochem Biophys Res Commun.*, 148, 99-105.

Hui, D.Y. & Kissel, J.A. (1990). Sequence identity between human pancreatic cholesterol esterase and bile salt-stimulated milk lipase. *FEBS Lett.*, 276, 131-134.

Ishii, I., Oka, M., Katto, N., Shirai, K., Saito, Y. & Hirose, S. (1992). Beta-VLDL-induced cholesterol ester deposition in macrophages may be regulated by neutral cholesterol esterase activity. *Arterioscler. Thromb.*, 12, 1139-1145.

Johnson, W.J., Jang, S.Y. & Bernard, D.W. (2000). Hormone sensitive lipase mRNA in both monocyte and macrophage forms of the human THP-1 cell line. *Comp Biochem Physiol B Biochem Mol Biol.*, 126, 543-52.

Kanda, H., Tateya, S., Tamori, Y., Kotani, K., Hiasa, K., Kitazawa, R., Kitazawa, S., Miyachi, H., Maeda, S., Egashira, K. & Kasuga, M. (2006). MCP-1 contributes to macrophage infiltration into adipose tissue, insulin resistance, and hepatic steatosis in obesity. *J Clin Invest.*, 116, 1494-505.

Khallou-Laschet, J., Varthaman, A., Fornasa, G., Compain, C., Gaston, A.T., Clement, M., Dussiot, M., Levillain, O., Graff-Dubois, S., Nicoletti, A. & Caligiuri G. (2010). Macrophage plasticity in experimental atherosclerosis. *PLoS One.*, 5, e8852.

Khoo, J.C., Reue, K., Steinberg, D. & Schotz, M.C. (1993). Expression of hormone-sensitive lipase mRNA in macrophages. *J Lipid Res.*, 34, 1969-1974.

Kim, D.H., Sandoval, D., Reed, J.A., Matter, E.K., Tolod, E.G., Woods, S.C. & Seeley, R.J. (2008). The role of GM-CSF in adipose tissue inflammation. *Am J Physiol Endocrinol Metab.*, 295, E1038-1046.

Kissel, J.A., Fontaine, R.N., Turck, C.W., Brockman, H.L. & Hui, D.Y. (1989). Molecular cloning and expression of cDNA for rat pancreatic cholesterol esterase. *Biochim Biophys Acta.*, 1006, 227-236.

Knolle, P., Löhr, H., Treichel, U., Dienes, H.P., Lohse, A., Schlaack, J. & Gerken, G. (1995). Parenchymal and nonparenchymal liver cells and their interaction in the local immune response. *Z Gastroenterol.*, 33, 613-620.

Kodvawala, A., Ghering, A.B., Davidson, W.S. & Hui, D.Y. (2005). Carboxyl ester lipase expression in macrophages increases cholesteryl ester accumulation and promotes atherosclerosis. *J Biol. Chem.*, 280, 38592-38598.

Koseki, M., Hirano, K., Masuda, D., Ikegami, C., Tanaka, M., Ota, A., Sandoval, J. C., Nakagawa-Toyama, Y., Sato, S. B., Kobayashi, T., Shimada, Y., Ohno-Iwashita, Y., Matsuura, F., Shimomura, I. & Yamashita, S. (2007). Increased lipid rafts and accelerated lipopolysaccharide-induced tumor necrosis factor-alpha secretion in Abca1-deficient macrophages. *J. Lipid Res.*, 48, 299–306.

Kozarsky, K.F., Donahee, M.H., Rigotti, A., Iqbal, S.N., Edelman, E.R. & Krieger, M. (1997). Overexpression of the HDL receptor SR-BI alters plasma HDL and bile cholesterol levels. Nature, 387, 414-417.

Levine, D.M., Parker, T.S., Donnelly, T.M., Walsh, A. & Rubin, A.L. (1993). In vivo protection against endotoxin by plasma high density lipoprotein. *Proc Natl Acad Sci U S A.*, 90, 12040-12044.

Li, F. & Hui, D.Y. (1997). Modified low density lipoprotein enhances the secretion of bile salt-stimulated cholesterol esterase by human monocyte-macrophages. Species-specific difference in macrophage cholesteryl ester hydrolase. *J. Biol. Chem.*, 272, 28666-28671.

Li, F. & Hui, D.Y. (1997). Modified low density lipoprotein enhances the secretion of bile salt-stimulated cholesterol esterase by human monocyte-macrophages. Species-specific difference in macrophage cholesteryl ester hydrolase. *J. Biol. Chem.*, 272, 28666-28671.

Mathur, S.N., Field, F.J., Megan, M.B. & Armstrong, H.L. (1985). A defect in mobilization of cholesteryl esters in rabbit macrophages. *Biochim. Biophys. Acta.*, 834, 48-57.

Matsuda, K. (1994). ACAT inhibitors as antiatherosclerotic agents. *Med. Res. Rev.* 14, 271-305.

Matsuo, M., Ito, F., Konto, A., Aketa, M., Tomoi, M. & Shimomura, K (1995). Effect of FR145237, a novel ACAT inhibitor on atherogenesis in cholesterol fed and WHHl rabbits. Evidence for a direct effect on the arterial wall. *Biochem. Biophys. Acta*, 1259, 254-260.

McGillicuddy, F.C., de la Llera Moya, M., Hinkle, C.C., Joshi, M.R., Chiquoine, E.H., Billheimer, J.T., Rothblat, G.H., & Reilly, M.P. (2009). Inflammation impairs reverse cholesterol transport in vivo. *Circulation.*, 119, 1135-1145.

Milosevic, N., Schawalder, H. & Maier, P. (1999). Kupffer cell-mediated differential down-regulation of cytochrome P450 metabolism in rat hepatocytes. *Eur J Pharmacol.*, 368, 75-87.

Natarajan, R., Ghosh, S. & Grogan, W.M. (1996). Age-related changes in mRNA, protein and catalytic activity of hepatic neutral cholesterol ester hydrolase in male rats: evidence for transcriptional regulation. *Biochim Biophys Acta.*, 1302 153-158 .

Natarajan, R., Ghosh, S. & Grogan, W.M. (1998). Molecular cloning of the promoter for rat hepatic neutral cholesterol ester hydrolase: evidence for transcriptional regulation by sterols. *Biochem Biophys Res Commun.*, 243, 349-355.

Nicolosi, R.J., Wilson, T.A. & Krause, B.R. (1998). The ACAT inhibitor, CI 1011 is effective in the prevention and regression of aortic fatty streak in hamsters. *Atherosclerosis*, 137, 77-85.

Nissen, S.E., Tsunoda, T., Tuzcu, E.M., Schoenhagen, P., Cooper, C.J., Yasin, M., Eaton, G.M., Lauer, M.A., Sheldon, W.S., Grines, C.L., Halpern, S., Crowe, T., Blankenship, J.C. & Kerensky, R. (2003). Effect of recombinant ApoA-I Milano on coronary atherosclerosis in patients with acute coronary syndromes: a randomized controlled trial. *JAMA.*, 290, 2292-2300.

Okazaki, H., Igarashi, M., Nishi, M., Sekiya, M., Tajima, M., Takase, S., Takanashi, M., Ohta, K., Tamura, Y., Okazaki, S., Yahagi, N., Ohashi, K., Amemiya-Kudo, M., Nakagawa, Y., Nagai, R., Kadowaki, T., Osuga, J. & Ishibashi, S. (2008). Identification of neutral cholesterol ester hydrolase, a key enzyme removing cholesterol from macrophages. J *Biol Chem.*, 283, 33357-33364.

Olefsky, J.M. & Glass, C.K. (2010). Macrophages, inflammation, and insulin resistance. *Annu Rev Physiol.*, 72, 219-246.

Osuga, J., Ishibashi, S., Oka, T., Yagyu, H., Tozawa, R., Fujimoto, A., Shionoiri, F., Yahagi, N., Kraemer, F.B., Tsutsumi, O. & Yamada, N. (2000). Targeted disruption of hormone-sensitive lipase results in male sterility and adipocyte hypertrophy, but not in obesity. *Proc. Natl. Acad. Sci USA*, 97, 787-792.

Patel, S., Drew, B.G., Nakhla, S., Duffy, S.J., Murphy, A.J., Barter, P.J., Rye, K.A., Chin-Dusting, J., Hoang, A., Sviridov, D., Celermajer, D.S. & Kingwell, B.A. (2009).

Reconstituted high-density lipoprotein increases plasma high-density lipoprotein anti-inflammatory properties and cholesterol efflux capacity in patients with type 2 diabetes. *J Am Coll Cardiol.*, 53, 962-971.

Perrey, S., Legendre, C., Matsuura, A., Guffroy, C., Binet, J., Ohbayashi, S., Tanaka, T., Ortuno, J.C., Matsukura, T., Laugel, T., Padovani, P., Bellamy, F. & Edgar, A.D. (2001). Preferential pharmacological inhibition of macrophage ACAT increases plaque formation in mouse and rabbit models of atherogenesis. *Atheroscler.*, 155, 359-370.

Persson, J., Nilsson, J. & Lindholm, M.W. (2008). Interleukin-1beta and tumour necrosis factor-alpha impede neutral lipid turnover in macrophage-derived foam cells. *BMC Immunol.*, 9, 70-75.

Reue, K., Cohen, R.D. & Schotz, M.C. (1997). Evidence for hormone-sensitive lipase mRNA expression in human monocyte/macrophages. *Arterioscler Thromb Vasc Biol.*, 17, 3428-32.

Ross, R. (1993). The pathogenesis of atherosclerosis: a perspective for the 1990s. *Nature*, 362, 801-809.

Ross, R., Glomset, J., & Harker, L. (1977). Response to injury and atherogenesis. *Am J Pathol.*, 86, 675-684.

Scott, M.J., Liu, S., Su, G.L., Vodovotz, Y. & Billiar, T.R. (2005). Hepatocytes enhance effects of lipopolysaccharide on liver nonparenchymal cells through close cell interactions. *Shock*, 23, 453-458.

Sekiya, M., Osuga, J. & Yahagi, N. (2008). Hormone-sensitive lipase is involved in hepatic cholesteryl ester hydrolysis. *J Lipid Res.*, 49,1829-3188.

Sliskovic, D.R. & White, A.D. (1991). Therapeutic potential of ACAT inhibitors as lipid lowering and anti-atherosclerotic agents. *Trends Pharmacol. Sci.*, 12, 194-199.

Small, C.A., Goodacre, J.A. & Yeaman, S.J. (1989). Hormone sensitive lipase is responsible for the neutral cholesteryl ester hydrolase activity in macrophages. *FEBS Lett.*, 247, 205-208.

Smythies, L.E., White, C.R., Maheshwari, A., Palgunachari, M.N., Anantharamaiah, G.M., Chaddha, M., Kurundkar, A.R. & Datta, G. (2010). Apolipoprotein A-I mimetic 4F alters the function of human monocyte-derived macrophages. *Am J Physiol Cell Physiol.*, 298, C1538-1548, 2010.

Subramanian, S., Han, C.Y., Chiba, T., McMillen, T.S., Wang, S.A., Haw, A. 3rd., Kirk, E.A., O'Brien, K.D. & Chait, A. (2008). Dietary cholesterol worsens adipose tissue macrophage accumulation and atherosclerosis in obese LDL receptor-deficient mice. *Arterioscler Thromb Vasc Biol.*, 28, 685-691.

Sun, Y., Ishibashi, M., Seimon, T., Lee, M., Sharma, S.M., Fitzgerald, K.A., Samokhin, A.O., Wang, Y., Sayers, S., Aikawa, M., Jerome, W.G., Ostrowski, M.C., Bromme, D., Libby, P., Tabas, I.A., Welch, C.L. & Tall, A.R. (2009). Free cholesterol accumulation in macrophage membranes activates Toll-like receptors and p38 mitogen-activated protein kinase and induces cathepsin K. *Circ Res.*, 104, 455-465.

Swirski, F.K., Libby, P., Aikawa, E., Alcaide, P., Luscinskas, F.W., Weissleder, R. & Pittet, M.J. (2007). Ly-6Chi monocytes dominate hypercholesterolemia-associated monocytosis and give rise to macrophages in atheromata. *J Clin Invest.* 117, 195-205.

Tang, C. & Oram, J.F. (2009). The cell cholesterol exporter ABCA1 as a protector from cardiovascular disease and diabetes. Biochim Biophys Acta. 1791, 563-572.

Tang, C., Liu, Y., Kessler, P.S., Vaughan, A.M. & Oram, J.F. (2009). The macrophage cholesterol exporter ABCA1 functions as an anti-inflammatory receptor. *J Biol Chem.*, 284, 32336-32343.

Trayhurn, P & Wood, I.S. (2004). Adipokines: inflammation and the pleiotropic role of white adipose tissue. *Br. J Nutr.*, 92, 347-355.

Williams, K.J. & Tabas I. (1995) The Response-to-Retention Hypothesis of Early Atherogenesis. *Arterioscle. Thromb. Vasc. Biol.*, 15, 551-561.

Wisse, B.E. (2004). The inflammatory syndrome: the role of adipose tissue cytokines in metabolic disorders linked to obesity. *J Am Soc Nephrol.*, 15, 2792-2800.

Yagu, H., Kitamine, T., Osuga, J., Tozawa, R., Chen, Z., Kaji, Y., Oka, T., Perry, S., Tamura, Y. & Ohyashi, K. (2000). Absence of ACAT-1 attenuates atherosclerosis but causes dry eye and cutaneous xanthomatosis in mice with congenital hyperlipidemia. *J. Biol. Chem.*, 275, 21324-21330.

Yancey, P.G. & St. Clair, R.W. (1994). Mechanism of the defect in cholesteryl ester clearance from macrophages of atherosclerosis-susceptible White Carneau pigeons. *J. Lipid Res.* 35, 2114-2129.

Yerkovich, S.T., Rigby, P.J., Fournier, P.A., Olynyk, J.K. & Yeoh GC. (2004). Kupffer cell cytokines interleukin-1beta and interleukin-10 combine to inhibit phosphoenolpyruvate carboxykinase and gluconeogenesis in cultured hepatocytes. *Int J Biochem Cell Biol.* 36, 1462-1472.

Yki-Jarvinen H (2005). Fat in the liver and insulin resistance. *Ann Med.*, 37:347-356.

Zhang, Y., Zanotti, I., Reilly, M.P., Glick, J.M., Rothblat, G.H. & Rader DJ (2003). Overexpression of apolipoprotein A-I promotes reverse transport of cholesterol from macrophages to feces in vivo. *Circulation.* 108, 661-663.

Zhao, B., Fisher, B.J., St Clair, R.W., Rudel, L.L. & Ghosh, S. (2005). Redistribution of macrophage cholesteryl ester hydrolase from cytoplasm to lipid droplets upon lipid loading. *J Lipid Res.*, 46, 2114-2121.

Zhao, B., Natarajan, R. & Ghosh, S. (2005). Human liver cholesteryl ester hydrolase: cloning, molecular characterization, and role in cellular cholesterol homeostasis. *Physiol Genomics.*, 23, 304-310.

Zhao, B., Song, J., & Ghosh, S. (2008). Hepatic overexpression of cholesteryl ester hydrolase enhances cholesterol elimination and in vivo reverse cholesterol transport. *J Lipid Res.*, 49, 2212-2217.

Zhao, B., Song, J., Chow, W.N., St Clair, R.W., Rudel, L.L. & Ghosh, S. (2007). Macrophage-specific transgenic expression of cholesteryl ester hydrolase significantly reduces atherosclerosis and lesion necrosis in Ldlr mice. *J Clin Invest.*, 117, 2983-2992.

# The Role of TGF-β and TGF-β Receptors in Atherosclerosis

Petr Nachtigal, Jana Rathouska, Lenka Vecerova and Zbynek Strasky
*Charles University in Prague/ Faculty of Pharmacy in Hradec Kralove,*
*Department of Biological and Medical Sciences*
*Czech Republic*

## 1. Introduction

Researchers discovered a new cytokine with the capability to transform fibroblasts in 1983 while studying epidermal and platelet derived growth factors in rat fibroblasts. Originally called sarcoma growth factor, TGFβ was first isolated from neoplastic mouse tissue by Moloney sarcoma virus (Assoian et al., 1983). After more than three decades TGF-β family comprise several members including - nodals, activins, bone morphogenic proteins (BMPs), myostatin, anti-Muellerian hormone (AMH) and others - control cell division, differentiation, migration, adhesion, organization and programmed cell death (Massague, 1998). There are three TGF-β isoforms currently described in humans, including TGF-β1, TGF-β2, and TGF-β3. Alignment of the amino acid sequences of the three mammalian TGF-β isoforms reveals that the different isoforms share a high level of similarity between the active domains; TGF- β3 is 86% similar to that of TGF- β1 while it shares 91% similarity with that of TGF-β2. However, despite TGF- β2 and - β3 sharing the highest level of sequence similarity of the three isoforms, TGF- β2 binds to the TGF-β receptor II (TβRII) in a different way from TGF β1 and - β3. Furthermore, while TGF-β1 and -β3 are both capable of binding directly to the type II receptor, presentation of TGF-β2 to the receptor requires the presence of a co-receptor (beta glycan or endoglin), which may explain the differences in activities of TGF-β2 and -β1 (Laverty et al., 2009). The importance of TGF-β isoforms in mammalian biology is highlighted by the lack of viability in TGF-$\beta^{-/-}$ mice. Targeted disruption of the TGF-β1 genes leads to hematopoietic and vasculogenic defects that result in death of about half of null embryos by 10 days gestation. Moreover, embryos that survive die within 3 weeks due to widespread inflammatory disease (Shull et al., 1992). TGF-β2 null mice die in the perinatal period due to cyanotic heart disease, pulmonary insufficiency, and another abnormalities in urogenital, visual, auditory, neural and skeletal systems (Sanford et al., 1997). Additionally, mice lacking TGF-β3 exhibit cleft palate with 100% penetration and die immediately after birth due to an inability to suckle effectively (Proetzel et al., 1995). In addition, other organs are not affected when compared with mice lacking TGF-β1 and TGF-β2.

Several other papers showed differences in postnatal effects of different TGF-β isoforms, including different role in neovascularization (Wu et al., 1997), collagen production and bone production (ten Dijke et al., 1990). Moreover, TGF-betas are released by immune cells and detected in wound fluid, especially during inflammation and tissue repair. Although all three TGF-β isoforms participate in wound healing TGF-β1 plays a dominant role in the wound repair process while TGF-β2 and TGF-β3 have been shown to play a key role in embryonic development and scarless wound healing (Tandon et al., 2010).

TGF-β1 (the first member of the family to be discovered and the best-studied member to date) is present at high levels in the healthy blood vessel wall, whereas TGF-β2 and TGF-β3 isoforms are either absent (β2) or present only at low levels (β3) (Lebrin et al., 2005). Moreover, TGF-β1 is a potent regulator of vascular development and vessel remodeling and plays key roles in atherosclerosis and restenosis, regulating endothelial, smooth muscle cell (SMC), macrophage, T-cell and probably vascular calcifying cell responses (Bobik, 2006).

Thus, in this review, we will focus on TGF-β1 cytokine and its receptors and transducers related mostly to *in vivo* atherogenesis, both in animals and humans.

## 2. TGF-β1 and atherogenesis

There are a number of studies which demonstrate the role of TGF-β1 cytokine in atherosclerosis. TGF-β1 is produced by both inflammatory and vascular cells and is expressed in human and mouse atherosclerotic plaques (Mallat et al., 2001).

There is some controversial information regarding the role of TGF-β1 in atherogenesis. One group of papers show anti-atherogenic role of TGF-β1 cytokine. Inhibition of TGF-β1 activity by various approaches results in pro-atherogenic changes in the vessel wall in animal models of atherosclerosis (Singh and Ramji, 2006). Deletion of a single allele of the TGF-β1 gene, which reduces the amount of TGF-β1 protein in the vessel media by ~ 50%, results in reduced SMC differentiation, and increased susceptibility to endothelial cell activation and vascular lipid lesion formation in response to pro-atherogenic stimuli such as a lipid-rich diet (Grainger et al., 2000). Moreover treatment with neutralizing anti-TGF-β1 antibodies led to increased vascular inflammation, accelerated lipid lesion formation and a shift in plaque morphology towards an unstable phenotype (Mallat et al., 2001). Inhibition of TGF-β1 with a recombinant soluble TGF-β receptor fusion protein was associated not only with increased inflammation but also with intraplaque hemorrhage (Lutgens et al., 2002). Additionally, TGF-β1 has been shown to increase bovine aortic endothelial cell (BAEC) and human umbilical vein endothelial cell (HUVEC) steady-state eNOS mRNA expression (Inoue et al., 1995), suggesting the protective role of this cytokine in the vessel endothelium. Moreover, smooth muscle cells in stable lesions express greater amounts of TGF-β1 than unstable lesions (Cipollone et al., 2004). Furthermore, disruption of TGF-β1 signaling specifically in T-cells also results in increased lesion size and development of an unstable phenotype (Li et al., 2006; Robertson et al., 2003). Additionally, TGF-β1 attenuates macrophage foam cell formation, increases cholesterol efflux (Panousis et al., 2001) and inhibits lipoprotein lipase expression (Irvine et al., 2005). Furthermore, TGF-β1 reduces cytokine-stimulated inducible nitric oxide synthase (iNOS) expression (Werner et al., 2000), promotes iNOS protein degradation (Mitani et al., 2005), and inhibits expression of cell adhesion molecules (DiChiara et al., 2000).

On the other hand, there have been some reports discussing a possible atherogenic activity of this cytokine. Elevated TGF-β1 levels have been found in vessel wall lesions (Majesky et al., 1991; Nikol et al., 1992). Moreover, TGF-β is a potent stimulator of proteoglycan biosynthesis in human SMCs (Chen et al., 1987), its presence in fatty lesions is likely to contribute to the synthesis of lipoprotein-trapping proteoglycans, which can contribute to accumulation of lipoproteins in the vessel wall (O'Brien et al., 1998) and their subsequent chemical modification (Grainger et al., 1995). Moreover TGF-β1 stimulates leukocyte chemotaxis (Ashcroft, 1999), suggesting that TGF-β contributes to early macrophage migration and lipid accumulation. When infused into rats with preexisting vascular lesions, TGF-β1 caused an 80% increase in lesion size due to extracellular matrix accumulation (Majesky et al., 1991). Localization of TGF-β1 correlated with areas of neointimal formation, where increase in expression of fibronectin and collagen types I and III was observed (Bahadori et al., 1995; Majesky et al., 1991). Antibodies against TGF-β1 suppressed intimal hyperplasia in a rat model (Wolf et al., 1994). Similarly, Schulick et al. demonstrated that overexpression of active TGF-β1 in uninjured rat arteries results in the development of a matrix-rich neointima (Schulick et al., 1998). All these data generally suggest a strong participation of TGF-β1 in the development of atherosclerosis.

In summary, TGF-β1 seems to participate in the development of atherosclerosis, but maybe more interestingly promote a stable lesion phenotype, suggesting its role in the protection of acute ischemic situations like myocardial infarction.

TGF-β1 is secreted in a latent form, where it is associated in a complex with latency-associated protein (LAP) and latent TGF-β1 binding protein-1 (LTBP). Latent TGF-β1 can be activated by a number of physical processes, including heat, acid, reactive oxygen species, and biological processes such as proteolysis or integrin - mediated activation. A number of proteases, including plasmin, thrombin, elastase, MMP-2 (matrix metalloproteinase-2) and MMP-9, have been shown to be capable of directly activating latent TGF-β1 *in vitro* (Jenkins, 2008). TGF-β1 can bind a heteromeric complex of type I and type II transmembrane serine/threonine kinase receptors. This complex is usually formed by ligand, one TGF-β type II receptor (TβR-II) and two TGF-β type I receptors called activin receptor-like kinase (ALK) (ten Dijke and Hill, 2004). This process can be affected by type III receptor known as endoglin (CD105) (Grainger, 2007). In the ligand-bound complex, the type II receptor phosphorylates serine and threonine residues in the GS region of the type I receptor. After that, conformational changes in the type I receptor appear and subsequently, phosphorylation of signaling molecules named Smads propagate the signal to the nucleus, where they finally regulate transcription of several genes, including those with importance in atherogenesis (Lebrin et al., 2005). Human genome encodes seven type I receptors (ALKs 1-7) and five type II receptors (ActR-IIA, ActR-IIB, BMPRII, AMHR-II and TβR-II) that are paired in different combinations as receptor complexes for various members of TGF-β family (Massague and Gomis, 2006). Moreover, there are also three distinct types of Smad proteins (Feinberg and Jain, 2005).

In the following part of this review we will discuss the role of TGF-β receptors in atherogenesis.

### 2.1 TGF-β receptors I and their role in atherogenesis

As mentioned above there are seven type I receptors, designated activin receptor-like kinases (ALK-1 to ALK-7) (de Caestecker, 2004; Miyazono et al., 2000). The decision which type I receptor is activated is determined by receptor expression and/or ligand concentration (Goumans et al., 2002). The most important and the most studied type I receptors with respect to atherogenesis are ALK-1 and ALK-5.

Many previously published *in vitro* studies demonstrated a large interplay and mostly opposite effects of ALK-1 and ALK-5 (Goumans et al., 2003). In endothelial cells, TGF-β type

II receptor can activate endothelial cell-restricted ALK-1 and/or broadly expressed ALK-5, which have opposite effects on endothelial cell behavior (Lebrin et al., 2005). Both ALK-1 and ALK-5 can activate various Smad proteins, which will be discussed later. ALK-5 was found to be important for recruitment of ALK-1 into a TGF-β receptor complex, and additionally, the kinase activity of ALK-5 is essential for efficient ALK-1 activation (Massague and Gomis, 2006).

Both ALK-1 and ALK-5 are important for endothelial cell regulation. The TGF-β/ALK-1 pathway stimulates endothelial cell proliferation and migration, whereas the TGF-β/ALK-5 pathway inhibits these processes. ALK-1 stimulates the expression of Id-1, an inhibitor of basic helix-loop-helix proteins, and promotes endothelial cell proliferation, migration and tube formation (Valdimarsdottir et al., 2002), whereas ALK-5 induces expression of fibronectin, an extracellular matrix protein (Lebrin et al., 2005), and plasminogen activator inhibitor-1, a negative regulator of endothelial cell migration and angiogenesis (Watabe et al., 2003).

Very little is known about changes in expression patterns of type I receptors during atherogenesis.

The study of Yao et al. showed that ALK-1 is minimally expressed in atherosclerosis-free segments of human coronary arteries. On the other hand, ALK-1 expression was strongly upregulated in atherosclerotic lesions. The expression was detected in neointima, coronary endothelium and in areas of the shoulder region that appeared to be a site of neoangiogenesis. In addition, the expression was detected in the core of the lesions and in areas that appeared to undergo cellular organization (Yao et al., 2007). Authors also suggested that ALK-1 signaling in the endothelium may be important in the initiation of the atherosclerotic lesion. Moreover, ALK-1 expression in atherosclerotic lesions may contribute to regulation of proliferation and promotion of SMC differentiation, both during development and progression of atherosclerosis (Yao et al., 2007). Another study showed that ALK-1 may stimulate expression of vascular endothelial growth factor (VEGF) in endothelial cells (Yao et al., 2008), which might represent a protective effect on vessel endothelium with respect to the development of endothelial dysfunction (Walshe et al., 2009). In line with these results, ALK-1 expression was related to decreased plaque size after both atorvastatin treatment (Rathouska et al., 2011) and reduction of cholesterol in apoE/LDLr-deficient mice (Strasky et al., 2011).

In many studies, ALK-5, usually named simply TGF-β receptors I, is weakly expressed in intimal cells in human non-atherosclerotic aortas. On the other hand, strong ALK-5 expression was detected in fatty streaks/fibrofatty lesions. Additionally, its expression was strongly decreased in fibrous plaques (Bobik et al., 1999), suggesting that ALK-5 might support TGF-β1 activity in the promotion of lipoprotein retention, activation of proteolytic systems of macrophages, and also limitation of SMC proliferation in fatty lesions (Bobik et al., 1999). On the other hand, ALK-5-mediated signaling plays an important role in keeping the endothelium quiescent by inhibiting EC proliferation, tube formation and migration, thus angiogenesis (Goumans et al., 2002). Additionally, most of the effects of TGF-β on SMC function appear to be mediated via ALK-5 (Bobik, 2006). All effects of ALK-5 are mediated by Smad2/3 proteins which will be discussed later.

### 2.2 TGF-β receptor II and its role in atherogenesis

As mentioned above, TβR-II interacts with various TβR-I, including ALK-1 and ALK-5. However, there are some studies focusing on the role TβR-II in atherosclerosis alone.

In general, it was shown that TβR-II expression is strong in non-atherosclerotic human vessels in the majority of cells in media and intima and also in fatty streaks, predominantly in smooth muscle cells and macrophages. On the other hand, the expression of TβR-II was reduced in fibrous plaque and associated media (Bobik et al., 1999). These data assume strong activity of TGF-β1/TβR-II system in fatty streaks/fibrofatty lesions. Moreover, Piao and Tokunaga observed in human aortic atherosclerotic lesions increased levels of TβR-II, mainly in intima, SMCs, and macrophages, as well as in endothelial cells, when compared with non-atherosclerotic vessels, proposing its participation in atherosclerosis (Piao and Tokunaga, 2006). On the other hand, papers showed that there are some differences in TGF-β receptor expression patterns in vascular SMCs derived from normal versus diseased arteries. It was demonstrated that the type II receptor is decreased in SMCs derived from atherosclerotic lesions, with little change in the type I or III receptors. Subsequent analysis of human lesion versus normal tissues confirmed that the type I receptor is consistently present in the lesion, while the type II receptor was much more variable and commonly absent in both coronary artery and carotid artery lesions (McCaffrey, 2000). Additionally, others suggested an important role of TβR-II expression with respect to plaque stability. In mouse, suppression of TGF-β signaling through expression of a dominant negative type II TGF-β receptor, either systemically (Lutgens et al., 2002) or selectively in T-cells (Gojova et al., 2003); (Robertson et al., 2003), results in accelerated lipid lesion formation, increased vascular inflammation and a shift to an unstable lesion phenotype, thus more macrophage and lymphocyte and less collagen content. In addition, Lutgens et al. showed that inhibition of TGF-β activity following systemic administration of a recombinant soluble TGF-β type II receptor leads to change of plaque morphology into inflammatory phenotype that is low in fibrosis (Lutgens et al., 2002).

In summary, these data suggest a protective role of TβR-II expression in atherosclerosis.

## 3. Endoglin, the accessory type III receptor

Endoglin (or CD105) is a homodimeric transmembrane glycoprotein, that interacts with TGF-β1 and TGF-β3, but only when it is associated with TβRII (Lastres et al., 1996). Endoglin is not the true receptor but it strongly modulates activities of TGF-βRII (Guerrero-Esteo et al., 2002), ALK-1 (Guerrero-Esteo et al., 2002; Lebrin et al., 2004) and ALK-5 (Guerrero-Esteo et al., 2002). Endoglin physically interacts with TGF-βRI and TGF-βRII, and this interaction is not modified by the presence of exogenous ligand or by the activation state of the signaling kinases (Wrana et al., 1994). Additionally, endoglin inhibits phosphorylation levels of TGF-βRII *in vivo* and *in vitro*. On the other hand, endoglin was found to affect not only the phosphorylation status of TGF-βRII but also that of TGF-βRI. The presence of endoglin also appears to affect signaling downstream of TGF-βRI-TGF-βRII complex (Lopez-Novoa and Bernabeu, 2010). In general, endoglin is highly expressed by vascular endothelial cells (Li et al., 2000), SMCs (Adam et al., 1998), macrophages (Lastres et al., 1992) and T-cells (Bobik, 2006), which are cells strongly participating in the atherogenesis.

There are some studies showing the expression of endoglin in atherosclerotic lesions, both in humans and experimental animals. Low levels of endoglin expression in endothelial cells, medial smooth muscle cells and adventitial fibroblasts were detected in normal porcine coronary arteries. However, balloon injury in these vessels significantly increased its expression in both endothelial cells and smooth muscle cells (Ma et al., 2000). Moreover, in atherosclerotic human coronary artery tissue, endoglin was overexpressed in SMCs, in smooth muscle alpha-actin (SM a-actin) positive cells of atherosclerotic plaques, but it was not expressed in normal vascular smooth muscle, suggesting that endoglin may play a role in the response of the vessel wall to injury, including the development of atherosclerosis (Conley et al., 2000). Also other studies showed higher expression of endoglin in atherosclerotic vessels when compared with non–diseased vessels, suggesting that endoglin participates in atherogenesis (Piao and Tokunaga, 2006; Tashiro et al., 2002). Additionally, endoglin expression was linked to neo-angiogenesis within atherosclerotic aortic and carotid plaques, supporting its role in this process (Krupinski et al., 2008). Moreover, endoglin serum levels were found to be elevated in patients with atherosclerosis and correlated with total cholesterol levels (Blann et al., 1996).

On the other hand, several papers suggested an important role of endoglin in regulation of expression and activity of endothelial NO synthase (eNOS). The levels of eNOS are strongly related to the amount of endoglin, both *in vivo* and *in vitro* (Jerkic et al., 2004; Toporsian et al., 2005). Toporsian et al. found that partial or total loss of endoglin in murine endothelial cells is associated with a 50% decrease in eNOS levels (Toporsian et al., 2005). In addition, eNOS - derived NO seems to play a major role in endoglin-dependent angiogenesis (Jerkic et al., 2006). Santibanez et al. demonstrated that endoglin-dependent induction of eNOS occurs at the transcriptional level and moreover that endoglin is able to regulate eNOS expression independently of TGF-β (Santibanez et al., 2007). Endoglin colocalization with eNOS in aortic endothelial cells in mice atherosclerosis was also demonstrated (Nachtigal et al., 2009b). More recently, it was demonstrated that endoglin serum levels are decreased by extracorporeal LDL-cholesterol elimination in patients with familial hypercholesterolemia, suggesting that endoglin can serve as a marker for evaluation of the treatment efficacy of these procedure (Blaha et al., 2008).

In the light of above mentioned data, it is suggested that endoglin plays a role in atherogenesis, however its role with respect to atherogenic and/or atheroprotective effects remains to be elucidated.

## 4. Smad proteins in atherogenesis

As mentioned above, TGF-β1 and its receptors activate intracellular signal transducers called Smad proteins (Derynck et al., 1996). Eight Smad proteins are encoded in the human and mouse genomes but only five of them are substrates for TGF-β receptors, which are commonly referred to as receptor-regulated Smads, or RSmads ( Smad1, Smad2, Smad3, Smad5, and Smad8) (Massague, 1998). Smad4, named Co-Smad, serves as a common partner for all RSmads. Moreover, there are inhibitory Smad6 and Smad7 (Miyazono et al., 2000).

In general, no expression of Smad2 and Smad3 was detected in healthy human non-atherosclerotic aorta. On the other hand, strong Smad2 and Smad3 expression was detected in macrophages after differentiation from monocytes in fatty streaks/fibrofatty lesions (Kalinina et al., 2004). Smads were not detected in smooth muscle cells in these lesions. On the contrary, strong SMAD2 and SMAD3 expression was detected in SMC in aortic fibrous plaques, suggesting their participation in collagen production in these lesions, which seems to be important for lesion stability (Kalinina et al., 2004). Several other, mostly *in vitro,* studies revealed the effects of various Smads on the cellular components of atherosclerotic lesions. Smad3 was shown to be important for suppressing the inflammatory response in macrophages, including inhibition of inducible nitric oxide synthase (iNOS), monocyte chemoattractant protein-1 (MCP-1), and MMP-9 (Feinberg et al., 2004a; Werner et al., 2000). These inhibitory effects of Smad3 were attributed to inhibition of transcription factors, including AP-1, and to competition with NF-κB for limiting quantities of the co-activator p300/CBP (Feinberg and Jain, 2005).

Moreover, Smad3 seems to be important also in the modification of T-cell activity related to atherosclerosis. CD4+ and CD8+ T-cells from Smad3-deficient mice had increased IL-2 production (McKarns and Schwartz, 2005). Moreover, it was demonstrated that Smad3 stimulates production of Th2 cytokine shown to have anti-inflammatory effects in various experimental atherosclerotic models (Blokzijl et al., 2002). Smad3 potentiated by Smad4 is also able to reduce expression of SMC activation markers IL-6 and iNOS (Feinberg et al., 2004b), which are also linked to the progression of atherosclerosis.

Smad2 was shown to be important in endothelial cells. Saura et al demonstrated that the overexpression of Smad2 induces expression of eNOS, a critical regulator of vascular function and response to inflammation (Saura et al., 2002). Potential role of Smad2 in regulation of vascular inflammation can be related to its inhibition of NF-κB via competition with NF-κB for limiting amounts of p300/CBP (DiChiara et al., 2000).

These data nicely demonstrate anti-inflammatory and endothelial-protective effects of Smad2 and Smad3 in atherogenesis.

Smad1 effects on atherogenesis are not well documented so far. In general, Smad1 can be activated by BMP ligands, as well as by TGF-β1/ALK-1 activation mostly in endothelial cells (Goumans et al., 2002). This activation is related to activation of cell proliferation and angiogenesis (Oh et al., 2000). Since the specific role of angiogenesis in atherosclerosis with respect to pro- or anti-atherogenic effects is still not clear, the role of Smad1 in atherosclerosis remains to be elucidated in the future (Khurana et al., 2005).

Smad4 can form a complex with other Smads, including Smad2 and/or Smad3, and participates in augmenting of several effects of these Smads in a variety of cell types important in vascular inflammation (Feinberg and Jain, 2005). Smad4 was expressed together with Smad2 and Smad3 in fibrous plaques participating in collagen production, suggesting its effects on stable plaque phenotype (Kalinina et al., 2004).

Smad6 and Smad7 are inhibitors of both Smad2 and Smad3 phosphorylation (Shi and Massague, 2003). However, their effects in different tissues are not the same. For example, Smad7 blocked the TGF-β1-induced growth inhibition in VSMCs, Smad6 did not possess this ability (Ikedo et al., 2003). NF-κB and IFN-γ signaling rapidly induce Smad7 expression. This results in an increased expression of pro-inflammatory cytokines (IL-1β or TNF-α) in macrophages and vascular SMCs, suggesting that Smad7 blocks anti-inflammatory effects of TGF-β1 at least *in vitro* (Kato et al., 2001).

Recently, a splice variant of Smad6 (Smad6s) expressed in endothelial cells has been shown to affect TGF-β signaling. Both isoforms were detected in both normal vessels and atherosclerotic lesions localized in endothelial cells of the intima and in vasa vasorum as well as in smooth muscle cells of media (Krishnan et al., 2001). However, functional roles of these two isoforms in the context of atherogenesis have not been determined.

It can be concluded that Smad proteins are expressed in atherosclerotic lesions, where Smad2 and Smad3 play potential anti-atherogenic roles. The role of other Smads in relation to *in vivo* atherogenesis remains to be elucidated.

## 5. TGF-β1 related signaling pathways and atherogenesis

In previous chapters, we described studies that focused on the role of one or two members of TGF-β pathway. In this part, we are going to focus on studies, in which at least 3 members were part of the study.

As mentioned previously, TGF-β1 activates TGF-β receptor II which is followed by activation of different TGF-β receptor I, e.g. ALK-1 and ALK-5, with subsequent phosphorylation of various Smad proteins (Goumans et al., 2009). All these pathways can be modified by accessory TGF-β III receptors, mainly by endoglin (Lopez-Novoa and Bernabeu, 2010).

In general, TGF-β/ALK-5 signaling induces Smad2/3 phosphorylation and blocks angiogenesis by inhibiting EC proliferation, tube formation and migration. TGF-β/ALK-5/Smad2/3 signaling plays an important role in keeping the endothelium quiescent (Goumans et al., 2009; Goumans et al., 2002).

In contrast to TGF-β/ALK-5, TGF-β/ALK-1 signaling induces Smad1/5 activation and has been shown to stimulate EC migration, proliferation and tube formation (Goumans et al., 2003). Strong interplay between both cascades has been demonstrated *in vitro*. ALK-5-deficient ECs are not only defective in TGF-β/ALK-5 signaling but also exhibit impaired TGF-β/ALK-1 responses. Furthermore, ALK-1 can directly antagonize ALK-5/Smad2/3 signaling at the level of Smads (Goumans et al., 2002; Oh et al., 2000).

Piao et al studied the expression of TGF-β1, endoglin and TGF-β receptor II in human aortic atherosclerotic lesions and non-atherosclerotic aortas. Immunohistochemical analysis revealed a weak expression of all studied markers in the vessel wall. On the other hand, they described simultaneous expression of TGF-β1, endoglin and TβR-II in most atherosclerotic aortas in endothelium, macrophages and smooth muscle cells, suggesting the participation of these proteins in atherosclerosis (Piao and Tokunaga, 2006).

In another *in vitro* study Santibanez et al revealed a mechanism in which endoglin regulates the expression of eNOS. They showed that endoglin strongly supports TGF-β/Smad2 signaling by increasing the levels of Smad2 protein as a consequence of enhancing Smad2 stability. Secondary to the increase in Smad2 protein levels, they observed increased association of Smad2 with the receptor complex, higher levels of Smad2 phosphorylation, and an increase in Smad2/Smad4 heteromeric complex formation which was followed by increased expression of eNOS (Santibanez et al., 2007). These data suggest an important role of TGF-β1/endoglin/Smad2/eNOS pathway in the function of endothelium and atherosclerosis.

Moreover, Chen et al also demonstrated an important role of TGF-β receptors and Smad2 with respect to cholesterol levels. They demonstrated that cholesterol inhibits TGF-β1/TβR-II/TβR-I/Smad2 signaling by lowering of TβR-II/TβR-I binding ratio in plasma membrane and decrease in Smad2 phosphorylation, which was related to progression of atherosclerosis (Chen et al., 2008; Chen et al., 2007). These data were supported recently by Strasky et al, who demonstrated that hypercholesterolemia decreases endoglin, phosphorylated Smad2 and endothelial protective VEGF expression simultaneously with increased atherosclerosis in mice aorta (Strasky et al., 2011). In addition, Bot et al, described endoglin/TGF-β1/Smad2/3 expression and signaling in human atherosclerotic lesions. These authors demonstrated that endoglin/TGF-β1/Smad2/3 expression and activity correlates with a fibrous plaque phenotype, increased collagen levels, less matrix degradation, more SMC proliferation, reduction in inflammatory cell number and decreased amount of intraplaque

thrombi. This suggests that these markers are associated with more stable plaque phenotype in human atherosclerosis (Bot et al., 2009).
In summary, activation of TGF-β1 signaling pathway, which includes endoglin and Smad2, seems to play a protective role in atherogenesis via protection of vascular endothelium and atherosclerotic plaque stabilization.

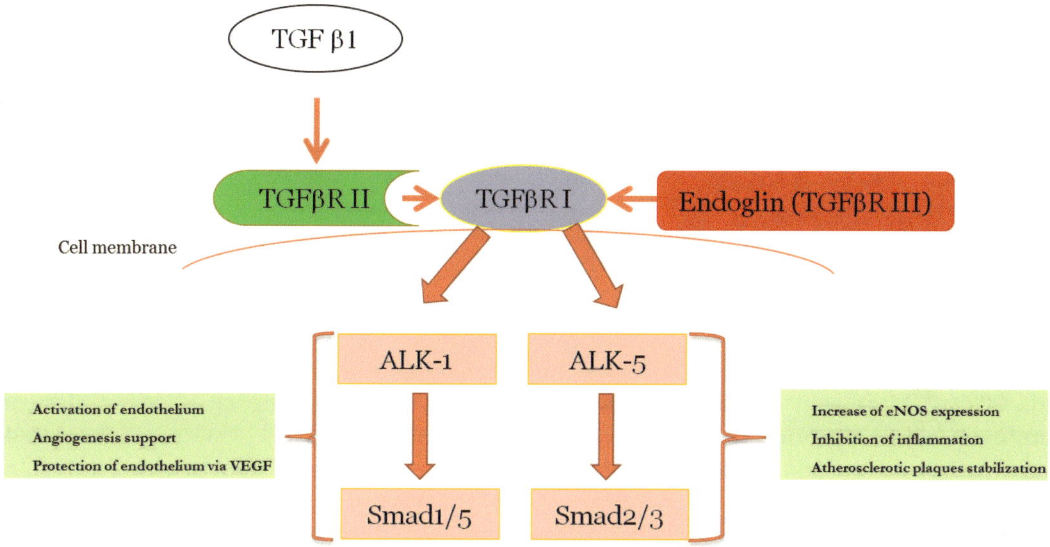


Fig. 1. TGF-β1 signaling pathway. TGF-β1 activates TβR-II, and the complex TGF-β1/TGF-RII is presented to TGF-R-I, which can represent several subtypes called activin-like kinases or ALKs. In atherogenesis, the activation of ALK-1 or ALK-5 under the control of endoglin is the most common. Activation of TGF-β1/TβR-II/endoglin/ALK-5/Smad2/3 signaling is related to several anti-atherogenic effects, including increased eNOS expression, increased collagen production (plaque stabilization), inhibition of inflammatory activities of macrophages, T-cells and inhibition of NF-κB signaling. On the other hand activation of TGF-β1/TβR-II/endoglin/ALK-1/Smad1 was related to increased VEGF production which was demonstrated to be important in angiogenesis and/or vascular endothelium protection.

### 5.1 TGF-β1 related pathways and statins

In this part we would like to discuss TGF-β1 pathway and possible effects of the most used hypolipidemic drugs in clinical practice. 3-hydroxy-3-methylglutaryl coenzyme A reductase (HMG CoA-reductase) inhibitors, commonly known as statins, inhibit the rate-limiting step of the cholesterol biosynthesis pathway. This hypolipidemic effect is very important, regarding the benefit of statin treatment in humans. However, statins also have non-lipid effects that were demonstrated in both humans and experimental models of atherosclerosis (Zhou and Liao, 2010). Statins regulate many of cellular responses, via the blockade of isoprenoid production and inhibition of intracellular signaling systems, including transcription factors, such as NF-κB, and kinases, like mitogen-activated protein kinases (MAPK) cascade and RhoA/ROCK pathway (Zhou and Liao, 2010).

Baccante et al showed that pravastatin induces TGF-β1 expression and down-regulates the expression of type A scavenger receptor in THP-1 cells (human macrophage cell line) by a TGF-β1-dependent mechanism, suggesting the protection against formation of foam cells (Baccante et al., 2004). Additionally, pravastatin treatment up-regulated TGF-β1 serum levels in hypercholesterolemic patients, and also TGF-β1 production *in vitro* in human monocytes (Porreca et al., 2002). Chen et al. showed that fluvastatin and lovastatin increase accumulation of TβR-II in non-lipid raft microdomains, and attenuate degradation of TβR-II which results in enhanced TGF-β1 signaling (Chen et al., 2008; Chen et al., 2007) in endothelial cells. Moreover, simvastatin and atorvastatin significantly increased TGF-β1 secretion, TβR-II expression and induced Smad2 and Smad3 phosphorylation in a dose-dependent manner in vascular smooth muscle cells (Rodriguez-Vita et al., 2008). Additionally, atorvastatin increased phosphorylation of Smad3 and expression of TβR-II in atherosclerotic lesions in apoE-deficient mice (Rodriguez-Vita et al., 2008). This increase was related to decreased plaque size and increased production of collagen in vascular smooth muscle cells. Further studies also confirmed atheroprotective effects of statin administration via TGF-β1 dependent pathway. Atorvastatin treatment significantly induced expression of endoglin, SMAD2, phosphorylated SMAD2/3 and eNOS in mice aortic atherosclerotic lesions (Nachtigal et al., 2009a). Moreover, in another study atorvastatin treatment increased expression of endoglin/ALK-1/p-Smad1/VEGF pathway simultaneously with decreased atherosclerosis in aorta of ApoE/LDLR double knockout mice (Rathouska et al., 2011). In addition, colocalization of all these proteins was demonstrated in endothelial cells, suggesting that activation of these pathways might contribute to TGF-β related protection of endothelial cells (Nachtigal et al., 2009b).

In summary, statin treatment activates TGF-β1 signaling cascades involving TβR-II, endoglin, Smad2/3 which results in reduced plaque size, increased collagen content and increased production of NO in endothelium.

## 6. Conclusion

In conclusion, the data presented in this chapter show the importance of TGF-β1 signaling in atherosclerosis in both animals and humans. Despite a few papers showing participation of TGF-β1 in early atherosclerosis, most of the papers demonstrate atheroprotective effects of TGF-β1 signaling. Activation of TGF-β1 signaling pathway results in anti-inflammatory effects, including decreased expression of cell adhesion molecules (with participation of Smad2 and endoglin), inhibition of inflammation in macrophages, T-cells (with participation of Smad3), increased expression of nitric oxide synthase (with participation of endoglin and Smad2), smooth muscle cells production of collagen and plaques stabilization (with participation of endoglin and Smad2/3). Moreover, reduction of cholesterol levels and/or statin treatment significantly enhances atheroprotective effects of TGF-β1 signaling.

## 7. Acknowledgments

This work was supported by grant from The Grant Agency of Charles University in Prague No. 300811/C, 137310/C Charles University in Prague project SVV/2011/263003 and Research project MZO 00179906.

## 8. References


Adam P. J., Clesham G. J. and Weissberg P. L. (1998) Expression of endoglin mRNA and protein in human vascular smooth muscle cells. *Biochem Biophys Res Commun* 247, 33-37.

Ashcroft G. S. (1999) Bidirectional regulation of macrophage function by TGF-beta. *Microbes Infect* 1, 1275-1282.

Assoian R. K., Komoriya A., Meyers C. A., Miller D. M. and Sporn M. B. (1983) Transforming growth factor-beta in human platelets. Identification of a major storage site, purification, and characterization. *J Biol Chem* 258, 7155-7160.

Baccante G., Mincione G., Di Marcantonio M. C., Piccirelli A., Cuccurullo F. and Porreca E. (2004) Pravastatin up-regulates transforming growth factor-beta1 in THP-1 human macrophages: effect on scavenger receptor class A expression. *Biochem Biophys Res Commun* 314, 704-710.

Bahadori L., Milder J., Gold L. and Botney M. (1995) Active macrophage-associated TGF-beta co-localizes with type I procollagen gene expression in atherosclerotic human pulmonary arteries. *Am J Pathol* 146, 1140-1149.

Blaha M., Cermanova M., Blaha V., Jarolim P., Andrys C., Blazek M., Maly J., Smolej L., Zajic J., Masin V., Zimova R. and Rehacek V. (2008) Elevated serum soluble endoglin (sCD105) decreased during extracorporeal elimination therapy for familial hypercholesterolemia. *Atherosclerosis* 197, 264-270.

Blann A. D., Wang J. M., Wilson P. B. and Kumar S. (1996) Serum levels of the TGF-beta receptor are increased in atherosclerosis. *Atherosclerosis* 120, 221-226.

Blokzijl A., ten Dijke P. and Ibanez C. F. (2002) Physical and functional interaction between GATA-3 and Smad3 allows TGF-beta regulation of GATA target genes. *Curr Biol* 12, 35-45.

Bobik A. (2006) Transforming growth factor-betas and vascular disorders. *Arterioscler Thromb Vasc Biol* 26, 1712-1720.

Bobik A., Agrotis A., Kanellakis P., Dilley R., Krushinsky A., Smirnov V., Tararak E., Condron M. and Kostolias G. (1999) Distinct patterns of transforming growth factor-beta isoform and receptor expression in human atherosclerotic lesions. Colocalization implicates TGF-beta in fibrofatty lesion development. *Circulation* 99, 2883-2891.

Bot P. T., Hoefer I. E., Sluijter J. P., van Vliet P., Smits A. M., Lebrin F., Moll F., de Vries J. P., Doevendans P., Piek J. J., Pasterkamp G. and Goumans M. J. (2009) Increased expression of the transforming growth factor-beta signaling pathway, endoglin, and early growth response-1 in stable plaques. *Stroke* 40, 439-447.

Cipollone F., Fazia M., Mincione G., Iezzi A., Pini B., Cuccurullo C., Ucchino S., Spigonardo F., Di Nisio M., Cuccurullo F., Mezzetti A. and Porreca E. (2004) Increased expression of transforming growth factor-beta1 as a stabilizing factor in human atherosclerotic plaques. *Stroke* 35, 2253-2257.

Conley B. A., Smith J. D., Guerrero-Esteo M., Bernabeu C. and Vary C. P. (2000) Endoglin, a TGF-beta receptor-associated protein, is expressed by smooth muscle cells in human atherosclerotic plaques. *Atherosclerosis* 153, 323-335.

de Caestecker M. (2004) The transforming growth factor-beta superfamily of receptors. *Cytokine Growth Factor Rev* 15, 1-11.

Derynck R., Gelbart W. M., Harland R. M., Heldin C. H., Kern S. E., Massague J., Melton D. A., Mlodzik M., Padgett R. W., Roberts A. B., Smith J., Thomsen G. H., Vogelstein B. and Wang X. F. (1996) Nomenclature: vertebrate mediators of TGFbeta family signals. *Cell* 87, 173.

DiChiara M. R., Kiely J. M., Gimbrone M. A., Jr., Lee M. E., Perrella M. A. and Topper J. N. (2000) Inhibition of E-selectin gene expression by transforming growth factor beta in endothelial cells involves coactivator integration of Smad and nuclear factor kappaB-mediated signals. *J Exp Med* 192, 695-704.

Feinberg M. W. and Jain M. K. (2005) Role of transforming growth factor-beta1/Smads in regulating vascular inflammation and atherogenesis. *Panminerva Med* 47, 169-186.

Feinberg M. W., Shimizu K., Lebedeva M., Haspel R., Takayama K., Chen Z., Frederick J. P., Wang X. F., Simon D. I., Libby P., Mitchell R. N. and Jain M. K. (2004a) Essential role for Smad3 in regulating MCP-1 expression and vascular inflammation. *Circ Res* 94, 601-608.

Feinberg M. W., Watanabe M., Lebedeva M. A., Depina A. S., Hanai J., Mammoto T., Frederick J. P., Wang X. F., Sukhatme V. P. and Jain M. K. (2004b) Transforming growth factor-beta1 inhibition of vascular smooth muscle cell activation is mediated via Smad3. *J Biol Chem* 279, 16388-16393.

Gojova A., Brun V., Esposito B., Cottrez F., Gourdy P., Ardouin P., Tedgui A., Mallat Z. and Groux H. (2003) Specific abrogation of transforming growth factor-beta signaling in T cells alters atherosclerotic lesion size and composition in mice. *Blood* 102, 4052-4058.

Goumans M. J., Liu Z. and ten Dijke P. (2009) TGF-beta signaling in vascular biology and dysfunction. *Cell Res* 19, 116-127.

Goumans M. J., Valdimarsdottir G., Itoh S., Lebrin F., Larsson J., Mummery C., Karlsson S. and ten Dijke P. (2003) Activin receptor-like kinase (ALK)1 is an antagonistic mediator of lateral TGFbeta/ALK5 signaling. *Mol Cell* 12, 817-828.

Goumans M. J., Valdimarsdottir G., Itoh S., Rosendahl A., Sideras P. and ten Dijke P. (2002) Balancing the activation state of the endothelium via two distinct TGF-beta type I receptors. *EMBO J* 21, 1743-1753.

Grainger D. J. (2007) TGF-beta and atherosclerosis in man. *Cardiovasc Res* 74, 213-222.

Grainger D. J., Kemp P. R., Metcalfe J. C., Liu A. C., Lawn R. M., Williams N. R., Grace A. A., Schofield P. M. and Chauhan A. (1995) The serum concentration of active transforming growth factor-beta is severely depressed in advanced atherosclerosis. *Nat Med* 1, 74-79.

Grainger D. J., Mosedale D. E., Metcalfe J. C. and Bottinger E. P. (2000) Dietary fat and reduced levels of TGFbeta1 act synergistically to promote activation of the vascular endothelium and formation of lipid lesions. *J Cell Sci* 113 ( Pt 13), 2355-2361.

Guerrero-Esteo M., Sanchez-Elsner T., Letamendia A. and Bernabeu C. (2002) Extracellular and cytoplasmic domains of endoglin interact with the transforming growth factor-beta receptors I and II. *J Biol Chem* 277, 29197-29209.

Chen C. L., Huang S. S. and Huang J. S. (2008) Cholesterol modulates cellular TGF-beta responsiveness by altering TGF-beta binding to TGF-beta receptors. *J Cell Physiol* 215, 223-233.

Chen C. L., Liu I. H., Fliesler S. J., Han X., Huang S. S. and Huang J. S. (2007) Cholesterol suppresses cellular TGF-beta responsiveness: implications in atherogenesis. *J Cell Sci* 120, 3509-3521.

Chen J. K., Hoshi H. and McKeehan W. L. (1987) Transforming growth factor type beta specifically stimulates synthesis of proteoglycan in human adult arterial smooth muscle cells. *Proc Natl Acad Sci U S A* 84, 5287-5291.

Ikedo H., Tamaki K., Ueda S., Kato S., Fujii M., Ten Dijke P. and Okuda S. (2003) Smad protein and TGF-beta signaling in vascular smooth muscle cells. *Int J Mol Med* 11, 645-650.

Inoue N., Venema R. C., Sayegh H. S., Ohara Y., Murphy T. J. and Harrison D. G. (1995) Molecular regulation of the bovine endothelial cell nitric oxide synthase by transforming growth factor-beta 1. *Arterioscler Thromb Vasc Biol* 15, 1255-1261.

Irvine S. A., Foka P., Rogers S. A., Mead J. R. and Ramji D. P. (2005) A critical role for the Sp1-binding sites in the transforming growth factor-beta-mediated inhibition of lipoprotein lipase gene expression in macrophages. *Nucleic Acids Res* 33, 1423-1434.

Jenkins G. (2008) The role of proteases in transforming growth factor-beta activation. *Int J Biochem Cell Biol* 40, 1068-1078.

Jerkic M., Rivas-Elena J. V., Prieto M., Carron R., Sanz-Rodriguez F., Perez-Barriocanal F., Rodriguez-Barbero A., Bernabeu C. and Lopez-Novoa J. M. (2004) Endoglin regulates nitric oxide-dependent vasodilatation. *Faseb J* 18, 609-611.

Jerkic M., Rodriguez-Barbero A., Prieto M., Toporsian M., Pericacho M., Rivas-Elena J. V., Obreo J., Wang A., Perez-Barriocanal F., Arevalo M., Bernabeu C., Letarte M. and Lopez-Novoa J. M. (2006) Reduced angiogenic responses in adult Endoglin heterozygous mice. *Cardiovasc Res* 69, 845-854.

Kalinina N., Agrotis A., Antropova Y., Ilyinskaya O., Smirnov V., Tararak E. and Bobik A. (2004) Smad expression in human atherosclerotic lesions: evidence for impaired TGF-beta/Smad signaling in smooth muscle cells of fibrofatty lesions. *Arterioscler Thromb Vasc Biol* 24, 1391-1396.

Kato S., Ueda S., Tamaki K., Fujii M., Miyazono K., ten Dijke P., Morimatsu M. and Okuda S. (2001) Ectopic expression of Smad7 inhibits transforming growth factor-beta responses in vascular smooth muscle cells. *Life Sci* 69, 2641-2652.

Khurana R., Simons M., Martin J. F. and Zachary I. C. (2005) Role of angiogenesis in cardiovascular disease: a critical appraisal. *Circulation* 112, 1813-1824.

Krishnan P., King M. W., Neff A. W., Sandusky G. E., Bierman K. L., Grinnell B. and Smith R. C. (2001) Human truncated Smad 6 (Smad 6s) inhibits the BMP pathway in Xenopus laevis. *Dev Growth Differ* 43, 115-132.

Krupinski J., Turu M. M., Luque A., Badimon L. and Slevin M. (2008) Increased PrPC expression correlates with endoglin (CD105) positive microvessels in advanced carotid lesions. *Acta Neuropathol* 116, 537-545.

Lastres P., Bellon T., Cabanas C., Sanchez-Madrid F., Acevedo A., Gougos A., Letarte M. and Bernabeu C. (1992) Regulated expression on human macrophages of endoglin, an Arg-Gly-Asp-containing surface antigen. *Eur J Immunol* 22, 393-397.

Lastres P., Letamendia A., Zhang H., Rius C., Almendro N., Raab U., Lopez L. A., Langa C., Fabra A., Letarte M. and Bernabeu C. (1996) Endoglin modulates cellular responses to TGF-beta 1. *J Cell Biol* 133, 1109-1121.

Laverty H. G., Wakefield L. M., Occleston N. L., O'Kane S. and Ferguson M. W. (2009) TGF-beta3 and cancer: a review. *Cytokine Growth Factor Rev* 20, 305-317.

Lebrin F., Deckers M., Bertolino P. and Ten Dijke P. (2005) TGF-beta receptor function in the endothelium. *Cardiovasc Res* 65, 599-608.

Lebrin F., Goumans M. J., Jonker L., Carvalho R. L., Valdimarsdottir G., Thorikay M., Mummery C., Arthur H. M. and ten Dijke P. (2004) Endoglin promotes endothelial cell proliferation and TGF-beta/ALK1 signal transduction. *EMBO J* 23, 4018-4028.

Li C., Hampson I. N., Hampson L., Kumar P., Bernabeu C. and Kumar S. (2000) CD105 antagonizes the inhibitory signaling of transforming growth factor beta1 on human vascular endothelial cells. *Faseb J* 14, 55-64.

Li C., Mollahan P., Baguneid M. S., McMahon R. F., Kumar P., Walker M. G., Freemont A. J. and Kumar S. (2006) A comparative study of neovascularisation in atherosclerotic plaques using CD31, CD105 and TGF beta 1. *Pathobiology* 73, 192-197.

Lopez-Novoa J. M. and Bernabeu C. (2010) The physiological role of endoglin in the cardiovascular system. *Am J Physiol Heart Circ Physiol* 299, H959-974.

Lutgens E., Gijbels M., Smook M., Heeringa P., Gotwals P., Koteliansky V. E. and Daemen M. J. (2002) Transforming growth factor-beta mediates balance between inflammation and fibrosis during plaque progression. *Arterioscler Thromb Vasc Biol* 22, 975-982.

Ma X., Labinaz M., Goldstein J., Miller H., Keon W. J., Letarte M. and O'Brien E. (2000) Endoglin is overexpressed after arterial injury and is required for transforming growth factor-beta-induced inhibition of smooth muscle cell migration. *Arterioscler Thromb Vasc Biol* 20, 2546-2552.

Majesky M. W., Lindner V., Twardzik D. R., Schwartz S. M. and Reidy M. A. (1991) Production of transforming growth factor beta 1 during repair of arterial injury. *J Clin Invest* 88, 904-910.

Mallat Z., Gojova A., Marchiol-Fournigault C., Esposito B., Kamate C., Merval R., Fradelizi D. and Tedgui A. (2001) Inhibition of transforming growth factor-beta signaling accelerates atherosclerosis and induces an unstable plaque phenotype in mice. *Circ Res* 89, 930-934.

Massague J. (1998) TGF-beta signal transduction. *Annu Rev Biochem* 67, 753-791.

Massague J. and Gomis R. R. (2006) The logic of TGFbeta signaling. *FEBS Lett* 580, 2811-2820.

McCaffrey T. A. (2000) TGF-betas and TGF-beta receptors in atherosclerosis. *Cytokine Growth Factor Rev* 11, 103-114.

McKarns S. C. and Schwartz R. H. (2005) Distinct effects of TGF-beta 1 on CD4+ and CD8+ T cell survival, division, and IL-2 production: a role for T cell intrinsic Smad3. *J Immunol* 174, 2071-2083.

Mitani T., Terashima M., Yoshimura H., Nariai Y. and Tanigawa Y. (2005) TGF-beta1 enhances degradation of IFN-gamma-induced iNOS protein via proteasomes in RAW 264.7 cells. *Nitric Oxide* 13, 78-87.

Miyazono K., ten Dijke P. and Heldin C. H. (2000) TGF-beta signaling by Smad proteins. *Adv Immunol* 75, 115-157.

Nachtigal P., Pospisilova N., Vecerova L., Micuda S., Brcakova E., Pospechova K. and Semecky V. (2009a) Atorvastatin Increases Endoglin, SMAD2, Phosphorylated SMAD2/3 and eNOS Expression in ApoE/LDLR Double Knockout Mice. *J Atheroscler Thromb* 16, 265-274.

Nachtigal P., Vecerova L., Pospisilova N., Micuda S., Brcakova E., Navarro Hernandez E., Pospechova K. and Semecky V. (2009b) Endoglin co-expression with eNOS, SMAD2 and phosphorylated SMAD2/3 in normocholesterolemic and hypercholesterolemic mice: an immunohistochemical study. *Histol Histopathol* 24, 1499-1506.

Nikol S., Isner J. M., Pickering J. G., Kearney M., Leclerc G. and Weir L. (1992) Expression of transforming growth factor-beta 1 is increased in human vascular restenosis lesions. *J Clin Invest* 90, 1582-1592.

O'Brien K. D., Olin K. L., Alpers C. E., Chiu W., Ferguson M., Hudkins K., Wight T. N. and Chait A. (1998) Comparison of apolipoprotein and proteoglycan deposits in human coronary atherosclerotic plaques: colocalization of biglycan with apolipoproteins. *Circulation* 98, 519-527.

Oh S. P., Seki T., Goss K. A., Imamura T., Yi Y., Donahoe P. K., Li L., Miyazono K., ten Dijke P., Kim S. and Li E. (2000) Activin receptor-like kinase 1 modulates transforming growth factor-beta 1 signaling in the regulation of angiogenesis. *Proc Natl Acad Sci U S A* 97, 2626-2631.

Panousis C. G., Evans G. and Zuckerman S. H. (2001) TGF-beta increases cholesterol efflux and ABC-1 expression in macrophage-derived foam cells: opposing the effects of IFN-gamma. *J Lipid Res* 42, 856-863.

Piao M. and Tokunaga O. (2006) Significant expression of endoglin (CD105), TGFbeta-1 and TGFbeta R-2 in the atherosclerotic aorta: an immunohistological study. *J Atheroscler Thromb* 13, 82-89.

Porreca E., Di Febbo C., Baccante G., Di Nisio M. and Cuccurullo F. (2002) Increased transforming growth factor-beta(1) circulating levels and production in human monocytes after 3-hydroxy-3-methyl-glutaryl-coenzyme a reductase inhibition with pravastatin. *J Am Coll Cardiol* 39, 1752-1757.

Proetzel G., Pawlowski S. A., Wiles M. V., Yin M., Boivin G. P., Howles P. N., Ding J., Ferguson M. W. and Doetschman T. (1995) Transforming growth factor-beta 3 is required for secondary palate fusion. *Nat Genet* 11, 409-414.

Rathouska J., Vecerova L., Strasky Z., Slanarova M., Brcakova E., Mullerova Z., Andrys C., Micuda S. and Nachtigal P. (2011) Endoglin as a possible marker of atorvastatin treatment benefit in atherosclerosis. *Pharmacol Res* 64, 53-59.

Robertson A. K., Rudling M., Zhou X., Gorelik L., Flavell R. A. and Hansson G. K. (2003) Disruption of TGF-beta signaling in T cells accelerates atherosclerosis. *J Clin Invest* 112, 1342-1350.

Rodriguez-Vita J., Sanchez-Galan E., Santamaria B., Sanchez-Lopez E., Rodrigues-Diez R., Blanco-Colio L. M., Egido J., Ortiz A. and Ruiz-Ortega M. (2008) Essential role of TGF-beta/Smad pathway on statin dependent vascular smooth muscle cell regulation. *PLoS One* 3, e3959.

Sanford L. P., Ormsby I., Gittenberger-de Groot A. C., Sariola H., Friedman R., Boivin G. P., Cardell E. L. and Doetschman T. (1997) TGFbeta2 knockout mice have multiple developmental defects that are non-overlapping with other TGFbeta knockout phenotypes. *Development* 124, 2659-2670.

Santibanez J. F., Letamendia A., Perez-Barriocanal F., Silvestri C., Saura M., Vary C. P., Lopez-Novoa J. M., Attisano L. and Bernabeu C. (2007) Endoglin increases eNOS expression by modulating Smad2 protein levels and Smad2-dependent TGF-beta signaling. *J Cell Physiol* 210, 456-468.

Saura M., Zaragoza C., Cao W., Bao C., Rodriguez-Puyol M., Rodriguez-Puyol D. and Lowenstein C. J. (2002) Smad2 mediates transforming growth factor-beta induction of endothelial nitric oxide synthase expression. *Circ Res* 91, 806-813.

Shi Y. and Massague J. (2003) Mechanisms of TGF-beta signaling from cell membrane to the nucleus. *Cell* 113, 685-700.

Shull M. M., Ormsby I., Kier A. B., Pawlowski S., Diebold R. J., Yin M., Allen R., Sidman C., Proetzel G., Calvin D. and et al. (1992) Targeted disruption of the mouse transforming growth factor-beta 1 gene results in multifocal inflammatory disease. *Nature* 359, 693-699.

Schulick A. H., Taylor A. J., Zuo W., Qiu C. B., Dong G., Woodward R. N., Agah R., Roberts A. B., Virmani R. and Dichek D. A. (1998) Overexpression of transforming growth factor beta1 in arterial endothelium causes hyperplasia, apoptosis, and cartilaginous metaplasia. *Proc Natl Acad Sci U S A* 95, 6983-6988.

Singh N. N. and Ramji D. P. (2006) The role of transforming growth factor-beta in atherosclerosis. *Cytokine Growth Factor Rev* 17, 487-499.

Strasky Z., Vecerova L., Rathouska J., Slanarova M., Brcakova E., Kudlackova Z., Andrys C., Micuda S. and Nachtigal P. (2011) Cholesterol Effects on Endoglin and Its Downstream Pathways in ApoE/LDLR Double Knockout Mice. *Circ J* 75, 1747-1755.

Tandon A., Tovey J. C., Sharma A., Gupta R. and Mohan R. R. (2010) Role of transforming growth factor Beta in corneal function, biology and pathology. *Curr Mol Med* 10, 565-578.

Tashiro H., Shimokawa H., Sadamatu K. and Yamamoto K. (2002) Prognostic significance of plasma concentrations of transforming growth factor-beta in patients with coronary artery disease. *Coron Artery Dis* 13, 139-143.

ten Dijke P. and Hill C. S. (2004) New insights into TGF-beta-Smad signalling. *Trends Biochem Sci* 29, 265-273.

ten Dijke P., Iwata K. K., Goddard C., Pieler C., Canalis E., McCarthy T. L. and Centrella M. (1990) Recombinant transforming growth factor type beta 3: biological activities and receptor-binding properties in isolated bone cells. *Mol Cell Biol* 10, 4473-4479.

Toporsian M., Gros R., Kabir M. G., Vera S., Govindaraju K., Eidelman D. H., Husain M. and Letarte M. (2005) A role for endoglin in coupling eNOS activity and regulating vascular tone revealed in hereditary hemorrhagic telangiectasia. *Circ Res* 96, 684-692.

Valdimarsdottir G., Goumans M. J., Rosendahl A., Brugman M., Itoh S., Lebrin F., Sideras P. and ten Dijke P. (2002) Stimulation of Id1 expression by bone morphogenetic protein is sufficient and necessary for bone morphogenetic protein-induced activation of endothelial cells. *Circulation* 106, 2263-2270.

Walshe T. E., Dole V. S., Maharaj A. S., Patten I. S., Wagner D. D. and D'Amore P. A. (2009) Inhibition of VEGF or TGF-{beta} signaling activates endothelium and increases leukocyte rolling. *Arterioscler Thromb Vasc Biol* 29, 1185-1192.

Watabe T., Nishihara A., Mishima K., Yamashita J., Shimizu K., Miyazawa K., Nishikawa S. and Miyazono K. (2003) TGF-beta receptor kinase inhibitor enhances growth and integrity of embryonic stem cell-derived endothelial cells. *J Cell Biol* 163, 1303-1311.

Werner F., Jain M. K., Feinberg M. W., Sibinga N. E., Pellacani A., Wiesel P., Chin M. T., Topper J. N., Perrella M. A. and Lee M. E. (2000) Transforming growth factor-beta 1 inhibition of macrophage activation is mediated via Smad3. *J Biol Chem* 275, 36653-36658.

Wolf Y. G., Rasmussen L. M. and Ruoslahti E. (1994) Antibodies against transforming growth factor-beta 1 suppress intimal hyperplasia in a rat model. *J Clin Invest* 93, 1172-1178.

Wrana J. L., Attisano L., Wieser R., Ventura F. and Massague J. (1994) Mechanism of activation of the TGF-beta receptor. *Nature* 370, 341-347.

Wu L., Siddiqui A., Morris D. E., Cox D. A., Roth S. I. and Mustoe T. A. (1997) Transforming growth factor beta 3 (TGF beta 3) accelerates wound healing without alteration of scar prominence. Histologic and competitive reverse-transcription-polymerase chain reaction studies. *Arch Surg* 132, 753-760.

Yao Y., Shao E. S., Jumabay M., Shahbazian A., Ji S. and Bostrom K. I. (2008) High-density lipoproteins affect endothelial BMP-signaling by modulating expression of the activin-like kinase receptor 1 and 2. *Arterioscler Thromb Vasc Biol* 28, 2266-2274.

Yao Y., Zebboudj A. F., Torres A., Shao E. and Bostrom K. (2007) Activin-like kinase receptor 1 (ALK1) in atherosclerotic lesions and vascular mesenchymal cells. *Cardiovasc Res* 74, 279-289.

Zhou Q. and Liao J. K. (2010) Pleiotropic effects of statins. - Basic research and clinical perspectives. *Circ J* 74, 818-826.

16

# CXCL4-Induced Macrophages: A Novel Therapeutic Target in Human Atherosclerosis?

Christian A. Gleissner and Christian Erbel
*University of Heidelberg*
*Germany*

## 1. Introduction

Atherosclerosis and its consequences (i.e. myocardial infarction and cardiac death) remain the major cause of morbidity and mortality in Western countries (Roger et al. 2011). Despite clinical advances that have substantially improved outcomes in patients suffering from coronary artery disease, including pharmacological interventions (e.g. novel anti platelet therapies, statins, etc.) as well as interventional and surgical therapies (e.g. drug-eluting stents), there is still a huge demand for improved diagnostic tools to identify patients at risk for adverse events as well as therapeutic means to prevent adverse events in these patients. Biomarkers such as high sensitivity CRP (Ridker 2007) or high sensitivity troponin T (Kurz et al. 2011) have brought some improvement in identifying patients requiring more intense treatment; however, the clinical need for better tools remains.

An important concept that may help to improve clinical care for patients with coronary artery disease is the inducement of plaque stability. Atherosclerotic lesions can show features of plaque stability or plaque instability (Naghavi et al. 2003a, Naghavi et al. 2003b). Stable plaques are characterized by a thick fibrous cap and a small necrotic core. By contrast, unstable plaques display a thin fibrous cap and a large necrotic core consisting of apoptotic macrophages, foam cells, and smooth muscle cells. Unstable plaques are more likely to rupture, and plaque rupture may subsequently result in thrombosis and occlusion of the vessel leading to a myocardial infarction or stroke.

A promising approach to identify potential markers of plaque instability may be the study of atherogenesis on a cellular and molecular level. During the development of atherosclerotic lesions, blood monocytes adhere to the activated endothelium, transmigrate into the subendothelial space, and differentiate towards macrophages, dendritic cells, or foam cells (Galkina & Ley 2009). Among the various leukocyte types involved in atherogenesis, monocytes and monocyte-derived macrophages represent the major fraction. The monocyte-macrophage differentiation process is affected by the extracellular matrix as well as by the combination of chemokines and cytokines representing the micromilieu of the plaque (Shashkin et al. 2005). In addition, cell-cell interactions may also affect the fate of monocytes within the atherosclerotic plaque. Monocyte-derived cells secrete chemokines, cytokines, and other mediators, leading to attraction of other immune cells and thereby promoting plaque progression and plaque instability (Shashkin et al. 2005). While it was initially thought that monocyte-derived macrophages represent a homogenous population of cells, substantial heterogeneity of human plaque macrophages has been recognized for almost two decades (Poston & Hussain 1993). However, only recently has the pathophysiological importance of macrophage heterogeneity aroused further scientific interest (Bouhlel et al. 2007, Boyle et al. 2009, Gleissner et al. 2010a, Waldo et al. 2008).

Platelets and platelet-derived mediators represent important players potentially promoting macrophage heterogeneity in atherosclerosis. It has been long known that platelets play an important role in inflammatory processes reaching far beyond their function in hemostasis (Ross 1999). Especially in the context of atherosclerosis, platelets and platelet-derived molecules are heavily involved. Thus, platelet-derived chemokines may interact with the endothelium as well as with various leukocyte types (Gleissner et al. 2008). Accordingly, activated platelets promote atherogenesis as shown in *Apoe*$^{-/-}$ mice (Huo et al. 2003). This effect may in part be chemokine-mediated by promotion of monocyte adherence to the endothelium (von Hundelshausen et al. 2001, von Hundelshausen et al. 2005), but it may also be a consequence of chemokine-induced monocyte-macrophage differentiation (Gleissner et al. 2010a, Gleissner et al. 2010b, Scheuerer et al. 2000).

The current review will discuss novel insights into the effects of CXCL4, one of the most abundant platelet chemokines, on macrophage differentiation in the context of atherogenesis. It attempts to summarize what is known about CXCL4-induced macrophages, put it into context with knowledge of macrophage heterogeneity in human atherosclerosis, and try to answer the question of whether specifically targeting these CXCL4-induced macrophages may be a promising approach to prevent or treat atherosclerosis in humans.

## 2. Macrophages and atherogenesis

### 2.1 Studying macrophages in human and murine models

Studying myeloid cells and especially monocyte-derived macrophages in humans is a difficult task. While monocytes can easily be isolated from human peripheral blood and differentiated towards macrophages in order to perform *in vitro* studies, the possibility of studying human macrophages within atherosclerotic lesions is restricted to the analysis of *post mortem* tissues or explanted tissues, e.g. of carotid endatherectomy specimens or explanted hearts after heart allograft transplantation. Even though these materials will allow studying macrophages within their pathophysiological environments, the systems may still be biased by post mortem processes or effects due to prolonged ischemic time resulting in changes that do not allow correctly assessing the *in vivo* situation.

On the other hand, using mouse models to study monocytes and monocyte-derived macrophages offers great potential by using differently-labeled or genetically modified monocyte subsets (e.g. using the CXC3CR1 FITC mice) that allow the generation impressive *in vivo* tracking models that have helped to identify differential roles of specific monocyte subsets (Auffray et al. 2007, Geissmann et al. 2003). However, these systems have one notable problem: it is extremely difficult to transfer the information gained from these mouse models to the human system. Thus, some of the markers used to identify murine monocyte subsets (e.g. Gr-1. Ly6C, etc.) do not exist in the human system or do not have a human marker that clearly corresponds to them. Furthermore, in many aspects, murine monocyte-derived macrophages behave differently from human macrophages. Thus, treating murine macrophages with lipopolysaccharide (LPS) leads to increased uptake of modified LDL (Fitzgerald et al. 2000). Conversely, treating human macrophages with LPS prevents uptake of modified LDL (own unpublished observation). Considering that uptake of modified LDL represents a crucial step during macrophage foam cell formation with great impact on atherogenesis, it becomes questionable as to how relevant results from murine experiments may be for the human situation.

A recent extremely valuable study has compared the transcriptomes of human and murine monocyte subsets (Ingersoll et al. 2010). In this study, the authors used CCR2 and CXC3CR1 to identify the two murine monocyte subsets, whereas CD14 and CD16 were used to differentiate between the human monocyte subsets. About 270 genes in humans and 550 genes in mice were differentially-expressed between the monocyte subsets. Interestingly, only about 130 were conserved between species and a substantial number of genes were found to be differentially-expressed in a cross-species comparison. Among those, the authors identified genes extremely important in atherogenesis, including the scavenger receptors CD36 or macrophage scavenger receptor-A, as well as other functionally important molecules such as receptors for apoptotic cells. Again, this supports the notion that there are considerable differences between the human and murine system, and that results from murine experiments should be taken with care when drawing conclusions for human atherosclerosis.

Based on these considerations, the current article will specifically focus on data derived from studies on human macrophages wherever possible. Murine data will only be referred to when no data on human cells are available.

## 2.2 Macrophage heterogeneity

### 2.2.1 General concept of macrophage plasticity and polarization

A central feature of macrophages is their plasticity. *Macrophage plasticity* is defined as the capacity of the cell to readily change its phenotypic and functional capacities depending on the external conditions. Thus, the repertoire of surface receptors, the ability to generate reactive oxygen species, and the potential to migrate towards specific chemoattractants can differ substantially depending on the external conditions. By contrast, the term *macrophage polarization* is used for defined states of macrophage plasticity, which can be induced by specific conditions (e.g. combination of cytokines) and is defined by the presence of specific surface markers or functional capacities.

*In vivo*, the conditions inducing or preventing macrophage plasticity and polarization are probably determined primarily by the micromilieu. In fact, the presence of differentially-polarized macrophages has been postulated early on (Poston & Hussain 1993) and has been confirmed within human atherosclerotic lesions by various groups including ourselves (Bouhlel et al. 2007, Boyle et al. 2009, Gleissner et al. 2010a, Waldo et al. 2008). These findings make clear that macrophages within one atherosclerotic plaque can not be considered to be a uniform cell population but may have different functions depending on their specific polarization type.

### 2.2.2 Accepted models of macrophage polarization

There is currently a well defined scheme of macrophage polarization in vitro and in vivo. The first to describe an "alternative" macrophage activation were Gordon et al., who demonstrated that upon stimulation with IL-4, macrophages express high levels of mannose receptor CD206 (Stein et al. 1992). Based on this finding, the paradigm of "classically" activated M1 macrophages and "alternatively" activated M2 macrophages became accepted (Fig.1).

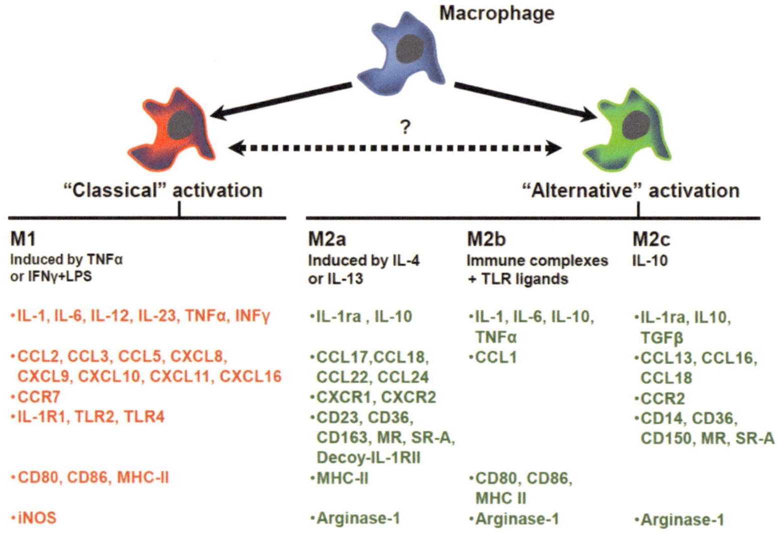


Fig. 1. The established paradigm of macrophage polarization. While M1 macrophages are thought to be involved in type I inflammation (bacterial killing or tumor resistance), M2 macrophages are associated with type II inflammation (allergy, parasital killing). For each polarization type, typical cytokines, chemokines, chemokine receptors, other receptors, surface molecules involved in antigen presentation, and intracellular enzymes are indicated.

According to this paradigm, M1 macrophages can be induced by a combination of interferon-γ and LPS or by tumor necrosis factor-α and are characterized by expression of pro-inflammatory cytokines like interleukin-1, interleukin-6, tumor necrosis factor-α, or interferon-γ. Furthermore, M1 macrophages express chemokines like CLL2 or CCL5, surface receptors like TLR2 or TLR4, and enzymes like iNOS. It is thought that M1 macrophage polarization mirrors the Th1 response of T cells, i.e. they represent a rather pro-inflammatory type of macrophage.

By contrast, M2 macrophages can be induced by Th2 cytokines like IL-4. They can express Th2 cytokines like IL-10 and are specifically characterized by the expression of surface receptors like CD163, CD206 (mannose receptor), or scavenger receptor-A and CD36. Since the first description of alternative macrophage activation has been published, several additional types of M2 macrophages have been identified, now defined as M2a (induced by IL-4 or Il-13), M2b (induced by immune complexes and TLR ligands), and M2c (induced by Il-10). Overall, M2 macrophages reflect the Th2 response and can be considered rather anti-inflammatory.

M1 and M2 macrophage polarization have been extensively studied including a comprehensive transcriptomic analysis of both macrophage polarization types (Martinez et al. 2006). In this gene array analysis, Martinez et al. confirmed the basic M1-M2 paradigm. Interestingly, monocyte-macrophage differentiation induced by MCSF alone leads to expression of many M2 genes, suggesting that basal conditions favour a default shift toward M2. Beyond this novel finding, the authors identified specific gene clusters involved in lipid metabolism, specific clusters of G protein-coupled receptors, and specific chemokines clusters in both M1 and M2 macrophages (Martinez et al. 2006). Both M1 and M2 macrophage polarization have been excellently reviewed by Gordon et al. as well as by Mantovani (Gordon 2003, Mantovani et al. 2009).

## 3. Platelet factor-4 (CXCL4), macrophages, and atherogenesis

### 3.1 CXCL4 – A platelet-derived chemokine in atherogenesis

Platelets and platelet-derived chemokines are important factors during atherogenesis (Gleissner et al. 2008, von Hundelshausen et al. 2007, Weber 2005, Weber 2008, Zernecke et al. 2008). In 2003, Ley et al. were able to demonstrate that activated platelets are able to promote atherogenesis (Huo et al. 2003). Upon activation, platelets release various chemokines from their alpha granules. Furthermore, activated platelets present or deposit chemokines and thereby induce recruitment of other cells to the arterial wall.

Among the plethora of chemokines released from activated platelets, CXCL4 (formerly known as platelet factor-4) is one of the most abundant. Accordingly, CXCL4 is released in human blood in micromolar concentrations upon platelet activation (Brandt et al. 2000). CXCL4 has been considered an "enigmatic" chemokine as it lacks the ELR domain typically seen in CXCL chemokines (Gear & Camerini 2003) and has been demonstrated to have effects on various cell types including endothelial cells, lymphocytes, neutrophils, and monocytes (Gleissner et al. 2008). However, the mechanisms by which CXCL4 exerts its effects, including receptors and signal transduction, have not fully been elucidated. Notably, CXCL4 has been demonstrated to induce monocyte adhesion to endothelial cells in conjunction with CCL5 (RANTES) (von Hundelshausen et al. 2005) and to promote macrophage differentiation from human peripheral blood monocytes (Scheuerer et al. 2000). Both mechanisms may be relevant during atherogenesis.

### 3.2 CXCL4 and macrophage differentiation

A role for CXCL4 for monoycte-macrophage differentiation has been suggested by Scheuerer et al. in 2000 (Scheuerer et al. 2000). Their data demonstrate that CXCL4 not only acts in an anti-apoptotic manner on human peripheral blood monocytes, but also promotes their differentiation towards macrophages in a dose-dependent manner as demonstrated by increased myeloperoxidase expression. The fact that these CXCL4-induced macrophages do not express any detectable CD86 levels on their cell surface suggested that they may be different from those induced by the typically used growth factor macrophage colony-stimulation factor MCSF (Scheuerer et al. 2000).

Interestingly, these first data had been abandoned for almost a decade. One reason for this may be the fact that up to now, nobody has been able to identify the CXCL4 receptor on human monocytes and macrophages. While on T cells and microvascular endothelial cells CXCR3 or splice variants thereof like CXCR3B (Lasagni et al. 2003) have been clearly identified, it is still not clear by which receptor and signal transduction CXCL4 acts on human myeloid cells. Accordingly, it was not until 2010 that our own group did a comprehensive gene expression screen on these cells revealing novel insights into the potential role of CXCL4-induced macrophages (Gleissner et al. 2010b).

### 3.3 Potential role of CXCL4-induced macrophages in human atherosclerosis

#### 3.3.1 General considerations

Monocyte-derived macrophages are present in atherosclerotic lesions at very early stages of the disease (Galkina & Ley 2009). Activated platelets have been demonstrated to promote atherogenesis, an effect mediated by chemokines released from their alpha granules (Huo et al. 2003). CXCL4 is one of these platelet chemokines and is released from platelets upon activation (Brandt et al. 2000). CXCL4 is known to prevent monocyte apoptosis (Scheuerer et al. 2000) and to promote differentiation of a specific macrophage phenotype distinct from previously identified macrophage polarizations (Gleissner et al. 2010b). Taking into account that the genetic deletion of CXCL4 in *Apoe*$^{-/-}$ mice is accompanied by reduced atherogenesis (Sachais et al. 2007), and that in human atherosclerotic lesions the presence of CXCL4 has been associated with plaque progression and clinical symptoms (Pitsilos et al. 2003), it seems extremely reasonable to hypothesize that CXCL4-induced macrophages significantly contribute to atherogenesis and progression of atherosclerosis. An important mechanisms of this action may represent the induction of CXCL4-specific, pro-atherogenic macrophages.

### 3.3.2 Features of CXCL4-induced macrophages – The M4 macrophage

To identify potential mechanisms by which CXCL4-induced macrophages are induced to act in a pro-atherogenic manner, we studied their transcriptome and compared it to that of MCSF-induced macrophages from the same donors. In this analysis, we found that both MCSF- and CXCL4-induced macrophages have strong phenotypic similarities. Thus, they both express similar mRNA and surface levels of CD45, CD14 or intracellular levels of CD68. Their transcriptomes show a strong correlation clearly indicating that they both represent macrophages (Gleissner et al. 2010b).

Interestingly, while CXCL4-treated human monocytes display phenotypic and functional characteristics of macrophages after six days in culture, they also have characteristics that clearly distinguish them from MCSF-induced macrophages. We found 375 genes differentially-expressed between MCSF- and CXCL4-induced macrophages, 206 of them being over-expressed in CXCL4-induced macrophages. Interestingly, CXCL4-induced macrophages displayed neither typical markers of M1 nor of M2 polarization (Gleissner et al. 2010b). Accordingly, using different statistical approaches including gene set enrichment analyses (Subramanian et al. 2005), modified principal components analysis (PCA), and hierarchical clustering (based on transcriptomic data from MCSF-treated, M1-polarized and M2-polarized macrophages (Martinez et al. 2006)), we were able to demonstrate that CXCL4 induces a transcriptome distinct from every macrophage polarization type described thus far (Gleissner et al. 2010b). In all statistical models, it turned out that in relation to their corresponding MCSF-control macrophages, M1 (induced by LPS and interferon-γ) and M2 macrophages (induced by IL-4) clustered together more closely than CXCL4-induced macrophages.

These findings suggest that CXCL4 induces a macrophage phenotype with specific phenotypic and functional characteristics, which will be discussed in more detail below. Based on these results, we have suggested calling these macrophages M4 - a term that we believe reflects both the fact that these cells are distinct from M1 and M2 macrophages and that they can be induced by CXCL4. Accordingly, in the following paragraphs CXCL4-induced macrophages will be referred to as M4 macrophages. Fig. 2 summarizes some of the findings described below in more detail.

### 3.3.3 Gene expression of matrix metalloproteinases in M4 macrophages

Considering that CXCL4 promotes atherogenesis in *Apoe*$^{-/-}$ mice, we hypothesized that M4 macrophages would over-express genes that are involved in atherogenesis as compared to their MCSF-induced counterparts. Therefore, it was a surprise to discover that M4 macrophages cannot generally be considered pro-atherogenic: some genes implicated in atherogenesis showed higher expression levels, others lower expression levels as compared to MCSF-induced macrophages.

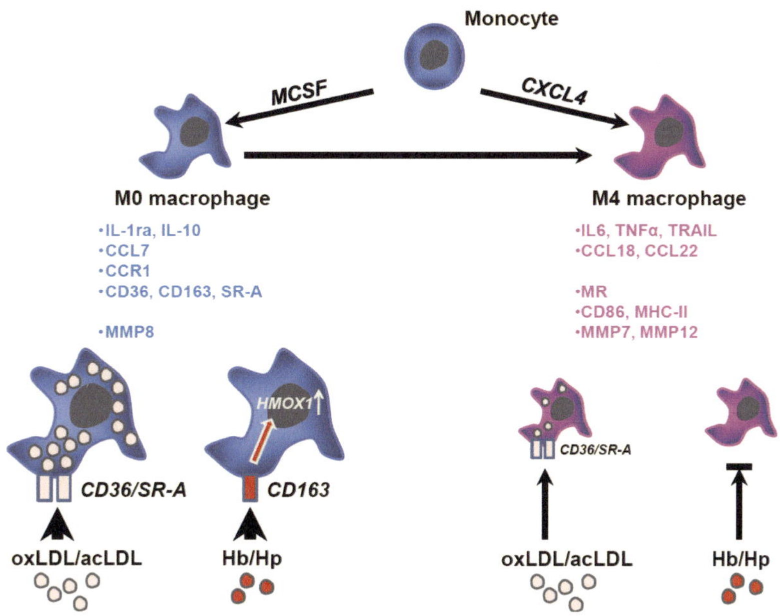


Fig. 2. Features of MCSF- and CXCL4-induced macrophage (M0 and M4 macrophages). For each polarization type, typical cytokines, chemokines, chemokine receptors, other receptors, surface molecules involved in antigen presentation, and intracellular enzymes are indicated. The figures at the bottom indicate functional differences regarding scavenger receptor expression, uptake of modified LDL and the differential potential to clear hemoglobin-haptoglobin complexes resulting in heme oxygenase-1 upregulation.

This ambiguous picture was also seen with matrix metalloproteinases (MMP), of which some showed higher expression in M4 macrophages (e.g. *MMP7* or *MMP12*) while others were expressed more highly in MCSF-induced macrophages (e.g. *MMP8*). Of course, gene expression data do not necessarily reflect protein expression and in the case of MMPs, enzyme activities may be also differentially-regulated; the regulation of MMPs is furthermore affected by activation through cathepsins, which in part are also differentially-regulated (cathepsin B and K significantly higher in M4 macrophages) (Newby 2008).

Taken together, due to the lack of functional data at this stage, it is impossible to judge whether differential-expression of MMPs and potentially different MMP activity in M4 macrophages represent a pro-atherogenic feature of M4 macrophages.

### 3.3.4 Foam cell formation in M4 macrophages

Based on previous data, that CXCL4 promotes atherogenesis in *Apoe*$^{-/-}$ mice, we hypothesized that CXCL4-induced macrophages would be more prone to foam cell formation induced by modified (i.e. acetylated or oxidized) low density lipoprotein (LDL). Interestingly, the opposite was the shown to be true. While cholesterol efflux transporter ABCA1 and ABCG1 were not differentially-expressed on the mRNA level, scavenger receptors involved in uptake of modified LDL showed significantly lower expression in CXCL4-induced macrophages. Specifically, CD36 and macrophage scavenger receptor-A (which both account for the vast majority of uptake of modified LDL during macrophage foam cell formation) showed significantly lower mRNA expression, while the differences measured by flow cytometry were only significant for CD36. Interestingly, both uptake of acetylated and oxidized LDL (acLDL and oxLDL) was significantly lower in M4 macrophages, suggesting that CXCL4-induced macrophages have a lower tendency to differentiate towards foam cells. This was somewhat unexpected and supports the notion that the pro-atherosclerotic effects of CXCL4 as shown in *Apoe*$^{-/-}$ likely reflects a multitude of different effects, including those on cells other than macrophages (i.e. endothelial cells, T cells, and potentially smooth muscle cells).

### 3.3.5 CD163 and heme oxygenase-1 in M4 macrophages

When analyzing the transcriptome of M4 macrophages, we found *CD163* mRNA coding for the hemoglobin-haptoglobin scavenger receptor to be significantly down-regulated as compared to MCSF-induced macrophages (Gleissner et al. 2010a). CD163 binds hemoglobin-haptoglobin complexes (and hemoglobin with lower affinity). Binding of the ligand to CD163 results in upregulation of heme oxygenase-1 (Schaer et al. 2006). Heme oxygenase-1 (and specifically heme oxygenase-1 expressed in bone marrow-derived cells like monocytes and monocyte-derived macrophages) is thought to be atheroprotective as demonstrated in several mouse models (Juan et al. 2001, Orozco et al. 2007, Yet et al. 2003).

Further experiments studying gene and protein expression in freshly isolated blood monocytes and macrophage induced either by MCSF or CXCL4 confirmed the significant differences. Thus, while MCSF treatment resulted in further up-regulation of CD163 expression, exposure to CXCL4 resulted in complete loss of the receptor within hours. This loss was not mediated by shedding of the receptor, which is one mechanism by which CD163 surface expression can be down-regulated (e.g. after treatment with LPS (Buechler et al. 2000)). Functionally, loss of CD163 resulted in loss of heme oxygenase-1 up-regulation upon exposure to hemoglobin-haptoglobin complexes confirming the functional relevance of our findings.

To assess whether these *in vitro* findings play a role *in vivo*, we studied CD163 protein expression in human atherosclerotic lesions and found that it is differentially-expressed on CD68$^+$ macrophages (Gleissner et al. 2010a). Furthermore, in a cohort of 18 consecutive patients undergoing carotid endatherectomy we found an inverse correlation between gene expression of *PF4* (coding for CXCL4) and *CD163*. Considering that *PF4* is exclusively expressed in megakaryocytes and platelets and *CD163* expression is restricted to myeloid cells, we concluded that the presence of large amounts of CXCL4 is associated with low levels of CD163 supporting that this mechanism does play a role *in vivo.*

## 3.4 M4 macrophages as therapeutic target in atherosclerosis?

As described above, macrophages present in human atherosclerotic lesions do not represent a homogeneous entity, but are composed of different subsets that are characterized by differential-expression of cytokines, chemokines, surface receptors and their enzymatic repertoire. We believe that the platelet-derived chemokine CXCL4 may represent an important inducer of macrophage heterogeneity as it (I) is present in the atherosclerotic lesions, (II) is associated with disease progression, and (III) promotes monocyte differentiation towards a distinct macrophage polarization type.

Based on these considerations, it was surprising to discover that CXCL4-induced M4 macrophages do not display a clearly pro-atherogenic phenotype. In fact, some of their features seem clearly pro-atherogenic (e.g. loss of CD163), while others are ambiguous (e.g.

MMP expression) or may even be anti-atherogenic (e.g. reduced uptake of modified LDL). However, many of these functional data have been obtained *in vitro* on isolated macrophages. Thus, it is possible that in the context of an atherosclerotic lesion consisting of extracellular matrix as well as various other cells types, CXCL4-induced macrophages may have a more clearly pro-atherogenic phenotype. On the other hand, it is possible that the pro-atherogenic effects of CXCL4 represent the summary of various effects on various cell types.

The possibility to specifically address the interaction between a chemokines and its partner (in this case CXCL4 and CCL5 (RANTES)) in the context of atherogenesis has been demonstrated in a very elegant study by Koenen et al., who have designed a small molecule that specifically inhibits the interaction between those two chemokines (Koenen et al. 2009). When treating *Apoe*$^{-/-}$ mice with this substance, lesion development was significantly reduced. Even though at this point it is unclear to what extent this effect was due to direct inhibition of CXCL4 effects on macrophages, it still demonstrates that tackling pro-atherogenic chemokines represents a promising approach to prevent or even treat atherosclerosis.

## 4. Macrophage heterogeneity and the novel M4 macrophage

### 4.1 Unresolved questions on macrophage heterogeneity

There are a number of unresolved questions regarding macrophage heterogeneity, which make it difficult to assess the specific role of M4 macrophages in this context. Firstly, in vitro models usually do not account for the diversity of peripheral blood monocytes. Thus, CD14$^+$ cells are used to generate macrophages and it is unknown whether certain monocyte subsets (Geissmann et al. 2010, Ziegler-Heitbrock 1989) may be more likely to differentiate towards a specifically polarized macrophage type than others. Secondly, the concept of macrophage polarization is somewhat artificial as it considers the effects of isolated soluble factors (like TNF-alpha or IL-4), whereas in vivo the local micromilieu may be composed of a combination of various cytokine and chemokines. Thirdly, when studying macrophage polarization *in vitro*, dynamics over time are rarely being taken into account. Even though Mantovani et al. have studied the transcriptomes of monocytes, and monocyte-derived macrophages after three or six days' treatment with MCSF (plus additional treatment with LPS/interferon-$\gamma$ (M1) or IL-4 (M2)) (Martinez et al. 2006), more detailed information on time courses are lacking at this point. Finally, we do not know exactly which of the thus far defined macrophage polarization types represent final states of differentiation and which of them are temporary, i.e. whether induction of a specific polarization type is reversible or not.

### 4.2 Macrophage polarization beyond M1 and M2

The recent data on macrophage heterogeneity in human atherosclerosis is interesting and puzzling at the same time. Thus, while Bouhlel *et al.* were able to demonstrate gene expression of both M1 and M2 markers in different areas of human atherosclerotic plaques suggesting that both polarization types may exist *in vivo* (Bouhlel et al. 2007), other groups including ourselves have described macrophage phenotypes *in vitro* and *in vivo* that do not necessarily fit into the established scheme of macrophage polarizations (Boyle et al. 2009, Gleissner et al. 2010a, Waldo et al. 2008).

Waldo et al. compared MCSF- and GMCSF-induced macrophages (even though the latter are sometimes considered dendritic cells) and found significant differences in the expression of CD14, which was virtually absent in GMCSF-induced cells (Waldo et al. 2008). Furthermore, these cells were less likely to spontaneously accumulate modified LDL. The authors were able to confirm the existence and the functional characteristics of these macrophages *in vitro* as well as in human atherosclerotic lesions.

Boyle et al. described a novel macrophage that is induced by haemoglobin-haptoglobin (Hb-Hp) complexes and is characterized by high levels of CD163 and low levels of HLA-DR (Boyle et al. 2009). *In vitro,* these cells cleared Hb-Hp complexes more efficiently and showed reduced oxidative stress (Boyle et al. 2009). Mechanistic data show, that this phenotype is induced by autocrine effects of IL-10 suggesting a certain similarity to M2c macrophages.

Our own group has studied the effects of oxidized LDL on human monocyte-derived macrophages and found that these cells express markers that have been associated with dendritic cells (Cho et al. 2007). Thus, these cells up-regulate genes coding for MHC-II, CD11c, and DC-STAMP, suggesting that there may be phenotypic and functional overlap between foam cells and dendritic cells within atherosclerotic lesions.

Finally, as mentioned above, we have studied the phenotypic and functional characteristics of CXCL4-induced macrophages and found features that clearly distinguish these macrophages from any polarization type described thus far (Gleissner et al. 2010b).

### 4.3 Suggestion for a novel nomenclature of macrophage polarization

Based on this evidence, we feel the necessity to develop a novel classification of macrophage polarization that includes the novel macrophage types described *in vitro* and *in vivo* over the past years. Therefore, we here propose a novel framework that tries to systematically cover those macrophage types that have been unequivocally identified in human atherosclerotic plaques. Many of these polarization types have been extensively characterized, sometimes including transcriptomic analysis. Accordingly, we suggest assigning the "novel" macrophage polarization types names that consist of "M" (for macrophage) and a second number, or letter, or combination of both that is related to the inducers of this polarization type.

Our proposed system has several advantages: Firstly, it allows keeping the established terms M1 and M2 and thereby not only respects the pioneering work by Gordon et al., but also avoids confusion associated with the introduction of new terms. Secondly, for "novel" macrophage polarization types the proposed names hint as to what inducers are involved. Finally, the system allows flexibility as based on the above-mentioned principles, so further addition of novel macrophage polarization types remains possible in the future.

Notably, the proposed nomenclature is restricted to monocyte-derived cells that occur during pathology, i.e. it does not cover tissue macrophages like Kupffer cells in the liver or alveolar macrophages in the lung. By including dendritic cells (DC) in the system, we specifically address myeloid dendritic cells derived from monocyte precursors. Plasmacytoid DCs or DCs constitutively present in certain tissues like Langerhans cells of the skin are again not covered by the proposed system. Accordingly, our system may have some overlap with other classifications of DCs. Table 1a and b give an overview of the proposed system.

| | M1 | M0 | M2a | M2b | M2c |
|---|---|---|---|---|---|
| Inducers | MCSF + IFNγ/ LPS *or* TNF-α | MCSF | IL-4 *or* IL-13 | Immune complexes + TLR ligands | IL-10 |
| Prominent markers (selection) | CCR7, TLR2, TLR4, MHC-II, iNOS | CD14, CD16, CD163 | CD36, CD163, MR, SR-A, MHC-II | CD80, CD86, MHC-II | CCR2, CD14, CD36, MR, SR-A |
| Functional characteristics | Pro-inflammatory | Inflammation resolution? | Inflammation resolution | Inflammation resolution | Tissue repair |
| Transcriptome | Yes | yes | yes | no | no |
| *In vivo* evidence in athero-sclerosis | Gene expression | Gene expression | Gene expression | no | no |
| References for transcriptomic analysis | (Martinez et al. 2006) | (Cho et al. 2007, Gleissner et al. 2010b, Martinez et al. 2006, Waldo et al. 2008) | (Martinez et al. 2006) | - | - |

Table 1a. Proposal for a novel macrophage classification (established polarization types). The columns are ordered in a way that reflects similarity based on transcriptomic analysis where available.

| | M-Hb | M4 | M-ox | M-GM | M-DC |
|---|---|---|---|---|---|
| Inducers | MCSF + hemoglobin/ haptoglobin | CXCL4 | MCSF + oxLDL | GMCSF | GMCSF + IL-4 |
| Prominent markers (selection) | CD163 MHC-II$^{low}$ | CD163$^{-}$ | CD206, MHC-II | CD1a, CD1c, CCR7 CD14$^{-}$ | CD206, MHC-II |
| Functional characteristics | High clearance of Hb/hp, reduced oxidative stress | Defective Hb/hp clearance, reduced foam cell formation | Ag presentation? | Less spontaneous cholesterol accumulation, unclear | Ag presentation, T cell activation |
| Transcriptome | No | Yes | Yes | Yes | Yes |
| *In vivo* evidence in athero-sclerosis | Histology | Gene expression, histology (CD163) | Histology | Histology (CD68) | Histology |
| References | (Boyle et al. 2009) | (Gleissner et al. 2010b) | (Cho et al. 2007) | (Waldo et al. 2008) | (Bobryshev & Lord 1995, Jeffrey et al. 2006) |

Table 1b. Proposal for a novel macrophage classification (novel polarization types). The columns are ordered in a way that reflects similarity based on transcriptomic analysis where available

## 5. Conclusions

In summary, we have discussed the role of the platelet-derived chemokine CXCL4 for macrophage differentiation in the general context of macrophage heterogeneity in atherogenesis. There is good evidence that CXCL4 promotes atherogenesis, even though at this point, the relevance of CXCL4-induced macrophages for this process is not entirely understood. While CXCL4-induced macrophages display some potentially pro-atherogenic features, their pro-atherogenic nature is not as evident as expected. Thus, we believe that it will be necessary to study these cells in more detail to elucidate the mechanisms involved in CXCL4-induced macrophage differentiation, but also to study these cells in their pathohpysiological environment, i.e. within the human atheroclerotic plaque.

As CXCL4 is not the only mediator of monocyte macrophage differentiation and as an increasing number of polarized macrophages clearly distinct from M1 and M2 macrophages with potential implication for atherogenesis have been identified *in vitro* and *in vivo*, we have proposed a novel macrophage classification schema, that both respects the established M1 and M2 paradigm and takes into account novel macrophage phenotypes and their inducers.

Taken together, even though our knowledge on macrophage heterogeneity in general and the impact of CXCL4 on macrophage heterogeneity in atherogenesis is growing, we still need more insight into the mechanisms involved in order to use this knowledge as the basis for novel, specific therapies for atherosclerosis.

## 6. Acknowledgments

The authors would like to thank Kristina M. Little, PhD, for critically reading the manuscript.

## 7. References

Auffray C, Fogg D, Garfa M, Elain G, Join-Lambert O, Kayal S, Sarnacki S, Cumano A, Lauvau G, Geissmann F. (2007) Monitoring of blood vessels and tissues by a population of monocytes with patrolling behavior. *Science,* Vol.317, No.5838, 2007, pp. 666-670, 1095-9203 (Electronic).

Bobryshev YV, Lord RS. (1995) Ultrastructural recognition of cells with dendritic cell morphology in human aortic intima. Contacting interactions of vascular dendritic cells in athero-resistant and athero-prone areas of the normal aorta. *Arch Histol Cytol,* Vol.58, No.3, 1995, pp. 307-322, 0914-9465 (Print).

Bouhlel MA, Derudas B, Rigamonti E, Dievart R, Brozek J, Haulon S, Zawadzki C, Jude B, Torpier G, Marx N, Staels B, Chinetti-Gbaguidi G. (2007) Ppargamma activation primes human monocytes into alternative m2 macrophages with anti-inflammatory properties. *Cell Metabolism,* Vol.6, No.2, 2007, pp. 137-143, 1550-4131 (Print).

Boyle JJ, Harrington HA, Piper E, Elderfield K, Stark J, Landis RC, Haskard DO. (2009) Coronary intraplaque hemorrhage evokes a novel atheroprotective macrophage phenotype. *American Journal of Pathology,* Vol.174, No.3, 2009, pp. 1097-1108, 1525-2191 (Electronic).

Brandt E, Petersen F, Ludwig A, Ehlert JE, Bock L, Flad HD. (2000) The beta-thromboglobulins and platelet factor 4: Blood platelet-derived cxc chemokines with divergent roles in early neutrophil regulation. *J Leukoc Biol,* Vol.67, No.4, 2000, pp. 471-478,

Buechler C, Ritter M, Orso E, Langmann T, Klucken J, Schmitz G. (2000) Regulation of scavenger receptor cd163 expression in human monocytes and macrophages by pro- and antiinflammatory stimuli. *J Leukoc Biol,* Vol.67, No.1, 2000, pp. 97-103,

Cho HJ, Shashkin P, Gleissner CA, Dunson D, Jain N, Lee JK, Miller Y, Ley K. (2007) Induction of dendritic cell-like phenotype in macrophages during foam cell formation. *Physiological Genomics,* Vol.29, No.2, 2007, pp. 149-160,

Fitzgerald ML, Moore KJ, Freeman MW, Reed GL. (2000) Lipopolysaccharide induces scavenger receptor a expression in mouse macrophages: A divergent response relative to human thp-1 monocyte/macrophages. *The Journal of Immunology,* Vol.164, No.5, 2000, pp. 2692-2700, 0022-1767 (Print).

Galkina EV, Ley K. (2009) Immune and inflammatory mechanisms of atherosclerosis. *Annual Reviews in Immunology,* Vol.27, No.27, 2009, pp. 165-197,

Gear AR, Camerini D. (2003) Platelet chemokines and chemokine receptors: Linking hemostasis, inflammation, and host defense. *Microcirculation,* Vol.10, No.3-4, 2003, pp. 335-350, 1073-9688 (Print).

Geissmann F, Jung S, Littman DR. (2003) Blood monocytes consist of two principal subsets with distinct migratory properties. *Immunity,* Vol.19, No.1, 2003, pp. 71-82, 1074-7613 (Print).

Geissmann F, Manz MG, Jung S, Sieweke MH, Merad M, Ley K. (2010) Development of monocytes, macrophages, and dendritic cells. *Science,* Vol.327, No.5966, 2010, pp. 656-661, 1095-9203 (Electronic).

Gleissner CA, von Hundelshausen P, Ley K. (2008) Platelet chemokines in vascular disease. *Arteriosclerosis, Thrombosis and Vascular Biology,* Vol.28, No.11, 2008, pp. 1920-1927, 1524-4636 (Electronic).

Gleissner CA, Shaked I, Erbel C, Bockler D, Katus HA, Ley K. (2010a) Cxcl4 downregulates the atheroprotective hemoglobin receptor cd163 in human macrophages. *Circulation Research,* Vol.106, No.1, 2010a, pp. 203-211, 1524-4571 (Electronic).

Gleissner CA, Shaked I, Little KM, Ley K. (2010b) Cxc chemokine ligand 4 induces a unique transcriptome in monocyte-derived macrophages. *The Journal of Immunology,* Vol.184, No.9, 2010b, pp. 4810-4818,

Gordon S. (2003) Alternative activation of macrophages. *Nat Rev Immunol,* Vol.3, No.1, 2003, pp. 23-35, 1474-1733 (Print).

Huo Y, Schober A, Forlow SB, Smith DF, Hyman MC, Jung S, Littman DR, Weber C, Ley K. (2003) Circulating activated platelets exacerbate atherosclerosis in mice deficient in apolipoprotein e. *Nature Medicine,* Vol.9, No.1, 2003, pp. 61-67,

Ingersoll MA, Spanbroek R, Lottaz C, Gautier EL, Frankenberger M, Hoffmann R, Lang R, Haniffa M, Collin M, Tacke F, Habenicht AJ, Ziegler-Heitbrock L, Randolph GJ. (2010) Comparison of gene expression profiles between human and mouse monocyte subsets. *Blood,* Vol.115, No.3, 2010, pp. e10-19, 1528-0020 (Electronic).

Jeffrey KL, Brummer T, Rolph MS, Liu SM, Callejas NA, Grumont RJ, Gillieron C, Mackay F, Grey S, Camps M, Rommel C, Gerondakis SD, Mackay CR. (2006) Positive regulation of immune cell function and inflammatory responses by phosphatase pac-1. *Nat Immunol,* Vol.7, No.3, 2006, pp. 274-283, 1529-2908 (Print).

Juan S-H, Lee T-S, Tseng K-W, Liou J-Y, Shyue S-K, Wu KK, Chau L-Y. (2001) Adenovirus-mediated heme oxygenase-1 gene transfer inhibits the development of atherosclerosis in apolipoprotein e-deficient mice. *Circulation,* Vol.104, No.13, 2001, pp. 1519-1525,

Koenen RR, von Hundelshausen P, Nesmelova IV, Zernecke A, Liehn EA, Sarabi A, Kramp BK, Piccinini AM, Paludan SR, Kowalska MA, Kungl AJ, Hackeng TM, Mayo KH, Weber C. (2009) Disrupting functional interactions between platelet chemokines inhibits atherosclerosis in hyperlipidemic mice. *Nat Med,* Vol.15, No.1, 2009, pp. 97-103, 1546-170X (Electronic).

Kurz K, Giannitsis E, Becker M, Hess G, Zdunek D, Katus H. (2011) Comparison of the new high sensitive cardiac troponin t with myoglobin, h-fabp and ctnt for early identification of myocardial necrosis in the acute coronary syndrome. *Clinical Research in Cardiology,* Vol.100, No.3, 2011, pp. 209-215, 1861-0684.

Lasagni L, Francalanci M, Annunziato F, Lazzeri E, Giannini S, Cosmi L, Sagrinati C, Mazzinghi B, Orlando C, Maggi E, Marra F, Romagnani S, Serio M, Romagnani P. (2003) An alternatively spliced variant of cxcr3 mediates the inhibition of endothelial cell growth induced by ip-10, mig, and I-tac, and acts as functional receptor for platelet factor 4. *J Exp Med,* Vol.197, No.11, 2003, pp. 1537-1549,

Mantovani A, Garlanda C, Locati M. (2009) Macrophage diversity and polarization in atherosclerosis: A question of balance. *Arteriosclerosis, Thrombosis and Vascular Biology,* Vol.29, No.10, 2009, pp. 1419-1423, 1524-4636 (Electronic).

Martinez FO, Gordon S, Locati M, Mantovani A. (2006) Transcriptional profiling of the human monocyte-to-macrophage differentiation and polarization: New molecules and patterns of gene expression. *J Immunol,* Vol.177, No.10, 2006, pp. 7303-7311,

Naghavi M, Libby P, Falk E, Casscells SW, Litovsky S, Rumberger J, Badimon JJ, Stefanadis C, Moreno P, Pasterkamp G, Fayad Z, Stone PH, Waxman S, Raggi P, Madjid M, Zarrabi A, Burke A, Yuan C, Fitzgerald PJ, Siscovick DS, de Korte CL, Aikawa M, Airaksinen KE, Assmann G, Becker CR, Chesebro JH, Farb A, Galis ZS, Jackson C, Jang IK, Koenig W, Lodder RA, March K, Demirovic J, Navab M, Priori SG, Rekhter MD, Bahr R, Grundy SM, Mehran R, Colombo A, Boerwinkle E, Ballantyne C, Insull W, Jr., Schwartz RS, Vogel R, Serruys PW, Hansson GK, Faxon DP, Kaul S, Drexler H, Greenland P, Muller JE, Virmani R, Ridker PM, Zipes DP, Shah PK, Willerson JT. (2003a) From vulnerable plaque to vulnerable patient: A call for new definitions and risk assessment strategies: Part II. *Circulation,* Vol.108, No.15, 2003a, pp. 1772-1778, 1524-4539 (Electronic).

Naghavi M, Libby P, Falk E, Casscells SW, Litovsky S, Rumberger J, Badimon JJ, Stefanadis C, Moreno P, Pasterkamp G, Fayad Z, Stone PH, Waxman S, Raggi P, Madjid M, Zarrabi A, Burke A, Yuan C, Fitzgerald PJ, Siscovick DS, de Korte CL, Aikawa M, Juhani Airaksinen KE, Assmann G, Becker CR, Chesebro JH, Farb A, Galis ZS, Jackson C, Jang IK, Koenig W, Lodder RA, March K, Demirovic J, Navab M, Priori SG, Rekhter MD, Bahr R, Grundy SM, Mehran R, Colombo A, Boerwinkle E, Ballantyne C, Insull W, Jr., Schwartz RS, Vogel R, Serruys PW, Hansson GK, Faxon DP, Kaul S, Drexler H, Greenland P, Muller JE, Virmani R, Ridker PM, Zipes DP, Shah PK, Willerson JT. (2003b) From vulnerable plaque to vulnerable patient: A call for new definitions and risk assessment strategies: Part I. *Circulation,* Vol.108, No.14, 2003b, pp. 1664-1672, 1524-4539 (Electronic).

Newby AC. (2008) Metalloproteinase expression in monocytes and macrophages and its relationship to atherosclerotic plaque instability. *Arterioscler Thromb Vasc Biol,* Vol.28, No.12, 2008, pp. 2108-2114, 1524-4636 (Electronic).

Orozco LD, Kapturczak MH, Barajas B, Wang X, Weinstein MM, Wong J, Deshane J, Bolisetty S, Shaposhnik Z, Shih DM, Agarwal A, Lusis AJ, Araujo JA. (2007) Heme oxygenase-1 expression in macrophages plays a beneficial role in atherosclerosis. *Circ Res,* Vol.100, No.12, 2007, pp. 1703-1711,

Pitsilos S, Hunt J, Mohler ER, Prabhakar AM, Poncz M, Dawicki J, Khalapyan TZ, Wolfe ML, Fairman R, Mitchell M, Carpenter J, Golden MA, Cines DB, Sachais BS. (2003) Platelet factor 4 localization in carotid atherosclerotic plaques: Correlation with clinical parameters. *Thromb Haemost,* Vol.90, No.6, 2003, pp. 1112-1120,

Poston RN, Hussain IF. (1993) The immunohistochemical heterogeneity of atheroma macrophages: Comparison with lymphoid tissues suggests that recently blood-derived macrophages can be distinguished from longer-resident cells. *J Histochem Cytochem,* Vol.41, No.10, 1993, pp. 1503-1512, 0022-1554 (Print).

Ridker PM. (2007) C-reactive protein and the prediction of cardiovascular events among those at intermediate risk: Moving an inflammatory hypothesis toward consensus. *Journal of the American College of Cardiology,* Vol.49, No.21, 2007, pp. 2129-2138, 0735-1097.

Roger VL, Go AS, Lloyd-Jones DM, Adams RJ, Berry JD, Brown TM, Carnethon MR, Dai S, de Simone G, Ford ES, Fox CS, Fullerton HJ, Gillespie C, Greenlund KJ, Hailpern SM, Heit JA, Ho PM, Howard VJ, Kissela BM, Kittner SJ, Lackland DT, Lichtman JH, Lisabeth LD, Makuc DM, Marcus GM, Marelli A, Matchar DB, McDermott MM, Meigs JB, Moy CS, Mozaffarian D, Mussolino ME, Nichol G, Paynter NP, Rosamond WD, Sorlie PD, Stafford RS, Turan TN, Turner MB, Wong ND, Wylie-Rosett J, Committee obotAHAS, Stroke Statistics Subcommittee, Disease ObotAHAH, Stroke Statistics Writing Group. (2011) Heart disease and stroke statistics--2011 update: A report from the american heart association. *Circulation,* Vol.123, No.4, 2011, pp. e18-209,

Ross R. (1999) Atherosclerosis--an inflammatory disease. *N Engl J Med,* Vol.340, No.2, 1999, pp. 115-126, 0028-4793 (Print).

Sachais BS, Turrentine T, Dawicki McKenna JM, Rux AH, Rader D, Kowalska MA. (2007) Elimination of platelet factor 4 (pf4) from platelets reduces atherosclerosis in c57bl/6 and apoe-/- mice. *Thromb Haemost,* Vol.98, No.5, 2007, pp. 1108-1113,

Schaer CA, Schoedon G, Imhof A, Kurrer MO, Schaer DJ. (2006) Constitutive endocytosis of cd163 mediates hemoglobin-heme uptake and determines the noninflammatory and protective transcriptional response of macrophages to hemoglobin. *Circ Res,* Vol.99, No.9, 2006, pp. 943-950,

Scheuerer B, Ernst M, Durrbaum-Landmann I, Fleischer J, Grage-Griebenow E, Brandt E, Flad HD, Petersen F. (2000) The cxc-chemokine platelet factor 4 promotes monocyte survival and induces monocyte differentiation into macrophages. *Blood,* Vol.95, No.4, 2000, pp. 1158-1166,

Shashkin P, Dragulev B, Ley K. (2005) Macrophage differentiation to foam cells. *Current Pharmaceutical Design,* Vol.11, No.23, 2005, pp. 3061-3072,

Stein M, Keshav S, Harris N, Gordon S. (1992) Interleukin 4 potently enhances murine macrophage mannose receptor activity: A marker of alternative immunologic macrophage activation. *J Exp Med,* Vol.176, No.1, 1992, pp. 287-292, 0022-1007 (Print).

Subramanian A, Tamayo P, Mootha VK, Mukherjee S, Ebert BL, Gillette MA, Paulovich A, Pomeroy SL, Golub TR, Lander ES, Mesirov JP. (2005) Gene set enrichment analysis: A knowledge-based approach for interpreting genome-wide expression profiles. *Proc Natl Acad Sci U S A,* Vol.102, No.43, 2005, pp. 15545-15550, 0027-8424 (Print).

von Hundelshausen P, Weber KS, Huo Y, Proudfoot AE, Nelson PJ, Ley K, Weber C. (2001) Rantes deposition by platelets triggers monocyte arrest on inflamed and atherosclerotic endothelium. *Circulation,* Vol.103, No.13, 2001, pp. 1772-1777,

von Hundelshausen P, Koenen RR, Sack M, Mause SF, Adriaens W, Proudfoot AE, Hackeng TM, Weber C. (2005) Heterophilic interactions of platelet factor 4 and rantes promote monocyte arrest on endothelium. *Blood,* Vol.105, No.3, 2005, pp. 924-930,

von Hundelshausen P, Petersen F, Brandt E. (2007) Platelet-derived chemokines in vascular biology. *Thromb Haemost,* Vol.97, No.5, 2007, pp. 704-713,

Waldo SW, Li Y, Buono C, Zhao B, Billings EM, Chang J, Kruth HS. (2008) Heterogeneity of human macrophages in culture and in atherosclerotic plaques. *American Journal of Pathology,* Vol.172, No.4, 2008, pp. 1112-1126, 0002-9440 (Print).

Weber C. (2005) Platelets and chemokines in atherosclerosis: Partners in crime. *Circ Res,* Vol.96, No.6, 2005, pp. 612-616, 1524-4571 (Electronic).

Weber C. (2008) Chemokines in atherosclerosis, thrombosis, and vascular biology. *Arterioscler Thromb Vasc Biol,* Vol.28, No.11, 2008, pp. 1896, 1524-4636 (Electronic).

Yet SF, Layne MD, Liu X, Chen YH, Ith B, Sibinga NE, Perrella MA. (2003) Absence of heme oxygenase-1 exacerbates atherosclerotic lesion formation and vascular remodeling. *FASEB J,* Vol.17, No.12, 2003, pp. 1759-1761, 1530-6860 (Electronic).

Zernecke A, Shagdarsuren E, Weber C. (2008) Chemokines in atherosclerosis: An update. *Arterioscler Thromb Vasc Biol,* Vol.28, No.11, 2008, pp. 1897-1908, 1524-4636 (Electronic).

Ziegler-Heitbrock HW. (1989) The biology of the monocyte system. *Eur J Cell Biol,* Vol.49, No.1, 1989, pp. 1-12, 0171-9335 (Print).

# 17

# The Role of IL-10 in Atherosclerosis

Xinbing Han[1] and William A. Boisvert[2]
[1]*Department of Medicine, Beth Israel Deaconess Medical Center, Harvard Medical School, Boston, MA,*
[2]*Center for Cardiovascular Research, John A. Burns School of Medicine, University of Hawaii, Honolulu, HI, USA*

## 1. Introduction

Cardiovascular diseases, including coronary artery disease (CAD), ischemic gangrene, abdominal aortic aneurysms, and many cases of heart failure and stroke currently account for the most number of deaths in the Western world (Hansson et al., 2006). The root cause of these diseases is atherosclerosis, which is widely accepted these days to be a chronic inflammatory disease in addition to the more recognized disorder of lipid metabolism. Although it was established long ago that high levels of low-density lipoprotein (LDL) cholesterol is a major risk factor for atherosclerosis, more recently both innate and adaptive immune systems have been accepted as major participants in the initiation and progression of atherosclerosis. Besides monocytes/macrophages, T cells and dendritic cells (DCs) can be detected within atherosclerotic lesions and have been implicated in the pathogenesis of atherosclerosis (Hansson and Libby, 2006) (Weber et al., 2008). Atherosclerotic lesion progression has been shown to depend on ongoing, chronic inflammation in the artery wall. Following hyperlipidemia, a rapid influx of circulating monocytes into the atherosclerosis-prone areas of the arterial intima occurs. These recruited inflammatory monocytes differentiate into macrophages and take up modified atherogenic cholesteryl ester (CE)- rich lipoproteins in the intima of the vessel wall (Lusis, 2000) (Ross, 1999) (Wang and Tall, 2003). The accumulation of cholesterol-loaded macrophages in the arterial wall called "foam cells" is a key feature of early atherosclerotic lesions (Brown and Goldstein, 1983).

Upon lipid uptake within the artery wall, macrophage foam cells activate a compensatory pathway for cholesterol efflux, mediated by the ATP-binding cassette (ABC) transporters ABCA1 and ABCG1 (Wang et al., 2007). During systemic hypercholesterolemia, however, this homeostatic mechanism is overwhelmed, leading to the accumulation of foam cells and the initiation of fatty streak lesions. The importance of these transporters is illustrated by the fact that a combined deficiency of ABCA1 and ABCG1 accelerates foam cell accumulation and atherosclerotic development in mice (Yvan-Charvet et al., 2007). Cholesterol loading of macrophages also stimulates the production of inflammatory mediators, which recruit other cell types and contribute to the development of a complex lesion (Hansson et al., 2002). Thus, processes that interfere with the intracellular cholesterol balance would be expected to exacerbate lesion formation.

Cholesterol is an essential structural component in the cell membrane and a precursor for steroid hormone and bile acid synthesis in metabolic pathways. Thus, cholesterol homeostasis needs to be strictly regulated. The intracellular cholesterol concentration is tightly controlled by feedback mechanisms that operate at both transcriptional and posttranscriptional levels (Brown and Goldstein, 1997). For example, the liver X receptor (LXR), belonging to the family of nuclear hormone receptors, contributes to cholesterol homeostasis by activating the transcription of genes involved in the response to cholesterol excess, including ABCA1 and ABCG1 (Beaven and Tontonoz, 2006). These transporters promote cellular cholesterol efflux to high-density lipoprotein (HDL) and its associated apolipoprotein (apo)-A1, a crucial step in the initiation of reverse cholesterol transport (RCT) to the liver for excretion (Tall et al., 2008).

Other ways in which lipid-loaded and activated macrophage foam cells can significantly contribute to the maintenance and progression of atherogenesis is by producing nitric oxide, reactive oxygen species, inflammatory lipids, growth factors, and pro-inflammatory cytokines such as interleukin (IL) -1, IL-6, interferon (IFN)-γ and tumor necrosis factor (TNF)-α (Hansson, 2001). Taken together, alterations in both lipid metabolism and the immune responses in macrophages play a significant role in promoting the development of atherosclerotic lesions. Knowledge of the mechanisms that regulate these responses could therefore be of considerable value with respect to the development of new approaches to prevention and treatment.

As a prototypic anti-inflammatory cytokine, IL-10 is made primarily by the macrophages and T lymphocytes of the Th2 subtype. Its major functions include inhibition of macrophage activation as well as inhibition of MMP, pro-inflammatory cytokines and cyclooxygenase-2 expression. IL-10 induces the proliferation of mast cells, B and T lymphocytes, and enhances T cell response to IL-2. Although it is clearly documented that IL-10 is expressed in the atherosclerotic plaque (de Vries, 1995) (de Waal Malefyt et al., 1991) (Gerard et al., 1993) it is not fully understood how IL-10 influences the atherogenic process. This chapter will highlight the current knowledge about the role of IL-10 in the initiation and progression of atherosclerosis. Inasmuch as macrophages play a critical role in the pathogenesis of atherosclerosis, the review will focus largely on how IL-10 stimulates and regulates the activities of macrophages that are important in the development of atherosclerosis.

## 2. Anti-atherogenic properties of IL-10

IL-10 exerts its atheroprotective effect on plaque progression, rupture, or thrombosis throughout the different stages of atherosclerosis by influencing the local inflammatory process within the atherosclerotic lesion. As an anti-inflammatory cytokine IL-10's athero-protective effects are exerted mainly by inhibiting various cell processes including the production of inflammatory mediators, matrix metalloproteinases (MMPs) and tissue factor (TF) production, and apoptosis. IL-10 is produced predominantly by macrophages within the local atherosclerotic lesion where it could play a significant role in the modulation of the local inflammatory response for both macrophages and T cells.

### 2.1 Influence on macrophage function

Macrophages play a central role during all stages of atherosclerosis (Moore and Tabas, 2011). Early in vivo studies using immunochemistry and PCR have indicated that macrophages in atherosclerotic lesion are the main source of IL-10 production in advanced atherosclerotic plaques (Mallat et al., 1999b). IL-10 plays an essential role in down-modulating adaptive and innate immune responses, partly by inhibiting the activation of human monocytes and monocyte-derived dendritic cells (Woszczek et al., 2008).

Atherogenesis is initiated with the recruitment of inflammatory cells to the intima. Following inflammatory activation, the recruited monocytes are differentiated into macrophages which take up modified LDL particles such as oxidized LDL (oxLDL), through scavenger receptors, thereby promoting cholesterol loading and foam cell formation in the plaque's core. Lipid-laden macrophages produce multiple pro-inflammatory mediators, reactive oxygen species (ROS), and TF pro-coagulant that promote local inflammation and promote thrombotic complications. The paradigm that macrophages play a critical and definitive role in human atherosclerosis has been evidenced by a large number of publications from various studies of experimental atherosclerosis. The morphological observation that macrophages are abundantly distributed from early stage lesion in fatty streak to the late stage within fibrous plaques indicates; macrophage-derived foam cells are absolutely critical for development of atheromas (Libby et al., 2011) (Little et al., 2011).

The mechanisms by which IL-10 may protect against atherogenesis can be categorized, albeit artificially, into 4 aspects of macrophage function: 1. anti-inflammatory properties 2. inhibition of MMPs and TF 3. anti-apoptotic feature 4. modulation of lipid metabolism.

### 2.1.1 Anti-inflammatory properties of IL-10

Atherosclerosis is a chronic inflammatory condition of the arterial wall characterized by progressive accumulation of lipids, cells (macrophages, T lymphocytes, and smooth muscle cells), and extracellular matrix (Ross, 1999) (Libby et al., 2011) (Charo and Taub, 2011) (Maskrey et al., 2011). During recent years, inflammation has emerged as a major driving force in atherosclerotic lesion development throughout the different stages of the disease (Libby et al., 2011) (Charo and Taub, 2011) (Moubayed et al., 2007) (Little et al., 2011), from early fatty streak to advanced fibro-fatty plaque formation. Of the cells participating in atherogenesis, monocyte-derived macrophages and T-lymphocytes are the most prominent cells that secrete various pro- or anti-atherogenic cytokines that can influence the disease development and affect plaque stability (Ferri et al., 2009) (Pasqui et al., 2006) (Kleemann et al., 2008) (Galkina and Ley, 2009) (Woollard and Geissmann, 2010) (Weber et al., 2008).

Being the most abundant inflammatory cell type in the plaque, macrophages are the most important source of cytokine production in atherosclerotic lesions (Tedgui and Mallat, 2006) and can produce pro-inflammatory cytokines such as TNF-$\alpha$, IL-1, IL-6, IL-12, IL-15, IL-18, as well as the anti-inflammatory cytokines like IL-10 and transforming growth factor-$\beta$ (TGF-$\beta$). It has been well documented that pro-inflammatory cytokines can promote development of atherosclerosis (Little et al., 2011) while anti-inflammatory cytokines like TGF-$\beta$ (Bobik et al., 1999) and IL-10 (Nishihira et al., 2006) can have an anti-atherogenic effect.

One of the earlier studies showed that IL-10 mRNA was detected by RT-PCR in 4 of 5 human atherosclerotic specimens but not in plaque-free aortic specimens (Uyemura et al., 1996). When human monocytes isolated from PBMC were incubated with oxLDL, IL-10 protein production was increased (Uyemura et al., 1996). The presence of IL-10 in advanced human atherosclerotic plaque was subsequently verified by another group (Mallat et al., 1999b). They showed also by using RT-PCR, that IL-10 mRNA was present in 12 of 17 atherosclerotic plaques, mainly in macrophages (Mallat et al., 1999b). These studies suggest that progressive inflammation during atherosclerosis causes macrophages to express IL-10.

IL-10 is a potent anti-inflammatory cytokine. Increased IL-10 serum level is a beneficial prognostic determinant in patients with acute coronary syndromes (Heeschen et al., 2003). A line of publications has shown that IL-10 expression by plaque macrophages limits the inflammatory response and promotes plaque healing (de Vries, 1995) (de Waal Malefyt et al., 1991) (Gerard et al., 1993) by inhibiting IL-12 (Uyemura et al., 1996) and inducible nitric oxide synthase (iNOS) production (Mallat et al., 1999b) (Ito and Ikeda, 2003). Attenuation of atherogenesis by IL-10 was attributed to its anti-inflammatory effects, most notably its ability to inhibit the release of several pro-inflammatory cytokines (including IL-1β, TNF-α, and IL-8) from monocytic cells, and to induce the production of IL-1 receptor antagonist (Terkeltaub, 1999) (van der Poll et al., 1994) (Wang et al., 1995). IL-10 also suppresses the production of the chemokine KC/GRO-α (Kishore et al., 1999) which is implicated in intimal macrophage accumulation and the progression of complex atherosclerotic lesions in advanced disease (Boisvert et al., 1998). MCP-1 is chemotactic for monocytes and highly expressed in macrophage-rich areas of the lesion. IL-10-induced inhibition of MCP-1 (Ajuebor et al., 1999) (Han et al., 2009) (Han et al., 2010) (Zimmerman et al., 2004), a key player in monocyte recruitment to early atherosclerotic lesions (Gosling et al., 1999), has been regarded as an important protective mechanism of atherogenesis by IL-10.

### 2.1.2 Inhibition of matrix metalloproteinases and tissue factor

Pathological studies have provided evidence that extracellular matrix content and its degradation are related to vulnerability and instability of plaques (Libby, 1995). It has been well documented that clinical instability of atherosclerosis is related to the activation of local inflammatory and immune cells with increased expression of MMPs (Libby, 1995) and TF (Ardissino et al., 1997) in the culprit plaque as well as increased systemic production of MMPs (Kai et al., 1998) and thrombin (Biasucci et al., 1996) (Caligiuri et al., 2003). Macrophages are important sources of MMPs within atherosclerostic lesions , including MMP-2, MMP-8, MMP-9, MMP-12, MMP-13, and MMP-14 (Gough et al., 2006) (Little et al., 2011). MMPs affect lesion development and progression by degrading extracellular matrix proteins, leading eventually to the development of unstable, rupture-prone atherosclerotic lesions (Boyle, 2005) (Little et al., 2011). Tissue factor is a prothrombotic molecule expressed by various cell types within atherosclerotic plaques and has been thought to play an essential role in thrombus formation after atherosclerotic plaque rupture (Kamimura et al., 2005). There is evidence that IL-10 may have protective effects against plaque rupture and thrombus formation (Waehre et al., 2002). IL-10 can inhibit the secretion of MMPs (Waehre et al., 2002) (Han et al., 2009) (Han et al., 2010) (Holven et al., 2006), the synthesis of TF (Kamimura et al., 2005) (Ramani et al., 1993), and the production of thrombin (Pajkrt et al., 1997) from PBMC and macrophages. Decreased collagen synthesis and increased activity of macrophage-derived matrix degrading metalloproteinases are responsible for fibrous cap thinning and fragility. Therefore, low levels of IL-10 may lead to augmented MMP activity which may in turn promote plaque instability to cause acute cardiovascular events in certain individuals (Holven et al., 2006) (Mallat et al., 1999a). In addition, the balance between Th1 (IFN-γ) and Th2 (IL-10) polarization in T helper cells may play an important role in atherogenesis. IFN-γ may destabilize plaques not only by inhibiting collagen production (Amento et al., 1991) in human vascular smooth muscle cells, but by stimulating MMP production in macrophages (Libby, 1995) (Saren et al., 1996) and modulating the fibrinolytic response of endothelial cells (Arnman et al., 1995) (Gallicchio et al., 1996).

### 2.1.3 Anti-apoptotic properties

Both IL-10 transgenic animal models and mice deficient in either IL-10 or IL-10 receptor have highlighted the anti-apoptotic feature of IL-10. Both apoptosis and necrosis occur in the atherosclerotic plaque (Geng and Libby, 1995) (Isner et al., 1995) (Han et al., 1995) (Bjorkerud and Bjorkerud, 1996; Cai et al., 1997; Geng and Libby, 1995; Han et al., 1995; Isner et al., 1995). IL-10's anti-apoptotic properties have been reported in cultured macrophages (Arai et al., 1995) (Han et al., 2009) (Han et al., 2010) and in T lymphocytes (Cohen et al., 1997). Inflammatory nitric oxide has apoptotic effects (Geng et al., 1996) (Albina et al., 1993) and can induce cell death, at least in part through local peroxynitrite formation (Luoma et al., 1998) (Kockx et al., 1998). One mechanism by which IL-10 can protect from excessive cell damage and death in the plaque is by inhibition of iNOS production (Cattaruzza et al., 2003). The production of ROS is increased in atherosclerotic arteries (Minor et al., 1990), leading to endothelial damage, oxidation of lipid components (Witztum and Steinberg, 2001), and recruitment of inflammatory cells to the site of injury. IL-10 may down-regulate immune responses in atherosclerosis by inhibiting antigen presentation to T cells (de Waal Malefyt et al., 1991), and by inhibiting production of reactive oxygen intermediates which result in oxidation of LDL (Bogdan et al., 1991). In addition, IL-10 activates signal transducer and activator of transcription 3 (STAT3), which suppresses endoplasmic reticulum (ER) stress-induced apoptosis in macrophages by inducing the expression of cell-survival molecules (Li et al., 2008). The increased expression of the anti-apoptotic genes Bfl-1 and Mcl-1 in response to IL-10 contributes to the suppression of apoptosis by IL-10 in lipid-laden foam cells (Halvorsen et al., 2005). Furthermore, because excessive accumulation of free cholesterol can cause apoptosis in cells, one other way in which IL-10 may exert its anti-apoptotic effects is by stimulating ABCA1/ABCG1 production which increases the cholesterol efflux from lipid laden foam cells (Rubic and Lorenz, 2006) (Han et al., 2009) (Han et al., 2010).

### 2.1.4 Polarization of macrophage by IL-10

In response to cytokines and microbial products, macrophages have the ability to be polarized into one of two subgroups: classically activated M1 and alternatively activated M2 form (Benoit et al., 2008). The concept of macrophage polarization has been widely accepted in recent years (Mantovani et al., 2005) (Martinez et al., 2008). M1 macrophages are induced by IFN-γ, microbial stimuli (e.g. LPS) or cytokines such as TNF-α and GM-CSF. M2 macrophages are induced by IL-4, IL-10, IL-13, immune complexes, glucocorticoid or secosteroid (vitamin D3) hormones (Mantovani et al., 2005; Martinez et al., 2008). One of the notable features of M1 macrophage is its low level of IL-10 expression and high levels of IL-12 and IL-23 expression. As efficient producers of reactive oxygen and nitrogen intermediates and inflammatory cytokines, M1 macrophages are associated with protection during acute infectious diseases, and can induce and polarize Th1 response as well as mediate immune response against intracellular parasites and tumors (Benoit et al., 2008).

By contrast, M2 macrophage phenotype is characterized by abundant expression of IL-10 and low levels of IL-12 and IL-23 production. By expressing high levels of scavenger, mannose and galactose-type receptors, M2 macrophages participate in polarized Th2 response and exert immunoregulatory functions (Martinez et al., 2008) (Mantovani et al., 2005) by promoting killing and encapsulation of parasites (Noel et al., 2004). They are actively involved in tumor progression, tissue repair and remodeling (Wynn, 2004). Chronic infectious diseases are associated with macrophage reprogramming towards an M2 profile (Benoit et al., 2008).

Both M1 and M2 macrophages are present in atherosclerotic lesions (Khallou-Laschet et al.). Exposure of macrophages to oxLDL renders M2 macrophages pro-inflammatory (van Tits et al., 2011). Compared with pro-inflammatory M1 macrophages, anti-inflammatory M2 macrophages are more susceptible to foam cell formation (van Tits et al., 2011). Interestingly, however, a recent report indicates that M2 phenotype may exert an athero-protective action in experimental atherosclerosis (Khallou-Laschet et al.). On the other hand, PPARγ activation plays an essential role in promoting polarization of circulating blood monocytes to become M2 macrophages (Bouhlel et al., 2007) (Charo, 2007) (Chinetti-Gbaguidi and Staels). Convincing clinical evidence and animal experiments from PPARγ-deficient mice and from the mice treated with PPARγ ligands have demonstrated the beneficial role of PPARγ activation in preventing atherosclerosis (Staels, 2005) (Ricote et al., 1998). Because IL-10 increases ABCA1-mediated cholesterol efflux through PPARγ activation (Han et al., 2009) (Han et al., 2010), it is likely that PPARγ-driven M2 macrophage formation plays an important role in athero-protective action by IL-10.

### 2.1.5 Modulation of lipid metabolism

The loading of macrophages with lipoprotein-derived cholesterol alters macrophage functions during atherogenic processes. The fact that IL-10 production is increased in lipid laden macrophages suggests that IL-10 may be involved in lipid metabolism in these cells. In fact, oxLDL can promote immune activation by inducing pro-inflammatory cytokines IL-12 and TNF-α, and anti-inflammatory cytokine IL-10 production by mononuclear leukocytes from human atherosclerotic plaque (Fei et al., 2003). During recent years, the involvement and importance of IL-10 in lipid metabolism, particularly in macrophages, has been increasingly recognized.

With regard to lipid metabolism and foam cell formation, two steps are critical in maintaining lipid homeostasis in macrophages: 1. cholesterol uptake mediated by scavenger receptors and 2. cholesterol efflux mediated by ABCA1/ABCG1. Scavenger receptors such as scavenger receptor A and CD36 on macrophages mediate the uptake of modified lipoproteins from the vessel wall (Nagy et al., 1998). In addition, reverse cholesterol transport through ABCA1 and ABCG1 is an important mechanism to export cytotoxic cellular free cholesterol to lipid poor apoAI and lapidated HDL particles (Chinetti et al., 2001; Kennedy et al., 2005) . It is well documented that cholesterol efflux via ABCA1 and ABCG1 is essential to slow the development of atherosclerosis by decreasing lipid loading (Yvan-Charvet et al., 2007) (Zhao et al., 2010) (Calkin and Tontonoz, 2010) (Fitzgerald et al., 2010) (Ye et al., 2011). Although the role of scavenger receptors appears complicated because of conflicting results from gene knockout or transgenic mouse studies (Hansson and Hermansson, 2011) the general consensus among recent publications is that these receptors are protective against atherosclerosis due to their ability to remove modified LDL from the vessel wall (Marleau et al., 2005) (Moore et al., 2005) (Van Eck et al., 2000) (Whitman et al., 2002) (Liao et al., 2000) (Teupser et al., 1999).

Recent in vivo results show that the role of IL-10 in regulating lipid metabolism remains elusive. Plasma lipoprotein levels including LDL, HDL and triglyceride have been measured in these animal models but the results appear controversial and are dependent on several factors such as the animal model used, route of administration and stage of atherosclerosis investigated. In C57BL/6J mice, total plasma cholesterol and HDL cholesterol levels were not affected by IL-10 deficiency (Mallat et al., 1999a) (Pinderski Oslund et al., 1999). Systemic IL-10 overexpression lowered plasma VLDL and LDL cholesterol levels in LDLR-/- mice (Von Der Thusen et al., 2001), but IL-10 overexpression in T cells did not alter circulating lipoprotein profiles (Pinderski et al., 2002). No changes in plasma (Namiki et al., 2004) or reduced cholesterol levels (Yoshioka et al., 2004) were observed in apoE-/- mice with intramuscular gene transfer of IL-10 cDNA. Interestingly, the lack of IL-10 led to increased LDL cholesterol whereas VLDL was reduced in apoE-/- mice with no significant changes observed in either total cholesterol or triglyceride levels (Caligiuri et al., 2003). However, systemic delivery of adeno-associated virus type 2-hIL-10 inhibited atherogenesis in LDLR knockout mice with no changes in plasma cholesterol levels (total cholesterol, LDL, HDL, and TG) compared with those with no treatment (Liu et al., 2006). In APOE*3-Leiden mice, IL-10 deficiency did not lead to significant changes in cholesterol levels but overexpression of IL-10 reduced cholesterol levels after feeding a high-fat, cholesterol-rich diet (Eefting et al., 2007). These confusing set of results suggest that IL-10-modulated lipid metabolism and plasma cholesterol levels vary widely and is dependent on the animal models utilized. The role of IL-10 in lipid metabolism needs to be rigorously elucidated, especially in relation to human atherosclerosis.

Recent publications provide convincing evidence that IL-10 can modulate cellular lipid metabolism, including cholesterol uptake and cholesterol efflux (reverse cholesterol transport). In 2005, Halvorsen et al. reported that IL-10 enhances oxLDL-induced formation of macrophage foam cells (Halvorsen et al., 2005). The authors propose that IL-10 not only enhances foam cell formation but also has anti-apoptotic effects by increasing the expression of anti-apoptotic genes Bfl-1 and Mcl-1 (Halvorsen et al., 2005). In 2006, Rubic and Lorenz showed that IL-10 can stimulate ABCA1/ABCG1 which increases the cholesterol efflux from lipid-laden foam cells. In addition, they observed a down-regulation of CD36-mediated oxLDL uptake in macrophages. According to their results IL-10 is able to decrease oxLDL uptake and increase reverse cholesterol transport in macrophages, thereby preventing foam cell formation (Rubic and Lorenz, 2006). These results appear to contradict the report by Halvorsen et al. in which IL-10 increases foam cell formation. These confusing findings were partially clarified by a study by Han et al. in 2009 in which they reported that IL-10 modulates lipid metabolism in macrophages by facilitating both cholesterol uptake and efflux (Han et al., 2009). This study clearly revealed that IL-10 not only can up-regulate ABCA1 in a PPAR-γ-dependent mechanism but can increase the expression of scavenger receptors (scavenger receptor A and CD36). In support of this Montoya et al. reported that IL-10 stimulates the expression of scavenger receptors and enhances foam cell formation (Montoya et al., 2009). These data support the hypothesis that increased cholesterol uptake by IL-10 may be athero-protective by actively removing the highly atherogenic lipoproteins from the artery wall. On the other hand, the increase in ABCA1-dependent cholesterol efflux by IL-10 is a crucial factor in the efficient disposal of cytotoxic free cholesterol through reverse cholesterol transport. Interestingly, a recent report indicated that anti-inflammatory M2 macrophages but not pro-inflammatory M1 macrophages rapidly accumulate oxidized LDL (van Tits et al., 2011). As IL-10 is one of the effectors that promote M2 macrophage polarization as mentioned above (Martinez et al., 2009) (Tabas, 2010), it is likely that IL-10 is involved in the lipid accumulation predominantly in M2 macrophages. These results present a comprehensive anti-atherogenic role of IL-10 in macrophages, along with a more traditional role of IL-10 in inhibiting inflammatory molecules (e.g. TNF-α, iCAM-1, and MMP9) and reducing apoptosis (Han et al., 2009) (Han et al., 2010) . A cartoon depicting the multi-faceted anti-atherogenic role of IL-10 in macrophages is shown in the figure below.

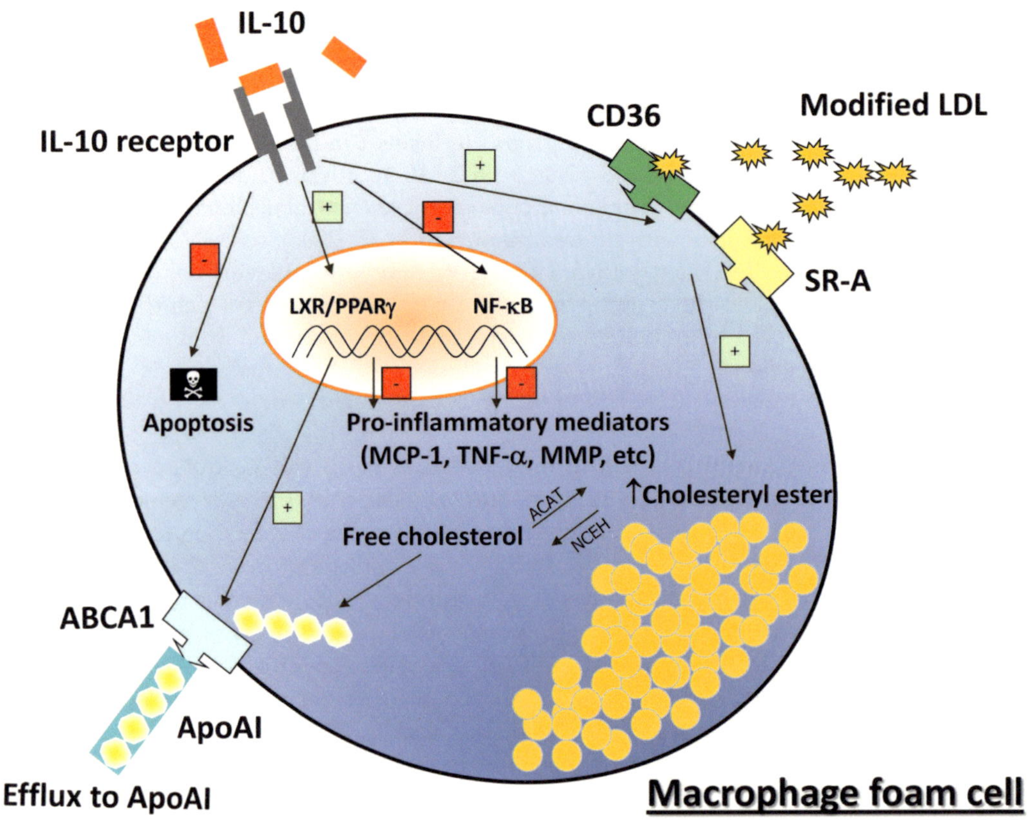


Fig. 1. Schematic overview of the protective role of IL-10 during atherosclerosis involving regulation of lipid metabolism in macrophages. Upon binding to its receptor, IL-10 up-regulates scavenger receptors, SR-A (SR-I and SR-II) and CD36, which account for an increase in modified LDL uptake by macrophages. This promotes cholesteryl ester accumulation and foam cell formation. IL-10 also promotes ABCA1-mediated free cholesterol efflux to apoAI in a PPARγ-dependent manner. In a more traditional role as an anti-inflammatory cytokine, IL-10 markedly suppresses the expression of pro-inflammatory molecules such as TNF-α, MCP-1 and MMPs, presumably through the inhibition of NF-κB activity as documented before (Wang et al., 1995), and diminishes apoptosis in the lipid-laden foam cells (Han et al., 2009).

### 2.2 Influence on T lymphocyte function

Recent publications have shown that, although T cell numbers are far fewer than mononuclear phagocytes, they are also recruited to the intima and play an important role in the development of atherogenesis. Therefore, the protective action of IL-10 in atherogenesis is likely to involve T cell immune response.

### 2.2.1 Polarization and balance of T helper cells

T lymphocytes are found in lesions in an activated state and coexist with lesion macrophages, particularly in early phases of atherosclerosis. The key role for Th1 cytokines, such as IL-12 (Lee et al., 1999) or IFN-γ (Gupta et al., 1997) as well as the general role of lesion T lymphocytes in atherogenesis have been reviewed elsewhere (Daugherty and Rateri, 2002). As a prototypic anti-inflammatory cytokine, IL-10 down-regulates Th1 cytokines such as IL-12 and IL-18 leading to inhibition of Th1-biased immune response (Moore et al., 2001), and polarization of the Th1:Th2 balances toward Th2 (Daugherty and Rateri, 2002). Induction of a regulatory T cell type 1 response attenuates the development of atherosclerosis in apoE-knockout mice by decreasing the Th1 response, decreasing the production of IFN-γ and increasing IL-10 production (Mallat et al., 2003). Also, it may be that the reduction in atherosclerotic lesion formation in FcγRIII (CD16) -/- mice crossed onto the LDLR-/- mice is associated with increased production of IL-10 by the expansion of CD4+ T cells (Kelly et al., 2010).

The imbalance between pro- and anti-inflammatory forces influences plaque disruption and recurrent cardiovascular events (Trompet et al., 2007) with a shift towards the Th1 dominance seen in atherosclerosis patients (Ait-Oufella et al., 2011). In support of this concept is the report that serum IL-18/IL-10 ratio is an independent predictor of in-hospital adverse events in patients with acute coronary syndrome (Chalikias et al., 2005). Furthermore, an anti-inflammatory marker such as IL-10 is a better prognostic marker than inflammatory markers such as CRP and IL-18 to predict cardiovascular events in ACS patients (Tziakas et al., 2007). Likewise, it has been demonstrated that CRP accentuates inflammation, which is pivotal in atherothrombosis, by lowering IL-10, thereby altering the anti-inflammatory/pro-inflammatory balance (Singh et al., 2006). There is an inverse correlation between pro-inflammatory CRP and anti-inflammatory IL-10 levels in patients with athersoclerosis (Seyrek et al., 2005). More recently, an inflammatory imbalance between the TNF-α system and IL-10 has been characterized in children with familial hypercholesterolemia (Narverud et al., 2011).

Th1 biased phenotype is responsible for clinical instability (Liuzzo et al., 2000) and atherogenesis (Jonsson et al., 2001) (Hurt-Camejo et al., 2001) (Laurat et al., 2001) (Zhou et al., 1998) (Caligiuri et al., 2003) (Mallat and Tedgui, 2004) (Mallat et al., 2005). Interestingly, in IL-10-/- ApoE-/- double KO mice, Th1-bias was accompanied by a higher susceptibility to atherosclerosis, but only at the early stage of the disease when macrophages dominate (which is when they are sensitive to Th1 and Th2 cytokines (Caligiuri et al., 2003)).

### 2.2.2 Regulatory T cells and Th17 cells

Recently, the role of regulatory T cells (Treg) and IL-17-producing T cells (Th17 cells) has been emphasized in atherosclerosis (Taleb et al., 2010) (Lahoute et al., 2011). Treg are important in protection against atherosclerosis at least in part through the production of IL-10 (Mor et al., 2007) (Taleb et al., 2010) (George, 2008) (Feng et al., 2009). It is also believed that the pro-atherogenic response by Th1 cells can be controlled by Treg (Binder et al., 2004).

IL-17-producing Th17 cells also play an important role in atherosclerosis (Hansson and Hermansson, 2011). Irradiated LDLR-/- mice transplanted with IL-17R deficient bone marrow exhibit reduced lesion size in aortic root, increased IL-10 production, and decreased IL-6 production (van Es et al., 2009). This suggests that signaling via the IL-17 receptor in bone marrow derived cells enhances atherosclerosis. Similarly, blockade of IL-17 results in reduced atherosclerosis in apoE-/- mice (Smith et al., 2010) (Erbel et al., 2009). However, the role of IL-

17 in atherogenesis is controversial in that increased level of IL-17 is associated with a stable human plaque phenotype while defective Th17 cell differentiation may be implicated in increased susceptibility to vascular inflammation (Taleb et al., 2009). In addition, Th17 response is protective against vascular inflammation and the progression of atherosclerosis (Taleb et al., 2010). Similarly, a deficiency of SOCS3 in T cells leads to IL-17-dependent reduction in lesion development and vascular inflammation by increasing IL-17 and IL-10 production, and by inducing an anti-inflammatory macrophage phenotype (Taleb et al., 2009)

## 3. Human studies and in vivo animal models

The role of IL-10 in atherosclerosis has been investigated using different animal models as listed on the table below. In 1996, Uyemura et al. (Uyemura et al., 1996) first described that IL-10 was produced in human atherosclerotic lesions and that ox-LDL induced IL-10 release from monocytes in vitro. The down-regulation of IL-12 by IL-10 (Sieling et al., 1994) (D'Andrea et al., 1993) (de Waal Malefyt et al., 1991) observed in this study and others suggest that the balance between IL-12 and IL-10 production contributes to the level of immune-mediated tissue injury in atherosclerosis. IL-12 and IL-10 are two important cytokines produced by activated monocytes that regulate the Th1 and Th2 responses, respectively (D'Andrea et al., 1992) (Gately et al., 1991) (Germann et al., 1993) (Hsieh et al., 1993) (Seder et al., 1993) (Sieling et al., 1994) (de Waal Malefyt et al., 1991) (Barnes et al., 1992). IL-12 is a T cell growth factor (Gately et al., 1991) that is primarily produced by activated monocytes (D'Andrea et al., 1992) which selectively induces the Th1 cytokine pattern (Gately et al., 1991) (Germann et al., 1993) (Hsieh et al., 1993) (Seder et al., 1993) (Sieling et al., 1994). One important mechanism of IL-10 action is that it inhibits the local production of IL-12 which may potentiate the chronic inflammatory Th1 cell and macrophage responses leading to tissue injury in atherosclerosis (Uyemura et al., 1996). The complicated issue of athero-regulation by both IL-12 and IL-10 was further exhibited by an observation that IL-12 is expressed at an earlier stage of atherosclerosis than IL-10 in apoE-/- mice (Lee et al., 1999). This suggests that IL-12 and IL-10 may play an active role in regulating the immune response during the different phases of atherosclerosis.

In 1999, Mallat et al. reported the expression and potential effects of IL-10 in advanced human atherosclerotic plaques (Mallat et al., 1999b). Immunohistochemical staining from this study indicated that macrophages in advanced human atherosclerotic plaques are the main source of IL-10. The local anti-inflammatory response of IL-10 and its effect on protection from excessive cell death in the plaque was supported by the data that high levels of IL-10 expression were associated with low levels of iNOS expression and cell death.

Studies involving IL-10-deficient and IL-10-overexpressing mouse models on either apoE-/- or LDLR -/- background have greatly advanced our understanding of the mechanism of IL-10 function in atherogenesis. In 1999, two labs independently reported that IL-10 is protective in atherosclerosis (Mallat et al., 1999a; Pinderski Oslund et al., 1999). Since then, more than ten groups utilized different animal models and various IL-10 delivery systems in an attempt to understand how IL-10 affects atherosclerosis. The first report using the IL-10-deficient mice fed an atherogenic diet showed an increased lipid accumulation, higher T-cell infiltration, abundant IFN-γ expression, and decreased collagen content in the lesion compared with wild-type mice (Mallat et al., 1999a). Transfer of murine

| Publication | Approach | Animal model | Underlying mechanism |
|---|---|---|---|
| Mallat et al. 1999, Circ Res (Mallat et al., 1999a) | IL-10-encoding plasmid transferred to muscle cells using electrotransfer procedures | C57BL/6 mice | Inhibit inflammation, plaque collagen content and stability |
| Pinderski Oslund et al. 1999, ATVB (Pinderski Oslund et al., 1999) | Systemic overexpression of IL-10 | C57BL/6J mice | Block monocyte adhesion to human aortic endothelial cells |
| Von der Thusen et al. 2001, FASEB J (Von Der Thusen et al., 2001) | Systemic adenovirus-mediated transfer of IL-10 | LDLR-/- mice | Monocyte deactivation by inhibition of TNF-α and lowering of serum cholesterol levels |
| Pinderski et al. 2002, Circ Res (Pinderski et al., 2002) | Murine IL-10 transgene under human IL-2 promoter, bone marrow transplantation (overexpression of IL-10 by T cells) | LDLR -/- mice | Polarization to Th2 phenotype; lowered activation of monocytes; decreased apoptosis of macrophage foam cells within lesion |
| Caligiuri G et al. 2003,<br>Mol Med (Caligiuri et al., 2003) | IL-10 deficiency | ApoE-/- mice | Increased Th1 response; increased TF and MMP activity; increase in LDL and decrease in vLDL in IL-10-/-ApoE-/- mice |
| Namiki M et al 2004<br>Atherosclerosis (Namiki et al., 2004) | Intramuscular gene transfer of IL-10 cDNA | ApoE-/- mice | Change in the Th1 response by inhibiting IL-12 and IFN-γ expression |
| Yoshioka et al. 2004, Gene Ther (Yoshioka et al., 2004) | Systemic delivery of adeno-associated virus vector (tibial muscle injection) | ApoE-/- mice | Inhibition of inflammation and oxidative stress |
| Liu et al. 2006, Atherosclerosis (Liu et al., 2006) | Systemic delivery (tail vein injection) | LDLR-/- mice | Anti-inflammatory (MCP-1) and cholesterol-lowering effects |
| Namiki et al. 2004, Atherosclerosis (Namiki et al., 2004) | Transfer of murine IL-10 cDNA plasmid to femoral muscle with Hemagglutinin virus of Japan (HVJ)-liposome | ApoE-/- mice | Reduced macrophage infiltration and altered Th1 response |
| Han X, et al.<br>2010, FASEB J (Han et al., 2010) | Overexpression of IL-10 by macrophages, bone marrow transplantation | LDLR-/- mice | Inhibition of inflammation and apoptosis; modulation of lipid metabolism in foam cells (both lipid uptake and cholesterol efflux) |
| Du L, et al.<br>2011, Human Gen Therapy (Du et al., 2011) | Expression of IL-10 in carotid arteries achieved with helper-dependent adenoviral vector | Rabbit | No athero-protective effect |

IL-10 through in vivo intramuscular electrotransfers of pCor-IL-10 plasmid DNA achieved a 60% reduction in lesion size in IL-10-deficient mice. In agreement with these findings, Pinderski Oslund et al. observed that diet-induced atherosclerotic lesions were larger in IL-10 null mice than in control mice (Pinderski Oslund et al., 1999). In addition, they also observed that transgenic murine IL-10 expression which was selectively driven in T cells by human IL-2 promoter decreased atherosclerotic lesion formation (Pinderski Oslund et al., 1999).

In 2001, von der Thusen and colleagues reported that increased plasma concentrations of IL-10 as a result of adenoviral gene transfer in LDLR-/- mice led to reduction in atherosclerotic lesion size by inhibiting the production of TNF-α (Han et al., 2010; Von Der Thusen et al., 2001). The mechanism involves the inhibition of anti-inflammatory TNF-α production by IL-10 (Han et al., 2010; Von Der Thusen et al., 2001). At the same time, Pinderski et al. demonstrated that overexpression of IL-10 by activated T lymphocytes attenuated lesion formation by driving the shift to a Th2 phenotype with decreased IFN-γ production (by peripheral blood lymphocytes, splenocytes, and circulating monocytes) (Pinderski et al., 2002). Alteration of macrophage function was exhibited by markedly decreased apoptosis in macrophage foam cells within the lesions of IL-10 transgenic mice (Pinderski et al., 2002).

The athero-protective results obtained with IL-10-deficient mice on the C57BL/6J background (Mallat et al., 1999a; Pinderski Oslund et al., 1999) were confirmed in IL-10 and apoE double knockout mice as demonstrated by Caligiuri et al. (Caligiuri et al., 2003). Several significant findings were revealed by this study: (1) Th-1 response and lesion size were dramatically increased in double knockout mice compared with apoE-/- controls at the early phase of lesion development; (2) the proteolytic and procoagulant activity was elevated in advanced lesions as indicated by an increase in TF and MMP activities, suggesting that IL-10 may reduce atherogenesis and improve the stability of plaques; and (3) lipid metabolism regulated by IL-10 was implicated in this study as LDL cholesterol was increased but VLDL was decreased in the double KO mice without significant changes in total cholesterol or triglyceride levels (Caligiuri et al., 2003).

In an attempt to utilize IL-10 as a therapeutic agent, several techniques have been used by different groups to deliver the IL-10 gene in vivo. One study showed that intramuscular gene transfer of IL-10 cDNA reduces atherosclerotic lesion formation in apoE-/- mice (Namiki et al., 2004). IL-10 gene transfer quelled the Th1 response by inhibiting IL-12 and IFN-γ expression in transgenic mice (Namiki et al., 2004). These results were confirmed in another study in which adeno-associated virus vector-mediated IL-10 gene transfer via intramuscular injection inhibited atherosclerosis in apoE-/- mice (Yoshioka et al., 2004) by lowering MCP-1 expression in both the vascular wall of the ascending aorta and serum. In agreement with these results, a systemic delivery of adeno-associated virus type 2-hIL-10 inhibited atherogenesis in LDLR-/- mice by combating inflammation and oxidative stress (Liu et al., 2006). Similar effects of IL-10 deficiency and overexpression on neointima formation were seen in the hypercholesterolemic apoE*3-Leiden mice as well (Eefting et al., 2007).

Anti-atherosclerotic properties of IL-10 were further displayed in high fat diet-fed LDLR -/- mice in which IL-10 was overexpressed in macrophages by utilizing a macrophage-specific retroviral vector that allows long-term in vivo expression of IL-10 in macrophages through transplantation of retrovirally transduced bone marrow cells (BMCs) (Han et al., 2010). The

IL-10 expressed by macrophages in the plaques derived from transduced BMCs inhibited atherosclerosis in these mice, at least in part by reducing the inflammation and apoptosis in IL-10-overexpressing macrophages. These results are consistent with previous findings (Han et al., 2009) and provided evidence that IL-10 production in macrophages is protective against atherosclerosis. Their results also highlight a novel therapeutic technique against atherosclerosis using an effective stem cell transduction system that allows prolonged production of IL-10 from macrophages.

It is worth emphasizing that most strategies mentioned above had systemic effects on multiple cells including T cells, monocytes and endothelium resulting from overexpression of IL-10 in circulation. For example, overexpression of IL-10 in activated T lymphocytes inhibited monocyte activation and led to a shift to either Th2 phenotype (Pinderski et al., 2002) or Th1 phenotype (Zhou et al., 1998). As a cytokine with diverse effects on most hematopoietic cell types, IL-10 can inhibit the activation and effector function of T cells, monocytes, and macrophages (Moore et al., 2001). In addition, IL-10 can regulate the growth and/or differentiation of B cells, NK cells, cytotoxic and helper T cells, mast cells, granulocytes, dendritic cells, keratinocytes, and endothelial cells (Moore et al., 2001). Therefore, alterations in circulating IL-10 levels can influence the function of other immune cells which may in turn influence atherosclerosis. In the study by Han et al. there was no detectable IL-10 in circulating plasma at any time point during the atherogenic diet feeding whereas IL-10 was readily detected in IL-10-overexpressing macrophages in atherosclerotic lesions. This suggests that IL-10 was expressed in differentiated macrophages but not in circulating monocytes. Therefore, their technique of overexpressing IL-10 only in differentiated macrophages is useful to evaluate the unique role of locally-produced IL-10 in atherogenesis, and clearly shows that IL-10 acting in the vessel wall can decrease the development of atherosclerosis despite ongoing hyperlipidemia.

However, a recent study using a rabbit model showed that prolonged and stable expression of IL-10 in rabbit carotid arteries achieved with a helper-dependent adenoviral vector had neither an atheroprotective effect nor any effect on adhesion molecules or any other atherogenic cytokines (Du et al., 2011). Possible explanation accounting for the discrepant results may be inadequate protein expression *in vivo* or lack of suitability of this rabbit model to detect IL-10's therapeutic effects. This study suggests that gene therapy involving IL-10 delivery may bring about different results in different species.

## 4. Therapeutic considerations

In light of the findings that systemic and intralesional delivery of IL-10 can be anti-atherogenic, it is tempting to speculate that IL-10 treatment may have the potential to be a novel therapeutic agent against atherosclerosis in the future. IL-10 expression after intramuscular DNA electrotransfer or other techniques leads to a persistent expression of this protective cytokine in circulation and in local lesion (Deleuze et al., 2002; Han et al., 2010; Pinderski et al., 2002). It is likely that systemic delivery of IL-10 will result in suppression of immune response and increase the opportunity of infection, particularly involving intracellular pathogens such as *Chlamydia* and *Listeria* monocytogenes (Terkeltaub, 1999). Compared with systemic delivery of IL-10, local expression of IL-10 in atherosclerotic lesions may have much less impact on the general immune response. On the other hand, a robust local expression driven by retrovirus or adenovirus makes it difficult to regulate IL-10 expression in a temporally and spatially controllable manner as desired. Accordingly, the safety and effectiveness of exogenous IL-10 administration utilizing these techniques will need to be evaluated in the future before they are adopted in human patients for the treatment of atherosclerosis.

## 5. References


Ait-Oufella, H., Taleb, S., Mallat, Z., and Tedgui, A. (2011). Recent advances on the role of cytokines in atherosclerosis. Arterioscler Thromb Vasc Biol *31*, 969-979.

Ajuebor, M.N., Das, A.M., Virag, L., Flower, R.J., Szabo, C., and Perretti, M. (1999). Role of resident peritoneal macrophages and mast cells in chemokine production and neutrophil migration in acute inflammation: evidence for an inhibitory loop involving endogenous IL-10. J Immunol *162*, 1685-1691.

Albina, J.E., Cui, S., Mateo, R.B., and Reichner, J.S. (1993). Nitric oxide-mediated apoptosis in murine peritoneal macrophages. J Immunol *150*, 5080-5085.

Amento, E.P., Ehsani, N., Palmer, H., and Libby, P. (1991). Cytokines and growth factors positively and negatively regulate interstitial collagen gene expression in human vascular smooth muscle cells. Arterioscler Thromb *11*, 1223-1230.

Arai, T., Hiromatsu, K., Nishimura, H., Kimura, Y., Kobayashi, N., Ishida, H., Nimura, Y., and Yoshikai, Y. (1995). Endogenous interleukin 10 prevents apoptosis in macrophages during Salmonella infection. Biochem Biophys Res Commun *213*, 600-607.

Ardissino, D., Merlini, P.A., Ariens, R., Coppola, R., Bramucci, E., and Mannucci, P.M. (1997). Tissue-factor antigen and activity in human coronary atherosclerotic plaques. Lancet *349*, 769-771.

Arnman, V., Stemme, S., Rymo, L., and Risberg, B. (1995). Interferon-gamma modulates the fibrinolytic response in cultured human endothelial cells. Thromb Res *77*, 431-440.

Barnes, P.F., Chatterjee, D., Abrams, J.S., Lu, S., Wang, E., Yamamura, M., Brennan, P.J., and Modlin, R.L. (1992). Cytokine production induced by Mycobacterium tuberculosis lipoarabinomannan. Relationship to chemical structure. J Immunol *149*, 541-547.

Beaven, S.W., and Tontonoz, P. (2006). Nuclear receptors in lipid metabolism: targeting the heart of dyslipidemia. Annu Rev Med *57*, 313-329.

Benoit, M., Desnues, B., and Mege, J.L. (2008). Macrophage polarization in bacterial infections. J Immunol *181*, 3733-3739.

Biasucci, L.M., Liuzzo, G., Caligiuri, G., Quaranta, G., Andreotti, F., Sperti, G., van de Greef, W., Rebuzzi, A.G., Kluft, C., and Maseri, A. (1996). Temporal relation between ischemic episodes and activation of the coagulation system in unstable angina. Circulation *93*, 2121-2127.

Binder, C.J., Hartvigsen, K., Chang, M.K., Miller, M., Broide, D., Palinski, W., Curtiss, L.K., Corr, M., and Witztum, J.L. (2004). IL-5 links adaptive and natural immunity specific for epitopes of oxidized LDL and protects from atherosclerosis. J Clin Invest *114*, 427-437.

Bjorkerud, S., and Bjorkerud, B. (1996). Apoptosis is abundant in human atherosclerotic lesions, especially in inflammatory cells (macrophages and T cells), and may contribute to the accumulation of gruel and plaque instability. Am J Pathol *149*, 367-380.

Bobik, A., Agrotis, A., Kanellakis, P., Dilley, R., Krushinsky, A., Smirnov, V., Tararak, E., Condron, M., and Kostolias, G. (1999). Distinct patterns of transforming growth factor-beta isoform and receptor expression in human atherosclerotic lesions. Colocalization implicates TGF-beta in fibrofatty lesion development. Circulation *99*, 2883-2891.

Bogdan, C., Vodovotz, Y., and Nathan, C. (1991). Macrophage deactivation by interleukin 10. J Exp Med *174*, 1549-1555.

Boisvert, W.A., Santiago, R., Curtiss, L.K., and Terkeltaub, R.A. (1998). A leukocyte homologue of the IL-8 receptor CXCR-2 mediates the accumulation of macrophages in atherosclerotic lesions of LDL receptor-deficient mice. J Clin Invest *101*, 353-363.

Bouhlel, M.A., Derudas, B., Rigamonti, E., Dievart, R., Brozek, J., Haulon, S., Zawadzki, C., Jude, B., Torpier, G., Marx, N., *et al.* (2007). PPARgamma activation primes human monocytes into alternative M2 macrophages with anti-inflammatory properties. Cell Metab *6*, 137-143.

Boyle, J.J. (2005). Macrophage activation in atherosclerosis: pathogenesis and pharmacology of plaque rupture. Curr Vasc Pharmacol *3*, 63-68.

Brown, M.S., and Goldstein, J.L. (1983). Lipoprotein metabolism in the macrophage: implications for cholesterol deposition in atherosclerosis. Annu Rev Biochem *52*, 223-261.

Brown, M.S., and Goldstein, J.L. (1997). The SREBP pathway: regulation of cholesterol metabolism by proteolysis of a membrane-bound transcription factor. Cell *89*, 331-340.

Cai, W., Devaux, B., Schaper, W., and Schaper, J. (1997). The role of Fas/APO 1 and apoptosis in the development of human atherosclerotic lesions. Atherosclerosis *131*, 177-186.

Caligiuri, G., Rudling, M., Ollivier, V., Jacob, M.P., Michel, J.B., Hansson, G.K., and Nicoletti, A. (2003). Interleukin-10 deficiency increases atherosclerosis, thrombosis, and low-density lipoproteins in apolipoprotein E knockout mice. Mol Med *9*, 10-17.

Calkin, A.C., and Tontonoz, P. (2010). Liver x receptor signaling pathways and atherosclerosis. Arterioscler Thromb Vasc Biol *30*, 1513-1518.

Cattaruzza, M., Slodowski, W., Stojakovic, M., Krzesz, R., and Hecker, M. (2003). Interleukin-10 induction of nitric-oxide synthase expression attenuates CD40-mediated interleukin-12 synthesis in human endothelial cells. J Biol Chem *278*, 37874-37880.

Chalikias, G.K., Tziakas, D.N., Kaski, J.C., Hatzinikolaou, E.I., Stakos, D.A., Tentes, I.K., Kortsaris, A., and Hatseras, D.I. (2005). Interleukin-18: interleukin-10 ratio and in-hospital adverse events in patients with acute coronary syndrome. Atherosclerosis *182*, 135-143.

Charo, I.F. (2007). Macrophage polarization and insulin resistance: PPARgamma in control. Cell Metab *6*, 96-98.

Charo, I.F., and Taub, R. (2011). Anti-inflammatory therapeutics for the treatment of atherosclerosis. Nat Rev Drug Discov *10*, 365-376.

Chinetti-Gbaguidi, G., and Staels, B. Macrophage polarization in metabolic disorders: functions and regulation. Curr Opin Lipidol.

Chinetti, G., Lestavel, S., Bocher, V., Remaley, A.T., Neve, B., Torra, I.P., Teissier, E., Minnich, A., Jaye, M., Duverger, N., *et al.* (2001). PPAR-alpha and PPAR-gamma activators induce cholesterol removal from human macrophage foam cells through stimulation of the ABCA1 pathway. Nat Med *7*, 53-58.

Cohen, S.B., Crawley, J.B., Kahan, M.C., Feldmann, M., and Foxwell, B.M. (1997). Interleukin-10 rescues T cells from apoptotic cell death: association with an upregulation of Bcl-2. Immunology *92*, 1-5.

D'Andrea, A., Aste-Amezaga, M., Valiante, N.M., Ma, X., Kubin, M., and Trinchieri, G. (1993). Interleukin 10 (IL-10) inhibits human lymphocyte interferon gamma-production by suppressing natural killer cell stimulatory factor/IL-12 synthesis in accessory cells. J Exp Med *178*, 1041-1048.

D'Andrea, A., Rengaraju, M., Valiante, N.M., Chehimi, J., Kubin, M., Aste, M., Chan, S.H., Kobayashi, M., Young, D., Nickbarg, E., *et al.* (1992). Production of natural killer cell stimulatory factor (interleukin 12) by peripheral blood mononuclear cells. J Exp Med *176*, 1387-1398.

Daugherty, A., and Rateri, D.L. (2002). T lymphocytes in atherosclerosis: the yin-yang of Th1 and Th2 influence on lesion formation. Circ Res *90*, 1039-1040.

de Vries, J.E. (1995). Immunosuppressive and anti-inflammatory properties of interleukin 10. Ann Med *27*, 537-541.

de Waal Malefyt, R., Abrams, J., Bennett, B., Figdor, C.G., and de Vries, J.E. (1991). Interleukin 10(IL-10) inhibits cytokine synthesis by human monocytes: an autoregulatory role of IL-10 produced by monocytes. J Exp Med *174*, 1209-1220.

Deleuze, V., Scherman, D., and Bureau, M.F. (2002). Interleukin-10 expression after intramuscular DNA electrotransfer: kinetic studies. Biochem Biophys Res Commun *299*, 29-34.

Du, L., Dronadula, N., Tanaka, S., and Dichek, D.A. (2011). Helper-Dependent Adenoviral Vector Achieves Prolonged, Stable Expression of Interleukin-10 in Rabbit Carotid Arteries but Does Not Limit Early Atherogenesis. Hum Gene Ther.

Eefting, D., Schepers, A., De Vries, M.R., Pires, N.M., Grimbergen, J.M., Lagerweij, T., Nagelkerken, L.M., Monraats, P.S., Jukema, J.W., van Bockel, J.H., *et al.* (2007). The effect of interleukin-10 knock-out and overexpression on neointima formation in hypercholesterolemic APOE*3-Leiden mice. Atherosclerosis *193*, 335-342.

Erbel, C., Chen, L., Bea, F., Wangler, S., Celik, S., Lasitschka, F., Wang, Y., Bockler, D., Katus, H.A., and Dengler, T.J. (2009). Inhibition of IL-17A attenuates atherosclerotic lesion development in apoE-deficient mice. J Immunol *183*, 8167-8175.

Fei, G.Z., Huang, Y.H., Swedenborg, J., and Frostegard, J. (2003). Oxidised LDL modulates immune-activation by an IL-12 dependent mechanism. Atherosclerosis *169*, 77-85.

Feng, J., Zhang, Z., Kong, W., Liu, B., Xu, Q., and Wang, X. (2009). Regulatory T cells ameliorate hyperhomocysteinaemia-accelerated atherosclerosis in apoE-/- mice. Cardiovasc Res *84*, 155-163.

Ferri, L.A., Maugeri, N., Rovere-Querini, P., Calabrese, A., Ammirati, E., Cianflone, D., Maseri, A., and Manfredi, A.A. (2009). Anti-inflammatory action of apoptotic cells in patients with acute coronary syndromes. Atherosclerosis *205*, 391-395.

Fitzgerald, M.L., Mujawar, Z., and Tamehiro, N. (2010). ABC transporters, atherosclerosis and inflammation. Atherosclerosis *211*, 361-370.

Galkina, E., and Ley, K. (2009). Immune and inflammatory mechanisms of atherosclerosis (*). Annu Rev Immunol *27*, 165-197.

Gallicchio, M., Hufnagl, P., Wojta, J., and Tipping, P. (1996). IFN-gamma inhibits thrombin- and endotoxin-induced plasminogen activator inhibitor type 1 in human endothelial cells. J Immunol *157*, 2610-2617.

Gately, M.K., Desai, B.B., Wolitzky, A.G., Quinn, P.M., Dwyer, C.M., Podlaski, F.J., Familletti, P.C., Sinigaglia, F., Chizonnite, R., Gubler, U., *et al.* (1991). Regulation of human lymphocyte proliferation by a heterodimeric cytokine, IL-12 (cytotoxic lymphocyte maturation factor). J Immunol *147*, 874-882.

Geng, Y.J., and Libby, P. (1995). Evidence for apoptosis in advanced human atheroma. Colocalization with interleukin-1 beta-converting enzyme. Am J Pathol *147*, 251-266.

Geng, Y.J., Wu, Q., Muszynski, M., Hansson, G.K., and Libby, P. (1996). Apoptosis of vascular smooth muscle cells induced by in vitro stimulation with interferon-gamma, tumor necrosis factor-alpha, and interleukin-1 beta. Arterioscler Thromb Vasc Biol *16*, 19-27.

George, J. (2008). Mechanisms of disease: the evolving role of regulatory T cells in atherosclerosis. Nat Clin Pract Cardiovasc Med *5*, 531-540.

Gerard, C., Bruyns, C., Marchant, A., Abramowicz, D., Vandenabeele, P., Delvaux, A., Fiers, W., Goldman, M., and Velu, T. (1993). Interleukin 10 reduces the release of tumor necrosis factor and prevents lethality in experimental endotoxemia. J Exp Med *177*, 547-550.

Germann, T., Gately, M.K., Schoenhaut, D.S., Lohoff, M., Mattner, F., Fischer, S., Jin, S.C., Schmitt, E., and Rude, E. (1993). Interleukin-12/T cell stimulating factor, a cytokine with multiple effects on T helper type 1 (Th1) but not on Th2 cells. Eur J Immunol *23*, 1762-1770.

Gosling, J., Slaymaker, S., Gu, L., Tseng, S., Zlot, C.H., Young, S.G., Rollins, B.J., and Charo, I.F. (1999). MCP-1 deficiency reduces susceptibility to atherosclerosis in mice that overexpress human apolipoprotein B. J Clin Invest *103*, 773-778.

Gough, P.J., Gomez, I.G., Wille, P.T., and Raines, E.W. (2006). Macrophage expression of active MMP-9 induces acute plaque disruption in apoE-deficient mice. J Clin Invest *116*, 59-69.

Gupta, S., Pablo, A.M., Jiang, X., Wang, N., Tall, A.R., and Schindler, C. (1997). IFN-gamma potentiates atherosclerosis in ApoE knock-out mice. J Clin Invest *99*, 2752-2761.

Halvorsen, B., Waehre, T., Scholz, H., Clausen, O.P., von der Thusen, J.H., Muller, F., Heimli, H., Tonstad, S., Hall, C., Froland, S.S., *et al.* (2005). Interleukin-10 enhances the oxidized LDL-induced foam cell formation of macrophages by antiapoptotic mechanisms. J Lipid Res *46*, 211-219.

Han, D.K., Haudenschild, C.C., Hong, M.K., Tinkle, B.T., Leon, M.B., and Liau, G. (1995). Evidence for apoptosis in human atherogenesis and in a rat vascular injury model. Am J Pathol *147*, 267-277.

Han, X., Kitamoto, S., Lian, Q., and Boisvert, W.A. (2009). Interleukin-10 facilitates both cholesterol uptake and efflux in macrophages. J Biol Chem *284*, 32950-32958.

Han, X., Kitamoto, S., Wang, H., and Boisvert, W.A. (2010). Interleukin-10 overexpression in macrophages suppresses atherosclerosis in hyperlipidemic mice. FASEB J *24*, 2869-2880.

Hansson, G.K. (2001). Immune mechanisms in atherosclerosis. Arterioscler Thromb Vasc Biol *21*, 1876-1890.

Hansson, G.K., and Hermansson, A. (2011). The immune system in atherosclerosis. Nat Immunol *12*, 204-212.

Hansson, G.K., and Libby, P. (2006). The immune response in atherosclerosis: a double-edged sword. Nat Rev Immunol *6*, 508-519.

Hansson, G.K., Libby, P., Schonbeck, U., and Yan, Z.Q. (2002). Innate and adaptive immunity in the pathogenesis of atherosclerosis. Circ Res *91*, 281-291.

Hansson, G.K., Robertson, A.K., and Soderberg-Naucler, C. (2006). Inflammation and atherosclerosis. Annu Rev Pathol *1*, 297-329.

Heeschen, C., Dimmeler, S., Hamm, C.W., Fichtlscherer, S., Boersma, E., Simoons, M.L., and Zeiher, A.M. (2003). Serum level of the antiinflammatory cytokine interleukin-10 is an important prognostic determinant in patients with acute coronary syndromes. Circulation *107*, 2109-2114.

Holven, K.B., Halvorsen, B., Bjerkeli, V., Damas, J.K., Retterstol, K., Morkrid, L., Ose, L., Aukrust, P., and Nenseter, M.S. (2006). Impaired inhibitory effect of interleukin-10 on the balance between matrix metalloproteinase-9 and its inhibitor in mononuclear cells from hyperhomocysteinemic subjects. Stroke *37*, 1731-1736.

Hsieh, C.S., Macatonia, S.E., Tripp, C.S., Wolf, S.F., O'Garra, A., and Murphy, K.M. (1993). Development of TH1 CD4+ T cells through IL-12 produced by Listeria-induced macrophages. Science *260*, 547-549.

Hurt-Camejo, E., Paredes, S., Masana, L., Camejo, G., Sartipy, P., Rosengren, B., Pedreno, J., Vallve, J.C., Benito, P., and Wiklund, O. (2001). Elevated levels of small, low-density lipoprotein with high affinity for arterial matrix components in patients with rheumatoid arthritis: possible contribution of phospholipase A2 to this atherogenic profile. Arthritis Rheum *44*, 2761-2767.

Isner, J.M., Kearney, M., Bortman, S., and Passeri, J. (1995). Apoptosis in human atherosclerosis and restenosis. Circulation *91*, 2703-2711.

Ito, T., and Ikeda, U. (2003). Inflammatory cytokines and cardiovascular disease. Curr Drug Targets Inflamm Allergy *2*, 257-265.

Jonsson, S.W., Backman, C., Johnson, O., Karp, K., Lundstrom, E., Sundqvist, K.G., and Dahlqvist, S.R. (2001). Increased prevalence of atherosclerosis in patients with medium term rheumatoid arthritis. J Rheumatol *28*, 2597-2602.

Kai, H., Ikeda, H., Yasukawa, H., Kai, M., Seki, Y., Kuwahara, F., Ueno, T., Sugi, K., and Imaizumi, T. (1998). Peripheral blood levels of matrix metalloproteases-2 and -9 are elevated in patients with acute coronary syndromes. J Am Coll Cardiol *32*, 368-372.

Kamimura, M., Viedt, C., Dalpke, A., Rosenfeld, M.E., Mackman, N., Cohen, D.M., Blessing, E., Preusch, M., Weber, C.M., Kreuzer, J., *et al.* (2005). Interleukin-10 suppresses tissue factor expression in lipopolysaccharide-stimulated macrophages via inhibition of Egr-1 and a serum response element/MEK-ERK1/2 pathway. Circ Res *97*, 305-313.

Kelly, J.A., Griffin, M.E., Fava, R.A., Wood, S.G., Bessette, K.A., Miller, E.R., Huber, S.A., Binder, C.J., Witztum, J.L., and Morganelli, P.M. (2010). Inhibition of arterial lesion progression in CD16-deficient mice: evidence for altered immunity and the role of IL-10. Cardiovasc Res *85*, 224-231.

Kennedy, M.A., Barrera, G.C., Nakamura, K., Baldan, A., Tarr, P., Fishbein, M.C., Frank, J., Francone, O.L., and Edwards, P.A. (2005). ABCG1 has a critical role in mediating cholesterol efflux to HDL and preventing cellular lipid accumulation. Cell Metab *1*, 121-131.

Khallou-Laschet, J., Varthaman, A., Fornasa, G., Compain, C., Gaston, A.T., Clement, M., Dussiot, M., Levillain, O., Graff-Dubois, S., Nicoletti, A., *et al.* Macrophage plasticity in experimental atherosclerosis. PLoS One *5*, e8852.

Kishore, R., Tebo, J.M., Kolosov, M., and Hamilton, T.A. (1999). Cutting edge: clustered AU-rich elements are the target of IL-10-mediated mRNA destabilization in mouse macrophages. J Immunol *162*, 2457-2461.

Kleemann, R., Zadelaar, S., and Kooistra, T. (2008). Cytokines and atherosclerosis: a comprehensive review of studies in mice. Cardiovasc Res *79*, 360-376.

Kockx, M.M., Muhring, J., Knaapen, M.W., and de Meyer, G.R. (1998). RNA synthesis and splicing interferes with DNA in situ end labeling techniques used to detect apoptosis. Am J Pathol *152*, 885-888.

Lahoute, C., Herbin, O., Mallat, Z., and Tedgui, A. (2011). Adaptive immunity in atherosclerosis: mechanisms and future therapeutic targets. Nat Rev Cardiol *8*, 348-358.

Laurat, E., Poirier, B., Tupin, E., Caligiuri, G., Hansson, G.K., Bariety, J., and Nicoletti, A. (2001). In vivo downregulation of T helper cell 1 immune responses reduces atherogenesis in apolipoprotein E-knockout mice. Circulation *104*, 197-202.

Lee, T.S., Yen, H.C., Pan, C.C., and Chau, L.Y. (1999). The role of interleukin 12 in the development of atherosclerosis in ApoE-deficient mice. Arterioscler Thromb Vasc Biol *19*, 734-742.

Li, Y., Zhang, Y., Dorweiler, B., Cui, D., Wang, T., Woo, C.W., Brunkan, C.S., Wolberger, C., Imai, S., and Tabas, I. (2008). Extracellular Nampt promotes macrophage survival via a nonenzymatic interleukin-6/STAT3 signaling mechanism. J Biol Chem *283*, 34833-34843.

Liao, H.S., Kodama, T., and Geng, Y.J. (2000). Expression of class A scavenger receptor inhibits apoptosis of macrophages triggered by oxidized low density lipoprotein and oxysterol. Arterioscler Thromb Vasc Biol *20*, 1968-1975.

Libby, P. (1995). Molecular bases of the acute coronary syndromes. Circulation *91*, 2844-2850.

Libby, P., Ridker, P.M., and Hansson, G.K. (2011). Progress and challenges in translating the biology of atherosclerosis. Nature *473*, 317-325.

Little, P.J., Chait, A., and Bobik, A. (2011). Cellular and cytokine-based inflammatory processes as novel therapeutic targets for the prevention and treatment of atherosclerosis. Pharmacol Ther *131*, 255-268.

Liu, Y., Li, D., Chen, J., Xie, J., Bandyopadhyay, S., Zhang, D., Nemarkommula, A.R., Liu, H., Mehta, J.L., and Hermonat, P.L. (2006). Inhibition of atherogenesis in LDLR knockout mice by systemic delivery of adeno-associated virus type 2-hIL-10. Atherosclerosis *188*, 19-27.

Liuzzo, G., Goronzy, J.J., Yang, H., Kopecky, S.L., Holmes, D.R., Frye, R.L., and Weyand, C.M. (2000). Monoclonal T-cell proliferation and plaque instability in acute coronary syndromes. Circulation *101*, 2883-2888.

Luoma, J.S., Stralin, P., Marklund, S.L., Hiltunen, T.P., Sarkioja, T., and Yla-Herttuala, S. (1998). Expression of extracellular SOD and iNOS in macrophages and smooth muscle cells in human and rabbit atherosclerotic lesions: colocalization with epitopes characteristic of oxidized LDL and peroxynitrite-modified proteins. Arterioscler Thromb Vasc Biol *18*, 157-167.

Lusis, A.J. (2000). Atherosclerosis. Nature *407*, 233-241.

Mallat, Z., Ait-Oufella, H., and Tedgui, A. (2005). Regulatory T cell responses: potential role in the control of atherosclerosis. Curr Opin Lipidol *16*, 518-524.

Mallat, Z., Besnard, S., Duriez, M., Deleuze, V., Emmanuel, F., Bureau, M.F., Soubrier, F., Esposito, B., Duez, H., Fievet, C., *et al.* (1999a). Protective role of interleukin-10 in atherosclerosis. Circ Res *85*, e17-24.

Mallat, Z., Gojova, A., Brun, V., Esposito, B., Fournier, N., Cottrez, F., Tedgui, A., and Groux, H. (2003). Induction of a regulatory T cell type 1 response reduces the development of atherosclerosis in apolipoprotein E-knockout mice. Circulation *108*, 1232-1237.

Mallat, Z., Heymes, C., Ohan, J., Faggin, E., Leseche, G., and Tedgui, A. (1999b). Expression of interleukin-10 in advanced human atherosclerotic plaques: relation to inducible nitric oxide synthase expression and cell death. Arterioscler Thromb Vasc Biol *19*, 611-616.

Mallat, Z., and Tedgui, A. (2004). Immunomodulation to combat atherosclerosis: the potential role of immune regulatory cells. Expert Opin Biol Ther *4*, 1387-1393.

Mantovani, A., Sica, A., and Locati, M. (2005). Macrophage polarization comes of age. Immunity *23*, 344-346.

Marleau, S., Harb, D., Bujold, K., Avallone, R., Iken, K., Wang, Y., Demers, A., Sirois, M.G., Febbraio, M., Silverstein, R.L., *et al.* (2005). EP 80317, a ligand of the CD36 scavenger receptor, protects apolipoprotein E-deficient mice from developing atherosclerotic lesions. FASEB J *19*, 1869-1871.

Martinez, F.O., Helming, L., and Gordon, S. (2009). Alternative activation of macrophages: an immunologic functional perspective. Annu Rev Immunol *27*, 451-483.

Martinez, F.O., Sica, A., Mantovani, A., and Locati, M. (2008). Macrophage activation and polarization. Front Biosci *13*, 453-461.

Maskrey, B.H., Megson, I.L., Whitfield, P.D., and Rossi, A.G. (2011). Mechanisms of resolution of inflammation: a focus on cardiovascular disease. Arterioscler Thromb Vasc Biol *31*, 1001-1006.

Minor, R.L., Jr., Myers, P.R., Guerra, R., Jr., Bates, J.N., and Harrison, D.G. (1990). Diet-induced atherosclerosis increases the release of nitrogen oxides from rabbit aorta. J Clin Invest *86*, 2109-2116.

Montoya, D., Cruz, D., Teles, R.M., Lee, D.J., Ochoa, M.T., Krutzik, S.R., Chun, R., Schenk, M., Zhang, X., Ferguson, B.G., *et al.* (2009). Divergence of macrophage phagocytic and antimicrobial programs in leprosy. Cell Host Microbe *6*, 343-353.

Moore, K.J., Kunjathoor, V.V., Koehn, S.L., Manning, J.J., Tseng, A.A., Silver, J.M., McKee, M., and Freeman, M.W. (2005). Loss of receptor-mediated lipid uptake via scavenger receptor A or CD36 pathways does not ameliorate atherosclerosis in hyperlipidemic mice. J Clin Invest *115*, 2192-2201.

Moore, K.J., and Tabas, I. (2011). Macrophages in the pathogenesis of atherosclerosis. Cell *145*, 341-355.

Moore, K.W., de Waal Malefyt, R., Coffman, R.L., and O'Garra, A. (2001). Interleukin-10 and the interleukin-10 receptor. Annu Rev Immunol *19*, 683-765.

Mor, A., Planer, D., Luboshits, G., Afek, A., Metzger, S., Chajek-Shaul, T., Keren, G., and George, J. (2007). Role of naturally occurring CD4+ CD25+ regulatory T cells in experimental atherosclerosis. Arterioscler Thromb Vasc Biol *27*, 893-900.

Moubayed, S.P., Heinonen, T.M., and Tardif, J.C. (2007). Anti-inflammatory drugs and atherosclerosis. Curr Opin Lipidol *18*, 638-644.

Nagy, L., Tontonoz, P., Alvarez, J.G., Chen, H., and Evans, R.M. (1998). Oxidized LDL regulates macrophage gene expression through ligand activation of PPARgamma. Cell *93*, 229-240.

Namiki, M., Kawashima, S., Yamashita, T., Ozaki, M., Sakoda, T., Inoue, N., Hirata, K., Morishita, R., Kaneda, Y., and Yokoyama, M. (2004). Intramuscular gene transfer of interleukin-10 cDNA reduces atherosclerosis in apolipoprotein E-knockout mice. Atherosclerosis *172*, 21-29.

Narverud, I., Ueland, T., Nenseter, M.S., Retterstol, K., Telle-Hansen, V.H., Halvorsen, B., Ose, L., Aukrust, P., and Holven, K.B. (2011). Children with familial hypercholesterolemia are characterized by an inflammatory imbalance between the tumor necrosis factor alpha system and interleukin-10. Atherosclerosis *214*, 163-168.

Nishihira, K., Imamura, T., Yamashita, A., Hatakeyama, K., Shibata, Y., Nagatomo, Y., Date, H., Kita, T., Eto, T., and Asada, Y. (2006). Increased expression of interleukin-10 in unstable plaque obtained by directional coronary atherectomy. Eur Heart J *27*, 1685-1689.

Noel, W., Raes, G., Hassanzadeh Ghassabeh, G., De Baetselier, P., and Beschin, A. (2004). Alternatively activated macrophages during parasite infections. Trends Parasitol *20*, 126-133.

Pajkrt, D., van der Poll, T., Levi, M., Cutler, D.L., Affrime, M.B., van den Ende, A., ten Cate, J.W., and van Deventer, S.J. (1997). Interleukin-10 inhibits activation of coagulation and fibrinolysis during human endotoxemia. Blood *89*, 2701-2705.

Pasqui, A.L., Di Renzo, M., Bova, G., Maffei, S., Pompella, G., Auteri, A., and Puccetti, L. (2006). Pro-inflammatory/anti-inflammatory cytokine imbalance in acute coronary syndromes. Clin Exp Med *6*, 38-44.

Pinderski, L.J., Fischbein, M.P., Subbanagounder, G., Fishbein, M.C., Kubo, N., Cheroutre, H., Curtiss, L.K., Berliner, J.A., and Boisvert, W.A. (2002). Overexpression of interleukin-10 by activated T lymphocytes inhibits atherosclerosis in LDL receptor-deficient Mice by altering lymphocyte and macrophage phenotypes. Circ Res *90*, 1064-1071.

Pinderski Oslund, L.J., Hedrick, C.C., Olvera, T., Hagenbaugh, A., Territo, M., Berliner, J.A., and Fyfe, A.I. (1999). Interleukin-10 blocks atherosclerotic events in vitro and in vivo. Arterioscler Thromb Vasc Biol *19*, 2847-2853.

Ramani, M., Ollivier, V., Khechai, F., Vu, T., Ternisien, C., Bridey, F., and de Prost, D. (1993). Interleukin-10 inhibits endotoxin-induced tissue factor mRNA production by human monocytes. FEBS Lett *334*, 114-116.

Ricote, M., Li, A.C., Willson, T.M., Kelly, C.J., and Glass, C.K. (1998). The peroxisome proliferator-activated receptor-gamma is a negative regulator of macrophage activation. Nature *391*, 79-82.

Ross, R. (1999). Atherosclerosis--an inflammatory disease. N Engl J Med *340*, 115-126.

Rubic, T., and Lorenz, R.L. (2006). Downregulated CD36 and oxLDL uptake and stimulated ABCA1/G1 and cholesterol efflux as anti-atherosclerotic mechanisms of interleukin-10. Cardiovasc Res *69*, 527-535.

Saren, P., Welgus, H.G., and Kovanen, P.T. (1996). TNF-alpha and IL-1beta selectively induce expression of 92-kDa gelatinase by human macrophages. J Immunol *157*, 4159-4165.

Seder, R.A., Gazzinelli, R., Sher, A., and Paul, W.E. (1993). Interleukin 12 acts directly on CD4+ T cells to enhance priming for interferon gamma production and diminishes interleukin 4 inhibition of such priming. Proc Natl Acad Sci U S A *90*, 10188-10192.

Seyrek, N., Karayaylali, I., Balal, M., Paydas, S., Aikimbaev, K., Cetiner, S., and Seydaoglu, G. (2005). Is there any relationship between serum levels of interleukin-10 and atherosclerosis in hemodialysis patients? Scand J Urol Nephrol *39*, 405-409.

Sieling, P.A., Wang, X.H., Gately, M.K., Oliveros, J.L., McHugh, T., Barnes, P.F., Wolf, S.F., Golkar, L., Yamamura, M., Yogi, Y., *et al.* (1994). IL-12 regulates T helper type 1 cytokine responses in human infectious disease. J Immunol *153*, 3639-3647.

Singh, U., Devaraj, S., Dasu, M.R., Ciobanu, D., Reusch, J., and Jialal, I. (2006). C-reactive protein decreases interleukin-10 secretion in activated human monocyte-derived macrophages via inhibition of cyclic AMP production. Arterioscler Thromb Vasc Biol *26*, 2469-2475.

Smith, E., Prasad, K.M., Butcher, M., Dobrian, A., Kolls, J.K., Ley, K., and Galkina, E. (2010). Blockade of interleukin-17A results in reduced atherosclerosis in apolipoprotein E-deficient mice. Circulation *121*, 1746-1755.

Staels, B. (2005). PPARgamma and atherosclerosis. Curr Med Res Opin *21 Suppl 1*, S13-20.

Tabas, I. (2010). Macrophage death and defective inflammation resolution in atherosclerosis. Nat Rev Immunol *10*, 36-46.

Taleb, S., Romain, M., Ramkhelawon, B., Uyttenhove, C., Pasterkamp, G., Herbin, O., Esposito, B., Perez, N., Yasukawa, H., Van Snick, J., *et al.* (2009). Loss of SOCS3 expression in T cells reveals a regulatory role for interleukin-17 in atherosclerosis. J Exp Med *206*, 2067-2077.

Taleb, S., Tedgui, A., and Mallat, Z. (2010). Adaptive T cell immune responses and atherogenesis. Curr Opin Pharmacol *10*, 197-202.

Tall, A.R., Yvan-Charvet, L., Terasaka, N., Pagler, T., and Wang, N. (2008). HDL, ABC transporters, and cholesterol efflux: implications for the treatment of atherosclerosis. Cell Metab *7*, 365-375.

Tedgui, A., and Mallat, Z. (2006). Cytokines in atherosclerosis: pathogenic and regulatory pathways. Physiol Rev *86*, 515-581.

Terkeltaub, R.A. (1999). IL-10: An "immunologic scalpel" for atherosclerosis? Arterioscler Thromb Vasc Biol *19*, 2823-2825.

Teupser, D., Stein, O., Burkhardt, R., Nebendahl, K., Stein, Y., and Thiery, J. (1999). Scavenger receptor activity is increased in macrophages from rabbits with low atherosclerotic response: studies in normocholesterolemic high and low atherosclerotic response rabbits. Arterioscler Thromb Vasc Biol *19*, 1299-1305.

Trompet, S., Pons, D., AJ, D.E.C., Slagboom, P., Shepherd, J., Blauw, G.J., Murphy, M.B., Cobbe, S.M., Bollen, E.L., Buckley, B.M., *et al.* (2007). Genetic variation in the interleukin-10 gene promoter and risk of coronary and cerebrovascular events: the PROSPER study. Ann N Y Acad Sci *1100*, 189-198.

Tziakas, D.N., Chalikias, G.K., Kaski, J.C., Kekes, A., Hatzinikolaou, E.I., Stakos, D.A., Tentes, I.K., Kortsaris, A.X., and Hatseras, D.I. (2007). Inflammatory and anti-inflammatory variable clusters and risk prediction in acute coronary syndrome patients: a factor analysis approach. Atherosclerosis *193*, 196-203.

Uyemura, K., Demer, L.L., Castle, S.C., Jullien, D., Berliner, J.A., Gately, M.K., Warrier, R.R., Pham, N., Fogelman, A.M., and Modlin, R.L. (1996). Cross-regulatory roles of interleukin (IL)-12 and IL-10 in atherosclerosis. J Clin Invest *97*, 2130-2138.

van der Poll, T., Jansen, J., Levi, M., ten Cate, H., ten Cate, J.W., and van Deventer, S.J. (1994). Regulation of interleukin 10 release by tumor necrosis factor in humans and chimpanzees. J Exp Med *180*, 1985-1988.

Van Eck, M., De Winther, M.P., Herijgers, N., Havekes, L.M., Hofker, M.H., Groot, P.H., and Van Berkel, T.J. (2000). Effect of human scavenger receptor class A overexpression in bone marrow-derived cells on cholesterol levels and atherosclerosis in ApoE-deficient mice. Arterioscler Thromb Vasc Biol *20*, 2600-2606.

van Es, T., van Puijvelde, G.H., Ramos, O.H., Segers, F.M., Joosten, L.A., van den Berg, W.B., Michon, I.M., de Vos, P., van Berkel, T.J., and Kuiper, J. (2009). Attenuated atherosclerosis upon IL-17R signaling disruption in LDLr deficient mice. Biochem Biophys Res Commun *388*, 261-265.

van Tits, L.J., Stienstra, R., van Lent, P.L., Netea, M.G., Joosten, L.A., and Stalenhoef, A.F. (2011). Oxidized LDL enhances pro-inflammatory responses of alternatively activated M2 macrophages: a crucial role for Kruppel-like factor 2. Atherosclerosis *214*, 345-349.

Von Der Thusen, J.H., Kuiper, J., Fekkes, M.L., De Vos, P., Van Berkel, T.J., and Biessen, E.A. (2001). Attenuation of atherogenesis by systemic and local adenovirus-mediated gene transfer of interleukin-10 in LDLr-/- mice. FASEB J *15*, 2730-2732.

Waehre, T., Halvorsen, B., Damas, J.K., Yndestad, A., Brosstad, F., Gullestad, L., Kjekshus, J., Froland, S.S., and Aukrust, P. (2002). Inflammatory imbalance between IL-10 and TNFalpha in unstable angina potential plaque stabilizing effects of IL-10. Eur J Clin Invest *32*, 803-810.

Wang, N., and Tall, A.R. (2003). Regulation and mechanisms of ATP-binding cassette transporter A1-mediated cellular cholesterol efflux. Arterioscler Thromb Vasc Biol *23*, 1178-1184.

Wang, P., Wu, P., Siegel, M.I., Egan, R.W., and Billah, M.M. (1995). Interleukin (IL)-10 inhibits nuclear factor kappa B (NF kappa B) activation in human monocytes. IL-10 and IL-4 suppress cytokine synthesis by different mechanisms. J Biol Chem *270*, 9558-9563.

Wang, X., Collins, H.L., Ranalletta, M., Fuki, I.V., Billheimer, J.T., Rothblat, G.H., Tall, A.R., and Rader, D.J. (2007). Macrophage ABCA1 and ABCG1, but not SR-BI, promote macrophage reverse cholesterol transport in vivo. J Clin Invest *117*, 2216-2224.

Weber, C., Zernecke, A., and Libby, P. (2008). The multifaceted contributions of leukocyte subsets to atherosclerosis: lessons from mouse models. Nat Rev Immunol *8*, 802-815.

Whitman, S.C., Rateri, D.L., Szilvassy, S.J., Cornicelli, J.A., and Daugherty, A. (2002). Macrophage-specific expression of class A scavenger receptors in LDL receptor(-/-) mice decreases atherosclerosis and changes spleen morphology. J Lipid Res *43*, 1201-1208.

Witztum, J.L., and Steinberg, D. (2001). The oxidative modification hypothesis of atherosclerosis: does it hold for humans? Trends Cardiovasc Med *11*, 93-102.

Woollard, K.J., and Geissmann, F. (2010). Monocytes in atherosclerosis: subsets and functions. Nat Rev Cardiol *7*, 77-86.

Woszczek, G., Chen, L.Y., Nagineni, S., and Shelhamer, J.H. (2008). IL-10 inhibits cysteinyl leukotriene-induced activation of human monocytes and monocyte-derived dendritic cells. J Immunol *180*, 7597-7603.

Wynn, T.A. (2004). Fibrotic disease and the T(H)1/T(H)2 paradigm. Nat Rev Immunol *4*, 583-594.

Ye, D., Lammers, B., Zhao, Y., Meurs, I., Van Berkel, T.J., and Van Eck, M. (2011). ATP-binding cassette transporters A1 and G1, HDL metabolism, cholesterol efflux, and inflammation: important targets for the treatment of atherosclerosis. Curr Drug Targets *12*, 647-660.

Yoshioka, T., Okada, T., Maeda, Y., Ikeda, U., Shimpo, M., Nomoto, T., Takeuchi, K., Nonaka-Sarukawa, M., Ito, T., Takahashi, M., *et al.* (2004). Adeno-associated virus vector-mediated interleukin-10 gene transfer inhibits atherosclerosis in apolipoprotein E-deficient mice. Gene Ther *11*, 1772-1779.

Yvan-Charvet, L., Ranalletta, M., Wang, N., Han, S., Terasaka, N., Li, R., Welch, C., and Tall, A.R. (2007). Combined deficiency of ABCA1 and ABCG1 promotes foam cell accumulation and accelerates atherosclerosis in mice. J Clin Invest *117*, 3900-3908.

Zhao, Y., Van Berkel, T.J., and Van Eck, M. (2010). Relative roles of various efflux pathways in net cholesterol efflux from macrophage foam cells in atherosclerotic lesions. Curr Opin Lipidol *21*, 441-453.

Zhou, X., Paulsson, G., Stemme, S., and Hansson, G.K. (1998). Hypercholesterolemia is associated with a T helper (Th) 1/Th2 switch of the autoimmune response in atherosclerotic apo E-knockout mice. J Clin Invest *101*, 1717-1725.

Zimmerman, M.A., Reznikov, L.L., Raeburn, C.D., and Selzman, C.H. (2004). Interleukin-10 attenuates the response to vascular injury. J Surg Res *121*, 206-213.

# 18

# The 18 kDa Translocator Protein as a Potential Participant in Atherosclerosis

Jasmina Dimitrova-Shumkovska[1], Leo Veenman[2] and Moshe Gavish[2]
*[1]Institute of Biology, Department of Experimental Biochemistry and Physiology, Faculty of Natural Sciences and Mathematics, Ss. Cyril and Methodius University, Skopje,*
*[2]Rappaport Family Institute for Research in the Medical Sciences, Technion-Israel Institute of Technology, Department of Molecular Pharmacology, Haifa,*
*[1]Republic of Macedonia*
*[2]Israel*

## 1. Introduction

### 1.1 Inflammation in atherosclerosis

Inflammation is a process integral to atherosclerosis, a concept that dates back from the studies by Ross (1999). Since then, circulating markers have been established as predictive to atherosclerosis and its clinical events (Hansson et al., 2005; Packard & Libby, 2008). Accumulated subendothelial lipid, particularly if oxidized, exacerbates the local inflammatory reaction and maintains activation of the overlying endothelium (Tiwari et al., 2008). Atheroma formation involves expression of selectins and adhesion molecules and also expression of chemokines, in particular monocyte chemoatractant proteins-1 (MCP-1). Chemokines are proinflammatory cytokines that function in leukocyte chemoattraction and activation. Atheroma prone mice lacking MCP-1 develop smaller atherosclerotic lesions than those expressing MCP-1. Once captured at the vascular wall, inflammatory cells migrate into the subendothelial space where, under the influence of local chemokines, they become activated. There the monocytes mature into macrophages and express the necessary scavenger receptors to ingest modified lipids and become macrophage foamy cells. The predominant role of the macrophages in atherosclerosis is to ingest and dispose of atherogenic lipids. However, activated macrophages and T cells also express a variety of proinflammatory cytokines and growth factors that may contribute to atherosclerotic plaque formation. The progression of an atherosclerotic plaque is best understood in terms of dynamic interaction between a subendothelial inflammatory stimulus and the local reactive "wound healing" response of surrounding vascular smooth muscle cells (VSMCs) (Clarke & Bennett, 2006).
Inflammation produces reactive oxygen species (ROS) as a by-product, and antioxidant therapeutic strategies may have proved disappointing possibly because oxidative events are a consequence, rather than a cause of atherosclerosis. In this scenario, ROS scavenging would have little impact on the disease process. This notion is consistent with the observation that the relationship between the risk factors of atherosclerosis and inflammation is tight, in that all of the established cardiovascular disease risk factors are predictive of circulating inflammation markers. Also, modification of atherosclerotic risk factors by lipid lowering therapies, cessation of smoking, weight loss, and improved glucose control reduces circulating markers

of inflammation. These and other findings suggest that inflammation is a primary process and oxidative stress is only secondary one in relation to atherosclerosis (Rodriguez-Moran et al., 2003). Nevertheless, traditional anti-inflammatory therapies do not add to the recovery process, moreover, they may even slightly exacerbate atherosclerotic events (Libby et al., 2011).

### 1.2 Therapeutic strategies in atherosclerosis

The presence and biological consequences of DNA damage in atherosclerosis imply that both prevention and reversal of damage are therapeutic aims. *In vitro,* antioxidants can ameliorate ROS-induced DNA damage, even though antioxidant trials in humans have been disappointing so far. Whereas high dietary intake of vitamin E and C is associated with reduced risk of cardiovascular disease (CVD), well powered clinical trials in atherosclerosis-related CVD have indicated that supplements with vitamin C or vitamin E alone do not provide sufficient benefit, in comparison to, for example, statins (Kunitomo et al., 2009). Specific antioxidants scavenge or metabolize some, but not all of the relevant oxidized species. For example, radical scavengers will limit lipid peroxidation, but will have no effects on protein modification by peroxinitrite ($ONOO^-$), cell signalling by $H_2O_2$, or HOCl mediated oxidation reaction. Thus, whenever a physiological process goes unchecked in case of disease, strategies that rely simply on scavenging the offending species must be employed with extreme caution (Stocker and Keaney, 2005).

In contrast, cholesterol lowering by diet is associated with a reduction in DNA damage, at least in animal models (Singh et al., 2009). Drugs that have been proven to alter plaque progression have also been shown to alter vascular oxidative stress. In particular, 3-hydroxy-3-methylglutaryl coenzyme A (HMGCoA ) reductase inhibitors (Statins) reduce NAD(P)H oxidase activation and superoxide production *in vitro,* in part because of their capability to inhibit membrane translocation (and thus activity) of the small GTP-binding protein Rac-1, which is a regulatory component of vascular NAD(P)H oxidase activation (Cosotpoulos et al., 2008). Another trial, which investigated the use of niacin combined with a prostaglandin D2 receptor antagonist, intended to reduce cutaneous flushing, and has shown durability of benefit (Insull, 2009; Libby et al., 2011). Namely, together with lipid lowering therapy acute clinical benefits were cumulative, but tolerability issues has limited its use. Understanding the non-lipid associated events in atherogenesis raises the prospect of developing drugs targeted at specific events in its pathogenesis which might act synergistically with lipid lowering drugs to enhance plaque stability (Singh et al., 2009).

### 1.3 Translocator Protein 18 kDa (TSPO) as a potential participant in atherosclerosis

It was shown previously that the 18 kDa translocator protein (TSPO) is present throughout the cardiovascular system and may be involved in cardiovascular disorders such as ischemia. At cellular levels TSPO is present in virtually all of the cells of the cardiovascular system, where they appear to take part in responses to various challenges that an organism and its cardiovascular system face (Veenman & Gavish, 2006), including atherosclerosis and accompanying symptoms (Onyimba et al., 2011; Bird et al., 2010; Dimitrova-Shumkovska et al., 2010a,b,c).

#### 1.3.1 TSPO - Structure and localization

TSPO can be found in various tissues (Gavish et al., 1992, 1999). The TSPO is also known as peripheral type benzodiazepine receptor (PBR), since it is capable of binding benzodiazepines and is found in most if not all peripheral tissues (Veenman et al., 2007).

Mitochondrial membranes form the primary location for TSPO (Anholt et al., 1985). The present name of the TSPO, translocator protein, was chosen because of the TSPO's capability to transport molecules over the outer the mitochondrial membrane (Papadopoulos et al., 2006). For example, TSPO is known to transport cholesterol over the outer the mitochondrial membrane. At the mitochondria, TSPO are closely associated with the 32 kDa voltage-dependent anion channel (VDAC) and the 30-kDa adenine nucleotide translocator (ANT) ( Mc Enery et al., 1992; Veenman et al., 2007; **Figure 1**). VDAC and ANT are considered to form the core components of the mitochondrial permeability transition pore (mPTP) (Galiegue et al., 2003). The ratio of TSPO to VDAC and ANT appears to be tissue- and treatment-dependent (Golani et al., 2001; Veenman et al., 2002). The mitochondrial location of the TSPO is interesting in relation to cardiovascular diseases, as it is well known that mitochondria are a main source of cellular ROS (Lenaz, 1998). Furthermore, several studies have shown that the TSPO appears to be a participant in ROS generation at mitochondrial levels (Veenman et al., 2008,2010a; Zeno et al., 2009; Choi et al., 2011). As discussed above, ROS may play a role in cardiovascular diseases.

Furthermore, by its interactions with the VDAC and the ANT, the TSPO is able to modulate the flow of electrolytes over the outer and inner mitochondrial membranes and participate in the collapse of the mitochondrial membrane potential (Kugler et al., 2008; Zeno et al., 2009). In this context, TSPO is a participant in the initiation of mitochondrial apoptosis cascade, including release of cytochrome c from the mitochondrial membrane potential (Levin et al., 2005; Kugler et al., 2008; Veenman et al., 2010). It has been suggested that the role of TSPO in importing proteins and cholesterol into the mitochondria may partake in mitochondrial membrane biogenesis, required for cell growth and proliferation (Papadopoulos et al., 2006; Veenman et al., 2007). Even though many functions were attributed to the TSPO, its primary roles are still discussed and the mechanisms whereby TSPO takes part in many of these functions still need further clarification (Veenman & Gavish, 2006; Veenman et al., 2010b). Because TSPO appear to be involved in a large variety of physical diseases, mental disorders and responses to stress, clinical benefit may be attainable by increasing knowledge regarding the TSPO. Including its involvement in cardiovascular disorders.

TSPO are found throughout the animal kingdom, including insects, mollusks, pisces, amphibians, aves and mammals (Peterson et al., 1988; Veenman et al., 2007), yet have not been found in reptiles as to date (Bolger et al., 1986). Widely expressed throughout the body, TSPO exhibit different patterns of tissue specific expression (Golani et al., 2001; Veenman et al., 2002). *In vivo* studies showed the rank order of TSPO binding density in rats to be adrenal >> kidney ~ heart ~ testis ~ ovary >> liver ~ brain (Awad & Gavish, 1987; Gavish et al., 1999). In humans and dogs, the heart appears to be one of the organs with high TSPO density (Veenman & Gavish, 2006).

The rat TSPO protein consists of 169 amino-acids, is highly hydrophobic, and is rich in tryptophan. TSPO appears to constitute a five α-helical transmembrane structure that stretches the outer mitochondrial membrane. The human homologous TSPO also consists of 169 amino-acids, including two cysteine residues that may allow for S-nitrosylation of the protein. (Gavish et al., 1999; Babbage, A. Direct Submission, GenBank: CAB55884.1, 2009). The TSPO gene is conserved from prokaryotes to plants and animals, including humans and appears to have the hallmarks of a typical housekeeping gene, suggesting that this gene's product has a basic cellular function (Gavish et al., 1999).

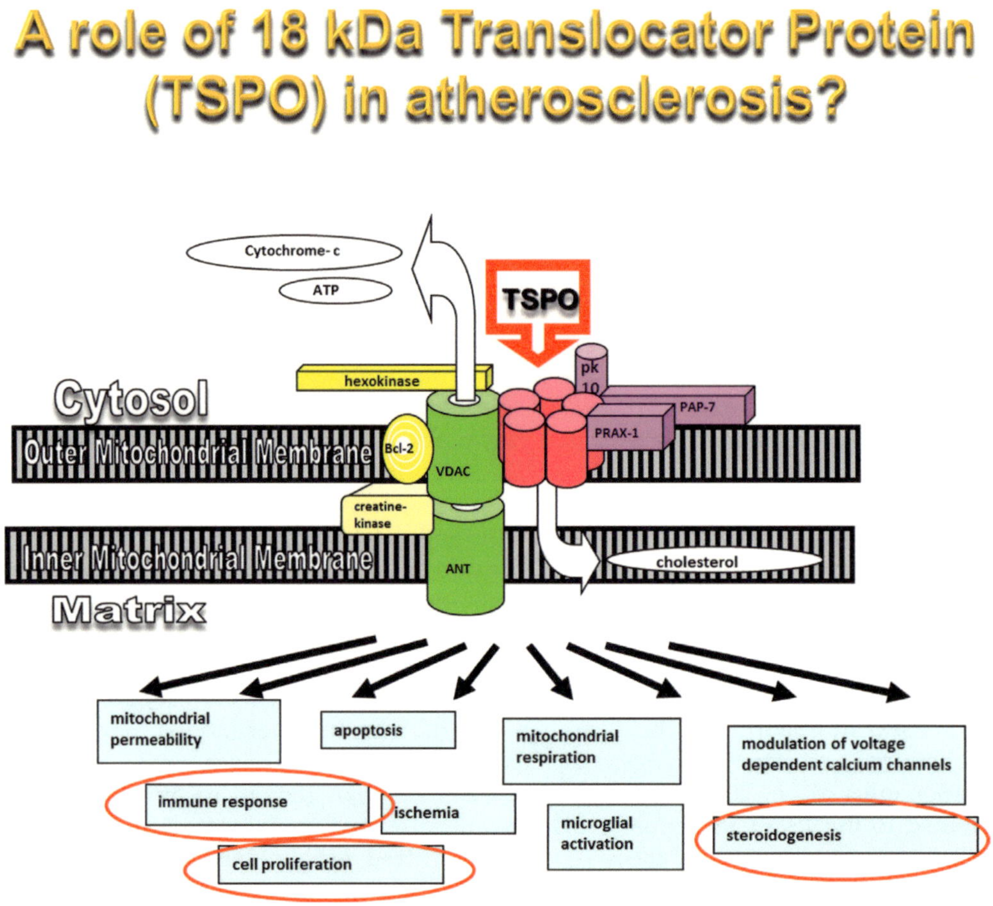


Fig. 1. TSPO structure, localization and functions. TSPO molecules are often found in groups and in conjugation with VDAC and ANT. As indicated in the figure, pk10, PRAX-1, and PAP7 face the cytosol. Furthermore, molecules of the Bcl-2 family and creatine kinase and hexokinase can be attached to VDAC and ANT. The TSPO is involved in various functions some of which are indicated towards the bottom of the figure. The encircled functions may relate to an association of the TSPO with cardiovascular pathology. Abbreviations: ANT, adenine nucleotide transporter; ATP, adenosine triphosphate; DBI, diazepam binding inhibitor; PAP7, PBR associated protein 7; PBR, peripheral-type benzodiazepine receptor; pk10, protein of 10 kiloDalton; PLA2, phospholipase A2; PRAX-1, PBR associated protein 1; TSPO, translocator protein (18-kDa); TTN, triakontatetra-neuropeptide; VDAC, voltage dependent anion channel (Veenman et al., 2007).

Recently, TSPO has been found to occur not only in the 18 kDa form, but also as 36-, 54-, and 72 kDa TSPO polymers (Delavoie et al., 2003). This topic has arisen from the electron microscopic observation that the 18 kDa TSPO protein was organized in clusters of 2-7 molecules on Leydig cell mitochondrial membranes (Papadopoulos et al., 1997). It was also suggested that free TSPO (meaning not in complex with VDAC and ANT) may be present in mitochondrial membranes (Veenman et al., 2002; Liu et al., 2003). This claim further takes into consideration that modulation of steroidogenesis only requires a mitochondrial channel that is formed by the mitochondrial TSPO, without participation of VDAC and ANT (Papadopoulos et al., 2006). It should be noted that, apart from mitochondria, TSPO can be found in various other subcellular locations (Veenman & Gavish, 2006). Nuclear/perinuclear-located TSPO, for example, is considered to play a part in cell proliferation (Brown et al., 2000). Other studies detected TSPO binding in plasma membrane and in mature human red blood cells, which lack mitochondria (Oke et al., 1992). It has been suggested that intracellular locations of the TSPO in human lymphocytes might be correlated with its capacity to bind to various endogenous TSPO ligands at these locations, and that this capability might be related to the ratio of TSPO to VDAC and ANT in such locations (Gavish et al., 1999).

### 1.3.2 General TSPO functions

TSPO have been implicated in various functions **(Figure 1)**, including apoptosis, steroidogenesis, oxidative stress, mitochondrial respiration, modulation of voltage dependent calcium channels, effects on the immune and phagocyte host-defence response, microglial activation related to brain damage, ischemia, regulation of the mitochondrial membrane potential, inflammation, cell growth and differentiation, and cancer cell proliferation (For reviews, see: Gavish et al., 1999; Veenman & Gavish, 2006, 2011; Veenman et al., 2007, 2008, 2010b, 2011). TSPO may potentially be involved in the regulation of several major stress systems, such as the Hypothalamic-Pituitary-Adrenal (HPA) axis, the sympathetic nervous system, the renin-angiotensin axis and the neuroendocrine-immune axis (Gavish et al., 1999; Veenman and Gavish, 2000, 2006). Thus, TSPO possibly plays a role in the mediation of organisms' various adaptations to stress and anxiety disorders.

In the endocrine system, TSPO is well known to participate in steroid production and may also play a role in the host-defence response (Papadopoulos et al., 2006). The presence of TSPO in glia of the central nervous system (CNS) has suggested that they might also be involved in glial functions in the brain. In neurodegenerative disorders, including Alzheimer's disease, TSPO ligand binding density is increased in the affected brain regions. Thus, it has been suggested that TSPO in glia may play a role in neurodegenerative processes and brain damage. In animal studies, both PK 11195 and Ro5-4864 presented neuroprotective effects against brain injury, which have been suggested to involve neurosteroid activation (Veenman et al., 2002; Veenman & Gavish, 2006, 2011; Soustiel et al., 2008). Alternatively, it has been suggested that enhanced levels of TSPO in neural cells (due to damage, disease, etc.) are inductive for apoptosis. In particular, activation of the TSPO may lead to a decrease of the mitochondrial membrane potential, mitochondrial dysfunction, and subsequent release of mitochondrial cytochrome c, followed by the activation of a caspase cascade leading to apoptosis (Levin et al., 2005).

Interestingly, as ROS generation accompanies in cardiovascular diseases, it has also been shown that oxidative stress modulates TSPO structure and function (Delavoie et al., 2003). Vice versa, TSPO appears to be an essential participant in ROS generation at mitochondrial levels induced by various agents (Veenman et al., 2008, 2010a; Zeno et al., 2009; Choi et al., 2011). In addition, Carayon et al. (1996) demonstrated that Jurkat cells transfected with human TSPO cDNA exhibited increased resistance to $H_2O_2$ toxicity, suggesting a function of these sites and their ligands in protecting cells against the toxicity of ROS produced during inflammatory processes. In the liver, the TSPO was found in co-localization with a ROS scavenger, the mitochondrial manganese-dependent superoxide dismutase (SOD) (Fischer et al., 2001). At present, no conclusive model is available to incorporate the various interactions between the TSPO and ROS.

### 1.3.3 Cholesterol translocation and steroidogenesis in relation to TSPO

TSPO has been reported to take part in the translocation of cholesterol from the outer to the inner mitochondrial membrane, which is the rate-limiting step in steroidogenesis (Papadopoulos et al., 1990). The fact that TSPO is abundant in steroidogenic endocrine organs (Benavides et al., 1983; Gavish et al., 1999; Papadopoulos et al., 2006), such as the adrenal gland and male and female gonads in rats, has been the first suggestion that TSPO may play a role in steroidogenesis.

The biosynthesis of steroids in all steroidogenic tissues begins with the enzymatic conversion of the precursor cholesterol to form pregnenolone. This reaction is catalyzed by the enzyme cholesterol side-chain-cleavage (P-450scc), which is located on the matrix side of the inner mitochondrial membrane and is dependent on an electron transport system comprised of adrenodoxin and adrenodoxin reductase. Pregnenolone leaves the mitochondrion to undergo enzymatic transformation in the endoplasmic reticulum, giving rise to the final steroid products (Papadopoulos et al., 2006; Veenman et al., 2007). The rate-limiting step in this process, is the transport of cholesterol from cellular stores across the aqueous intermembrane space of the mitochondria to the inner mitochondrial membrane and P-450.

It has been suggested that TSPO and StAR (steroidogenic acute regulatory protein), the latter which is involved in the acute trophic hormone regulation of steroid synthesis, work together in the cholesterol transport into the mitochondria (Stocco & Clark, 1996). Steroids have also been shown to be able to affect TSPO ligand-binding characteristics (Veenman et al., 2007), for example, as demonstrated by a 10-day estradiol treatment of rats that resulted in a marked reduction in TSPO binding in the rat testis, and up regulation of these sites in the kidney (Gavish & Weizman, 1997). Other observations were provided by the removal of the testes, which caused a significant decrease in TSPO density in Cowper's glands and the adrenal gland, while administration of testosterone acetate prevented this castration induced TSPO depletion (Weizman et al., 1992). Furthermore, removal of the pituitary gland, which resulted in the elimination of corticotrophin (ACTH) secretion, caused a significant reduction in the adrenal TSPO density (Anholt et al., 1985). Recently, it has been shown that steroid treatment can regulate gene expression of the TSPO (Mazurika et al., 2009).

Three-dimensional models of the channel formed by the five α-helices of the TSPO indicated that it would be able to accommodate a cholesterol molecule in the space delineated by the five helices. According to these models, the inner surface of the channel formed by the TSPO molecule would present a hydrophilic but uncharged pathway, allowing amphiphilic cholesterol molecules to cross the outer mitochondrial membrane (Papadopoulos et al., 2006; Veenman et al., 2007).

TSPO ligands are reported to induce TSPO-mediated translocation of cholesterol from the outer mitochondrial membrane to the inner mitochondrial membrane (Papadopoulos et al., 1997). Moreover, PK 11195 and Ro5-4864 (the classical specific TSPO ligands) increased cholesterol transport into the mitochondria and subsequent steroid synthesis in gonadal, adrenal, brain, and liver cells (Delavoie et al., 2003). Ro5-4864 directly stimulated the release of corticotrophin releasing hormone (CRH) in rats, whereas PK 11195 directly stimulated the secretion of ACTH. In various models of induced stress in rats, the increase in CRH and ACTH was attenuated by treatment with diazepam. It was reported that the presence of the endogenous ligand DBI was vital for steroidogenesis and stimulated cholesterol transport. DBI regulated steroidogenesis activated by ACTH and luteinizing hormone via binding to TSPO, and thus controlled mitochondrial cholesterol transport (Papadopoulos et al., 1991; Brown et al., 1992).

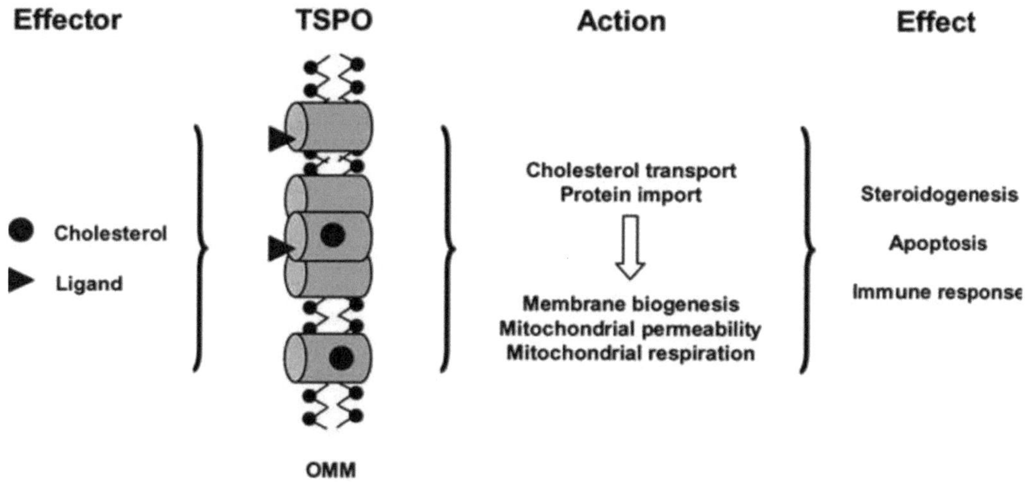


Fig. 2. Proposed model of cholesterol and ligand binding to TSPO. TSPO is found either as a monomer or polymer in the outer mitochondrial membrane. Binding of cholesterol and TSPO ligands to TSPO at this site may result in import of cholesterol or protein into the mitochondria. This may support cellular functions such as membrane biogenesis, mitochondrial permeability, and mitochondrial respiration. The final effects may include steroidogenesis, apoptosis, and immune responses. Abbreviation: OMM, outer mitochondrial membrane (Veenman et al., 2007).

The actual participation of TSPO in mitochondrial cholesterol translocation was demonstrated by disruption of the TSPO gene in Leydig cells, which resulted in the arrest of cholesterol transport into the mitochondria as well as steroid formation, while the reintroduction of TSPO by cDNA rescued steroidogenesis (Papadopoulos et al., 1997). The suggestion of TSPO involvement in steroidogenesis modulated by TSPO ligands was further supported by TSPO antisense knockdowns in MA-10 Leydig cells, which reduced steroid production (Hauet et al., 2005).

It has been proposed that TSPO polymerization modulates the function of this receptor in cholesterol transport, since polymer formation induced by ROS increased both TSPO ligand binding and cholesterol-binding capacities (Delavoie et al., 2003). The monomer binds cholesterol with high affinity but not so with TSPO ligands. The presence of cholesterol on the TSPO monomer prevents the ROS - induced polymer formation. The polymer binds TSPO ligands with high affinity and ligand binding induces rapid cholesterol binding. This process would allow a membrane that contains TSPO to import high levels of cholesterol in a time and ligand dependent manner. Apart from the significance of cholesterol transport by TSPO for steroidogenesis, it may also be relevant for membrane biogenesis and metabolic needs required for cell survival (Veenman et al., 2007). TSPO's interactions with cholesterol may be suggestive of a role of TSPO in atherosclerosis.

### 1.3.4 TSPO and responses to cardiovascular damage

In the cardiovascular lumen, TSPO are present in platelets, erythrocytes, lymphocytes, and mononuclear cells (Maeda et al., 1998). In the walls of the cardiovascular system, TSPO can be found in the endothelium, the striated cardiac muscle, the vascular smooth muscles, and the mast cells (Taniguchi et al., 1980; Veenman & Gavish, 2006). Regarding cardiovascular diseases, the TSPO has been found to be involved in ischemic processes, including oxidative stress and apoptosis (Kunduzova et al., 2004). Furthermore, TSPO may be involved in aortic damage due to diet and toxins (Dimitrova-Shumkovska et al., 2010a,b,c).

TSPO in the cardiovascular system appears to play roles in several aspects of the immune response, such as phagocytosis and the secretion of interleukin-2, interleukin-3, and immunoglobulin A (Veenman & Gavish, 2006). Mast cells have been implicated in immune responses to pathogens, in the regulation of thrombosis and inflammation, and in cardiovascular disease processes such as atherosclerosis, as well as in neoplastic conditions (Wojta et al., 2003; Marshall, 2004). Studies have shown that the benzodiazepines' inhibition of serotonin release in mast cells could reduce the blood brain permeability and influence pain levels and decrease vascular smooth muscle contractions (Veenman et al., 2006). Benzodiazepines have been found to bind to specific receptors on macrophages and to modulate in vitro their metabolic oxidative responsiveness (Lenfant et al., 1985). Since these tissues and cells possess TSPO, but not CBR, it is most likely that these benzodiazepines cause their effects via the TSPO present in these tissues and cells.

Recently, we have established that the TSPO appears to be an active participant in the generation of ROS at mitochondrial levels and maintenance of the mitochondrial membrane potential, in relation to apoptosis (Kugler et al., 2008; Zeno et al., 2009). In turn, ROS levels also affect TSPO function (Delavoie et al., 2003). As a result of this, we suggest that the TSPO may be involved in oxidative stress related to cardiovascular disorders.

### 1.3.5 TSPO ligands

A wide variety of endogenous molecules with affinity for the TSPO have been identified, including Diazepam Binding Inhibitor (DBI), which is an 11 kDa polypeptide of 86 amino acids. As its name suggests, DBI was originally shown to inhibit the binding of [$^3$H] diazepam to brain membranes and gamma aminobutyric acid (GABA) activated Cl - channel activation. DBI has the same low (μM) affinity for both the TSPO and the CBR. Other putative endogenous ligands for TSPO include the porphyrins (protoporphyrin IX, mesoporphyrin IX, deuteroporphyrin IX and haemin), which are known to modulate enzymatic activity of several enzymes and are involved with several mitochondrial proteins (Gavish et al., 1999; Zeno et al., in press). These compounds exhibit a very high (nM) affinity for TSPO, and hence are considered as putative endogenous TSPO ligands (Verma et al., 1987). Regarding synthetic ligands, the TSPO exhibits nanomolar affinity to the benzodiazepine Ro5-4864 (4'- chlorodiazepam, **Figure 3**), but low affinity to most other benzodiazepines species (Le Fur et al., 1983). Furthermore, it has been reported that isoquinolines, such as 1-(2- chlorophenyl)-N-methyl-N-(1-methyl-prop 1)-3 isoquinoline-carboxamide (PK 11195, **Figure 3**) interact specifically with TSPO (Le Fur et al., 1983; Gavish, 2006Veenman &) and that PK 11195 is currently the most widely used TSPO ligand, in part due to its high affinity for TSPO for all of the studied species (Le Fur et al., 1983; Veenman & Gavish, 2006).

PK 11195 and Ro5-4864 compete with each other in binding experiments, suggesting overlapping but not necessarily identical binding sites. It has been suggested that they interact with two different conformations or domains of the mitochondrial TSPO (Awad & Gavish, 1987). Behavioral studies have demonstrated that Ro5-4864 possesses anxiogenic and convulsant properties, whereas PK 11195 has been found to be anxiolytic and anticonvulsant (Gavish et al., 1999). Other studies have shown that Ro5-4864 and PK 11195 have identical effects, for example inhibition of apoptosis (Kugler et al., 2008). These effects are similar to, albeit less strong than TSPO knockdown, implying that these TSPO ligands block the pro-apoptotic functions of the TSPO (Levin et al., 2005; Zeno et al., 2009).

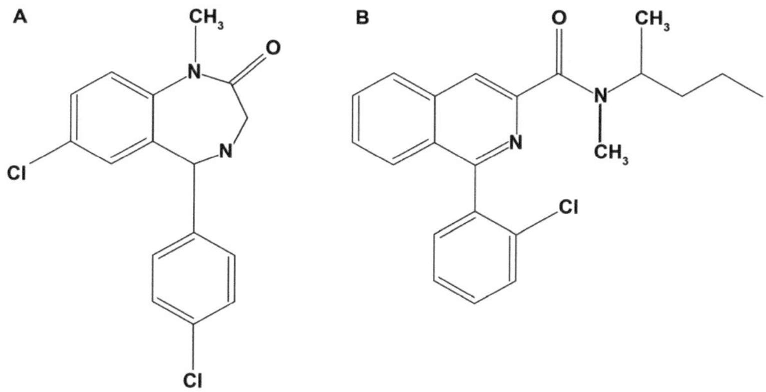


Fig. 3. Chemical structures of the two archetypical TSPO ligands: (A) the benzodiazepine, Ro5-4864; and (B) the isoquinoline carboxamide, PK 11195.

In some cases, various effects of TSPO ligands have been observed in TSPO deficient and TSPO knockdown cells (Hans et al., 2005), raising the issue of the possible presence of TSPO-independent mechanisms of action of these ligands (Falchi et al., 2007).
The effects induced by TSPO ligands have been widely investigated in steroidogenic cells (Gavish et al., 1999; Casellas et al., 2002). In addition, effects of TSPO ligands have been studied in non-steroidogenic cells, including cardiovascular tissues: 1) they were shown to modulate physiological mechanisms such as cellular respiration in heart, kidney, and liver (Moreno-Sanchez et al., 1991; Veenman & Gavish, 2006), 2) generation of ROS in neurons and HL60 human leukaemia cells (Fennell et al., 2001; Jayakumar et al., 2002), 3) anion transport in kidney (Basile et al., 1998), 4) mitochondrial permeability transition in cardiomyocytes (Chelli et al., 2001), 5) inhibition of cell proliferation in human fibroblasts (Kletsas et al., 2004), and 6) apoptosis in various cell lines (Decaudin et al., 2002; Chelli et al., 2004).
Numerous findings have suggested that TSPO ligands might act as potential therapeutic agents that may be useful for the treatment of a large spectrum of diseases. TSPO drug ligands are evaluated regarding their ability to regulate neurosteroid synthesis and brain function, to detect tumor cells *in vivo*, and to modulate apoptotic rates, with major potential therapeutic implications for cancer therapy (Galiegue et al., 2003). PK 11195 has been administrated safely to patients, and has been suggested to be included in clinical trials as a chemo sensitizing agent. In addition, alternative TSPO ligands with potential therapeutic effects are being developed in various laboratories.

## 2. TSPO binding density decreases in aorta due to atherogenic challenges

By its very nature, plaque rupture is difficult to study directly in humans. Therefore, animal models have been developed to study atherosclerosis, including plaque rupture and thrombus formation, and also how to take measures to prevent these from happening. However, all of the existing models (biological or mechanical triggering models, the Watanabe heritable hyperlipidemic (WHHL) rabbit model, the apolipoprotein E (ApoE) mouse model, and the LDL-receptor mouse model) suffer the drawback of lacking an end-stage atherosclerosis that would show plaque rupture accompanied by platelet and fibrin-rich occlusive thrombus at the rupture site (Singh et al., 2009). This is a very important limitation. There are additional disadvantages of the existing models, such as long preparatory activities, complicated manipulation, high cost of development, low yield of triggering, and high mortality, which hamper the execution of large-scale studies. Also, the study of human tissue in *in vitro* cell systems is limited by the obvious fact that these are not whole organisms, accompanied by the inherent problem of drifting phenotypes.

For the present study, regarding the potential involvement of the TSPO in atherosclerosis, we used outbred rats (*Wistar*) to study dietary factors applied by us that contribute to cardiovascular damage. We chose these outbred rats since they are atherosclerotic non - prone animals and under normal circumstances they typically do not show cardiovascular damage within the time-frame we applied. Although the use of rodents as a model may have some limitations to achieve complete understanding of the diet - disease relations in humans, it presents a unique opportunity to simultaneously explore several underlying mechanisms *in vivo* in the whole organism which is otherwise difficult to achieve with other approaches (Dorfman et al., 2003).

Classes of risk factors for cardiovascular disorders (CVD), also named "cardiovascular toxins", are presented by environmental pollutants with very well known carcinogenic effects (Iwano et al., 2006). Not only may pollutants exacerbate and accelerate CVD, risk factors associated with CVD could predispose and sensitize for pollutant toxicity. Chronic hypercholesterolemia, for instance, could significantly affect xenobiotic metabolism and disposition by either altering the expression of detoxification enzymes in liver and peripheral tissues, or by providing additional circulating nucleophylic binding sites, e.g., lysine residues of apolipoprotein and ethanolamine phospholipids (Miyata et al., 2001; Miller and Ramos, 2001). Realizing the need to study cardiovascular toxicity as a significant consequence of exposure to environmental pollutants, one of the aims of our research was to highlight the effects and cell responses due to exposure to carcinogen and air pollutant 7, 12 dimethylbenz [α]anthracene (DMBA) on hyperlipidemic rats chronically exposed on high fat high cholesterol (HFHC) diet. In previous studies we showed that HFHC diet as well as DMBA exposure caused oxidative stress in the aorta, in association with damage to this organ, as well as reduced TSPO binding density in this organ (Dimitrova-Shumkovska et al., 2010a,b,c). To further illustrate these effects, we present here data from a recent study combining HFHC diet with DMBA exposure.

To determine the effects of an HFHC diet in combination with DMBA exposure in our paradigm of cardiovascular damage, rats received a custom tailored HFHC diet (Dimitrova-Shumkovska et al., 2010a). Before application of the HFHC diet, the rats were randomized into 2 general groups: 1) control rats **(C-rats)** receiving commercial standard pellet feed for a period of 18 weeks (n = 18); 2) experimental rats **(HFHC+DMBA)** (n = 12) receiving HFHC diet for a period of 18 weeks, and then a single administration of 10 mg DMBA / 1 mL sesame oil applied by gavage), followed by an additional 4 weeks with HFHC diet. After 22 weeks in total, animals were sacrificed by exsanguination, and procedures related to TSPO binding characteristics, ROS parameters in aorta and histopathology were done, as described in detail previously (Dimitrova-Shumkovska et al., 2010 a,b,c). Specimens of aorta and plasma were collected for lipid analysis and analysis of parameters of oxidative stress. The parameters of oxidative injury that we studied included lipid peroxidation (TBARs assay described by Okhawa et al., 1989, modified by Draper and Hadley, 1990);

protein carbonylation (Levine et al., 1990, adopted by Reznick et al., 1994 and modified by Shacter, 2000), and advanced oxidized protein products (AOPP, Witko-Sarsat et al., 1996). Furthermore, anatomical observation and histopathology of aorta were performed. To determine TSPO binding characteristics in this paradigm we applied binding assays with [$^3$H]PK 11195. The effects of HFHC diet and of DMBA application by themselves were analyzed previously (Dimitrova-Shumkovska et al., 2010 a,b,c). Building on these previous studies, the present study seeks to determine whether the toxin DMBA may exacerbate the oxidative stress due to atherogenic diet.

In the endothelium of the aorta wall of the **HFHC+DMBA** rats, we observed the appearance of foamy cells (20-25% of the lumen circumference, visible among 5 animals from 8 analyzed). Early mild fibrosis, was observed in 2 of the 8 rats. All the control aortas remained negative for these changed, as described before (Dimitrova-Shumkovska et al., 2010 a, b, c). These present results indicate that combining the HFHC diet with the DMBA exposure do not cause more damage to the aorta of rats than previously found with HFHC diet alone (Dimitrova-Shumkovska et al., 2010a,b,c). These previous studies also did show that HFHC diet was more damaging to the aorta than DMBA exposure (Dimitrova-Shumkovska et al., 2010a,b,c)

Regarding protein oxidation and lipid peroxidation in the aorta (**Table 1**), in the HFHC + DMBA rats significant increases in TBARs, AOPP and PC levels could be observed, compared to vehicle control. In detail, regarding lipid peroxidation, TBARs production was significantly increased more than 2 fold (+129%, $p < 0.05$) in comparison to control (Table 1). Regarding protein oxidation, AOPP levels showed a significant more than 3 fold increase compared to control (+216%, $p < 0.001$). Protein carbonyls (PC) in the aorta showed an increase of 47% compared to control. The obtained results were similar to those of the HFHC diet only group (Dimitrova-Shumkovska et al., 2010a), but the observed effect of enhanced oxidative stress was higher than in DMBA only treated rats (Dimitrova-Shumkovska et al., 2010b). In the control tissue (kidney) such effects differences between the HFHC-DMBA and vehicle groups not observed **(data not shown)**.

| Variables / Aorta | Control | HFHC + DMBA |
|---|---|---|
| TBARs nmol/mg | 1.22 ± 0.2 (n=8) | 2.8 ± 1.4* (n=7) |
| AOPP nmol/mg | 12.5 ± 4.5 (n=8) | 39.5 ± 13.0** (n=7) |
| PC pmol/mg | 63.5 ± 24.0 (n=8) | 93.5 ± 24.1* (n=7) |

Table 1. Effects of HFHC diet combined with a DMBA exposure (HFHC + DMBA) on aorta oxidative stress parameters in rats. Mann Whitney non-parametric test, * $p < 0.05$, ** $p < 0.01$.

Binding assays of the aorta with the TSPO specific ligand [$^3$H]PK 11195 were done to determine potential effects on TSPO binding characteristics in HFHC + DMBA treated rats. For representative examples, see Figure 4. The kidney was used as a control tissue, where no changes were expected. The $B_{max}$ and $K_d$ values for TSPO in the aorta and kidney of control rats (**Table 2**) were in the range of previous described results (Gavish et al., 1999; Dimitrova-Shumkovska et al., 2010a,b,c). In the present study TSPO binding characteristics of the aorta of untreated vehicle rats were as follows: $B_{max} = 4100 \pm 1400$ fmol/mg and $K_d = 1.2 \pm 0.4$ nM (**Table 2**). Regarding the effect of HFHC+DMBA, we observed significantly reduced TSPO binding capacity in aorta by 49% compared to vehicle control (**Table 2, Figure 4**).

The TSPO $B_{max}$ in aorta of the HFHC+DMBA group (Bmax = 2092 ± 670 fmol/mg) was not significantly different from those subjected to HFHC diet alone as reported previously (Dimitrova-Shumkovska et al., 2010a,b) or DMBA exposure alone. No significant differences were observed between experimental and control groups regarding the $K_d$ (Table 2).
In contrast to aorta, a highly significant enhancement in the $B_{max}$ of TSPO (+ 41%) determined with [$^3$H]PK 11195 binding was observed in testis tissue due to the HFHC + DMBA treatment, compared to control (**data not shown**). This was similar to the effects seen with HFHC diet alone and DMBA treatment alone (Dimitrova-Shumkovska et al., 2010a,b,c). [$^3$H]PK 11195 binding levels in kidney appeared not to be significantly affected by the HFHC + DMBA treatment **(Table 2)**. For all tissues, both in the HFHC + DMBA group and control group, $K_d$ values determined with [$^3$H]PK 11195 binding were in the nM range (0.8 - 1.9 nM, which is in the range typically observed for [3H]PK 11195 binding (Awad & Gavish, 1987; Dimitrova-Shumkovska et al., 2010a,b). This implies also that all of these $K_d$ values were not affected by HFHC and DMBA exposure.

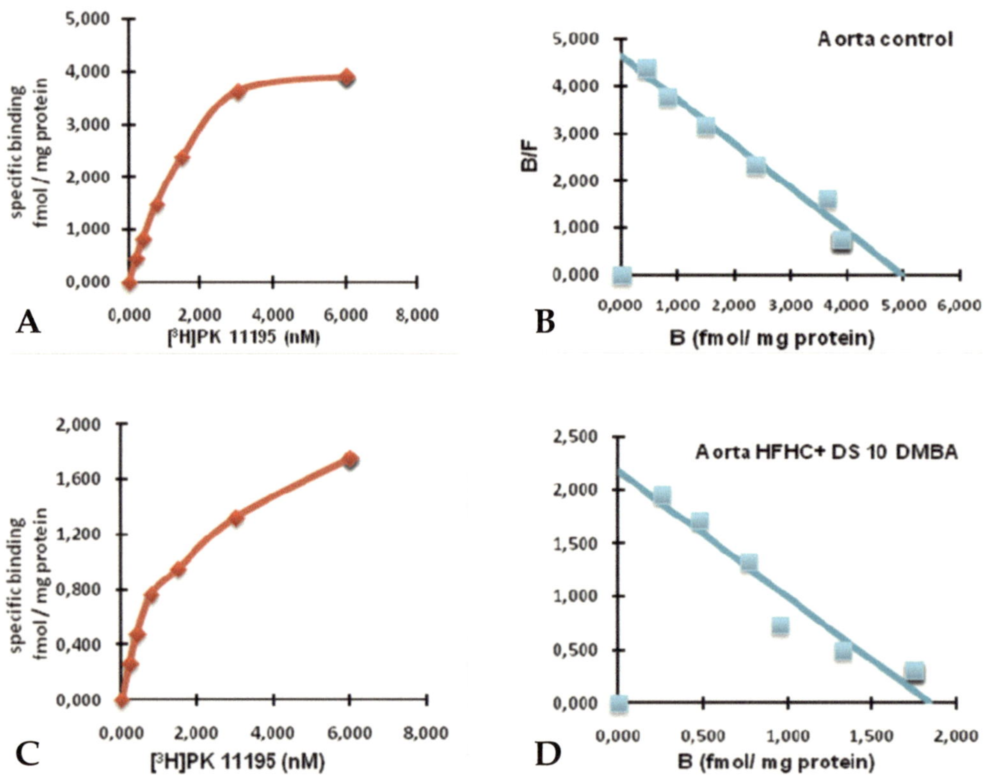


Fig. 4. Representative examples of Scatchard plots **(B, D)** and saturation curves **(A,C)** of [$^3$H]PK 11195 binding to membrane homogenates of aorta, respectively of vehicle control rats **(A,B)** and of rats exposed to HFHC and DMBA **(C,D)**. Abbreviations: C = vehicle control; The experimental group of HFHC+DMBA treatment (HFHC + DS 10 DMBA) is as described in the text. B: bound; B/F: bound over free.

| | C - Control | | | HFHC+DMBA | | |
|---|---|---|---|---|---|---|
| Tissue | n | B max (fmol / mg) | Kd (nmol) | n | B max (fmol / mg) | Kd (nmol) |
| Aorta | 10 | 4100 ± 1400 | 1.2 ± 0.4 | 6 | 2092 ± 670 * | 1.4 ± 0.8 |
| Kidney | 7 | 4270 ± 900 | 1.9 ± 0.9 | 7 | 4543 ± 870 | 2.8 ± 0.8 |

Table 2. Average $B_{max}$ values fmoles / mg protein and $K_d$ values (nM) of [$^3$H]PK 11195 binding to TSPO of aorta and kidney of HFHC+DMBA exposed rats versus vehicle control (C-Control). Kruskal-Wallis non-parametric, one-way analysis of variance ANOVA was used, with Mann-Whitney as the post-hoc, non-parametric test, * $p < 0.05$.

## 3. Discussion

It is well known that the TSPO is involved in tumorigenicity and also appears to be involved in atherosclerosis (Veenman & Gavish, 2006; Veenman et al., 2008; Dimitrova-Shumkovska et al., 2010a,b,c). Research over the past 30 years has suggested striking similarities between the pathways leading to atherosclerosis and cancer (reviews: Ross et al., 2001; Ramos and Partridge, 2005). Benditt and Benditt (1973) proposed that atherosclerotic plaque could be seen as neoplasm of smooth muscle cell origin, thereby paving the way for further research on the parallels between atherosclerosis and cancer. In accordance to this hypothesis, there is a body of evidence showing that established mutagenic and carcinogenic polycyclic aromatic hydrocarbons (PAHs), including methylcholantrene, benzopyrene, and DMBA, cause DNA-adducts in atherosclerotic lesions in humans or atherosclerotic prone animals (Izzoti et al., 2001; Iwano et al., 2005; Knaapen et al., 2007). Furthermore, smoking represents major risk factors for both cardiovascular disease and cancer (Knaapen et al., 2007; Catanzaro et al., 2007; Chiang et al., 2009). In addition, several animal studies have shown that components in tobacco smoke accelerate atherosclerosis in atherosclerotic prone animals, because of an increase in inflammatory cell content in atherosclerotic plaques (Izotti et al., 2001; Curfs et al., 2005).

For this study a HFHC diet was used in order to determine relations between systemic hypercholesterolemia, atherogenic pathology and oxidative stress in the cardiovascular system, in correlation with modulations in TSPO binding characteristics in these organs (Dimitrova-Shumkovska, 2010a). To observe the development of atherosclerosis in various animal models, atherogenic diets containing cholesterol, saturated fat, cocoa butter, and chocolate have been applied to vertebrates, including rodents (Faggiotto et al., 1984; Dimitrova, 2002; Kitade et al., 2006). Since the rat presents a resistant animal model for provoking atherosclerosis, relatively long time-courses are required to induce even moderate hypercholesterolemia and triglyceridemia (Nakamura et al., 1989; Lorkowska et al., 2006). Previous studies applying 1 - 2% cholesterol diets did not affect the endothelium, even though increased density of lipid loading at the adventitial vasa vasorum could be observed (Pisulewski et al., 2006; Lorkowska et al., 2006). Generally, HDL cholesterol is the dominating form in rats. Interestingly, increased expression of inflammatory cytokines (TNF, IL-1, IL-8 and VCAM-1) and augmented foamy cell formation can be found during chronic infection induced by Chlamydia pneumonia in white rats (Aziz, 2006). Furthermore, rats show augmented thrombotic response under hypertensive and hyperlipidemic conditions (Singh et al., 2009). These previous studies suggested that rats could present a useful model for studying hypercholesterolemia along with hypertension, but not a suitable model for atherosclerosis. Our diet containing 3% cholesterol not only was able to overcome at least in part the rats' resistance to elevation of plasma cholesterol levels but also initiated moderate cardiovascular damage (Dimitrova-Shumkovska et al., 2010a).

As a further indication of the validity of the HFHC diet (with 3% cholesterol) applied by us, the rats in our study showed obesity as well as hyperlipidemia and steatohepatitis (Dimitrova-Shumkovska et al., 2010a). Parameters for enhanced oxidative stress, as we detected in plasma of our HFHC rats may correlate with inflammatory processes, including atherogenic effects observed by us and others (Witko-Sarsat et al., 1998; Liu et al., 2006; Dimitrova-Shumkovska et al., 2010a). In particular the high AOPP levels observed in the liver, plasma, and aorta, as induced by the HFHC diet, may present factors reflecting liver pathology and atherogenesis (Watanabe et al., 2004; Oettl et al., 2008; Dimitrova-Shumkovska et al., 2010a).). In general, the involvement of oxidized proteins in atherosclerosis has been studied less than oxidized lipids. However, protein oxidation products have been found in the extracellular matrix of human and animal atherosclerotic plaques (Woods et al., 2003; Li et al., 2007). The study by Liu et al. (2006) was the first to our knowledge to provide *in vivo* evidence for a causal relationship between chronic AOPPs accumulation and atherosclerosis. This research suggests that increases in plasma AOPP, particularly in a hypercholesterolemic environment, accelerate atherosclerosis. Interestingly, a study from Wong et al. (2008) showed that protein carbonyls are not merely damaging, but can also serve as a second messenger for signal transduction in vascular smooth muscle cells.

Previous studies have shown that the TSPO is present throughout the cardiovascular system (Veenman & Gavish, 2006). Furthermore, the TSPO has been reported to be involved in oxidative stress and inflammation. In more detail, the TSPO is involved in various mechanisms that also have been found to play a role in atherosclerosis, including oxidative stress, ROS generation, inflammation, immune responses, apoptosis, and mitochondrial cholesterol transport (Papadopoulos et al., 1997, 2006). Most recent experimental data suggest that TSPO plays regulatory roles in adhesion to the extracellular matrix, vascularization, heme metabolism, and processes affected by nitrosylation of various proteins (Veenman and Gavish, 2011; Zeno et al., 2011; Bode et al., submitted). Thus, we assumed that the TSPO may be involved in cardiovascular disorders as induced in our paradigm.

Oxidative damage mediated by DMBA exposure and HFHC diet presents two examples of the plethora of risk factors in provoking atherosclerosis. Different forms of oxidative stress may give rise to different oxidation products, several of which were elevated in the aorta of our model induced by DMBA exposure and HFHC applied to the rats of this research (**Table 1**). As we used outbred Wistar rats, genetic disposition apparently is not a precondition for cardiovascular damage induced by DMBA. Histopathological analysis of the aorta showed that the HFHC + DMBA treatment induced foamy cells and fibrinoid connective tissue accumulation, as reported also for the separate treatments of HFHC and DMBA by themselves (Dimitrova-Shumkovska et al., 2010a,b,c). Furthermore, in the aorta the TSPO expression was inversely correlated with aggravated oxidative stress **(Table 2)**.

Previous *in vitro* studies of rat liver have shown as well that particular forms of oxidative stress can reduce TSPO binding density in this organ. For example, 0.001 mM Fe [$^{2+}$] in combination with 1 mM ascorbate reduced TSPO binding density by half (Courtiere et al., 1995). Interestingly, it was also shown that in response to UV irradiation-induced ROS covalent TSPO polymers were formed in Leydig and breast cancer cells *in vitro* and *in vivo,* resulting in increased binding affinity of the TSPO (Delavoie et al., 2003). Other evidence for TSPO's participation in oxidative processes has been indicated in a study by Carayon et al. (1996), where a correlation between the levels of TSPO expression and the resistance to $H_2O_2$ toxicity was demonstrated in hematopoietic cell lines. It may be considered that the reduction in TSPO binding density determined in the present research and other studies may impair such protective, anti-oxidative functions of the TSPO (Dimitrova-Shumkovska et al., 2010a,b,c). Alternatively, the reduced levels of TSPO may be a compensatory response to the challenges posed by the HFHC diet and DMBA exposure, i.e. reduced ROS generation otherwise due to TSPO activation and protection against the triggering of cell death, as for example was also found in various studies applying knockdown of TSPO by genetic manipulation *in vitro* (Levin et al., 2005; Zeno et al., 2009). Possibly, the enhanced levels of AOPP found in liver and aorta may be a contributing factor to the reduced binding density of TSPO in these organs (Dimitrova-Shumkovska et al., 2010a, b,c). As an alternative explanation, regulation of TSPO binding density can take place via modulations of gene expression (Giatzakis and Papadopoulos, 2004). With various studies we have demonstrated that steroids and stress are able to regulate TSPO binding density (for example, Veenman & Gavish, 2006; Veenman et al., 2007, 2009; Mazurika et al., 2009). As mentioned, growth hormone may take part in the effects of obesity. Similarly, testosterone levels may also be involved in the effects of atherogenic diet as discussed further below.

Our previous studies indicated the HFHC diet alone had more profound effects than DMBA exposure with a single dose of 10 mg in regard to aortic damage, histopathological changes in the liver, and oxidative stress measured in blood plasma and liver of rats (Dimitrova-Shumkovska et al., 2010a,b,c,). In the present study, also regarding oxidative stress in aorta, effects of HFHC combined with DMBA were more pronounced than of DMBA alone with a dose of 10 mg, but not more pronounced than of HFHC alone. The combination of HFHC diet and DMBA exposure did not appear to present a major synergetic effect on TSPO binding characteristics in the aorta. Possibly TSPO responses in the aorta may be part of a protective mechanism against lipid overload. Others have also suggested a role for TSPO in vascular inflammatory responses, for example in vascular permeability caused by carrageenin (Lazzarini et al., 2001). Presently, it is not known which components of the vascular wall, i.e. mast cells, smooth muscular, or dermal vascular endothelial cells, would be important for the potential correlation between TSPO expression and atherosclerosis (Morgan et al., 2004; Veenman & Gavish, 2006). Also, the importance of TSPO in relation to other mechanisms potentially associated with cardiovascular damage needs further research.

As TSPO may be modulated by ROS, and can modulate ROS generation itself (Courtiere et al., 1995; Papadopoulos et al., 1997, 2006; Delavoie et al., 2003; Veenman et al., 2007, 2008; Zeno et al., 2009), it can be postulated that the oxidative stress detected in aorta of our HFHC +DMBA rats may be associated directly with a reduction in TSPO binding density in these organs. While we did not see synergetic effects of HFHC and DMBA in rat aorta, preliminary data by us suggest that the combined effect of HFHC and DMBA in rat liver may lead to enhanced reductions in TSPO binding densities in this organ, compared to each treatment alone (unpublished results). At present it is not clear whether the TSPO levels modulate oxidative stress, or whether TSPO levels are only affected by oxidative stress. More studies are needed to resolve these questions.

As our studies showed an increase in the Bmax of TSPO binding in the testes, it would be interesting to study by which mechanisms this may occur. As discussed above, steroid hormones can have an effect on TSPO expression. Interestingly, several studies reported important positive correlations between high fat saturated supplementation and the levels of urinary excretion of testosterone (Hammoud et al., 2006). This is an important point to consider in evaluating levels of testosterone bioactivity in the body (Hill et al., 1980). Another approach to increase bioavailable testosterone would be to decrease the levels of sex-hormone binding globulin (SHBG). Reed et al. (1987) noted that normal men fed with a high fat diet showed increased SHBG levels, whereas a diet low in fat resulted in decreased in SHBG levels. It has been reported that decreased SHBG levels result in elevated testosterone bioactivity (Longcope et al., 2000). As with previous studies, showing increased TSPO binding density in the testes after DMBA and HFHC exposure (Dimitrova-Shumkovska et al., 2010a,b,c), also the combination of DMBA and HFHC exposures increased TSPO binding density in the testes (unpublished results). Potentially, this may be due to changes in testosterone levels, as previous studies have shown that increased testosterone can increase TSPO binding levels (Weizman et al., 1992).

Regarding future studies, it would be interesting indeed to find out whether modulation of TSPO responses by TSPO ligands would be able to counteract or enhance the effects of HFHC alone or with DMBA exposure. Similarly, it would be interesting to study in this paradigm the effects of hormones, as they are known to affect TSPO expression. For example, it is known that testosterone levels are reduced in humans as well as in rats as a consequence of a fattening diet and obesity (MacDonald et al., 2010). Since reduced testosterone levels are correlated with reduced TSPO levels in various tissues (Weizman et al., 1992), this may very well present part of the mechanism whereby the HFHC diet and the obesity of the rats of this research may lead to reduced TSPO levels in the aorta and liver. Alternatively, if enhanced oxidative stress in our paradigm contributes to changes in TSPO levels in various types of tissue, it will be interesting to study TSPO homomer polymerization, a phenomenon that has been reported by Delavoie et al. (2003). The potential appearance of TSPO multimers would suggest whether changes in TSPO binding capacity in some of the tissues studied may be due to the oxidative stress caused by the HFHC diet.

## 4. Conclusions

Our studies have shown that HFHC diet as well as DMBA exposure of rats can lead to oxidative stress in the aorta, as well as a reduction of TSPO binding density. The combination of HFHC diet plus an exposure to DMBA of rats did not affect the studied parameters regarding histopathological damage, oxidative stress and TSPO binding characteristics in aorta more than the maximal effects achieved by HFHC diet (Dimitrova-Shumkovska et al., 2010a), although they were higher than with DMBA treatment alone (Dimitrova-Shumkovska et al., 2010b). As addition of DMBA to HFHC treatment does not enhance levels of oxidative stress or changes in TSPO binding density in the aorta elicited by HFHC alone, this may indicate that HFHC treatment by itself already elicit maximal response from the TSPO / oxidative stress "system" in the aorta. Potentially, as the effects are not further enhanced, this may mean that the TSPO responses in the aorta indeed are a physiological response and do not simply represent damage to the TSPO protein (due to oxidative stress or otherwise).

We consider that the TSPO responses in aorta may present compensatory functions to deal with the oxidative stress induced by HFHC diet and DMBA exposure. Alternatively, the TSPO response may either be part of the oxidative stress mechanisms, or result from it. As discussed, TSPO function is not restricted to oxidative stress, but also encompasses adhesion to the extracellular matrix, angiogenesis, heme metabolism, protein nitrosylation, apoptosis, and immune responses.

Our research does show that exposure to irritants of the vascular endothelium (metabolical of chemical) decreases 18kDa TSPO binding capacity in the aorta. These decreases in TSPO binding capacity are potentially related to the oxidative stress in this organ. The data of this study suggest that TSPO may present a target for novel therapies designed to reduce the risk of atherosclerosis, including its component of oxidative stress.

## 5. Summary

The 18 kDa translocator protein (TSPO) is present throughout the cardiovascular system and may be involved in cardiovascular disorders. At cellular levels TSPO is present in virtually all of the cells of the cardiovascular system, where they appear to take part in the responses to various challenges that an organism and its cardiovascular system face, including atherosclerosis and accompanying symptoms. Several studies have shown that the TSPO appears to be a participant in reactive oxygen species (ROS) generation at mitochondrial levels. This may be part of oxidative stress challenges a cell may face. This potentially may play a role in cardiovascular diseases. In this context, TSPO modulates the initiation of mitochondrial apoptosis cascade. Furthermore, TSPO may be a participant in processes related to adhesion to the extracellular matrix, vascularisation, heme metabolism, and processes affected by nitrosylation of various proteins. Oxidative damage mediated by DMBA exposure and HFHC diet presents two examples of the plethora of risk factors in provoking atherosclerosis. Our studies have shown that a high fat, high cholesterol (HFHC) diet as well as 7, 12 dimethylbenz[α]anthracene (DMBA) exposure of rats can lead to oxidative stress in the aorta, in association with damage to the aorta wall, as well as a reduction of TSPO binding density. We consider that the TSPO responses in aorta may present compensatory functions to deal with the oxidative stress induced by HFHC diet and DMBA exposure. Alternatively, the TSPO response may either be part of the oxidative stress mechanisms, or result from it. The reviewed studies suggest that TSPO may present a target for novel therapies designed to reduce the risk of atherosclerosis, including its component of oxidative stress.

## 6. Explanation of abbreviations and symbols

ACTH, adrenocorticotropic hormone; ANOVA, analysis of variance; ANT, 30kDa adenine nucleotide translocator; (AOPPs), advanced oxidation protein products; Apo E-/- KO, apolipoprotein E knockout mice; cAMP, adenosine 3,5-cyclic monophosphate; CBR, central-type benzodiazepine receptor; DBI, Diazepam Binding Inhibitor CVD, cardiovascular disease; DMBA, 7, 12 Dimethylbenz[*a*]anthracene; DS 10 - single dose of 10 mg DMBA administered (10 mg/ 1ml of sesame oil); GABA, gamma-amino butyric acid; HDL, high-density lipoprotein; HFHC- high fat high cholesterol diet; HMGCoA, 3-hydroxy-3-methylglutaryl coenzyme A reductase; $H_2O_2$, hydrogen peroxide; Hb, hemoglobin; IL-1, interleukin-1 (IL-2, etc.); kDa, kilodalton; Kd, equilibrium dissociation constant; *Km*, equilibrium constant related to Michaelis-Menten kinetics (similarly, *Kd*, *Ka*, *Keq*, *Ks*); LDL, low density lipoproteins; mPTP, mitochondrial permeability transition pore; MCP-1, monocyte chemoatractant proteins-1; NADP, nicotinamide adenine dinucleotide phosphate;

NADH, reduced nicotinamide adenine dinucleotide; PAHs, polycyclic aromatic hydrocarbons; PBR, peripheral-type benzodiazepine receptor; PC protein carbonyls; PK 11195, 1-(2- chlorophenyl)-N-methyl-N-(1-methyl-prop 1)-3 isoquinolinecarboxamide; $ONOO^-$, peroxinitrite ; Ro5-4864, (4'- chlorodiazepam); ROS , reactive oxygen species; Sa$\beta$G, senescence-associated $\beta$ galactosidase; SOD, superoxide dismutase activity; TBARs, thiobarbituric acid reactive substances; TNF, tumor necrosis factor; TSPO, 18 kDa translocator protein; VCAM, vascular cell adhesion molecule; VDAC, 32 kDa voltage-dependent anion channel; VSMCs, vascular smooth muscle cells.

**Author Contributions:** Jasmina Dimitrova-Shumkovska and Leo Veenman contributed equally to this book chapter.

## 7. Acknowledgements

The contributing authors received research support from: Niedersachsen - Israel Project (MG, LV), Johnson & Johnson (MG, LV), L. Aronberg Research Fund in Neurology (MG, LV), E. & S. Schwarzbach Medical Research Fund (MG).

## 8. References

Amiri, Z., Weizman, R., Katz, Y., Burstein, O., Edoute, Y., Lochner, A., Gavish, M. (1991). Testosterone and cyproterone acetate modulate peripheral but not central benzodiazepine receptors in rats. *Brain Res.* 553, 155-8.

Anholt, R.R., De Souza, E.B., Kuhar, M.J., Snyder, S.H. (1985). Depletion of peripheral-type benzodiazepine receptors after hypophysectomy in rat adrenal gland and testis. *Eur J Pharmacol.* 110:41-6.

Awad, M., Gavish, M. (1987). Binding of [3H] Ro5-4864 and [3H] PK 11195 to cerebral cortex and peripheral tissues of various species: species differences and heterogeneity in peripheral benzodiazepine binding sites. *J Neurochem.* 495, 1407-1414.

Aziz, A. (2006). A study on immunopathogenetic mechanisms of atherosclerotic process caused by chronic infection of Chlamydia pneumoniae in rats. *Acta Med Indones.,* 38, 206-12.

Basile, A.S., Lueddens, H.W., Skolnick, P. (1988). Regulation of renal peripheral benzodiazepine receptors by anion transport inhibitors. *Life Sci.* 42(6):715-26.

Benditt, E.P., Benditt, J.M., 1973. Evidence for monoclonal origin of human atherosclerotic plaques. *Proc. Natl.Acad.Sci. USA.* 70, 1753-1756.

Bird, J.L., Izquierdo-Garcia, D., Davies, J.R., Rudd, J.H., Probst, K.C., Figg, N, Clark, J.C., Weissberg, P.L., Davenport, A.P., Warburton, E.A. (2010). Evaluation of translocator protein quantification as a tool for characterising macrophage burden in human carotid atherosclerosis. *Atherosclerosis.* 210(2):388-91.

Bode, J., Veenman, L., Kugler, W., Lakomek, L., Gavish, M. The 18 kDa Translocator Protein influences angiogenesis, as well as aggressiveness, adhesion, migration and proliferation of glioblastoma cells. *Pharmacogenetics and Genomics.* Submitted

Carayon, P., Portier, M., Dussossoy, D., Bord, A., Petitpretre, G., Canat, X., Le Fur, G., Casellas, P., 1996. Involvement of peripheral benzodiazepine receptors in the protection of hematopoietic cells against oxygen radical damage. *Blood* 87, 3170–8.

Casellas, P., Galiegue, S., Basile, A.S. (2002) Peripheral benzodiazepine receptors and mitochondrial function. Neurochem Int.40: 475-86.

Catanzaro, D.F., Zhou, Y., Chen, R., Yu, F., Catanzaro, S.E., De Lorenzo, M.S., Subbaramaiah, K., Zhou, X.K., Pratico, D., Dannenberg, A.J., Weksler, B.B. (2007). Potentially reduced exposure cigarettes accelerate atherosclerosis: evidence for the role of nicotine. *Cardiovasc Toxicol.* 7:192-201.

Choi, J., Ifuku, M., Noda, M., Guilarte, T.R. (2011). Translocator protein (18 kDa)/peripheral benzodiazepine receptor specific ligands induce microglia functions consistent with an activated state. *Glia.* 59(2):219-30.

Chelli, B, Falleni, A, Salvetti, F, Gremigni, V, Lucacchini, A, Martini C. (2001).Peripheral-type benzodiazepine receptor ligands: mitochondrial permeability transition induction in rat cardiac tissue. *Biochem Pharmacol.* 61: 695-705.

Chelli, B., Lena, A., Vanacore, R., Da Pozzo, E., Costa, B., Rossi, L., Salvetti, A., Scatena, F., Ceruti, S., Abbracchio, M.P., Gremigni, V., Martini, C. (2004). Peripheral benzodiazepine receptor ligands: mitochondrial transmembrane potential depolarization and apoptosis induction in rat C6 glioma cells. *Biochem Pharmacol.* 68: 125-34.

Chiang, P., Chang, T., Chen, J. (2009). Synergistic effect of fatty liver and smoking on metabolic syndrome. *World Journal of Gastroenterol.* 15, 5334-5339.

Clarke, M & Bennett, M. (2006).The Emerging Role of Vascular Smooth Muscle Cell Apoptosis in Atherosclerosis and Plaque Stability. *Am J Nephrol.,* 26:531-535.

Courtiere, A., Molard, F., Reybaud, J. (1995). Differential effects of in vitro peroxidation on peripheral - and central-type benzodiazepine receptors. Protection by diverse antioxidants. *Biochem Pharmacol.* 50, 1815-1822.

Curfs, D.M.J., Knaapen, A.M., Pachen, D.M.F.A., Gijbels, M.M.J., Lutgens, E., Smook, M.L.F., Kockx, M.M., Daemen, M.J.A.P., Van Schooten, F.J. (2005). Polycyclic aromatic hydrocarbons induce an inflammatory atherosclerotic plaque phenotype irrespective of their DNA binding properties. *Faseb J* 19, 1290-1292.

Decaudin, D., Castedo, M., Nemati, F., Beurdeley-Thomas, A., De Pinieux, G., Caron, A., Pouillart, P., Wijdenes, J., Rouillard, D., Kroemer, G., Poupon, M.F. (2002). Peripheral benzodiazepine receptor ligands reverse apoptosis resistance of cancer cells in vitro and in vivo. *Cancer Res.* 62(5):1388-93.

Delavoie, F., Li, H., Hardwick, M., Robert, J., Giatzakis, C., Peranzi, G., Maccario, J., Lacapere, J., Papadopoulos, V., (2003). In vivo and in vitro peripheral-type benzodiazepine receptor polymerization: functional significance in drug ligand and cholesterol binding. *Biochem.* 42, 4506-19.

Dimitrova, J. (2002). The Impact of Dietary Unsaturates and L-Arginine Administration upon Lipoprotein Metabolism in Mildly Hypercholesterolemic *Wistar*-Rats. Master thesis, Skopje (in Macedonian)

Dimitrova-Shumkovska, J., Veenman, L., Ristoski, T., Leschiner, S., Gavish, M. (2010a). Chronic High Fat, High Cholesterol Supplementation Decreases 18 kDa Translocator Protein Binding Capacity in Association with Increased Oxidative Stress in Rat Liver and Aorta. *Food and Chem. Toxicol.* 48, 910-921.

Dimitrova-Shumkovska, J., Veenman, L., Ristoski, T., Leschiner, S., Gavish, M. (2010b). Dimethylbenz [alpha] anthracene induces oxidative stress and reduces the binding capacity of the mitochondrial 18-kDa translocator protein in rat aorta. *Drug Chem. Toxicol.* 33, 337-47.

Dimitrova-Shumkovska, J., Veenman, L., Ristoski, T., Leschiner, S., Gavish, M. (2010c). Decreases in Binding Capacity of the Mitochondrial 18 kDa Translocator Protein Accompany Oxidative Stress and Pathological Signs in Rat Liver after DMBA Exposure. *Toxicol Pathol.*, 38:957-68.

Faggiotto, A., Ross, R., Harker, L. (1984). Studies of hypercholesterolemia in the nonhuman primate. Changes that lead to fatty streak formation. *Arteriosclerosis.* 4, 323-40.

Fennell, D.A., Corbo, M., Pallaska, A, Cotter, F.E. (2001).Bcl-2 resistant mitochondrial toxicity mediated by the isoquinoline carboxamide PK11195 involves de novo generation of reactive oxygen species. *Br J Cancer* 84(10):1397- 404.

Fischer, R., Schmitt, M., Bode, J.G., Häussinger, D., 2001. Expression of the peripheral-type benzodiazepine receptor and apoptosis induction in hepatic stellate cells. *Gastroenterology.*120, 1212-26.

Galiegue, S, Tinel, N., Casellas, P. (2003). The peripheral benzodiazepine receptor: a promising therapeutic drug target. *Curr Med Chem.* 10:1563-72.

Gavish, M., Bar-Ami, S., Weizman, R. (1992). The endocrine system and mitochondrial benzodiazepine receptors. *Mol Cell Endocrinol.* 88, 1-13.

Gavish, M., Weizman, R. (1997). Role of peripheral-type benzodiazepine receptors in steroidogenesis. *Clin Neuropharmacol.* 20:473-81.

Gavish, M., Bachman, I., Shoukrun, R., Katz, Y., Veenman, L., Weisinger, G. and Weizman, A. (1999). Enigma of the peripheral benzodiazepine receptor. *Pharmacol. Review.* 51, 630-646.

Giatzakis, C., Papadopoulos, V. (2004). Differential utilization of the promoter of peripheral-type benzodiazepine receptor by steroidogenic versus nonsteroidogenic cell lines and the role of Sp1 and Sp3 in the regulation of basal activity. *Endocrinology.* 145, 1113-23.

Goldstein, J.L. & Brown, M.S. (2009). The LDL receptor. *Arterioscl.Thromb.Vasc.Biol.*, 29:431-438.

Hammoud, A.O., Gibson, M., Peterson, C.M., Hamilton, B.D., Carrell, D.T. (2006). Obesity and male reproductive potential. (Review) *J Andrology.* 27, 619-626.

Hansson, G.K. (2005). Inflammation, Atherosclerosis and Coronary Artery Disease. *N Engl J Med.* 352, 2685-95.

Hauet, T., Yao, Z.H., Bose, H.S., Wall, C.T., Han,Z., Li, W., Hales, D.B., Miller, W.L., Culty,M. and Papadopoulos.V. (2005). Peripheral-Type Benzodiazepine Receptor-Mediated Action of Steroidogenic Acute Regulatory Protein on Cholesterol Entry into Leydig Cell Mitochondria. *Mol Endocrinol.*, 19:540-554.

Hill, P.B., Wynder, E.L. & Garbaczewski, L. (1980). Plasma hormones and lipids in men at different risk for coronary heart disease. *Amer. J of Clin. Nutr.* 33, 1010-1018.

Iwano, S., Shibahara, N., Saito, T., Kamataki, T. (2006). Activation of p53 as a causal step for atherosclerosis induced by polycyclic aromatic hydrocarbons. *FEBS Letters.* 580, 890-893.

Izzoti, A., Camoirano, C., Cariglia, C., Tampa, E., De Flora, S. (2001). Formation of DNA adducts in the aorta of smoke-exposed rats, and modulation by chemopreventive agents. *Mutat Res.* 494, 97-106.

Jayakumar, A.R., Panickar, K.S., Norenberg , M.D. (2002). Effects on free radical generation by ligands of the peripheral benzodiazepine receptor in cultured neural cells. *J Neurochem.* 83:1226-34.

Kelly-Hershkovitz, E., Weizman, R., Spanier, I., Leschiner, S., Lahav, M., Weisinger, G., Gavish, M. (1998). Effects of Peripheral-type Benzodiazepine Receptor Antisense Knockout on MA-10 Leydig Cell Proliferation and Steroidogenesis *J. Biol. Chem.* 273, 5478-5483.

Kitade, M., Yoshiji, H., Kojima, H., Ikenaka, Y., Noguchi, R., Kaji, K., Yoshii, J., Yanase, K., Namisaki, T., Asada, K., Yamazaki, M., Tsujimoto, T., Akahane, T., Uemura, M and Fukui, H. (2006). Leptin-Mediated Neovascularisation Is a Prerequisite for Progression of Non-alcoholic Steatohepatitis in Rats. *Hepathology.* 44, 983-991.

Kletsas, D., Li ,W., Han, Z., Papadopoulos, V. (2004). Peripheral-type benzodiazepine receptor (PBR) and PBR drug ligands in fibroblast and fibrosarcoma cell proliferation: role of ERK, c-Jun and ligand-activated PBR-independent pathways. *Biochem Pharmacol.* 67:1927-32.

Knaapen, A.M., Curfs, D.M., Pachen, D.M., Gottschalk, R.W., de Winther, M.P., Daemen, M.J., Van Schooten, F.J. (2007).The environmental carcinogen benzo[a]pyrene induces expression of monocyte-chemoattractant protein-1 in vascular tissue: a possible role in atherogenesis. *Mutat Res.* 621(1-2):31-41.

Krieger, M. (1997). The Other Side of Scavenger Receptors: Pattern Recognition for the Host Defence. *Curr Opin Lipidol.* 8, 257-80.

Kugler, W., Veenman, L., Shandalov, Y., Leschiner, S., Spanier, I., Lakomek, M., Gavish, M. (2008). Ligands of the mitochondrial 18 kDa Translocator Protein attenuate apoptosis in human glioblastoma cells exposed to erucylphosphohomocholine. *Cell. Oncol.* 30, 435-450.

Kunduzova, O. R., Escourrou, G, De La Farge, F., Salvayre, R., Seguelas, M. H., Leducq, N., Bono, F., Herbert , J.M., Parini, A. (2004). Involvement of peripheral benzodiazepine receptor in the oxidative stress, death-signalling pathways, and renal injury induced by ischemia-reperfusion. *J Am Soc Nephrol.* 15, 2152-2160.

Kunitomo, M., Yamaguchi, Y., Kagota, S., Yoshikawa, N., Nakamura, K., Shinozuka, K. (2009). Biochemical Evidence of Atherosclerosis Progression Mediated by Increased Oxidative Stress in Apolipoprotein E-Deficient Spontaneously Hyperlipidemic Mice Exposed to Chronic Cigarette Smoke. *J Pharmacol. Sci.* 110, 354-361

Lacapère, J.J. & Papadopoulos, V. (2003). Peripheral-type benzodiazepine receptor: structure and function of a cholesterol-binding protein in steroid and bile acid biosynthesis. *Steroids.* 68:569-85.

Laine, F., Bendavid, C., Moirand, R., Tessier, S., Perrin, M., Guillygomarch, A., Guyader, D., Calon, E., Renault, A., Brissot, P., Turlin, B., Deugnier, Y. (2004). Prediction of liver fibrosis in patients with features of the metabolic syndrome regardless of alcohol consumption. *Hepathology.* 39, 1639-1646.

Lazzarini, R., Malucelli, B.E. & Palermo-Neto, J. (2001). Reduction of acute inflammation in rats by diazepam: role of peripheral benzodiazepine receptors and corticosterone. *Immuno Pharmacol Immunotoxicol*. 23, 253-65.

Le Fur, G., Vaucher, N., Perrier, M.L., Flamier, A., Benavides, J., Renault, C., Dubroeucq, M.C., Guérémy, C., Uzan, A. (1983). Differentiation between two ligands for peripheral benzodiazepine binding sites, [3H] RO5-4864 and [3H] PK 11195, by thermodynamic studies. *Life Sci.* 33:449-57.

Lenaz, G. (1998). Role of mitochondria in oxidative stress and aging. *Biochim Biophys Acta.* 1366, 53-67.

Levin, E., Premkumar, A., Veenman, L., Kugler, W., Leschiner, S., Spanier, I., Weisinger, G., Lakomek, M., Weizman, A., Snyder, S.H., Pasternak, G.W., Gavish, M. (2005). The peripheral-type benzodiazepine receptor and tumorigenicity: isoquinoline binding protein (IBP) antisense knockdown in the C6 glioma Cell Line. *Biochemistry.* 44, 9924-9935.

Levine, R. L., Garland, D., Oliver, C.N., Amici, A., Climent, I., Lenz, A.G., Ahn, B.W., Shaltiel, S., Stadman, E.R. (1990). Determination of carbonyl content in oxidatively modified proteins. *Methods in Enzymol.* 186, 464-478.

Libby, P., Ridker, P.M., Hansson, G.K. (2009). Inflamation in Atherosclerosis. *J Amer College of Cardiol.* 2129-38.

Libby, P., Ridker, P.M. & Hansson, G.K. (2011). Progress and challenges in translating the biology of atherosclerosis. Review. *Nature* 473:317-325

Liu, J., Li, H., Papadopoulos, V. (2003) PAP7, a PBR/PKA - RI alpha-associated protein: a new element in the relay of the hormonal induction of steroidogenesis. *J Steroid Biochem Mol Biol.* 85:275-83.

Liu S.X., Hou, F.F., Guo, Z. J., Nagai, R., Zhang, W.R., Liu, Z.Q., Zhou, Z.M., Di Xie, Wang, G.B., Zhang, X. (2006). Advanced Oxidation Protein Products Accelerate Atherosclerosis Through Promoting Oxidative Stress and Inflammation. *Arterioscler Thromb Vasc Biol.* 26, 1156-1162.

Lizardi-Cervera, J. & Aquilar-Zapata, D. (2009). Nonalcoholic fatty liver disease and its association with cardiovascular disease. *Annals of Hepatol.*, 8, S 40-43.

Lorkowska, B., Bartus, M., Franczyk, M., Kostogrys, R.B., Jawien, J., Pisulewski, P.M., Chlopicki, S. (2006). Hypercholesterolemia does not alter endothelial function in spontaneously hypertensive rats. *J Pharmacol Exp Ther.* 317, 1019-1026.

Maeda, S., Miyawaki, T., Nakanishi, T., Takigawa, M., Shimada, M. (1998). Peripheral type benzodiazepine receptor in T lymphocyte rich preparation. *Life Sci.* 63, 1423-1430.

MacDonald, A.A., Herbison, G.P., Showell, M. and C.M. Farquhar, C.M. (2010) The impact of body mass index on semen parameters and reproductive hormones in human males: a systematic review with meta-analysis. *Hum.Reprod.Update.*16:293-311.

Matsuzawa, N., Takamura, T., Kurita, S., Misu, H., Ota, T., Ando, H., Yokoyama, M., Honda, M., Zen, Y., Nakanuma, Y., Miyamoto, K.I., Kaneko, S. (2007). Lipid-induced oxidative stress causes steatohepatitis in mice fed and atherogenic diet. *Hepathology.* 46, 1392-1403.

Mazurika, C., Veenman, L., Weizman, R., Bidder, M., Leschiner ,S., Golani, I., Spanier, I., Weisinger, G., Gavish, M. (2009). Estradiol modulates uterine 18 kDa translocator protein gene expression in uterus and kidney of rats. *Mol Cell Endocrinol.* 307, 43-49.

McEnery, M.W., Snowman, A.M., Trifiletti, R.R., Snyder , S.H. (1992). Isolation of the mitochondrial benzodiazepine receptor: association with the voltage-dependent anion channel and the adenine nucleotide carrier. *Proc Natl Acad Sci U S A.* 89:3170-4.

Michel, J.B., Virmani, R., Arbustini, E.,Pasterkamp, G. (2011). Intraplaque haemorrhages as the trigger of plaque vulnerability. *Eur Heart J.*Ehr 054.

Miller, K.P., and Ramos, K.S. (2001). Impact of cellular metabolism on the biological effects of benzo[a]pyrene and related hydrocarbons. *Drug Metabol Rev.* 33, 1-35.

Miyata, M., Furukawa, M., Takahashi, K., Gonzalez, F.J., Yamazoe, Y. (2001). Mechanism of 7,12-dimethylbenz[a]anthracene -induced immunotoxicity: role of metabolic activation at the target organ. *Jpn. J Pharmacol.* 86, 302-309.

Moreno-Sánchez, R., Bravo, C., Gutiérrez, J., Newman, A.H., Chiang, P.K. (1991). Release of Ca2+ from heart and kidney mitochondria by peripheral-type benzodiazepine receptor ligands. *Int J Biochem.* 23:207-13.

Morgan, J., Oseroff, A.R., Cheney, R.T. (2004). Expression of the peripheral benzodiazepine receptor is decreased in skin cancers in comparison with normal skin. *Br J Dermatol.* 151, 846-56.

Munck, A., Guyre, P.M. and Holbrook, N. (1984). Physiological functions of glucocorticoids in stress and their relation to pharmacological actions. *Endocr. Rev.* 5:25–44.

Nakamura, H., Izumiyama, N., Nakamura, K., Ohtsubo, K. (1989). Age-associated ultrastructural changes in the aortic intimae of rats with diet-induced hypercholesterolemia. *Atherosclerosis.* 79, (2-3):101-11

Oke, B.O., Suarez-Quian, C.A., Riond, J., Ferrara, P., Papadopoulos, V. (1992). Cell surface localization of the peripheral-type benzodiazepine receptor (PBR) in adrenal cortex. *Mol Cell Endocrinol.* 87:R1-6.

Onyimba, J.A., Coronado, M.J., Garton, A.E., Kim, J.B., Bucek, A., Bedja, D., Gabrielson, K.L., Guilarte, T.R., Fairweather, D. (2011). The innate immune response to coxsackievirus B3 predicts progression to cardiovascular disease and heart failure in male mice. *Biol Sex Differ.* 21; 2:2.

Packard, R.R. & Libby, P. (2008). Inflammation in atherosclerosis: from vascular biology to biomarker discovery and risk prediction. *Clin Chem.* 54, 24-38.

Papadopoulos, V., Berkovich, A., Krueger, K.E., Costa, E., Guidotti, A. (1991). Diazepam binding inhibitor and its processing products stimulate mitochondrial steroid biosynthesis via an interaction with mitochondrial benzodiazepine receptors. *Endocrinology.* 129:1481-8.

Papadopoulos, V., Amri, H., Boujrad, N., Cascio, C., Culty, M., Garnier, M., Hardwick, M., Li, H., Vidic, B., Brown, A.S., Reversa, J.L., Bernassau, J.M., Drieu, K (1997). Peripheral benzodiazepine receptor in cholesterol transport and steroidogenesis. *Steroid.*, 62, 21–28

Papadopoulos, V., Baraldi, M., Guilarte, T.R., Knudsen, T.B., Lacapère, J.J., Lindemann, P., Norenberg, M.D., Nutt, D., Weizman, A., Zhang, M.R., Gavish, M. (2006).

Translocator protein (18kDa). New nomenclature for the peripheral-type benzodiazepine receptor based on its structure and molecular function. *Trends Pharmacol Sci.* 27, 402-9.

Pisulewski, P.M., Franczyk, M., Kostogrys, R.B., Lorkowska, B., Bartus, M., Chlopicki, S. (2006). Spontaneously hypertensive rats are resistant to hypercholesterolemia-induced atherosclerosis. *J Animal and Food Sci* 15, 103-114.

Raa, A., Stainsberg, C., Steen, V. M., Bjerkvig, R., Reed, R.K., Stuhr, L.E.B. (2007). Hyperoxia retards growth and induces apoptosis and loss of glands and blood vessels in DMBA-induced rat mammary tumours. *BMC Cancer*, 7-23.

Ramos, K.S., Partridge, C.R. (2005). Atherosclerosis and Cancer: flip sides of the neoplastic response in mammalian cells? *Cardiovasc Toxicol* 5, 245-255.

Ross, R & Glomset, J.A. (1973). Atherosclerosis and the arterial smooth muscle cell: Proliferation of smooth muscle is a key event in the genesis of the lesions of atherosclerosis. *Science* 180: 1332-1339.

Ross, R., 1999. Atherosclerosis an Inflammatory Disease. *N Engl J Med.* 340, 115-26.

Ross, J.S., Stagliano, N.E., Donovan, M.J., Breitbart, R.E., Ginsburg, G.S. (2001). Atherosclerosis And Cancer: Common Molecular Pathways Of Disease Development And Progression. *Ann NY Acad Sci.* 947, 271–292

Singh, V., Tiwari, R.L., Dikshit, M., Barthwal, M.K. (2009). Models to Study Atherosclerosis: A Mechanistic Insight. *Curr Vasc Pharmacol.* 7, 75-109.

Steinberg, D., Parthasarathy, S., Carew, T. E., Khoo, J. C. & Witztum, J. L., 1989. Beyond cholesterol: modifications of low density lipoprotein that increase its atherogenicity. *N. Engl. J. Med.* 320, 915-924.

Stocco, D.M., Clark, B.J. (1996) Regulation of the acute production of steroids in steroidogenic cells. *Endocr Rev.* 17:221-44.

Stocker, R & Keaney, J.F. Jr. (2005). New insights on oxidative stress in the artery wall. *J Thromb Haemost* 3, 1825-1834.

Soustiel, J.F., Zaaroor, M., Vlodavsky, E., Veenman, L., Weizman, A., Gavish, M. (2008). Neuroprotective effect of Ro5-4864 following brain injury. *Exp Neurol.* 214(2):201-8.

Taniguchi, T., Wang, J.K, Spector, S. (1980). Properties of [$^3$H] diazepam binding to rat peritoneal mast cells. *Life Sci.* 27, 171-178.

Tannenbaum, B.M., Brindley, D.N., Tannenbaum, G.S., Dallman, M.F., McArthur, M.D. and Meaney.M.J. (1997). High-fat feeding alters both basal and stress-induced hypothalamic-pituitary-adrenal activity in the rat. *Am. J. Physiol. Endocrinol. Metab.* 36: E1168–E1177.

Tiwari, R.P., Singh, V., Bathwal, M.K., 2008. Macrophages: An elusive yet emerging therapeutic target of atherosclerosis. *Med Res Rev* 28, 483-544.

Upston, J.M., Terentis, A.C., Morris, K., Keaney, Jr J.F., Stocker, R. (2002).Oxidized lipid accumulates in the presence of α-tocopherol in atherosclerosis. *Biochem J.* 363: 753–760.

Varga, B., Markó, K., Hádinger, N., Jelitai, M., Demeter, K., Tihanyi, K., Vas, A., Madarász, E. (2009). Translocator protein (TSPO 18kDa) is expressed by neural stem and neuronal precursor cells. *Neurosci Lett.* 462(3):257-62.

Veenman, L. & Gavish, M. (2000). Peripheral-type benzodiazepine receptors: Their implication in Brain Disease. *Drug Dev Res* 50:355-370

Veenman, L., Leschiner, S., Spanier, I., Weisinger, G., Weizman, A., Gavish, M. (2002). PK 11195 attenuates kainic acid-induced seizures and alterations in peripheral-type benzodiazepine receptor (PBR) protein components in the rat brain. *J Neurochem.* 80(5):917-27.

Veenman, L., Gavish, M. (2006). The peripheral-type benzodiazepine receptor and the cardiovascular system. Implications for drug development. *Pharmacol Ther.*110, 503-24.

Veenman, L., Papadopoulos, V., Gavish, M. (2007). Channel-like functions of the 18-kDa translocator protein (TSPO): regulation of apoptosis and steroidogenesis as part of the host-defence response. *Curr Pharm Des.* 13, 2385-405.

Veenman, L., Shandalov, Y., Gavish, M. (2008). VDAC activation by the 18 kDa translocator protein (TSPO), implications for apoptosis. *J Bioenerg Biomembr.* 40(3):199-205.

Veenman, L., Weizman, A., Weisinger, G., Gavish, M. (2010). Expression and Functions of the 18 kDa Mitochondrial Translocator Protein TSPO in Health and Disease. *Targeted Drug Delivery in Cancer Therapeutics*, in press.

Veenman, L., Alten, J., Linnemannstöns, K., Shandalov, Y., Zeno, S., Lakomek, M., Gavish, M., Kugler, W. (2010a) Potential involvement of F0F1-ATP(synth)ase and reactive oxygen species in apoptosis induction by the antineoplastic agent erucylphosphohomocholine in glioblastoma cell lines: a mechanism for induction of apoptosis via the 18 kDa mitochondrial translocator protein. *Apoptosis.* (7):753-68.

Veenman, L., Weizman, A., Weisinger, G., Gavish, M. (2010b) "Expression and Functions of the 18 kDa Mitochondrial Translocator Protein (TSPO) in Health and Disease." *Targeted Drug Delivery in Cancer Therapeutics.* Editor: Michael A. Firer: Transworld Research Network: Kerala, India, pp. 49-84.

Veenman, L., Gavish, M. (2011). The role of 18 kDa mitochondrial Translocator Protein (TSPO) in programmed cell death, and effects of steroids on TSPO expression. *Current Molecular Medicine.* In press.

Veenman, L., Kugler, W., Lakomek, L., Gavish, M, Bode, J. The 18 kDa Translocator Protein influences angiogenesis, as well as aggressiveness, adhesion, migration and proliferation of glioblastoma cells. *Pharmacogenetics and Genomics.* Submitted

Verma, A., Nye, J.S., Snyder, S.H. (1987). Porphyrins are endogenous ligands for the mitochondrial (peripheral-type) benzodiazepine receptor. *Proc Natl Acad Sci U S A.* 84(8):2256-60.

Weizman, A, Amiri Z, Katz, Y., Snyder, S.H., Gavish, M. (1992).Testosterone prevents castration-induced reduction in peripheral benzodiazepine receptors in Cowper's gland and adrenal. *Brain Res.* 572:72-5.

Witko-Sarsat, V., M. Friedlander, C., Nguyen-Khoa, A. T., Nguyen, J., Zingraff, P., Jungers, and Descamps-Latscha, B. (1998). Advanced oxidation protein products as novel mediators of inflammation and monocyte activation in chronic renal failure. *J Immunol.* 161, 2524-2532.

Wong, C.M., Cheema, A.K., Zhang, L., Suzuki, Y.J.(2008). Protein Carbonylation as a novel mechanism in red ox signalling. *Circ Res.* 102, 310-318.

Zeno, S., Zaaroor, M., Leschiner, S., Veenman, L., Gavish, M. (2009). CoCl(2) induces apoptosis via the 18kDa translocator protein in U118MG human glioblastoma cells. *Biochem.* 48, 4652-61.

Zeno, S., Veenman, L., Katz, Y., Bode, J., Gavish, M., Zaaroor, M. (2011). The 18 kDa mitochondrial Translocator Protein (TSPO) prevents accumulation of protoporphyrin IX. A TSPO knockdown study. *Curr Molecular Medicine.* In press.

# Part 3

## Oxidative Stress in Atherosclerosis

# 19

# Are CVD Patients Under Oxidative Stress?

Yedidya Dotan, Dov Lichtenberg and Ilya Pinchuk
*Dept. of Physiology and Pharmacology, Sackler Medical School, Tel Aviv University*
*Israel*

## 1. Introduction

Oxidative stress has long been associated with cardiovascular disease (CVD) (Abuja & Albertini, 2001; Halliwell & Gutteridge, 1990; Parthasarathy et al., 2001; Steinbrecher et al., 1984). It was even assumed that the prevalence of CVD alone indicates the prevalence of oxidative stress (Witztum, 1994). Moreover, cross-sectional studies indicated that supplementation of low molecular weight antioxidants is associated with a relatively low incidence of CVD (Jha et al., 1995). By contrast, in most of the interventional studies the antioxidant supplementation did not prevent the progression of CVD nor did it improve any of the many clinical endpoints (Shekelle et al., 2004; Vivekananthan et al., 2003; Miller 2005; Bjelakovic, 2007; Dotan, 2009a; Dotan, 2009b). Based on these findings, Witztum (Witztum, 1998) and Morrow (Morrow, 2003) hypothesized that only individuals under oxidative stress may benefit from antioxidant supplementation. This, of course, implies that only people under oxidative stress should be treated with antioxidants. This, in turn, means that a criterion must be established for the ill-defined, intuitively understood term "oxidative stress".

This issue is of special importance in light of our previous study that demonstrated that no single index can be used as a universal criterion, indicating that there are several types of oxidative stress (Dotan et al., 2004). Hence, the question remains which criterion (or criteria) can be used to identify who is likely to benefit from antioxidant supplementation. The answer to this question can, theoretically, be based either on a criterion for the relevant type of oxidative stress (e.g. lipid peroxidation, as assessed by the concentrations of MDA or isoprostanes) or/and on diagnosis of specific diseases for which there is sufficient evidence for benefit of antioxidant supplementation.

In the current study, we present the results of a meta-analysis of case-control studies used to assess the association between CVD and oxidative stress, as evaluated on the basis of different criteria. Unlike previous meta-analyses, we analyzed the association between CVD and criteria for each of the types of OS. We hope that eventually this analysis will enable us to define threshold values of relevant indices of the relevant type of oxidative stress for treatment with antioxidants (Deeks, 2001; Deeks & Altman, 2004).

## 2. Methods

This work was performed according to the guidelines outlined by the Meta-analysis Of Observational Studies in Epidemiology (MOOSE) group (Stroup et al., 2000). A detailed description of the data retrieval process, the selection criteria and the analyses of the data is given in the following subsections.

## 2.1 Retrieval and selection of studies to be included in the analysis

First, we had to define criteria to be used in our search for clinical trials to be included in our meta-analysis (Fig. 1). The following criteria were defined for our search:

i. Design: only case-control or nested case control studies were included.
ii. Methods: for a clinical study to be included in our meta-analysis it had to use only generally accepted methods for the evaluation of oxidative stress (Dotan et al., 2004).
iii. Size: to be included in our meta-analysis, the study had to involve at least 20 CVD patients and at least 20 "CVD-free" individuals, serving as a control group.

The latter demand requires further definition of the two populations that can be regarded as being "CVD patients" and their respective controls. We included in the control group only "pathology-free" individuals. To be included in the group of "CVD patients", a person had to be diagnosed with one of the following conditions: (i) either stable angina pectoris (STP) or unstable angina pectoris (UTP), diagnosed either by angiogram or by physical examination, (ii) patients suffering from any of the stages of coronary stenosis and (iii) a recorded history of CVD (e.g. myocardial infraction).

With these criteria in mind, we searched through two major databases, namely, the Medline database (http://www.ncbi.nlm.nih.gov/entrez/query.fcgi?CMD=search&DB=pubmed) and the Thomson Reuters ISI Web of Science. Reference mining was conducted to find an arbitrarily predefined number of studies (20) that fit all the above selection criteria. We defined a list of keywords to search and conducted a simple keyword search, similar to that described by Shekelle et al. (Shekelle et al., 2004).

Data of case-control studies may be biased towards the prevailing paradigm and the findings of other recent trials (French et al., 2005; Moher & Tsertsvadze, 2006). Such bias must be considered when conducting a search for studies to be included in meta-analyses because it may cause a change in the significance of the pooled variables (French et al., 2005; Moher & Tsertsvadze, 2006). This is of special importance in the present meta-analysis because the prevailing paradigm changed from viewing "oxidative stress" as a cause of atherosclerosis (Witztum, 1994) to viewing it as being merely a result of questionable significance (Witztum & Steinberg, 2001). In addition, we had to assess the completeness of the retrieved data and its validity with respect to the complete body of published data (Bennett et al., 2004). Towards this end, we have devised an algorithm similar to the "capture-recapture technique" proposed by Spoor et al. (Spoor et al., 1996). Spoor et al. used different methods of data retrieval to assess their results. We used, for the same purpose, different time frames. Briefly, to achieve as random as possible subset of studies (Furukawa et al., 2002), we searched the Medline database to identify studies published between 1.1.1990 and 1.8.2003 and used studies dating from 1.8.2003 until 1.2.2006 to reassert our findings, as proposed by Moher & Tsertsvadze (Moher & Tsertsvadze, 2006). By that, we have minimized the bias towards recent publications.

## 2.2 Data analysis

The difference between individuals with prevalent CVD and their controls, as observed in each of the selected studies, was expressed in terms of two factors: (i) the standard mean difference (SMD), which is a composite index, and (ii) the 95% confidence interval of the

SMD, which reflects both the mean difference and the standard deviation. Our study required the use of SMD for two reasons: (i) it allows pooling of results obtained from different studies and (ii) its use compensates, at least partially, for the use of different methods, different units of measurement and inter-lab differences (Deeks et al., 2001). We implemented SMD by using "Hedges' adjusted g" because it contains a correction for small sample bias (Bennett et al., 2004).

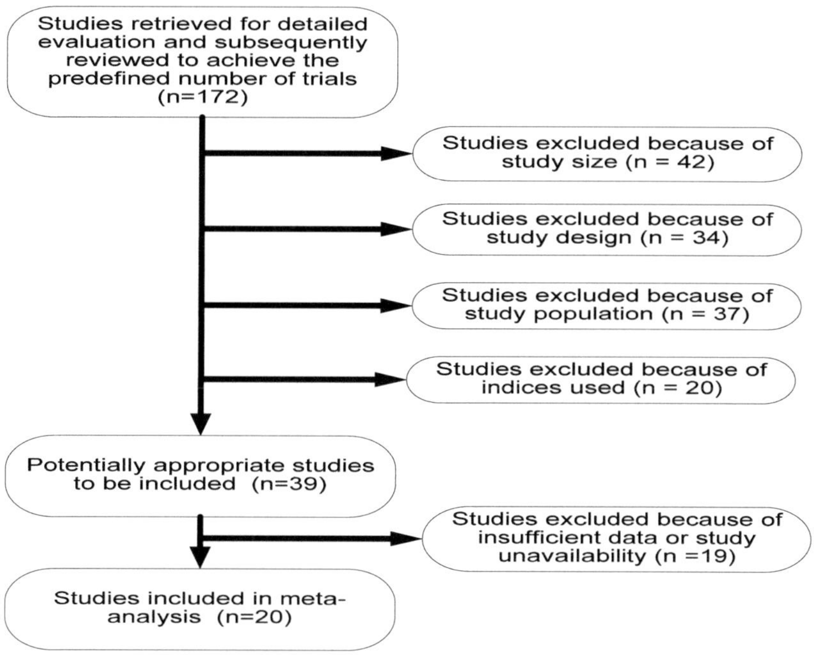


Fig. 1. An outline of the flow of studies in the meta-analyses. We identified many publications that contained the required sets of keywords (e.g. [CVD or CHD] and oxidative stress).

To pool our results, we have considered two possible models, namely the "fixed effect model", which assumes that all the studies and trials are the repeating of the same experiment (Lau et al., 1998) or the "random effects model" of DerSimonian and Laird, which assumes that the clinical trials estimate a different, yet related, variables with a common distribution (Higgins et al., 2002; Lau et al., 1998). From these two models, we chose to use the random effects model, because we expected heterogeneous results from observational studies (Egger et al., 1998). In our view, the "fixed effect model" oversimplifies the problem and its accuracy has been questioned by others in the same context (Lau et al., 1998), particularly when there was a need to pool results of heterogeneous populations (Lau et al., 1998).
In our analyses of the data, we relate not only to the mean value of the pooled variables. We also used the collected data to assess the credibility of the results as previously proposed by Smith et al. (Smith et al., 1997). Assessment of heterogeneity in a meta-analysis of observational studies is as important as the mean results (Egger et al., 1998; Egger et al., 1997a). We assessed the heterogeneity in terms of the following indices as proposed by Song

(Song et al., 2001): (i) $\chi^2$ (Deeks et al., 2001), (ii) $i^2$ (used by the RevMan 4.2.8 software) and (iii) $\log(\chi^2/DF+1)$, where DF is the number of degrees of freedom (Deeks et al., 2001), for comparing the degree of heterogeneity between heterogeneous results.

To detect variables that affect our models, we used stratification, clustering of associated variables and meta-regression models (Smith et al., 1997; Song et al., 2001). Yet, unlike in the case of clinical trials, we analyzed either the complete trial or a specific subgroup within the trial (Lau et al., 1998). We also analyzed the correlations between indices of oxidative stress and various stages of CVD, to determine causality (Egger et al., 1998; Mulrow, 1994; Smith et al., 1997). To assess the effects of exposure variables on the outcome, we used stratification for common risk-related variables such as age (in subgroups), gender and history of smoking (Smith et al., 1997; Sterne, et al., 2001). We also used stratification for variables specific to the pathology (e.g. stable and unstable angina pectoris in CVD), as proposed by Smith et al (Smith et al., 1997). We used meta-regression (logistic and multiple linear) to model the increase in continuous and ordinal SMD, as well as the annual event rates (Lau et al., 1998). We used the observed SMD as our dependent variable and the covariates of interest (independent variables) to assess the sources of heterogeneity (Lau et al., 1998). A mixed stepwise regression was used to detect trends and factors affecting SMD of MDA concentration in CVD (Lau et al., 1998).

To detect (and assess) the degree of bias in our meta-analyses, we have used both the "Trim and Fill method" (Duval & Tweedie , 2000) and a simple funnel plots (Sutton et al., 2000). A funnel plot is a regression of each trial's effect size against a measure of its size (e.g. 1/standard error) (Sutton et al., 2000). An asymmetry in a forest plot is attributed to the high probability that smaller studies with less statistical power are not published. Asymmetric publications were "trimmed" and then the number of studies missing was calculated. We used a simulation to fill the missing studies as described by Duval & Tweedie (Duval & Tweedie, 2000), thus verifying our initial assumption. We used additional methods to assess the relations between study size and results, mainly because publication-bias is not the only reason for asymmetry in funnel plots, and because this method may be subjective and have a relatively high false-positive rate of detecting bias (Sterne et al., 2001). We compensated for the subjective nature of graphical assessment by using the rank correlation method (Thornton and Lee, 2000) and an adjustment of the "Egger's method" (Egger et al., 1997b). Rank correlation is the statistical analogue of the funnel plot, namely a regression of the effect size (SMD) against both sizes of study and 1/SE (Thornton and Lee, 2000). We used an adjustment of the "Egger's method" to detect publication bias and its direction. We defined the standard normal deviate (SND) as the mean difference, divided by its standard error regressed against the estimate's precision (Bennett et al., 2004). We defined the threshold p-value for the intercept at a value of 0.1 to detect possible bias (Bennett et al., 2004).

## 3. Results

As depicted in Fig. 1, we reviewed 172 studies, of which 20 were selected for analysis. These chosen 20 studies compared 1068 CVD patients to 2128 matched controls, using 15 common indices to assess oxidative stress. A summary of the results is given in Fig. 2 (Akkus et al., 1996; Cavalca et al., 2001; Chiu et al., 1994; Cipollone et al., 2000; Clejan et al., 2002; Delanty et al., 1997; Durak et al., 2001; Ferns et al., 2000; Gackowski et al., 2001; Haidari et al., 2001; Halevy et al., 1997; Karmansky et al., 1996; Kesavulu et al., 2001; Kostner et al., 1997;

McMurray et al., 1992; Schisterman et al., 2002; Singh et al., 1995; Tamer et al., 2002; Turgan et al., 1999; Weinbrenner et al., 2003).

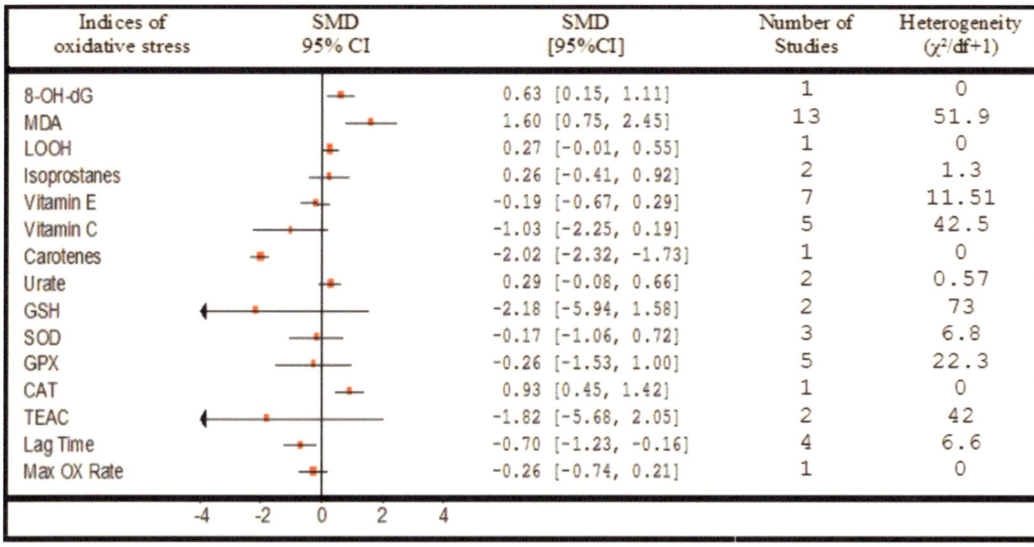


| Indices of oxidative stress | SMD [95%CI] | Number of Studies | Heterogeneity ($\chi^2$/df+1) |
|---|---|---|---|
| 8-OH-dG | 0.63 [0.15, 1.11] | 1 | 0 |
| MDA | 1.60 [0.75, 2.45] | 13 | 51.9 |
| LOOH | 0.27 [-0.01, 0.55] | 1 | 0 |
| Isoprostanes | 0.26 [-0.41, 0.92] | 2 | 1.3 |
| Vitamin E | -0.19 [-0.67, 0.29] | 7 | 11.51 |
| Vitamin C | -1.03 [-2.25, 0.19] | 5 | 42.5 |
| Carotenes | -2.02 [-2.32, -1.73] | 1 | 0 |
| Urate | 0.29 [-0.08, 0.66] | 2 | 0.57 |
| GSH | -2.18 [-5.94, 1.58] | 2 | 73 |
| SOD | -0.17 [-1.06, 0.72] | 3 | 6.8 |
| GPX | -0.26 [-1.53, 1.00] | 5 | 22.3 |
| CAT | 0.93 [0.45, 1.42] | 1 | 0 |
| TEAC | -1.82 [-5.68, 2.05] | 2 | 42 |
| Lag Time | -0.70 [-1.23, -0.16] | 4 | 6.6 |
| Max OX Rate | -0.26 [-0.74, 0.21] | 1 | 0 |

Fig. 2. Indices of oxidative stress in cardiovascular disease. We present both graphically and numerically the pooled standardized mean difference (SMD) and the 95% confidence interval. Also given is the heterogeneity, as defined by $\chi^2$/df + 1, of the studies regarding each index. Note that MDA is the only accepted index of oxidative stress that shows a mean difference greater the 1SMD.

Given the prevailing paradigm regarding the association between atherosclerosis and lipid peroxidation (Witztum & Steinberg, 2001), it is not surprising that MDA was the most frequently used index utilized to assess oxidative stress (13/20 studies). Furthermore, only MDA exhibited a strong effect size, given by a SMD of 1.60 (0.75 to 2.45). Using the "Trim and Fill" method (Duval & Tweedie, 2000) revealed that at least three studies were missing from the funnel plot. Adjusting for the latter finding resulted in a much lower SMD of 0.71 (0.37 to 1.05). The "Egger method" (Egger et al., 1997b) identified an intercept that was significant and positive, supporting the conclusion that the previously observed differences were overestimated.

We performed a mixed stepwise regression for MDA concentrations, factoring in age, gender, smoking habits, severity of CVD, prevalence of hypertension and diabetes mellitus as well as the use of NSAIDs. This analysis indicated that the inclusion of smokers in both CVD patients and control groups (estimate[1] = -1.3, p =0.04), results in an underestimation of the association between CVD and oxidative stress. By contrast, the inclusion of patients with both acute (severe CVD) and chronic (mild CVD) coronary syndromes (estimate =3.1, p=0.01), results in an overestimation of the latter associations.

We stratified the results from those studies that assessed MDA concentrations into three groups: (i) patients with unstable angina pectoris (UAP), (ii) patients with stable angina

[1]**Estimate:** A numerical value obtained from a statistical sample and assigned to a population parameter.

pectoris (SAP) and (iii) healthy controls. As seen in Fig. 3, the MDA concentrations of patients with SAP are not different from matched controls, whereas UAP patients have significantly higher MDA concentrations than both healthy controls and patients with SAP.
We also stratified the results from two types of studies, those that had acute coronary conditions (MI, UAP) and those CVD patients who had chronic coronary conditions (SAP and occlusions). As seen in Fig. 4, patients with acute coronary conditions had marked and significantly higher MDA concentrations (SMD = 2.30, 0.93 to 3.67) than matched controls. By contrast, patients with chronic coronary conditions had only slightly higher MDA concentrations (SMD = 0.60, 0.18 to 1.01) as compared with matched controls.
The concentrations of beta-carotene, as evaluated by Singh et al. (Singh et al., 1995), were significantly lower in CVD patients than in matched controls. The difference between the concentrations all other low molecular weight antioxidants (LMWA) in patients with CVD and healthy controls were not statistically significant (Fig. 2). In six of the seven studies vitamin E concentration in CVD patients and controls was similar (SMD = 0.02, -0.17 to 0.21).
Significantly lower concentrations were observed only by Singh et al. Furthermore, pooling the results from all the seven studies failed to achieve statistically significant differences (SMD = -0.19, -0.67 to 0.29), although the heterogeneity index substantially increased from 1.35 to 11.51. The differences between the results of Singh et al. and all other studies cannot be attributed either to publication bias or to small-sample bias. A viable possibility is that the difference is due to selection bias, particularly by a biased selection of controls. Indeed, the major difference between the results obtained by Singh et al. and the results observed in all the other studies assessing LMWA was that Singh et al. selected their control group to exclude most, if not all of the CVD-related risk factors (smoking, DM and glucose intolerance), whereas the CVD patients were not devoid of these risk factors.

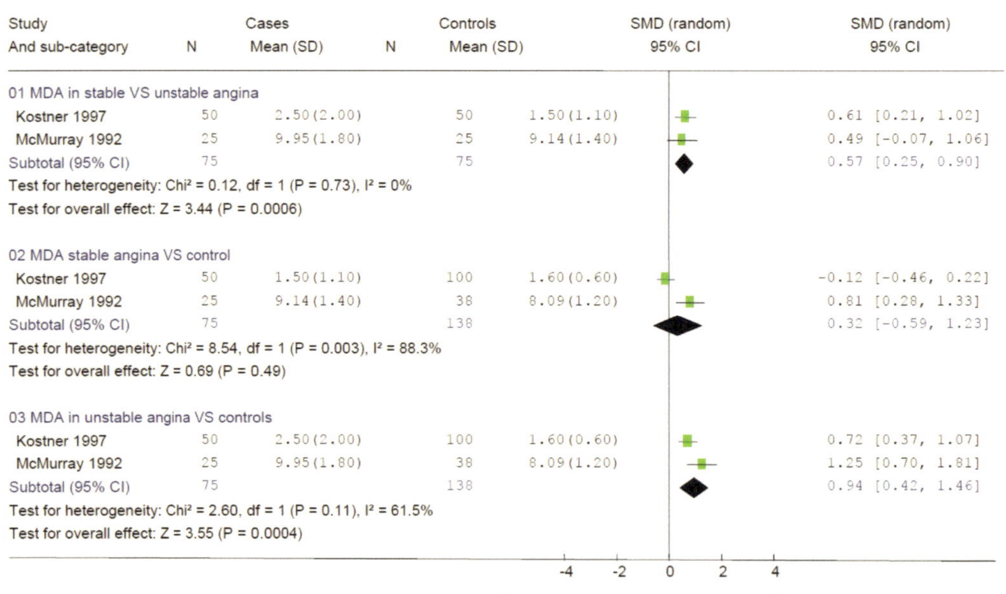


Fig. 3. A forest plot of studies assessing the differences between patients with stable angina pectoris and patients with unstable angina pectoris (upper panel) and comparison of each of these groups with controls (two lower panels).

Unfortunately, those studies that used either DNA damage or total antioxidant capacity (TEAC) to assess oxidative stress in patients with CVD in comparison to healthy controls (Fig. 2) were too few and too small to enable any conclusions.

## 4. Discussion

Based on many lines of indirect evidence, oxidative stress has long been associated with CVD. The following findings have been considered to lend support to the oxidative theory of CVD: (i) oxidized LDL may cause formation of foam cell in-vitro (Chisolm & Steinberg, 2000), (ii) the development of atherosclerosis is preceded by an increase of the levels of many indicators of oxidative stress in lab animals (Chisolm & Steinberg, 2000) and (iii) the incidence of CVD in individuals with low concentrations of antioxidants is relatively high (Chisolm and Steinberg, 2000). These (and other) findings and clinical trials led researchers to two assumptions: (i) oxidative stress plays a pivotal role in the formation of atherogenic plaque and (ii) individuals with prevalent CVD are likely to be under oxidative stress and therefore have high plasma concentrations of lipid peroxidation products and loss of LMWA.

The first assumption has long been disputed and is currently under scrutiny (Williams & Fisher, 2005). The second assumption is weakened by the results of our current meta-analysis, which shows that the prevalence of CVD is only slightly associated with OS, as defined on the basis MDA concentration. By contrast, no evidence is available for association between CVD and OS, as determined on the basis of all other indices of oxidative stress. Specifically, the concentrations of almost all the micronutrients in the plasma of CVD patients are within normal ranges (Fig. 2), the activities of relevant enzymes did not differ from those observed in matched controls (Fig. 2). The same results were observed for most of the indices of lipid peroxidation. The only index that is significantly different with the prevalence of CVD is the plasma concentration of MDA. Even if we choose to ignore the reservations regarding the use of MDA as an index of lipid peroxidation (Draper et al., 1993), the possibility of publication bias should not be ignored. Hence, we think that the existing evidence for association between oxidative stress and the prevalence of CVD is quite weak. In other words, it appears that the role of oxidative stress in atherogenesis has been overestimated. In accordance with this conclusion, is the viewpoint of the recent review, regarding association of several more OS indices (circulation levels of oxidized LDL and myeloperoxidase) with CVD (Strobel et al., 2011). The authors conclude that "results of studies using Ox-LDL have been equivocal" and that "the ability of oxidative stress biomarkers to predict CVD has yet to be established".

The latter considerations accord with the current trend in cardiovascular disease research, which views atherosclerosis as mostly an inflammatory disease (Ross, 1999) and implies that oxidative stress is a result and not the cause for atherosclerosis. This trend also accords with and therefore is strengthened by two of our findings: (i) we observed that patients with UAP, a condition commonly associated with acute inflammation, are under higher "oxidative stress", as assessed by the serum concentration of MDA, than both patients with SAP and matched controls (Fig. 3) and (ii) we observed that studies including more acute conditions are under higher "oxidative stress" than matched controls (Fig. 4).

In our opinion, these findings are of little relevance to the possibility that many individuals may benefit from antioxidant supplementation.

Our ongoing research is aimed at developing such an assay (or assays) that can serve as a basis for selective antioxidant supplementation. Our working hypothesis is a two step approach of identifying those individuals that may benefit from antioxidant supplementation. The first step is an initial, short-term treatment with vitamin E. The second step should be to assess plasma concentrations of lipid peroxidation products and to continue treatment with vitamin E only to individuals, responding to treatment by reducing significantly plasma concentration of lipid peroxidation products. In conclusion, we have no evidence that justify indiscriminate supplementation of vitamin E, nor do we have sufficient evidence to ban it, as recommended by the authors of the Cache County Study (Hayden et al., 2007). At present we have no assay that can be used to identify patients that are likely to benefit from Vitamin E supplementation.

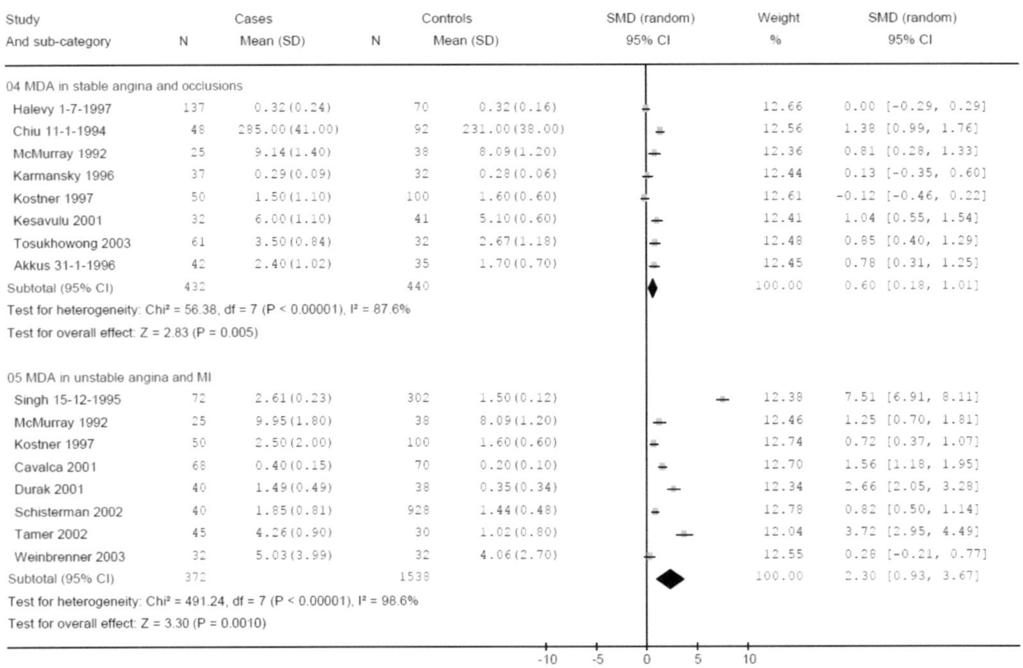


Fig. 4. A forest plot comparing two strata of studies. The first stratum compares the differences between patients with either stable angina pectoris or mild occlusions of the coronary arteries and healthy controls. The second stratum compares the differences between patients with either unstable angina pectoris or MI and healthy controls. Notably, while the first stratum of patients with SAP varies slightly from healthy controls, the second stratum of patients with UAP shows a significant difference. The two strata differ significantly (p = 0.02).

## 5. Conclusion

Our meta-analysis shows that the commonly accepted paradigm regarding the role of OS in the pathogenesis of CVD appears to be overestimated. CVD is associated with OS only when the evaluation of OS is based on plasma concentrations of MDA. Notably, even this

association is questionable due to (i) poor reliability of the laboratory assay of MDA and (ii) publication bias.
Most of the clinical trials that were designed to reduce OS by means of antioxidant supplementation yielded disappointing results. The latter results are consistent with the results of our meta-analysis. Hence, oxidative stress is only weakly associated with the prevalence of cardiovascular disease.

## 6. Acknowledgments

We thank the Lady Davis foundation and Israel Science Foundation (research grant 362/02-18) for financial support. We would also like to thank Dr. Yariv Gerber and Prof. Uri Goldburt for their sound guidance and Mrs. Ariela Bor for her skillful technical assistance.

## 7. References

Abuja, P.M. and Albertini, R., 2001. Methods for monitoring oxidative stress, lipid peroxidation and oxidation resistance of lipoproteins. Clin.Chim.Acta 306, 1-17.

Akkus, I., Saglam, N.I., Caglayan, O., Vural, H., Kalak, S., and Saglam, M., 1996. Investigation of erythrocyte membrane lipid peroxidation and antioxidant defense systems of patients with coronary artery disease (CAD) documented by angiography. Clin.Chim.Acta 244, 173-180.

Bennett, D.A., Latham, N.K., Stretton, C., and Anderson, C.S., 2004. Capture-recapture is a potentially useful method for assessing publication bias. Journal of Clinical Epidemiology 57, 349-357.

Bjelakovic, G., Nikolova D., Gluud L.L. et al, 2007. Mortality in randomized trials of antioxidant supplements for primary and secondary prevention: systematic review and meta-analysis. JAMA 297, 842- 857.

Cavalca, V., Cighetti, G., Bamonti, F., Loaldi, A., Bortone, L., Novembrino, C., De Franceschi, M., Belardinelli, R., and Guazzi, M.D., 2001. Oxidative stress and homocysteine in coronary artery disease. Clin.Chem. 47, 887-892.

Chisolm, G.M. and Steinberg, D., 2000. The oxidative modification hypothesis of atherogenesis: an overview. Free Radical Biology and Medicine 28, 1815-1826.

Chiu, H.C., Jeng, J.R., and Shieh, S.M., 1994. Increased oxidizability of plasma low density lipoprotein from patients with coronary artery disease. Biochim.Biophys.Acta 1225, 200-208.

Cipollone, F., Ciabattoni, G., Patrignani, P., Pasquale, M., Di Gregorio, D., Bucciarelli, T., Davi, G., Cuccurullo, F., and Patrono, C., 2000. Oxidant Stress and Aspirin-Insensitive Thromboxane Biosynthesis in Severe Unstable Angina. Circulation 102, 1007.

Clejan, S., Japa, S., Clemetson, C., Hasabnis, S.S., David, O., and Talano, J.V., 2002. Blood histamine is associated with coronary artery disease, cardiac events and severity of inflammation and atherosclerosis. J Cell Mol.Med 6, 583-592.

Deeks, J.J., 2001. Systematic reviews in health care: Systematic reviews of evaluations of diagnostic and screening tests. BMJ 323, 157-162.

Deeks, J.J. and Altman, D.G., 2004. Diagnostic tests 4: likelihood ratios. BMJ 329, 168-169.

Deeks, J.J., Altman, D.G., and Bradburn, M.J., 2001. Statistical methods for examining heterogeneity and combing results from several studies in meta-analysis.

Systematic reviews in health care Meta-analysis in context, Second ed. BMJ Publishing Group , pp. 285-312.

Delanty, N., Reilly, M.P., Pratico, D., Lawson, J.A., McCarthy, J.F., Wood, A.E., Ohnishi, S.T., Fitzgerald, D.J., and FitzGerald, G.A., 1997. 8-Epi PGF2{alpha} Generation During Coronary Reperfusion: A Potential Quantitative Marker of Oxidant Stress In Vivo. Circulation 95, 2492.

Dotan, Y., Lichtenberg, D., and Pinchuk, I., 2004. Lipid peroxidation cannot be used as a universal criterion of oxidative stress. Progress in Lipid Research 43, 200-227.

Dotan, Y., Lichtenberg, D., Pinchuk, I., 2009a. No evidence supports vitamin E indiscriminate supplementation. BioFactors 35, 469-473.

Dotan, Y., Pinchuk, I., Lichtenberg, D., Leshno, M., 2009b. Decision analysis supports the paradigm that indiscriminate supplementation of vitamin E does more harm than good. *ATVB* 29, 1304-1309.

Draper, H.H., Squires, E.J., Mahmoodi, H., Wu, J., Agarwal, S., and Hadley, M., 1993. A comparative evaluation of thiobarbituric acid methods for the determination of malondialdehyde in biological materials. Free Radic.Biol.Med. 15, 353-363.

Durak, I., Kacmaz, M., Cimen, M.Y., Buyukkocak, U., and Ozturk, H.S., 2001. Blood oxidant/antioxidant status of atherosclerotic patients. Int.J.Cardiol. 77, 293-297.

Duval, S. and Tweedie, R., 2000. Trim and Fill: A Simple Funnel-Plot-Based Method of Testing and Adjusting for Publication Bias in Meta-Analysis. Biometrics 56, 455-463.

Egger, M., Schneider, M., and Smith, G.D., 1998. Meta-analysis Spurious precision? Meta-analysis of observational studies. BMJ 316, 140-144.

Egger, M., Smith, G.D., and Phillips, A.N., 1997a. Meta-analysis: Principles and procedures. BMJ 315, 1533-1537.

Egger, M., Smith, G.D., Schneider, M., and Minder, C., 1997b. Bias in meta-analysis detected by a simple, graphical test. BMJ 315, 629-634.

Ferns, G., Williams, J., Forster, L., Tull, S., Starkey, B., and Gershlick, A., 2000. Cholesterol standardized plasma vitamin E levels are reduced in patients with severe angina pectoris. Int.J Exp Pathol. 81, 57-62.

French, S., McDonald, S., McKenzie, J., and Green, S., 2005. Investing in updating: how do conclusions change when Cochrane systematic reviews are updated? BMC Medical Research Methodology 5, 33.

Furukawa, T.A., Guyatt, G.H., and Griffith, L.E., 2002. Can we individualize the 'number needed to treat'? An empirical study of summary effect measures in meta-analyses. Int.J.Epidemiol. 31, 72-76.

Gackowski, D., Kruszewski, M., Jawien, A., Ciecierski, M., and Olinski, R., 2001. Further evidence that oxidative stress may be a risk factor responsible for the development of atherosclerosis. Free Radic.Biol.Med. 31, 542-547.

Haidari, M., Javadi, E., Kadkhodaee, M., and Sanati, A., 2001. Enhanced Susceptibility to Oxidation and Diminished Vitamin E Content of LDL from Patients with Stable Coronary Artery Disease. Clin Chem 47, 1234.

Halevy, D., Thiery, J., Nagel, D., Arnold, S., Erdmann, E., Hofling, B., Cremer, P., and Seidel, D., 1997. Increased Oxidation of LDL in Patients With Coronary Artery Disease Is Independent From Dietary Vitamins E and C. Arterioscler Thromb Vasc Biol 17, 1432.

Halliwell, B. and Gutteridge, J.M., 1990. Role of free radicals and catalytic metal ions in human disease: an overview. Methods Enzymol. 186, 1-85.

Hayden, K.M., Welsh-Bohmer, K.A., Wengreen, H.J., Zandi, P.P., Lyketsos, C.G., and Breitner, J.C.S., 2007. Risk of Mortality with Vitamin E Supplements: The Cache County Study. The American Journal of Medicine 120, 180-184.

Higgins, J., Thompson, S., Deeks, J., and Altman, D., 2002. Statistical heterogeneity in systematic reviews of clinical trials: a critical appraisal of guidelines and practice. J Health Serv.Res Policy 7, 51-61.

Jha, P., Flather, M., Lonn, E., Farkouh, M., and Yusuf, S., 1995. The Antioxidant Vitamins and Cardiovascular Disease: A Critical Review of Epidemiologic and Clinical Trial Data. Ann Intern Med 123, 860-872.

Karmansky, I., Shnaider, H., Palant, A., and Gruener, N., 1996. Plasma Lipid Oxidation and Susceptibility of Low-Density Lipoproteins to Oxidation in Male Patients With Stable Coronary Artery Disease. Clinical Biochemistry 29, 573-579.

Kesavulu, M.M., Rao, B.K., Giri, R., Vijaya, J., Subramanyam, G., and Apparao, C., 2001. Lipid peroxidation and antioxidant enzyme status in Type 2 diabetics with coronary heart disease. Diabetes Res.Clin.Pract. 53, 33-39.

Kostner, K., Hornykewycz, S., Yang, P., Neunteufl, T., Glogar, D., Weidinger, F., Maurer, G., and Huber, K., 1997. Is oxidative stress causally linked to unstable angina pectoris? A study in 100 CAD patients and matched controls. Cardiovasc.Res. 36, 330-336.

Lau, J., Ioannidis, J.P., and Schmid, C.H., 1998. Summing up evidence: one answer is not always enough. The Lancet 351, 123-127.

McMurray, J., Chopra, M., Abdullah, I., Smith, W.E., and Dargie, H.J., 1992. Evidence for oxidative stress in unstable angina. Br.Heart J 68, 454-457.

Miller, E.R. III, Pastor-Barriuso, R., Dalal, D. et al., 2005. Meta-analysis: high-dosage vitamin E supplementation may increase all-cause mortality. Ann Intern Med 142, 37- 46.

Moher, D. and Tsertsvadze, A., 2006. Systematic reviews: when is an update an update? The Lancet 367, 881-883.

Morrow, J.D., 2003. Is Oxidant Stress a Connection Between Obesity and Atherosclerosis? Arterioscler Thromb Vasc Biol 23, 368-370.

Mulrow, C.D., 1994. Systematic Reviews: Rationale for systematic reviews. BMJ 309, 597.

Parthasarathy, S., Khan-Merchant, N., Penumetcha, M., and Santanam, N., 2001. Oxidative stress in cardiovascular disease. J Nucl.Cardiol. 8, 379-389.

Ross, R., 1999. Atherosclerosis -- An Inflammatory Disease. N Engl J Med 340, 115-126.

Schisterman, E.F., Faraggi, D., Browne, R., Freudenheim, J., Dorn, J., Muti, P., Armstrong, D., Reiser, B., and Trevisan, M., 2002. Minimal and best linear combination of oxidative stress and antioxidant biomarkers to discriminate cardiovascular disease. Nutr Metab Cardiovasc.Dis. 12, 259-266.

Shekelle, P.G., Morton, S.C., Jungvig, L.K., Udani, J., Spar, M., Tu, W., Suttorp, J., Coulter, I., Newberry, S.J., and Hardy, M., 2004. Effect of supplemental vitamin E for the prevention and treatment of cardiovascular disease. J.Gen.Intern.Med. 19, 380-389.

Singh, R.B., Ghosh, S., Niaz, M.A., Singh, R., Beegum, R., Chibo, H., Shoumin, Z., and Postiglione, A., 1995. Dietary Intake, Plasma Levels of Antioxidant Vitamins, and Oxidative Stress in Relation to Coronary Artery Disease in Elderly Subjects. The American Journal of Cardiology 76, 1233-1238.

Smith, G.D., Egger, M., and Phillips, A.N., 1997. Meta-analysis: Beyond the grand mean? BMJ 315, 1610.

Song, F., Sheldon, T.A., Sutton, A.J., Abrams, K.R., and Jones, D.R., 2001. Methods for Exploring Heterogeneity in Meta-Analysis. Eval Health Prof 24, 126-151.

Spoor, P., Airey, M., Bennett, C., Greensill, J., and Williams, R., 1996. Use of the capture-recapture technique to evaluate the completeness of systematic literature searches. BMJ 313, 342-343.

Steinbrecher, U.P., Parthasarathy, S., Leake, D.S., Witztum, J.L., and Steinberg, D., 1984. Modification of Low-Density Lipoprotein by Endothelial-Cells Involves Lipid-Peroxidation and Degradation of Low-Density Lipoprotein Phospholipids. Proceedings of the National Academy of Sciences of the United States of America-Biological Sciences 81, 3883-3887.

Sterne, J.A.C., Egger, M., and Smith, G.D., 2001. Systematic reviews in health care: Investigating and dealing with publication and other biases in meta-analysis. BMJ 323, 101-105.

Strobel, N.A., Fassett R.G., Marsh S.A., Coombes J.S., 2011. Oxidative stress biomarkers as predictors of cardiovascular disease International Journal of Cardiology 147, 191–201.

Stroup, D.F., Berlin, J.A., Morton, S.C., Olkin, I., Williamson, G.D., Rennie, D., Moher, D., Becker, B.J., Sipe, T.A., Thacker, S.B., and for the Meta-analysis Of Observational Studies in Epidemiology Group, 2000. Meta-analysis of Observational Studies in Epidemiology: A Proposal for Reporting. JAMA 283, 2008-2012.

Sutton, A.J., Duval, S.J., Tweedie, R.L., Abrams, K.R., and Jones, D.R., 2000. Empirical assessment of effect of publication bias on meta-analyses. BMJ 320, 1574-1577.

Tamer, L., Sucu, N., Polat, G., Ercan, B., Aytacoglu, B., Yucebilgic, G., Unlu, A., Dikmengil, M., and Atik, U., 2002. Decreased serum total antioxidant status and erythrocyte-reduced glutathione levels are associated with increased serum malondialdehyde in atherosclerotic patients. Arch.Med.Res. 33, 257-260.

Thornton, A. and Lee, P., 2000. Publication bias in meta-analysis: its causes and consequences. Journal of Clinical Epidemiology 53, 207-216.

Turgan, N., Boydak, B., Habif, S., Gulter, C., Senol, B., Mutaf, I., Ozmen, D., and Bayindir, O., 1999. Urinary hypoxanthine and xanthine levels in acute coronary syndromes. Int.J Clin Lab Res. 29, 162-165.

Vivekananthan, D.P., Penn, M.S., Sapp, S.K., Hsu, A., and Topol, E.J., 2003. Use of antioxidant vitamins for the prevention of cardiovascular disease: meta-analysis of randomised trials. Lancet 361, 2017-2023.

Weinbrenner, T., Cladellas, M., Isabel Covas, M., Fito, M., Tomas, M., Senti, M., Bruguera, J., and Marrugat, J., 2003. High oxidative stress in patients with stable coronary heart disease. Atherosclerosis 168, 99-106.

Williams KJ, Fisher EA, 2005. Oxidation, lipoproteins, and atherosclerosis: which is wrong, the antioxidants or the theory? Curr Opin Clin Nutr Metab Care 8, 139 –146.

Witztum, J.L., 1994. The oxidation hypothesis of atherosclerosis. The Lancet 344, 793-795.

Witztum, J.L., 1998. To E or Not To E—How Do We Tell? Circulation 98, 2785.

Witztum, J.L. and Steinberg, D., 2001. The Oxidative Modification Hypothesis of Atherosclerosis; Does It Hold for Humans? Trends in Cardiovascular Medicine 11, 93-102.

# Vascular Biology of Reactive Oxygen Species and NADPH Oxidases: Role in Atherogenesis

Adrian Manea[1,2]
[1]"Petru Poni"Institute of Macromolecular Chemistry, Iasi
[2]"Nicolae Simionescu" Institute of Cellular Biology and Pathology, Bucharest
Romania

## 1. Introduction

Eukaryotic cells face constantly the formation of reactive oxygen species (ROS) as a result of their aerobic metabolism. ROS play an important role in the regulation of signal transduction pathways and gene expression but its over-production is acutely harmful to cells, particularly in cardiovascular diseases (CVD) by a mechanism that is not fully understood. Most CVD (the leading cause of mortality in developed countries) entail the focal development of atherosclerotic plaques in response to various deleterious insults that affect the artery wall's cells (Simionescu, 2007). Atheroma may occlude partially or totally the arterial lumen and ultimately, rupture of the vulnerable plaques results in thrombus formation and obstruction of the vessels of vital organs like heart, brain, lung, and kidney. Atheroma formation is characterized by progressive lipid accumulation in the vessel's intima, dysfunctions of endothelial cells (EC) and smooth muscle cells (SMC), and a strong inflammatory reaction with the participation of extravasated immune cells (Fearon & Faux, 2009). Compelling evidence (including ours) revealed that oxidative stress and NADPH oxidase - derived ROS play the key role in all stages of atherosclerosis and that genetic ablation of various oxidase components protects the cells against the detrimental effects of oxidative stress (Simionescu et al., 2009). Therefore, understanding the molecular mechanisms of ROS formation and function is a prerequisite of an effective anti-oxidative stress therapy.

## 2. Reactive oxygen species formation in the vasculature

As the name indicates, ROS are a class of highly reactive molecules derived from chemical conversion of molecular oxygen ($O_2$). ROS are formed in all the aerobic cells and organisms as by-products of metabolic and respiration processes, under the influence of ionizing radiation or produced deliberately by specialized enzyme systems. ROS formation is initiated by reduction of $O_2$ with one electron leading to the formation of short-lived and highly reactive superoxide anion ($O_2^{\bullet-}$). Successive reduction of $O_2^{\bullet-}$, protonation or interaction with various converting enzymes gives rise to a large spectrum of molecules with diverse physicochemical characteristics such as $H_2O_2$ and $HO^{\bullet}$. The dismutation of $O_2^{\bullet-}$ to $H_2O_2$ can be either spontaneous or catalyzed by specialized enzymes namely, members of the superoxide dismutase family. $H_2O_2$ may be completely reduced to $H_2O$ by means of various peroxidases such as catalase and glutathione peroxidase or partially reduced to HO•, one of the most powerful oxidizing agent identified in biological systems. The generation of HO• is mediated by various free transition metal ions (e.g., $Fe^{2+}$, $Cu^{2+}$) via the Haber-Weiss reaction (Manea, 2010).

Apart from the aforementioned chemical processing of $O_2$, superoxide can react with other molecular species including nitrogen species such as nitric oxide (NO) or polyunsaturated fatty acids. The reaction between $O_2^{\bullet -}$ and NO is tightly controlled by the rate of diffusion of both radicals, and result in the formation of ONOO- a potent oxidant. Alternative reactions may led to the generation of mixed reactive oxygen and nitrogen radicals such as nitrogen dioxide radical (•$NO_2$) and nitryl chloride ($NO_2Cl$) (Turrens, 2003).

Lipid peroxidation products formation represents an important mechanism whereby ROS elicit physiological and pathophysiological function in the living cells. ROS (especially HO•, •$NO_2$, and ONOO-) may react with polyunsaturated fatty acids present on biological membranes or circulating/infiltrated lipoproteins, a condition that facilitate the formation of fatty acid peroxyl radical (R-COO-) that can further attack adjacent fatty acid chains and trigger the production of other lipid radicals by a chain reaction mechanism (Negre-Salvayre et al., 2010; Riahi et al., 2010; Shao & Heinecke, 2009).

Tyrosyl radicals produced by myeloperoxidase (MPO) have also been shown to be involved in the initiation of lipid peroxidation (Hazen et al., 1997). *In vitro* studies revealed that lipid peroxidation occurred only in the presence of free L-tyrosine suggesting that tyrosyl radicals formation by MPO are essential mediators for the initiation of lipid peroxidation and subsequent LDL oxidation by activated human neutrophils, which contain abundant MPO and $H_2O_2$ (Savenkova et al., 1994). Tyrosyl radicals have also been shown to play a role in LDL oxidation *in vivo* and in atherogenesis. Analysis of LDL isolated from human vascular tissue demonstrated that *o,o'*-dityrosine levels were 100 times greater than that observed in circulating LDL. Similarly, *o,o'*-dityrosine formation was found to be robust increased in atherosclerotic fatty streaks and in advanced atheromas compared to normal aortic tissue, indicating that tyrosyl radical formation was capable of protein damage *in vivo* (Leeuwenburgh et al., 1997).

## 3. Molecular targets of ROS

The biological function of ROS is highly regulated by their basic physicochemical properties, cellular compartmentalization and the formation rate. Since $O_2^{\bullet -}$ is a short-lived charged species, it cannot diffuse through biological membranes and acts closeness of the formation site. Nevertheless, an anion channel-dependent plasma membrane transport mechanisms has been demonstrated to play an important role in mediating cell-to-cell communication. Notably, $O_2^{\bullet -}$ is water-soluble and functions either as an oxidizing agent (e.g., one-electron reduction of $O_2^{\bullet -}$ yields $H_2O_2$) or as a reducing agent (e.g., ONOO- formation). HO• is extremely reactive and does not diffuse more that a few molecular diameters from its site of formation (Touyz, 2003). In contrast, $H_2O_2$ is highly stable under physiological conditions. Being an uncharged molecule, $H_2O_2$ is membrane-permeable and able of activating downstream signalling molecules relatively far from the site of formation.

At low, physiological concentration, ROS modulate key signalling processes initiated by hormones, cytokines, vasoactive agents, blood coagulation factors, and hemodynamic shear stress. Reactive oxygen intermediates react at near-diffusion rate and influence the activity of numerous of signalling molecules including receptors, protein kinases/phosphatases, transcription factors, peptides, ion channels and transporters, lipids, carbohydrates, and other oxygen-based species, a process that influence dramatically the cell behavior (Shao & Heinecke, 2009). The affinity of ROS for a specific substrate is dictated by both physicochemical features of the reactive oxygen intermediates and also of the targeted molecules. In addition, the occurrence and the abundance of specific functional groups, such as iron-sulfur centers, disulfide-bonds, amino and hydroxyl groups or fatty acids double-bonds, greatly influence the chemical interactions between ROS and redox-sensitive biological molecules. As initially showed in microorganisms, eukaryotic cells respond to increased generation of $O_2^{\bullet-}$ and $H_2O_2$ by the up-regulation of various gene products, largely antioxidant enzymes and molecules implicated in the preservation of cellular homeostasis, self-renewal, and reparatory processes. In terms of selectivity, $O_2^{\bullet-}$ reacts preferentially with the transcription factors and electron transporters in respiratory chains containing iron-sulfur clusters. In contrast, $H_2O_2$ reacts mainly with the disulfide-bonds present on the protein kinases/phosphatases, transcription factors, and ion channels. Additional compelling evidence highlights that the redox-regulation of cell function represents an evolutionary conserved mechanism that alter directly or indirectly the activities of a large spectrum of signaling molecules (Liu et al., 2005).

Protein tyrosine phosphatases (PTPs) are probably the best characterized signaling molecules targeted directly by ROS, especially of $H_2O_2$, owing to the existence of a highly conserved 230-amino-acid domain that contains reactive cysteine, which catalyzes the hydrolysis of protein phosphotyrosine residues. Consequently, a key mechanism whereby $H_2O_2$ controls various cellular processes is determined by the reversible oxidation of PTPs catalytic cysteines that blocks protein dephosphorylation causing transient inhibition of PTPs.

Notably, several members of the protein tyrosine kinases (PTKs) family, including non-receptor protein tyrosine kinases (i.e., Src, Jak, Pyk) have been shown to be activated in response to cellular redox variations (Tonks, 2006). Nevertheless, the precise molecular mechanisms of PTKs redox regulation are not entirely understood, and it is not clear if the PTK activities are directly correlated with the alterations induced by ROS action on enzyme structures Still, most of the available date suggests that the majority of the effects are attributable to PTP inhibition by ROS rather than PTK oxidation (Tabet et al., 2008).

Another important class of molecules regulated by redox-dependent mechanisms is represented by the mitogen-activated protein kinase (MAPKs) family, that control key physiological processes such as mitosis, differentiation, proliferation, cell survival, and apoptosis. MAPKs are serine/threonine-specific protein kinases which activities are tightly regulated by complex phosphorylation pathways. Emerging evidence demonstrates that in the cardiovascular system, the functions of MAPKs are also influenced by extracellular and intracellular ROS by yet incompletely defined mechanisms (Wu et al., 2008). Apparently, the upstream regulators of MAPKs, namely MAPK kinases (MEKs), PTKs, and PTPs, might be the actual molecular targets of ROS and the genuine sensors of the intracellular redox state changes (Sedeek et al., 2009).

Similar to PTPs, MAPK phosphatases (MKPs) display a highly conserved redox-sensitive cysteine in their catalytic core. Thus, the oxidative inhibition of MKPs may results in the persistent activation of MAPKs, as observed in various developmental or pathological states. Taken together, redox-dependent and as well as redox-independent activation of MAPKs cascades congregate to activate downstream signaling pathway in response to hormones, growth factors, pro-inflammatory mediators, and vasoactive agents. Besides MAPKs, the activity of serine/threonine protein kinases Akt and Rho has been indicated to be redox-sensitive and to play a central role in cellular survival pathways (Lee & Griendling, 2008). Apart from protein kinases/phosphatases and transcription factors, ROS are important regulators calcium homeostasis, by mechanisms that engages reversible thiol oxidation of the cysteine residues present on ion channels and transporters. In the vascular cells ROS, particularly $O_2^{\bullet-}$ and $H_2O_2$, also enhance intracellular $Ca^{2+}$ concentrations by increasing the extracellular influx through the plasma membrane channels and mobilization from intracellular stores, and by the inhibition of Ca2+-ATPases located in the plasma membrane and endoplasmic reticulum. The plasma membrane K+ channels have been shown to be redox-sensitive, a process that mediates hyperpolarization-dependent vascular relaxation (Belia et al., 2009; Briones &Touyz, 2010). These data indicates that the redox status of ion channels and transporters plays an essential role in cell physiology and represents an important determinant of vascular pathology under conditions of the altered production of ROS.

## 4. Antioxidant mechanisms in the cardiovascular cells

ROS are physiologically produced at low concentration during metabolic processes in non-phagocytic cells, by the mitochondrial respiratory chain, cyclooxygenases, lipoxygesases, cytochrome P450 reductase, xanthine oxidase.

Almost three decades ago, the commonly accepted assumption was that the antioxidant system has developed to defend the cells against the damaging and unavoidable effects of ROS, which are capable to produce irreversible, structural, and functional oxidative damage of DNA, proteins, lipids, and carbohydrates. This theory was supported by many experimental evidence regarding the strategic tissular distribution, expression/concentration levels, and localization of the antioxidants within cellular compartments. Nevertheless, soon after the discovery of enzyme systems that deliberately generates ROS (e.g., NADPH oxidases) under physiological and pathological states, it has become apparent that ROS are not just the by-products of aerobic metabolism, but also important signalling molecules (Forman et al., 2010; Go & Jones 2010). Therefore, the subtle relationship among oxidizing and reducing agents permits ROS to function as second messengers and to regulate various cellular functions. Thus, besides neutralization of ROS, the antioxidant system has emerged as a critical regulator of the redox-sensitive processes.

The concentration of various oxygen-based reactive intermediates is maintained in physiological range by a very complex antioxidant system comprising both enzymatic ROS scavengers, namely superoxide dismutase, catalase, glutathione peroxidase, thioredoxin, glutaredoxin, peroxiredoxin, heme oxygenase, and paraoxonase, and non-enzymatic ROS quenchers, such as glutathione, vitamins, lipoate, urate, and ubiquinone (Zadák et al., 2009).

Superoxide dismutases (SOD) represent a family of enzymes that catalyze the dismutation of $O_2^{\bullet-}$ into $O_2$ and $H_2O_2$. Three SOD isoforms are expressed concomitantly in different cellular compartments, including the cytosol (SOD1; Cu/ZnSOD), mitochondria (SOD2; MnSOD), and the extracellular space (SOD3; ecSOD) (Valdivia et al., 2009). Catalase (CAT) is found in peroxisomes where it decomposes $H_2O_2$ to $H_2O$ and $O_2$. Glutathione peroxidases (GPx) represent a family of isoenzymes encoded by separate genes that differ in cellular distribution pattern and substrate specificity. GPx1, the most abundant isoform, is expressed in the cytosol and has $H_2O_2$ as its main substrate. GPx2 is an extracellular space enzyme, while GPx3 is particularly abundant in the plasma. GPx4 has as substrates lipid hydroperoxides and is present at a low level in nearly every cell type. Thioredoxins (TRx) and glutaredoxins (GRx) are proteins that function as antioxidants by enabling the reduction of other proteins by cysteine thioldisulfide exchange. Apart from being involved in antioxidant defense, different isoforms of the TRx and GRx families have been shown to play an important role in regulation of gene expression by redox-dependent processes. Peroxiredoxins (PRx) represent a ubiquitous family of antioxidant enzymes whose activities are tightly regulated by phosphorylation cascades and by changes in the redox and oligomerization states. PRx controls intracellular peroxide levels and mediate signal transduction in cardiovascular cells (Woo et al., 2010).

## 5. Role of oxidative stress in atherogenesis

Physiological production of ROS contribute to the preservation of vascular homeostasis by regulating important biological processes such as cell growth, proliferation, differentiation, apoptosis, cytoskeletal organization, and cell migration. Still, in the last few decades, it has become apparent that overproduction of ROS correlated with alterations of the antioxidant system, vascular inflammation and metabolic dysfunction are key pathological initiators of cardiovascular disorders. Generated in excess, ROS react randomly with all of biological molecules inducing the irreversible alterations of DNA, proteins, carbohydrates, and lipids components, thus altering cell functions (Martinet et al., 2001). As a result, extensive studies have concentrated on the role of oxidative stress-induced cellular dysfunction, redox control of vascular response to inflammatory and metabolic insults, the molecular mechanisms of ROS generation and the means that this class of molecules contributes to vascular damage.

Oxidative stress represents a pathological condition characterized by the incapacity of antioxidant mechanisms to neutralize the deleterious effects of ROS and their metabolites. The means of oxidative stress onset and progression in vascular pathological states, include the overproduction of ROS, changes in the endogenous antioxidant system, and the production of various oxygen intermediates such as ONOO- and HO• that cannot be efficiently buffered by the naturally occurring antioxidant mechanisms. In addition, spatial and temporal co-expression and co-localization of various enzymatic and non-enzymatic ROS-producing sources at the site of vascular insults may potentially exacerbate predispose to vascular insults and dysfunction (Kondo et al., 2009; Lee et al., 2009).

The importance of oxidative stress in onset and development of atherosclerosis is commonly accepted (Fearon & Faux, 2009). Still, numerous clinical trials failed to demonstrate that the antioxidant therapy improve the health of patients with cardiovascular diseases (Yusuf et al., 2000). Consequently, many questions arise relative to our current knowledge of the molecular processes implicated in ROS formation and action. Hitherto, different pharmacological approaches have been employed to counteract oxidative stress-induced injury in the cardiovascular system i.e. antioxidant supplements containing vitamins C and E, polyphenols or selective inhibitors of distinct sources of ROS (Olukman et al., 2010). Nevertheless, these pharmacological interventions have many disadvantages such as inadequate concentration of active compounds at the site of ROS formation, or vitamins themselves becoming radicals with pro-oxidant activity or not being effective scavengers for various reactive oxygen/nitrogen intermediates, namely hydrogen peroxide ($H_2O_2$), peroxynitrite anion (ONOO-), hydroxyl anion (HO•), and hypochlorous acid (HOCl).

Excessive ROS formation in atherogenesis triggers a chain of critical events such as EC dysfunction, oxidation of macromolecules especially LDL and extracellular matrix constituents, phenotypic alterations of SMC and macrophage/SMC-derived foam cell and modulate the function of signalling molecules in fibroblasts, which promotes inflammation of vascular adventitia (Sima et al., 2009). Vascular resident cells and transvasated immune cells are important sources of ROS within the atheroma (Heistad et al., 2009). These particularities show that atherosclerosis represents a multifactorial vascular disorder characterized by complex interactions and cross talk between the resident cells of the vascular wall, the cells of the immune system and the factors they produce.

As shown in various animal models of atherosclerosis, oxidative stress is a primary occurrence and a key contributor to endothelial dysfunction portrayed by diminished endothelial NO bioavailability, enhanced endothelial transcytosis, up-regulation of pro-inflammatory molecules, and the alteration of EC fibrinolytic activity (Dejana et al., 2009; Vendrov et al., 2007). In addition, oxidation of macromolecules especially of LDL (oxLDL) plays a key role in all stages of atherogenesis such as fatty streak formation, development of complex lesion, and plaque rupture. Of particular importance is that oxidative stress contributes, at least in part in the modulation of SMC phenotype switching and ultimately contributes to artery wall thickening. In atherosclerosis, SMCs undergo hypertrophy, produce excess extracellular matrix and inflammatory cytokines, proliferate and migrate from the media towards the vessel's intima.

Clinical evidence highlights that oxidative stress is a characteristic feature of many pathological conditions that predispose to atherosclerotic lesion formation such as hypercholesterolemia, hypertension, and diabetes. However, the precise pathological mechanisms accountable for the installation of oxidative stress are still an unsettled subject. In this context, although not completely validated in humans, oxidative stress may not be the sole causative effect of atherosclerosis and one has to consider the diversity of enzymatic and non-enzymatic sources of ROS, their vascular distribution pattern and subcellular compartmentalization, and complex regulation during various stages of the disease progression (Förstermann, 2008).

## 6. Vascular sources of ROS: Role of NADPH oxidases

Various pathways of ROS generation that can potentially contribute to oxidative stress have been described in the cardiovascular system including non-enzymatic decomposition of various compounds and metabolites (e.g., glucose autoxidation), production of ROS as byproducts of cellular respiration and metabolism (i.e., mitochondrial respiratory chain, lipo-/cyclooxygenases, dysfunctional nitric oxide (NO) synthases, cytochrome P450 reductases, xanthine oxidase), lysosomal enzymes or generated in a highly regulated manner by specialized enzymes (e.g., NADPH oxidases) (Gu et al., 2001; Harrison et al., 2003; Madamanchi et al., 2005; Martinez-Hervas et al., 2010; Zalba et al., 2007).

NADPH oxidases (Nox) represent a family of multi-component enzymes, whose unique biological function is the production of ROS both in physiological and pathological states (Lambeth, 2004). Nox was originally identified and characterized as being a "burst" enzyme in professional phagocytes such as neutrophils and macrophages. In phagocytes, in cooperation with MPO, Nox plays a major role in host defense process against invading pathogens through the production of toxic hypochlorous acid (HOCl), a highly reactive oxidant. During phagocytosis, macrophages also generate significant amounts of NO. As a result, the Nox-derived $O_2^{\bullet -}$ reacts with NO thus producing ONOO-, an extremely cytotoxic chemical species which directly affect and oxidize biological molecules in invading microorganisms, resulting in molecular alteration and microbial death (El-Benna et al., 2007). The phagocyte-type Nox consists of five subunits: a membrane-associated cytochrome b558, comprising a heavily glycosylated 91-kDa protein (gp91phox; Nox2) and non-glycosylated 22-kDa subunit (p22phox), and three cytosolic regulatory components, p40phox, p47phox, and p67phox. Besides "Phox" components, assembly of Nox in an active complex requires the contribution of a low-molecular-weight GTP-binding protein, Rac1/2 or Rap 1A. In latent cells, the Nox complex is dissociated but is rapidly assembled and activated following the exposure to pathogens or inflammatory mediators. Serine phosphorylation of p47phox represents the limiting step of Nox activation and triggers complex formation of cytosolic subunits followed by translocation to the membrane and association with cytochrome b558 (Hoyal et al., 2003; Lassègue & Griendling 2002; Li & Shah 2003;). Other than Nox2, macrophages also express Nox1 and Nox4 as inducible isoforms that, reportedly mediate LDL oxidation in the vascular wall (Lee et al., 2009; Maitra et al., 2009).

The expression of functionally active Nox subtypes has been reported in non-phagocytes, including cardiovascular cells. Thus far, the members of the Nox enzyme family consists of seven isoforms (Nox1-5, Duox1/2), each with a particular cell and tissue distribution. Nox enzymes are broadly divided into three major categories, as a function of the extra catalytic domains to the phagocyte-type subunit Nox2. The first group includes Nox1, Nox3, and Nox4 isoforms, which display a number of similarities with Nox2, for instance their structural organization and molecular weight. Besides Nox2-type catalytic core, Nox5, the second group of the Nox family, possess an extra amino-terminal calmodulin-like domain that contains four $Ca^{2+}$-binding EF-hands structures (Lambeth, 2007). Thus far, four splice variants of Nox5, namely Nox5α, Nox5β, Nox5γ, and Nox5δ, have been identified in humans. In particular, the *Nox5* gene is not present in the rodents' genome. A third class of of Nox is represented by the Nox5-like dual oxidases (Duox) which possess, in addition to the Nox5-type structure, an extracellular peroxidase domain that uses the $H_2O_2$ generated by its Nox catalytic core. For their function, all the Nox1-4 subtypes necessitate the p22phox component, while Nox5 and Duox are activated directly by calcium. As shown in aortic SMCs, activation of Nox1 requires the participation of a ClC-3 anion transporter. The anion transporter co-expresses with Nox1 in early endosomes and is required for charge neutralization of the electron flow generated by Nox1 across the membrane of signalling vesicles (Miller et al., 2007). Nox4 is constitutively active and its activity is supported by the association with p22phox, required for the electron transfer, and polymerase delta interacting-protein 2 (Polidp2), that apparently may serve to stabilize the enzymatic complex (Lyle et al., 2009). The activities of Nox1, Nox2, and Nox3 isoforms are highly controlled by phosphorylation reactions involving regulatory subunits that initiate the assembly of Nox into an active enzymatic complex. Other than p40phox, p47phox, and p67phox cytosolic regulatory components, two different structurally related proteins have been discovered in non-phagocyte, specifically Nox organizer 1 (Noxo1), which is an analog of p47phox, and Nox activator 1 (Noxa1), which is an analog of p67phox. Despite the structural similarities, dissimilar functional aspects are involved in the regulation of enzyme activity. For instance, different to p47phox, which in the resting cells is located in the cytosol, Noxo1 is pre-localized at the membrane jointly with Nox1 and p22phox (Lambeth,

2004). Different subtypes of the Nox enzyme family along with their regulatory proteins are expressed in the cardiovascular cells (i.e., ECs, SMCs, vascular and cardiac fibroblasts, cardiac myocytes, and pericytes), and in circulating immune cells interacting with the blood vessels (i.e., monocytes/macrophages, neutrophils, lymphocytes, platelets, dendritic cells) (Manea et al., 2005).

Nox subtypes are differentially located within the cellular compartments, suggesting a specific correlation between Nox subtypes, subcellular distribution and their specific function to control precise ROS-mediated signal transduction cascades. For instance, Nox1 and Nox2 were detected in caveolae, in the plasma membrane, and endosomes. Nox4 has been detected in focal adhesions, mitochondria endoplasmic reticulum, and the nucleus (Ago et al., 2010; Kuroda & Sadoshima, 2010). Nox5 is present in the perinuclear regions, endoplasmic reticulum, and in the plasma membrane (BelAiba et al., 2007; Fulton, 2009).

## 7. Involvement of Nox enzymes in atherogenresis

Studies in cell culture and transgenic/knockout mice provided most of the existing data concerning the role of Nox-dependent oxidative stress in atherosclerosis. Nox activity is up-regulated by numerous factors linked to atherosclerotic lesion formation and progression namely, inflammatory cytokines (tumor necrosis factor α, interferon γ), vasoactive agents (angiotensin II, endothelin 1), metabolic factors (high glucose, modified proteins/lipoproteins/lipids, homocysteine), growth factors (platelet-derived growth factor), coagulation factors (thrombin), and pathological shear stress (Chung et al., 2010; Hwang et al., 2003). Apart from direct detrimental effects, compelling data exists that Nox-derived ROS interact and stimulate other enzymatic sources of oxygen/nitrogen reactive intermediates, and generally amplify the initial response to insults (Cohena & Tong, 2010; Schrader & Fahimi, 2006).

It is generally accepted that Nox-derived ROS cooperate, and act in concert with other pathological factors leading to vascular inflammation and injury, and that genetic ablation of various Nox subunits (i.e., p47phox, Nox1, Nox2) defends the vascular cells against the harmful effects of oxidative stress. ApoE-/- mice, which develop atherosclerotic lesions that cover the entire range of human lesions (i.e., fatty streaks, intermediate lesions, fibrous plaques, and vulnerable plaques exhibiting necrotic core and intra-plaque hemorrhage) have been extensively used to investigate the role of Nox enzymes in atherogenesis (Nakashima et al., 1994). Using this animal model, it has become evident that enhances in Nox activity and expression occur early in atherogenesis, and hyperactivity of Nox associated with the up-regulation of various isoforms marks all the stages of the plaque formation (Fenyo et al., 2011).

In contrast, ApoE/p47phox double-knockout mice display significantly less atherosclerotic lesions compared with ApoE-/- mice. In the same line, aortic $O_2^{\bullet -}$ levels have been shown to be are lower in p47phox-/- mice than in wild-type mice. In addition, aortic SMCs from p47phox-/- mice exhibit a decreased proliferative response to growth factors compared with that of the SMCs of wild-type mice (Vendrov et al., 2007).

Accelerated atherosclerosis represents a major vascular complication of diabetes mellitus and is responsible for 70-80% of deaths in diabetic patients in developed and developing countries. Numerous reports revealed that the Nox expression and activity are significantly up-regulated in the vasculature of diabetic subjects, and are associated with the development of atherosclerosis and microvascular diseases (retinopathy, neuropathy, and nephropathy). In addition, Nox1, Nox2, and Nox4 are activated and up-regulated in the blood vessels of diabetic animals (Ding et al., 2007; Xu et al., 2007).

Hyperglycemia, the primary clinical manifestation of diabetes, contributes at least in part to diabetic complications by inducing Nox and the ensuing oxidative stress. Moreover, advanced glycation end-products (AGEs), a direct consequence of the high and persistent blood glucose level, are also important inducers of Nox-derived ROS in vascular cells in diabetes. Besides hyperglycemia, hyperinsulinemia contribute to aberrant ROS production and vascular wall dysfunction. Since Nox is one of the main triggers of oxidative stress, it has a prominent role in the pathology of diabetes-induced vasculopathy (Gao & Mann, 2009). These data make Nox enzymes potential therapeutic targets to counteract the deleterious effects of ROS in diabetes.

Hypertension represents a major risk factor for atherosclerosis and its complications and several reports highlight that oxidative stress is both cause and consequence of hypertension (Briones & Touyz, 2010). Nox1 deficiency in mice reduces angiotensin II (Ang II) -dependent blood pressure, media hypertrophy, and extracellular matrix deposition, but not cell proliferation (Gavazzi et al., 2007; Matsuno et al., 2005). In agreement with these data, AngII-treated mice overexpressing Nox1 in vascular smooth muscle cells exhibit an increase of blood pressure, a condition that is associated with medial hypertrophy and significant production of ROS (Dikalova et al., 2005). Furthermore, overexpression of Nox1 in vascular SMCs leads to enhanced responsiveness to Ang II causing up-regulation of ROS, eNOS uncoupling and the consequent decline in NO bioavailability, followed by impaired vascular relaxation (Dikalova et al., 2010).

Consistent with these reports, compared with wild-type mice, Nox2 ablation (Nox2-/-) diminishes robustly ROS-mediated protein oxidation, neointimal formation, SMCs proliferation and leukocyte accumulation, indicating that Nox2-mediated signalling and oxidation has a requisite role in the cell response to injury (Chen et al., 2004).

The role of Nox4 and Nox5 enzymes in atherogenesis is less investigated and consequently, not entirely elucidated, since there are few atherosclerosis-related studies conducted on Nox4 deficient mice, and the *Nox5* gene is not present in the rodent's genome. Thus, most of the current data are provided by studies performed *in vitro* on various cell-types and isolated tissues.

Recently, a Nox4 deficient mouse model and a cardiomyocyte-targeted Nox4-transgenic model have been developed to investigate the role of Nox4 during cardiac stress. (Zhang et al., 2010). One of the main breakthroughs of this study is that in contrast to the effects of generated by activated Nox1 or Nox2, the up-regulation cardiomyocyte Nox4 results in protection against pressure overload-induced adverse cardiac remodeling. The authors conclude that Nox4 facilitates the maintenance of myocardial capillary density during pressure overload by regulating stress-induced cardiomyocyte hypoxia inducible factor-1 activation and release of vascular endothelial growth factor, resulting in increased paracrine angiogenic activity. In addition, unlike Nox1, Nox2 or Nox5, it seems that Nox4 produces directly $H_2O_2$ and thus is incapable of scavenging NO or producing ONOO-.

The beneficial effects of Nox4-derived ROS were also reported by means of a newly developed transgenic mouse with endothelial-specific Nox4 overexpression (Ray et al., 2011). The authors showed that vascular segments and endothelial cells of these animals had a significant increase in $H_2O_2$ generation rather that $O_2^{\bullet-}$ and a significant augmentation of the pro-oxidative status. Despite of these aspects, the blood pressure of the animals was lower under basal conditions and after angiotensin II treatment. Interestingly, endothelium-dependent relaxation was significantly improved compared with wild-type animals. Notably, these effects were sensitive to the *ex vivo* addition of catalase and *in vivo* administration of *N*-acetylcysteine, indicating that they were mediated by peroxide-type, namely $H_2O_2$, mechanisms. Mechanistically, it seems that an $H_2O_2$ action on potassium channels may be responsible for the elaboration of endothelium-derived hyperpolarizing factor (EDHF) type. Thus, one has to ponder that the type of ROS released in the vascular system determines their biological function.

As mentioned above, less is know about the role of Nox5 in atherogenesis, and this is due mainly to the absence of *Nox5* gene in the rodents' genome and therefore to the lack of a reliable animal model., Still, it has been reported a significant correlation between Nox5 expression and atherosclerotic lesion progression. Interestingly, a specific expression pattern was reported; with Nox5 being expressed mainly by the endothelium in the early stages of the disease while its expression is significantly increased in SMCs underlying fibro-lipid atherosclerotic lesions (Guzik et al., 2008).

## 8. Mechanisms of Nox regulation

### 8.1 Phosphorylation pathways and transcription factors

Nox activity and expression is highly regulated at multiple levels by various physiologic and pathological factors which, by this means, dictate the enzyme complex function. The activities of both Nox1 and Nox2 isoforms are primarily regulated by complex networking of phosphorylation cascades involving regulatory components (i.e., p40phox, p47phox, p67phox, Noxo1, Noxa1) which induce the assembly of the enzyme complex. Nox4 is constitutively active and does not necessitate phosphorylation of regulatory proteins, whereas Nox5 has been demonstrated to be $Ca^{2+}$-responsivenes. Yet, activation mechanisms involving protein kinase C and the proto-oncogenic tyrosine kinase c-Abl phosphorylation of Nox5 have been reported (El Jamali et al., 2008; Serrander et al., 2007).

The phosphorylation mechanisms responsible for Nox1 and Nox2 activation consist of a large spectrum of signalling molecules such as protein kinase C (PKC), phosphatidylinositol 3-kinase (PI3K), GTP-binding proteins (Ras, Rac1/2), members of the mitogen-activated protein kinase (MAPK) family (p38MAPK, ERK1/2), phospholipases (PLCβ/γ, PLD), arachidonic acid metabolites, and non-receptor protein tyrosine kinases (Kilpatrick et al., 2010; Yamamori et al., 2004). Besides the aforementioned kinases, chaperone proteins (e.g., protein disulfide isomerase) have been proved to be important regulators on Nox function (Janiszewski et al., 2005).

In addition to the phosphorylation of cytosolic regulatory subunits, alterations of the Nox isoforms expression have been shown to be critical for their activity. Multiple transcription factors are coordinately implicated in the modulation of Nox expression and function. PU.1, Elf-1, IRF-1 (interferon regulatory factor-1), and ICSBP (interferon consensus sequence binding protein) are important transcriptional regulators of Nox2 in the myelomonocytic cell lineage (Kakar et al., 2005). In human colon epithelial Caco-2 cells, GATA-binding factors are critical for Nox1 transcriptional activity (Brewer et al., 2006), whereas in murine macrophages, the up-regulation of Nox1 in response to lipopolysaccharide (LPS) stimulation is mediated at least in part, by pro-inflammatory transcription factors CCAAT/enhancer-binding protein (C/EBP)β and C/EBPδ (Maitra et al., 2009).

In previous studies, we have shown that in human aortic SMCs exposed angiotensin II or tumor necrosis factor-α, the pro-inflammatory transcription factor AP-1 is an essential regulator of the genes coding for p22phox, Nox1, and Nox4 components (Manea et al., 2008; Raicu & Manea, 2010). Other than, activator protein -1 (AP-1), the vascular inflammation-related and growth-promoting transcription factors signal transducer and activator of transcription (STAT1 and STAT3) proteins physically interact with the promoters of human Nox1 and Nox4 genes in SMCs exposed to interferon (IFN) γ and a Jauns kinase (Jak)/STAT-dependent mechanisms are implicated in the ensuing $O_2^{\bullet -}$ production. Moreover, the promoter activities of the genes coding for p22phox, p47phox, and p67phox, have been demonstrated to be considerably augmented in SMCs overexpressing STAT1/STAT3, a result that suggests the existence of functionally gamma activated sequence (GAS)/interferon-stimulated response element (ISRE) consensus sequences (Manea et al., 2010a). In human aortic SMCs, Ets1, a critical mediator of vascular inflammation and remodelling, regulates p47phox expression in response to AngII (Ni et al., 2007). Similar observations were made in A7r5 cells and primary mouse aortic SMCs, in which the growth-promoting transcription factor E2F actually interacts and controls the Nox4 transcriptional program (Zhang et al., 2008).

In atherosclerosis, and other major cardiovascular disorders, nuclear factor kB (NF-kB) signalling represents a critical regulating mechanism involved in disease onset and progression, including inflammation, cell proliferation, migration, differentiation and apoptosis. Several line of evidence indicate that NF-kB is a redox-sensitive transcription factor which is robustly activated by ROS possible generated by activated Nox. Interestingly, a positive feed-back loop of Nox activation by NF-kB has been proposed in several studies. Thus, a new integrative concept has emergedthe "vicious cycle", to describe the interconnection between metabolic dysfunction, inflammation, and oxidative stress that converges to vascular disorders (Manea, 2010). In murine monocytes, the expression of the Nox2 is induced by NF-kB. Moreover, the up-regulation of p47phox and p22phox expression by LPS/IFNγ was blunted in IkBα-overexpressing cells suggesting the involvement of the NF-kB signaling in the regulation of the Nox components (Anrather et al. 2006). Similar finding were reported in human monocytes/macrophages exposed to TNFα (Gauss et al., 2007). Moreover, in previous studies we have shown that, NF-kB is an important transcriptional regulator of the genes coding for p22phox, Nox1, and Nox4, and has a profound impact in the up-regulation of Nox activity in TNFα-treated human aortic SMCs (Manea et al., 2007; Manea et al., 2010b).

The molecular mechanisms that facilitate hypoxia sensing and related signalling events are critical for the maintenance of vascular cell homeostasis. Compelling data depicts that hypoxic conditions up-regulate the expression and activity various Nox subtypes (Goyal et al., 2004). It has been demonstrated that persistent hypoxia induces Nox4 gene and protein expression levels in pulmonary artery SMCs and in pulmonary vessels in mice exposed to hypoxic conditions (Diebold et al., 2010). Mechanistically, the response is dependent on hypoxia inducible factor-1α (HIF-1α), which interacts with the corresponding elements in the Nox4 promoter. As a result, the HIF-1α dependent up-regulation of Nox4 by may be an essential mechanism to preserve ROS level after hypoxia and the hypoxia-induced proliferation of pulmonary artery SMCs. Furthermore, activating transcription factor-1 (ATF-1), a transcription factor of the CREB (CRE-binding protein)/ATF family, proved to play a key role in the induction of Nox1 in rat vascular SMCs (Katsuyama et al., 2005).

Nuclear factor (erythroid-derived 2)-like 2, also known as Nrf2 represents a master modulator of the antioxidant responses by inducing genes (e.g., *Sod* genes) with important function in combating oxidative stress. Interestingly, it has been demonstrated that Nrf2, also controls Nox4 expression in mouse lung and human lung endothelium in response to hyperoxia (Pendyala & Natarajan, 2010).

### 8.2 Genetic and epigenetic mechanisms of Nox regulation

Genetic studies highlight that several Nox-related polymorphisms are closely associated with an increased susceptibility for cardiovascular disorders. One of the most investigated genes from the Nox complex is *CYBA* which encodes the p22phox essential subunit. The p22phox is ubiquitously expressed in cardiovascular cells and forms stable and functional heterodimers with Nox1, Nox2 or Nox4, a critical structure for enzyme activity as shown by studies employing siRNA technology to knock-down p22phox expression (Kawahara et al., 2005). Moreover, it has been demonstrated that p22phox is more abundant in advanced atherosclerotic plaques than in nonatherosclerotic arteries, suggesting a correlation between p22phox expression, $O_2^{\bullet -}$ production, and the severity of atherosclerosis (Azumi et al., 1999).

The occurrence of particular polymorphisms of the *CYBA* gene has been shown to predispose to oxidative stress and to be independently correlated with cardiovascular risk factors and disease occurrence namely hypertension, coronary artery disease, myocardial infarction, cerebrovascular disease, diabetic and non-diabetic nephropathy) (San José et al., 2008). Various *CYBA* allelic variants were detected in both exonic sequences such as C242T, A640G, C549T (Dinauer et al., 1990; Guzik et al., 2000; Inoue et al., 1998), and promoter regions namely -930A/G, -675A/T, -852C/G, -536C/T (Lim et al., 2006; Moreno et al., 2007), which potentially affect the p22phox expression and consequently the Nox activity. Thus far, data indicating the existence of functional Nox1-5 polymorphisms with a relevant impact on vascular pathology are not available yet.

Emerging evidence demonstrates that epigenetic events such as DNA methylation and modifications of histone tails are important processes of oxidative stress onset. DNA methylation mechanisms of the promoter CpG islands has been shown to be involved in the up-regulation of 15-lipoxygenase, a pro-oxidative enzyme with implications in plaque formation and vulnerability, and down-regulation of superoxide dismutase 3, endothelial NO synthase, and various anti-proliferative genes (estrogen receptor-α), a condition that leads to oxidative stress, impaired vascular relaxation, and aberrant SMC hyperplasia (Fernandez et al., 2010). Hitherto, data about the role of epigenetics in the regulation of Nox subtypes are missing. Nevertheless, using both *in vitro* (e,g., human aortic SMCs exposed to pro-inflammatory conditions) and *in vivo* (ApoE-/- mice fed a high fat, cholesterol rich diet) models, we have found recently that an aberrant methylation of the Nox1 promoter may be responsible for the up-regulated expression and activity of this enzyme (Manea et al., unpublished data).

A schematic representation of the key molecular pathways implicated in the up-regulation of Nox enzymes as well as the potential pharmacological targets intended to counteract oxidative stress are presented in the figure below.

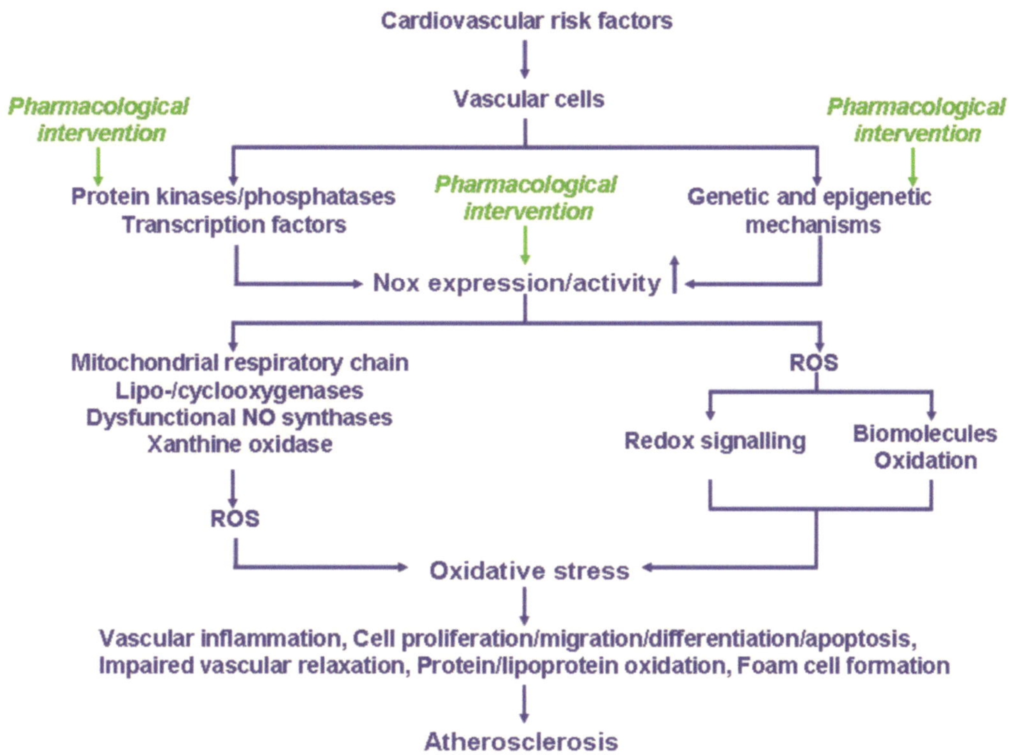


Fig. 1. Schematic depiction of the major mechanisms responsible for the up-regulation of Nox enzymes and installation of oxidative stress in atherosclerosis. In response to cardiovascular risk factors, vascular cells through their receptors activate a range of signalling pathways that up-regulate Nox expression, activity, and the ensuing ROS production. This triggers a chain of critical events that generally amplify the initial response to vascular insults (i.e., activation of other cellular sources of ROS and redox-sensitive signalling effectors). Persistent Nox activation leads to oxidative stress that is a major contributor to the initiation and the development of atherosclerotic lesions. The diagram highlights that genetic, epigenetic, as well as genetic/non-epigenetic-independent mechanisms linked to Nox up-regulation and hyperactivity in atherosclerosis may be used to target and control pharmacologically the Nox-derived oxidative stress (green text).

## 9. Conclusion

The Nox-derived ROS may have both beneficial and deleterious effects. Thus, we can safely assume that these effects are function of the expression pattern and regulation of various Nox isoforms, their subcellular compartmentalization, and the rate of ROS generation. Despite of the numerous existing data, the precise mechanisms of Nox regulation in atherosclerosis and the stream of signalling molecules (up-, or down-regulated) responsible for the increased oxidative stress that is associated with the onset and development of cardiovascular dysfunction, is poorly understood. Thus, a complex interplay of genetic, epigenetic and non-epigenetic factors, transcription factors, co-activators, and/or co-repressors may be coordinately involved in the up-regulation of Nox activity in atherogenesis. Therefore, elucidation of the complex interactions among different mechanisms that control Nox subtypes expression/activity and subcellular compartmentalization of ROS production and its subsequent biological meaning, may lead to a more focused and effective antioxidant therapies. The expected impact of these pharmacological strategies goes well beyond the atherosclerosis field. Oxidative stress is a common occurrence in most pathologies i.e. diabetes, neurodegenerative diseases, cancer, etc. The knowledge gained will be applicable to all these pathologies since controlling oxidative stress ought to have a beneficial knock-on effect on these diseases. Identifying the basic molecular mechanism regulating the oxidative stress will be used to find ways to manage its occurrence and correct its adverse effects.

## 10. Acknowledgement

This work was supported by grants from the Romanian Ministry of Education, and Research (CNCSIS-UEFISCSU project numbers PNII-IDEI 1005/2009 and PNII-TE 65/2010), and from the European Foundation for the Study of Diabetes - New Horizons. The financial support of European Social Fund - „Cristofor I. Simionescu" Postdoctoral Fellowship Programme (ID POSDRU/89/1.5/S/55216), Sectoral Operational Programme Human Resources Development 2007 - 2013 is acknowledged.

## 11. References

Ago, T., Kuroda, J., Pain, J., Fu, C., Li, H. & Sadoshima, J. (2010). Upregulation of Nox4 by hypertrophic stimuli promotes apoptosis and mitochondrial dysfunction in cardiac myocytes. *Circulation Research,* 106, 1253–1264, ISSN 0009-7330

Anrather, J., Racchumi, G. & Iadecola, C. (2006). NF-kappaB regulates phagocytic NADPH oxidase by inducing the expression of gp91phox. *Journal of Biological Chemistry,* 281, 5657-5667, ISSN 0021-9258

Azumi, H., Inoue, N., Takeshita, S., Rikitake, Y., Kawashima, S., Hayashi, Y., Itoh, H. & Yokoyama, M. (1999). Expression of NADH/NADPH oxidase p22phox in human coronary arteries. *Circulation,* 100, 1494-1498, ISSN 0009-7322

BelAiba, R.S., Djordjevic, T., Petry, A., Diemer, K., Bonello, S., Banfi, B., Hess, J., Pogrebniak, A., Bickel, C. & Görlach, A. (2007). NOX5 variants are functionally active in endothelial cells. *Free Radical Biology and Medicine,* 42, 446–459, ISSN 0891-5849

Belia, S., Santilli, F., Beccafico, S., De Feudis, L., Morabito, C., Davi, G., Fanò, G. & Mariggiò, M.A. (2009). Oxidative-induced membrane damage in diabetes lymphocytes: effects on intracellular Ca(2+) homeostasis. *Free Radical Biology and Medicine,* 43, 138–148, ISSN 0891-5849

Brewer, A.C., Sparks, E.C. & Shah, A.M. (2006). Transcriptional regulation of the NADPH oxidase isoform, Nox1, in colon epithelial cells: role of GATA-binding factor(s). *Free Radical Biology and Medicine,* 40, 260-274, ISSN 0891-5849

Briones, A.M. & Touyz, R.M. (2010). Oxidative stress and hypertension: current concepts. *Current Hypertension Reports,* 12, 135-142, ISSN 1522-6417

Chen, Z., Keaney, J.F. Jr., Schulz, E., Levison, B., Shan, L., Sakuma, M., Zhang, X., Shi, C., Hazen, S.L. & Simon, D.I. (2004). Decreased neointimal formation in Nox2-deficient mice reveals a direct role for NADPH oxidase in the response to arterial injury.

*Proceedings of the National Academy of Sciences USA,* 101, 13014-13019, ISSN 0027-8424

Chung, S.W., Park, J.W., Lee, S.A., Eo, S.K. & Kim, K. (2010). Thrombin promotes proinflammatory phenotype in human vascular smooth muscle cell. *Biochemical and Biophysical Research Communications,* 396, 748-754, ISSN 0006-291X

Dejana, E., Simionescu, M. & Wolburg, H. (2009). Endothelial cell biology and pathology. *Cell and Tissue Research,* 335, 1-3, ISSN 0302-766X

Diebold, I., Petry, A., Hess, J. & Görlach, A. (2010). The NADPH oxidase subunit NOX4 is a new target gene of the hypoxia-inducible factor-1. *Molecular Biology of the Cell,* 21, 2087-2096, ISSN 1059-1524

Dikalova, A., Clempus, R., Lassègue, B., Cheng, G., McCoy, J., Dikalov, S., San Martin, A., Lyle, A., Weber, D.S., Weiss, D., Taylor, W.R., Schmidt, H.H., Owens, G.K., Lambeth, J.D. & Griendling, K.K. (2005). Nox1 overexpression potentiates angiotensin II-induced hypertension and vascular smooth muscle hypertrophy in transgenic mice. *Circulation,* 112, 2668-2676, ISSN 0009-7322

Dikalova, A.E., Gόngora, M.C., Harrison, D.G., Lambeth, J.D., Dikalov, S. & Griendling, K.K. (2010). Upregulation of Nox1 in vascular smooth muscle leads to impaired endothelium-dependent relaxation via eNOS uncoupling. *American Journal of Physiology Heart and Circulatory Physiology,* 299, 673-679, ISSN 0363-6135

Dinauer, M.C., Pierce, E.A., Bruns, G.A., Curnutte, J.T. & Orkin, S.H. (1990). Human neutrophil cytochrome b light chain (p22-phox). Gene structure, chromosomal location, and mutations in cytochrome-negative autosomal recessive chronic granulomatous disease. *Journal of Clinical Investigation,* 86, 1729–1737, ISSN 0021-9738

Ding, H., Hashem, M. & Triggle, C. (2007). Increased oxidative stress in the streptozotocin-induced diabetic apoE-deficient mouse: changes in expression of NADPH oxidase subunits and eNOS. *European Journal of Pharmacology,* 561, 121-128, ISSN 0014-2999

El Jamali, A., Valente, A.J., Lechleiter, J.D., Gamez, M.J., Pearson, D.W., Nauseef, W.M. & Clark, R.A. (2008). Novel redox-dependent regulation of NOX5 by the tyrosine kinase c-Abl. *Free Radical Biology and Medicine,* 44, 868-881, ISSN 0891-5849

El-Benna, J., Dang, P.M. & Gougerot-Pocidalo, M.A. (2007). Role of the NADPH oxidase systems Nox and Duox in host defense and inflammation. *Expert Review of Clinical Immunology.* 3, 111-115, ISSN 1744-666X

Fearon, I.M. & Faux, S.P. (2009). Oxidative stress and cardiovascular disease: novel tools give (free) radical insight. *Journal of Molecular and Cellular Cardiology,* 47, 372-381, ISSN 0022-2828

Fenyo, I.M., Florea, I.C., Raicu, M. & Manea, A. (2011). Tyrphostin AG490 reduces NAPDH oxidase activity and expression in the aorta of hypercholesterolemic apolipoprotein E-deficient mice. *Vascular Pharmacology,* 54, 100-106, ISSN 1537-1891

Fernandez, Z., Siebel, A.L. & El-Osta, A. (2010). Atherogenic factors and their epigenetic relationships. *International Journal of Vascular Medicine,* doi:10.1155/2010/437809

Forman, H.J., Maiorino, M. & Ursini, F. (2010). Signaling functions of reactive oxygen species. *Biochemistry,* 49, 835–842, ISSN 0006-2960

Förstermann, U. (2008). Oxidative stress in vascular disease: causes, defense mechanisms and potential therapies. *Nature Clinical Practice Cardiovascular Medicine,* 5, 338-349, ISSN 1743-4297

Fulton, D.J. (2009). Nox5 and the regulation of cellular function. *Antioxidants and Redox Signaling,* 11, 2443–2452

Gao, L. & Mann, G.E. (2009). Vascular NAD(P)H oxidase activation in diabetes: a double-edged sword in redox signalling. *Cardiovascular Research,* 82, 9–20, ISSN 0008-6363

Gauss, K.A., Nelson-Overton, L.K., Siemsen, D.W., Gao, Y., DeLeo, F.R. & Quinn, M.T. (2007). Role of NF-kappaB in transcriptional regulation of the phagocyte NADPH oxidase by tumor necrosis factor-alpha. *Journal of Leukocyte Biology,* 82, 729-741, ISSN 0741-5400

Gavazzi, G., Deffert, C., Trocme, C., Schäppi, M., Herrmann, F.R. & Krause, K.H. (2007). NOX1 deficiency protects from aortic dissection in response to angiotensin II. *Hypertension,* 50, 189-196, ISSN 0194-911X

Go, Y.M. & Jones, D.P. (2010) Redox control systems in the nucleus: mechanisms and functions. *Antioxidants and Redox Signaling,* 13, 489–509

Goyal, P., Weissmann, N., Grimminger, F., Hegel, C., Bader, L., Rose, F., Fink, L., Ghofrani, H.A., Schermuly, R.T., Schmidt, H.H., Seeger, W. & Hänze, J. (2004). Upregulation of NAD(P)H oxidase 1 in hypoxia activates hypoxia-inducible factor 1 via increase in reactive oxygen species. *Free Radical Biology and Medicine,* 36, 1279-1288, ISSN 0891-5849

Gu, J.L., Pei, H., Thomas, L., Nadler, J.L., Rossi, J.J., Lanting, L. & Natarajan R. (2001). Ribozyme-mediated inhibition of rat leukocyte-type 12-lipoxygenase prevents intimal hyperplasia in balloon-injured rat carotid arteries. *Circulation,* 103, 1446 - 1452, ISSN 0009-7330

Guzik, T.J., Chen, W., Gongora, M.C., Guzik, B., Lob, H.E., Mangalat, D., Hoch, N., Dikalov, S., Rudzinski, P., Kapelak, B., Sadowski, J. & Harrison, D.G. (2008). Calcium-dependent NOX5 nicotinamide adenine dinucleotide phosphate oxidase contributes to vascular oxidative stress in human coronary artery disease. *Journal of the American College of Cardiology,* 52, 1803-1809, ISSN 0735-1097

Guzik, T.J., West, N.E., Black, E., McDonald, D., Ratnatunga, C., Pillai, R. & Channon, K.M. (2000). Functional effect of the C242T polymorphism in the NAD(P)H oxidase p22phox gene on vascular superoxide production in atherosclerosis. *Circulation,* 102, 1744-1747, ISSN 0009-7322

Harrison, D., Griendling, K.K., Landmesser, U., Hornig, B. & Drexler H. (2003). Role of oxidative stress in atherosclerosis. *American Journal of Cardiology,* 91, 7A–11A, ISSN ISSN 0002-9149

Hazen, S.L., Gaut, J.P., Hsu, F.F., Crowley, J.R., d'Avignon, A. & Heinecke, J.W. (1997). p-Hydroxyphenylacetaldehyde, the major product of L-tyrosine oxidation by the myeloperoxidase-$H_2O_2$-chloride system of phagocytes, covalently modifies epsilon-amino groups of protein lysine residues. *Journal of Biological Chemistry,* 272, 16990–16998, ISSN 0021-9258

Heistad, D.D., Wakisaka, Y., Miller, J., Chu, Y. & Pena-Silva, R. (2009). Novel aspects of oxidative stress in cardiovascular diseases. *Circulation Journal* 73, 201-207, ISSN 1346-9843

Hoyal, C.R., Gutierrez, A., Young, B.M., Catz, S.D., Lin, J.H., Tsichlis, P.N. & Babior, B.M. (2003). Modulation of p47PHOX activity by sitespecific phosphorylation: Akt-dependent activation of the NADPH oxidase. *Proceedings of the National Academy of Sciences USA,* 100, 5130–5135, ISSN 0027-8424

Hwang, J., Saha, A., Boo, Y.C., Sorescu, G.P., McNally, J.S., Holland, S.M., Dikalov, S., Giddens, D.P., Griendling, K.K., Harrison, D.G. & Jo, H. (2003). Oscillatory shear stress stimulates endothelial production of O2- from p47phox-dependent NAD(P)H oxidases, leading to monocyte adhesion. *Journal of Biological Chemistry,* 278, 47291-47298, ISSN 0021-9258

Inoue, N., Kawashima, S., Kanazawa, K., Yamada, S., Akita, H. & Yokoyama, M. (1998). Polymorphism of the NADH/NADPH oxidase p22phox gene in patients with coronary artery disease. *Circulation,* 97, 135–137, ISSN 0009-7322

Janiszewski, M., Lopes, L.R., Carmo, A.O., Pedro, M.A., Brandes, R.P., Santos, C.X. & Laurindo, F.R. (2005). Regulation of NAD(P)H oxidase by associated protein disulfide isomerase in vascular smooth muscle cells. *Journal of Biological Chemistry,* 280, 40813-40819, ISSN 0021-9258

Kakar, R., Kautz, B. & Eklund, E.A. (2005). JAK2 is necessary and sufficient for interferon-gamma-induced transcription of the gene encoding gp91PHOX. *Journal of Leukocyte Biology,* 77, 120-127, ISSN 0741-5400

Katsuyama, M., Fan, C., Arakawa, N., Nishinaka, T., Miyagishi, M., Taira, K. & Yabe-Nishimura, C. (2005). Essential role of ATF-1 in induction of NOX1, a catalytic subunit of NADPH oxidase: involvement of mitochondrial respiratory chain. *Biochemical Journal,* 386, 255-261, ISSN 0264-6021

Kawahara, T., Ritsick, D., Cheng, G. & Lambeth, J.D. (2005). Point mutations in the proline-rich region of p22phox are dominant inhibitors of Nox1- and Nox2-dependent reactive oxygen generation. *Journal of Biological Chemistry,* 280, 31859-31869, ISSN 0021-9258

Kilpatrick, L. E., Sun S., Li, H., Vary, T.C. & Korchak, H.M. (2010). Regulation of TNF-induced oxygen radical production in human neutrophils: role of delta-PKC. *Journal of Leukocyte Biology,* 87, 153-164, ISSN 0741-5400

Kondo, T., Hirose, M. & Kageyama, K. (2009). Roles of oxidative stress and redox regulation in atherosclerosis. *Journal of Atherosclerosis and Thrombosis,* 16, 532-538

Kuroda, J. & Sadoshima, J. (2010). NADPH oxidase and cardiac failure. *Journal of Cardiovascular Translational Research,* 3, 314–320

Lambeth J. D. (2004). NOX enzymes and the biology of reactive oxygen. *Nature Reviews Immunology,* 4, 181-189, ISSN 1474-1733

Lambeth, J.D. (2007). Nox enzymes, ROS, and chronic disease: an example of antagonistic pleiotropy. *Free Radical Biology and Medicine,* 43, 332–347, ISSN 0891-5849

Lassègue, B. & Griendling, K.K. (2002). Out phoxing the endothelium: what's left without p47? *Circulation Research,* 90, 123–124, ISSN 0009-7330

Lee, M.Y. & Griendling, K.K. (2008). Redox signaling, vascular function, and hypertension. *Antioxidant and Redox Signaling*, 10, 1045–1059

Lee, M.Y., San Martin, A., Mehta, P.K., Dikalova, A.E., Garrido, A.M., Datla, S.R., Lyons, E., Krause, K.H., Banfi, B., Lambeth, J.D., Lassègue, B. & Griendling, K.K. (2009). Mechanisms of vascular smooth muscle NADPH oxidase 1 (Nox1) contribution to injury-induced neointimal formation. *Arteriosclerosis Thrombosis and Vascular Biology*, 29, 480-487, ISSN 1079-5642

Leeuwenburgh, C., Rasmussen, J.E., Hsu, F.F., Mueller, D.M., Pennathur, S. & Heinecke, J.W. (1997). Mass spectrometric quantification of markers for protein oxidation by tyrosyl radical, copper, and hydroxyl radical in low density lipoprotein isolated from human atherosclerotic plaques. *Journal of Biological Chemistry*, 272, 3520–3526, ISSN 0021-9258

Li, J.M. & Shah, A.M. (2003). Mechanism of endothelial cell NADPH oxidase activation by angiotensin II. Role of the p47phox subunit. *Journal of Biological Chemistry*, 278, 12094–12100, ISSN 0021-9258

Lim, S.C., Goh, S.K., Lai, Y.R., Tee, W.W., Koh, A., Xu, X.H., Wu, Y.S., Yap, E., Subramaniam, T. & Sum, C.F. (2006). Relationship between common functional polymorphisms of the p22phox gene (-930A > G and +242C > T) and nephropathy as a result of Type 2 diabetes in a Chinese population. *Diabetic Medicine*, 23, 1037-1041, ISSN 0742-3071

Liu, H., Colavitti, R., Rovira, I.I. & Finkel, T. (2005). Redox-dependent transcriptional regulation. *Circulation Research*, 97, 967–974, ISSN 0009-7330

Lyle, A.N., Deshpande, N.N., Taniyama, Y., Seidel-Rogol, B., Pounkova, L., Du, P., Papaharalambus, C., Lassègue, B. & Griendling, K.K. (2009). Poldip2, a novel regulator of Nox4 and cytoskeletal integrity in vascular smooth muscle cells. *Circulation Research*, 105, 249-259, ISSN 0009-7330

Madamanchi N.R., Vendrov, A. & Runge M.S. (2005). Oxidative stress and vascular disease. *Arteriosclerosis Thrombosis and Vascular Biology*, 25, 29-38, ISSN 1079-5642

Maitra, U., Singh, N., Gan, L., Ringwood, L. & Li, L. (2009) IRAK-1 contributes to lipopolysaccharide-induced reactive oxygen species generation in macrophages by inducing NOX-1 transcription and Rac1 activation and suppressing the expression of antioxidative enzymes. *Journal of Biological Chemistry*, 284, 35403-35411, ISSN ISSN 0021-9258

Manea, A. (2010). NADPH oxidase-derived reactive oxygen species: involvement in vascular physiology and pathology. *Cell and Tissue Research*, 342, 325-339, ISSN 0302-766X

Manea, A., Manea, S.A., Gafencu, A.V. & Raicu, M. (2007). Regulation of NADPH oxidase subunit p22(phox) by NF-kB in human aortic smooth muscle cells. *Archives of Physiology and Biochemistry*, 113, 163-172, ISSN

Manea, A., Manea, S.A., Gafencu, A.V., Raicu, M. & Simionescu, M. (2008). AP-1-dependent transcriptional regulation of NADPH oxidase in human aortic smooth muscle cells: role of p22phox subunit. *Arteriosclerosis Thrombosis and Vascular Biology*, 28, 878-885, ISSN 1079-5642

Manea, A., Manea, S.A., Gafencu, A.V., Raicu, M. & Simionescu, M. (2008). AP-1-dependent transcriptional regulation of NADPH oxidase in human aortic smooth muscle cells:

role of p22phox subunit. *Arteriosclerosis Thrombosis and Vascular Biology*, 28, 878-885, ISSN 1079-5642

Manea, A., Raicu, M. & Simionescu, M. (2005). Expression of functionally phagocyte-type NAD(P)H oxidase in pericytes: effect of angiotensin II and high glucose. *Biology of the Cell*, 97, 723–734, ISSN 1059-1524

Manea, A., Tanase, L.I., Raicu, M. & Simionescu, M. (2010b). Transcriptional regulation of NADPH oxidase isoforms, Nox1 and Nox4, by nuclear factor-kappaB in human aortic smooth muscle cells. *Biochemical and Biophysical Research Communications*, 396, 901-907, ISSN 0006-291X

Manea, A., Tanase, L.I., Raicu, M. & Simionescu, M. (2010a). Jak/STAT signaling pathway regulates Nox1 and Nox4-based NADPH oxidase in human aortic smooth muscle cells. *Arteriosclerosis Thrombosis and Vascular Biology*, 30, 105-112, ISSN 1079-5642

Martinet, W., Knaapen, M.W., De Meyer, G.R., Herman, A.G. & Kockx, M.M. (2001). Oxidative DNA damage and repair in experimental atherosclerosis are reversed by dietary lipid lowering. *Circulation Research*, 88, 733–739, ISSN 0009-7330

Martinez-Hervas, S., Real, J.T., Ivorra, C., Priego, A., Chaves, F.J., Pallardo, F.V., Viña, J.R., Redon, J., Carmena, R. & Ascaso J.F. (2010). Increased plasma xanthine oxidase activity is related to nuclear factor kappa beta activation and inflammatory markers in familial combined hyperlipidemia. *Nutrition, Metabolism & Cardiovascular Diseases*, 20, 734-739, ISSN 0939-4753

Matsuno, K., Yamada, H., Iwata, K., Jin, D., Katsuyama, M., Matsuki, M., Takai, S., Yamanishi, K., Miyazaki, M., Matsubara, H. & Yabe-Nishimura, C. (2005). Nox1 is involved in angiotensin II-mediated hypertension: a study in Nox1-deficient mice. *Circulation*, 112, 2677-2685, ISSN

Miller, F.J. Jr., Filali, M., Huss, G.J., Stanic, B., Chamseddine, A., Barna, T.J. & Lamb, F.S. (2007). Cytokine activation of nuclear factor kappa B in vascular smooth muscle cells requires signaling endosomes containing Nox1 and ClC-3. *Circulation Research*, 101, 663–671, ISSN 0009-7330

Moreno, M.U., San José, G., Fortuño, A., Beloqui, O., Redón, J., Chaves, F.J., Corella, D., Díez, J. & Zalba, G. (2007). A novel CYBA variant, the -675A/T polymorphism, is associated with essential hypertension. *Journal of Hypertension*, 25, 1620-1626, ISSN

Nakashima, Y., Plump, A.S., Raines, E.W., Breslow, J.L. & Ross, R. (1994). ApoE-deficient mice develop lesions of all phases of atherosclerosis throughout the arterial tree. *Arteriosclerosis, Thrombosis, and Vascular Biology*, 14, 133-140, ISSN

Negre-Salvayre, A., Auge, N., Ayala, V., Basaga, H., Boada, J., Brenke, R., Chapple, S., Cohen, G., Feher, J., Grune, T., Lengyel, G., Mann, G.E., Pamplona, R., Poli, G., Portero-Otin, M., Riahi, Y., Salvayre, R., Sasson, S., Serrano, J., Shamni, O., Siems, W., Siow, R.C., Wiswedel, I., Zarkovic K. & Zarkovic, N. (2010). Pathological aspects of lipid peroxidation. *Free Radical Research*, 44, 1125-1171, ISSN 1071-5762

Ni, W., Zhan, Y., He, H., Maynard, E., Balschi, J.A. & Oettgen, P. (2007). Ets-1 is a critical transcriptional regulator of reactive oxygen species and p47(phox) gene expression in response to angiotensin II. *Circulation Research*, 101, 985-994, ISSN 0009-7330

Olukman, M., Orhan, C.E., Celenk, F.G. & Ulker, S. (2010). Apocynin restores endothelial dysfunction in streptozotocin diabetic rats through regulation of nitric oxide synthase and NADPH oxidase expressions. *Journal of Diabetes and its Complications,* 24, 415-423, ISSN 1056-8727

Pendyala, S. & Natarajan, V. (2010). Redox regulation of Nox proteins. Respiratory *Physiology &* Neurobiology,174, 265-271, ISSN 1569-9048

Raicu, M. & Manea, A. (2010). Activator protein-1 regulates Nox1 and Nox4-containing NADPH oxidase transcription in human vascular smooth muscle cells. *Annals of RSCB*, XV, 11-17

Ray, R., Murdoch, C.E., Wang, M., Santos, C.X., Zhang, M., Alom-Ruiz, S., Anilkumar, N., Ouattara, A., Cave, A.C., Walker, S.J., Grieve, D.J., Charles, R.L., Eaton, P., Brewer, A.C. & Shah, A.M. (2011). Endothelial Nox4 NADPH oxidase enhances vasodilatation and reduces blood pressure in vivo. *Arteriosclerosis Thrombosis and Vascular Biology,* 31, 1368-1376, ISSN 1079-5642

Riahi, Y., Cohen, G., Shamni, O. & Sasson, S. (2010). Signaling and cytotoxic functions of 4-hydroxyalkenals. *American Journal of Physiology Endocrinology and Metabolism,* 299, 879-886, ISSN 0193-1849

San José, G., Fortuño, A., Beloqui, O., Díez, J. & Zalba, G. (2008). NADPH oxidase CYBA polymorphisms, oxidative stress and cardiovascular diseases. *Clinical Science (Lond),* 114, 173-182, ISSN 0143-5221

Savenkova, M.L., Mueller, D.M. & Heinecke, J.W. (1994). Tyrosyl radical generated by myeloperoxidase is a physiological catalyst for the initiation of lipid peroxidation in low density lipoprotein. *Journal of Biological Chemistry,* 269, 20394–20400, ISSN 0021-9258

Sedeek, M., Hébert, R.L., Kennedy, C.R., Burns, K.D. & Touyz, R.M. (2009). Molecular mechanisms of hypertension: role of Nox family NADPH oxidases. *Current Opinion in Nephrology and Hypertension,* 18, 122–127, ISSN 0194-911X

Serrander, L., Jaquet, V., Bedard, K., Plastre, O., Hartley, O., Arnaudeau, S., Demaurex, N., Schlegel, W. & Krause, K.H. (2007). NOX5 is expressed at the plasma membrane and generates superoxide in response to protein kinase C activation. *Biochimie,* 89, 1159-1167, ISSN 0300-9084

Shao, B. & Heinecke, J.W. (2009). HDL, lipid peroxidation, and atherosclerosis. *Journal of Lipid Research,* 50, 599-601, ISSN 0022-2275

Shao, B. & Heinecke, J.W. (2009). HDL, lipid peroxidation, and atherosclerosis. *Journal of Lipid Research* 50, 599-601, ISSN 0022-2275

Sima, A.V., Stancu, C.S. & Simionescu, M. (2009). Vascular endothelium in atherosclerosis. *Cell and Tissue Research,* 335, 191-203, ISSN 0302-766X

Simionescu, M. (2007). Implications of early structural-functional changes in the endothelium for vascular disease. *Arteriosclerosis Thrombosis and Vascular Biology*, 27, 266-274, ISSN 1079-5642

Simionescu, M., Popov, D. & Sima, A. (2009). Endothelial transcytosis in health and disease. *Cell and Tissue Research,* 335, 27-40, ISSN 0302-766X

Tabet, F., Schiffrin, E.L., Callera, G.E., He, Y., Yao, G., Ostman, A., Kappert, K., Tonks, N.K. & Touyz, R.M. (2008). Redox-sensitive signaling by angiotensin II involves oxidative inactivation and blunted phosphorylation of protein tyrosine phosphatase SHP-2 in vascular smooth muscle cells from SHR. *Circulation Research*, 103, 149–158, ISSN 0009-7330

Tonks, N.K. (2006). Protein tyrosine phosphatases: from genes, to function, to disease. *Nature Reviews Molecular Cell Biology*, 7, 833-846, ISSN 1471-0072

Touyz, R.M. (2003) Reactive oxygen species in vascular biology: role in arterial hypertension. Expert Review *of Cardiovascular Therapy*, 1, 91-106

Turrens, J.F. (2003). Mitochondrial formation of reactive oxygen species. *Journal of Physiology*, 552, 335-344, ISSN 0022-3751

Valdivia, A., Pérez-Alvarez, S., Aroca-Aguilar, J.D., Ikuta, I. & Jordán, J. (2009). Superoxide dismutases: a physiopharmacological update. *Journal of Physiology and Biochemistry*, 65, 195–208, ISSN 1138-7548

Vendrov, A.E., Hakim, Z.S., Madamanchi, N.R., Rojas, M., Madamanchi, C. & Runge, M.S. (2007). Atherosclerosis is attenuated by limiting superoxide generation in both macrophages and vessel wall cells. *Arteriosclerosis Thrombosis and Vascular Biology*, 27, 2714-2721, ISSN 1079-5642

Vendrov, A.E., Hakim, Z.S., Madamanchi, N.R., Rojas, M., Madamanchi, C. & Runge, M.S. (2007). Atherosclerosis is attenuated by limiting superoxide generation in both macrophages and vessel wall cells. *Arteriosclerosis Thrombosis and Vascular Biology*, 27, 2714-2721, ISSN 1079-5642

Woo, H.A., Yim, S.H., Shin, D.H., Kang, D., Yu, D.Y. & Rhee, S.G. (2010). Inactivation of peroxiredoxin I by phosphorylation allows localized H(2)O(2) accumulation for cell signaling. *Cell*, 140, 517–528, ISSN 0092-8674

Wu, W.S., Wu, J.R. & Hu, C.T. (2008). Signal cross talks for sustained MAPK activation and cell migration: the potential role of reactive oxygen species. *Cancer Metastasis Rev*, 27, 303–314

Xu, X., Gao, X., Potter, B.J., Cao, J.M. & Zhang, C. (2007). Anti-LOX-1 rescues endothelial function in coronary arterioles in atherosclerotic ApoE knockout mice. *Arteriosclerosis Thrombosis and Vascular Biology*, 27, 871-877, ISSN 1079-5642

Yamamori, T., Inanami, O., Nagahata, H. & Kuwabara, M. (2004). Phosphoinositide 3-kinase regulates the phosphorylation of NADPH oxidase component p47(phox) by controlling cPKC/PKCdelta but not Akt. *Biochemical and Biophysical Research Communications*, 316, 720-730, ISSN 0006-291X

Yusuf, S., Dagenais, G., Pogue, J., Bosch, J., & Sleight, P. (2000) Vitamin E supplementation and cardiovascular events in high-risk patients. The Heart Outcomes Prevention Evaluation Study Investigators. *New England Journal of Medicine*, 342, 154-160, ISSN 0028-4793

Zadák, Z., Hyspler, R., Tichá, A., Hronek, M., Fikrová, P., Rathouská, J., Hrnciariková, D. & Stetina, R. (2009). Antioxidants and vitamins in clinical conditions. *Physiological Research*, 58, 13–17, ISSN 0862-8408

Zalba, G., Fortuño, A., San José, G., Moreno, M.U., Beloqui, O. & Díez, J. (2007). Oxidative stress, endothelial dysfunction and cerebrovascular disease. *Cerebrovascular Diseases* 24, 24-29, ISSN 1015-9770

Zhang, L., Sheppard, O.R., Shah, A.M. & Brewer, A.C. (2008). Positive regulation of the NADPH oxidase NOX4 promoter in vascular smooth muscle cells by E2F. *Free Radical Biology and Medicine,* 45, 679-685, ISSN 0891-5849

Zhang, M., Brewer, A.C., Schröder, K., Santos, C.X., Grieve, D.J., Wang, M., Anilkumar, N., Yu, B., Dong, X., Walker, S.J., Brandes, R.P. & Shah, A.M. (2010). NADPH oxidase-4 mediates protection against chronic load-induced stress in mouse hearts by enhancing angiogenesis. *Proceedings of the National Academy of Sciences USA,* 107, 18121-18126, ISSN 0027-8424

# 21

# Modified Forms of LDL in Plasma

José Luis Sánchez-Quesada[1] and Sandra Villegas[2]
[1]*Biomedical Research Institute Sant Pau (IIB Sant Pau), Barcelona*
[2]*Biochemistry and Molecular Biology Department, Universitat Autonoma de Barcelona*
*Spain*

## 1. Introduction

High blood concentration of low-density lipoprotein (LDL) cholesterol is a major risk factor for early development of atherosclerosis. Massive accumulation of cholesterol in the arterial wall and formation of lipid-laden cells (foam cells) typical of the atheromatous plaque occur after LDL entrapment in the subendothelial space. However, there is a general agreement that native non-modified LDL does not present any of the typical features of an atherogenic lipoprotein; native LDL does not promote foam cell formation and has no inflammatory, proliferative or apoptotic capacity. It is therefore assumed that when LDL is trapped in the arterial wall it is modified by several mechanisms such as lipoperoxidation, non-enzymatic glycosylation, enzymatic lipolysis and/or proteolysis. As a consequence, modified LDL particles acquire inflammatory and apoptotic capacity and are recognizable by scavenger receptors to promote foam cell formation. Although most studies on LDL modification have focused on mechanisms that could occur in the vessel wall, modified LDL particles have been reported in blood. The concentration of these particles is increased in subjects with high cardiovascular risk. The present chapter reviews the possible mechanisms leading to LDL modification. It then focuses on a subfraction of modified LDL particles detected in plasma, named electronegative LDL.

## 2. Modification of LDL as a key event for atherosclerosis

Pioneering studies by Goldstein and Brown demonstrated the involvement of LDL receptor (LDLr) in the plasma clearance of LDL and its major role in the development of atherosclerosis (Goldstein & Brown, 1985). However, these authors' outstanding observations gave rise to what was called the "cholesterol paradox" (Brown & Goldstein, 1983). Patients with homozygous familial hypercholesterolemia lack functional LDLr. Moreover, LDLr expression is negatively regulated by the intracellular cholesterol content, which results in a tight control of the concentration of esterified cholesterol in the cytoplasm (Brown & Goldstein, 1986). However, atherosclerosis is characterized by an abundance of foam cells loaded with esterified cholesterol droplets. Hence, there must be an alternative pathway leading to the massive accumulation of cholesterol in foam cells of the atherosclerotic lesion. This alternative pathway was discovered through the study of the scavenger receptors (SR) expressed by monocyte-derived macrophages (Krieger, 1992). These receptors have the ability to bind an unusual variety of ligands with the common characteristic of high electronegative charge. The first SR described was the type A SR (SRA) (Goldstein, 1979). SRA do not recognize native LDL but is able to bind modified forms of LDL; indeed, SRA expression is not regulated by the cytoplasm concentration of cholesterol. Early studies were performed using acetylated LDL (acLDL), a good ligand for SRA. However, acetylation does not occur spontaneously "in vivo". Soon, researchers looked for further modifications of LDL that would increase its negative charge and were able to occur "in vivo". The finding that oxidized LDL (oxLDL) could be internalized through SR and promote the formation of foam cells opened a vast field of research (Steinberg, 1989).

### 2.1 Oxidative modification of LDL

Oxidative modifications of lipid and proteins are frequent in many pathophysiological processes "in vivo" and it is now well-established that LDL undergoes oxidative modifications that confer to these modified particles a number of atherogenic properties (Witztum & Steinberg, 1991). In the early 80s several researchers independently observed that the incubation of LDL with endothelial cells in culture drastically altered these particles, transforming them into more electronegative LDL, after which they become a ligand for macrophages SR (Henriksen, 1981; Hessler, 1979). These studies concluded that the changes induced by endothelial cells on LDL were due to free radical modification. This was the origin of the oxidative modification hypothesis of atherogenesis (Steinberg, 1989). This hypothesis was gradually strengthened by subsequent findings regarding the properties of oxLDL obtained over the ensuing years. Table 1 summarizes the atherogenic properties observed in oxLDL and their contribution to atherosclerosis.

| Characteristic | Consequence in atherosclerosis |
|---|---|
| Impaired binding to the LDL receptor | Decreased plasma clearance |
| Recognition by SR | Foam cell formation |
| Increase in the expression of cytokines, chemokines and vascular adhesion molecules | Leukocyte recruitment, inflammation |
| Increase in the expression of growth factors | Cell proliferation and collagen secretion |
| Promotion of apoptosis and cytotoxicity | Formation of necrotic core |
| Immunogenicity | Immunogenic component of atherosclerosis |
| Inhibition of NO release and function | Vasoconstriction |
| Increase of tissue factor activity | Thombosis |

Table 1. Atherogenic characteristics of oxLDL

Oxidation of LDL primarily attacks the double bonds of unsaturated fatty acids in phospholipids and generates a plethora of lipid-derived compounds, including oxidized cholesterol (oxysterols), oxidized-fragmented phospholipids, lysophosphatidylcholine, hydroperoxids, aldehydes and ketones (Esterbauer, 1990). The protein moiety of LDL can be modified by reacting with lipid-oxidation products. Both aldehydes and ketones, for example, malondialdehyde (MDA) or 4-hydroxynonenal (HNE), have the ability to derivatize lysine and arginine residues in apoB (Fogelman, 1980). This reaction forms an adduct that eliminates the positive charge of these aminoacids and increases the negative charge of the particle, favouring its recognition by SRA (Goldstein, 1979). In addition to SRA, further SRs and other receptors which bind different forms of modified LDLs have been described in the last two decades (SRBI, CD36, LOX-1, CD68, LRP1, TLR4) (Adachi & Tsujimoto, 2006; Llorente-Cortes & Badimon, 2005; Miller, 2003; Van Berkel, 2000). These receptors play a role in innate immunity, scavenging a number of ligands and extracellular debris. Some of these are also expressed in endothelial cells or in smooth muscle cells (Adachi & Tsujimoto, 2006). The derivatization of lysines has an additional effect on LDL; since a lysine-rich cluster is the LDLr binding site of apoB (residues 3359-3369), the loss of their positive charge abolishes the interaction between oxLDL and LDLr (Boren, 1998a).

Besides lipid accumulation, other phenomena occur during the evolution of the disease. Atherosclerosis is a chronic inflammatory process that begins with leukocyte recruitment to the lesion area (Ross, 1999). A number of inflammation mediators, such as cytokines (IL6), chemokines (IL8, MCP1) or vascular adhesion molecules (VCAM, ICAM1, e-selectin) are hyperexpressed in response to oxLDL by all cells involved in atherogenesis, including endothelial cells, monocytes/macrophages, lymphocytes and smooth muscle cells (Berliner, 1997; Tedgui & Mallat, 2006). Related to the inflammatory activity of oxLDL is its ability to promote the expression of growth factors and colony stimulating factors. This proliferative activity is mediated by oxidation-derived lipids, and in smooth muscle cells it induces the change of the normal contractile phenotype to a proliferative phenotype (Auge, 2002). The proliferative phenotype of smooth muscle cells is characterized by the high production of collagen that will contribute decisively to the thickening of the arterial wall (Negishi, 2004).

Another hallmark of the atheromatous plaque in its advanced stages is the presence of a necrotic core formed by debris from dead cells (Stary, 2000). OxLDL also contributes to the formation of this necrotic core, because when the content of esterified cholesterol exceeds the storage capacity of foam cells apoptotic processes are induced (Hessler, 1983). Another mechanism of cytotoxicity is the high content of lysophosphatidylcholine in oxLDL that disrupts the integrity of cytoplasmatic membrane and promotes cell death (Naito, 1994).

OxLDL is immunogenic, and autoantibodies against oxidation-specific epitopes are detected in normal and hyperlipemic subjects (Lopes-Virella & Virella, 2010). The role of these autoantibodies is not well defined and published results are divergent; positive or negative associations between autoantibodies and atherosclerosis have been reported. In general, antibodies of IgG class are presumed to be pro-atherogenic, whereas IgM antibodies would play a protective role (Frostegard, 2010). Further deleterious properties of oxLDL are its capacity to increase the tissue factor activity (Petit, 1999), favouring thrombosis, or the inhibition of the release of nitric oxide (Minuz, 1995), promoting vasoconstriction.

The lipoperoxidative process is sequential and lipids degrade to produce new products which in turn form other molecules (Quehenberger, 1988). As a consequence, oxLDL comprises an extremely heterogeneous group of particles that have different atherogenic characteristics depending on the relative content of each molecule (Esterbauer, 1993). For instance, minimally oxidized LDL (mmLDL) has a high inflammatory activity due to its high content in oxidized phospholipids formed during the early phases of oxidation. However, mmLDL has normal affinity to the LDLr and is not recognized by SR. In contrast, extensively oxidized LDL has relatively low inflammatory activity but it is a major inductor of cytotoxicity due to its high content of oxysterols. Indeed, the more oxidized the LDL the more these particles promote foam cell formation.

### 2.2 Further modifications of LDL occurring in the arterial wall

Oxidative modification is not the only process affecting the native properties of lipoproteins in the arterial wall. Disappointing results from large-antioxidant trials have led to the concept that alternative mechanisms of modification could be involved (Steinberg, 2009). Current knowledge indicates that although oxidation is still relevant, other processes could contribute substantially to the development of atherosclerosis. A number of modifications have been studied over the past three decades.

Enzymes that are hyperexpressed in the microenvironment of the lesion area, such as lipases (cholesterol esterase (CEase), sphingomyelinase (SMase) or secretary phospholipase $A_2$ ($sPLA_2$)) or proteases (matrix metalloproteases or cathepsins) can modify LDL (Pentikainen, 2000). In the case of diabetes, non-enzymatic glycosylation could have a major role in LDL modification (Witztum, 1997). The interaction of LDL with the proteoglycans (PG) could modify apoB conformation, destabilizing its conformation and promoting aggregation (Pentikainen, 1997). Other putative physiological processes that could modify LDL are carbamylation (Basnakian, 2010) or desialylation (Tertov, 1990). Table 2 summarizes several possible physiological mechanisms leading to LDL modification.

| Mechanisms of modification | Foam cell formation | Inflammation/ proliferation | Cytotoxicity/ apoptosis |
|---|---|---|---|
| Oxidation[1] | +++ | +++ | +++ |
| Modification by CEase and protease | -/+ | ++ | ++ |
| Lipolysis by SMase | + | - | -/+ |
| Lipolysis by $PLA_2$ | -/+ | ++ | + |
| Non-enzymatic glycosylation | -/+ | -/+ | -/+ |
| Binding to PG | ++ | - | - |
| Carbamylation | ++ | ++ | ++ |
| Desialylation | ++ | + | ++ |

Table 2. Atherogenic properties of several modified LDLs. [1] The characteristics of oxLDL, and also those of the other modifications, depend on the extent of modification

#### 2.2.1 Enzymatically-modified LDL (E-LDL)

In an attempt to find a modified LDL alternative to oxLDL, Bhakdi and coworkers performed a series of studies using LDL that was modified by means of one protease and CEase. They found that this "enzymatically-modified LDL" (E-LDL) acquired a number of atherogenic properties (Bhakdi, 1995). As a result of the enzymatic treatment, E-LDL presents mild apoB fragmentation, and it has high free cholesterol and non-esterified fatty acids (NEFA) content (Klouche, 1998). E-LDL induces inflammation, proliferation and apoptosis (Dersch, 2005; Klouche, 1999; Klouche, 2000). The high content of NEFA seems to be major factor responsible for these atherogenic properties (Suriyaphol, 2002). E-LDL adds further atherogenic characteristics because it binds to C-reactive protein and activates the classical complement pathway (Bhakdi, 2004). The activation of complement by E-LDL concurs with the emerging concept of the innate immune response as a potentially important factor in atherosclerosis (Hartvigsen, 2009).

### 2.2.2 Phospholipase $A_2$-modified LDL ($PLA_2$-LDL)

Several studies have focused on the atherogenic effects of LDL modified with different types of secreted phospholipase $A_2$ ($sPLA_2$) (Divchev & Schieffer, 2008). Some $sPLA_2$ have been detected in atherosclerotic lesions and their products, lysophosphatidylcholine (LPC) and NEFA, induce cytotoxicity at relatively high concentrations by disrupting membrane integrity (Dersch, 2005; Naito, 1994). Moreover, both molecules have inflammatory potential by stimulating the expression of cytokines and chemokines (Sonoki, 2003). In addition, extensively lipolyzed LDL with some (type X), but not all (type IIA or V), $sPLA_2$ are able to induce foam cell formation (Curfs, 2008). An interesting approach was performed by Sparrow and coworkers, which combined $sPLA_2$ and lipoxygenase to modify LDL (Sparrow, 1988). This combination of lipoperoxidation and phospholipolysis generated LDL particles with similar properties to those promoted by endothelial cell-induced oxidative modification. Another atherogenic characteristic of $sPLA_2$-modified LDL is its increased affinity for PG binding due to the exposition of an alternative binding site in apoB that specifically recognizes PG (Boren, 1998b). As occurs with SMase-modified LDL, this would lead to increased subendothelial retention.

PAF-acetylhydrolase (PAF-AH), another $PLA_2$ with relevance in the metabolism of LDL, merits special mention. This enzyme is transported in plasma bound to lipoproteins (approximately 70% in LDL and 25% in HDL) but, in contrast to $sPLA_2$, its substrate is not native phospholipids but fragmented phospholipids that have been generated by oxidation (Tjoelker & Stafforini, 2000). Thus, LPC content is high in oxLDL due to the action of PAF-AH. However, there is controversy regarding the pro- or anti-atherogenic role of PAF-AH (Tellis & Tselepis, 2009). On one hand, its function should be atheroprotective since it degrades highly-inflammatory fragmented phospholipids. On the other hand, however, the by-products formed are LPC and short-chain NEFA, which also have inflammatory potential, though to a lesser extent than oxidized phospholipids (MacPhee, 1999).

### 2.2.3 Sphingomyelinase-modified LDL (SMase-LDL)

The hyperexpression of acid and neutral SMases in atherosclerotic lesions has been known for several years (Tabas, 1999). SMase hydrolyzes sphingomyelin (SM) yielding phosphorylcholine and ceramide. Ceramide directly exerts several biological effects, but its main action is to elicit the production of bioactive sphingolipids, such as sphingosine-1-phosphate that plays a major role in apoptosis (van Blitterswijk, 2003). Another action of SMase is to promote extensive LDL aggregation (Oorni, 2000). Aggregation of LDL confers several atherogenic properties. First, aggregated LDL (agLDL) is able to induce foam cell formation, not through SR in this case but through the LDL-receptor related protein 1 (LRP1), a receptor of aggregated lipoproteins highly expressed in smooth muscle cells (Llorente-Cortes & Badimon, 2005). Second, agLDL binds with higher affinity to PG (Oorni, 1998). As discussed below, this binding promotes structural changes in apoB. The association of agLDL to PG precludes the exit of this lipoprotein from the subendothelial space, and consequently favours that agLDL could undergo further modifications.

### 2.2.4 Glycated LDL (glLDL)

Although non-enzymatic glycosylation of LDL occurs in all subjects, it has stronger consequences in people with diabetes mellitus. Glucose can interact with the free amino groups of lysines and arginines in apoB, forming a Schiff base that rearranges to yield an

Amadori product (Brownlee, 1992). This modification leads to a loss of electropositive charges in glycated LDL (glLDL), decreasing its affinity to the LDLr and consequently prolonging its mean lifetime in plasma (Witztum, 1982). The increase in lifetime can result in further modification of LDL forming advanced glycation end-products (AGE) and producing a form of LDL named AGE-LDL (Menzel, 1997). AGE-LDL can also be internalized by specific receptors (RAGE) (Bucala, 1996). AGE-LDL and glLDL increase chemotactic activity in monocytes, stimulate cell proliferation and enhance platelet aggregation, although the relative contribution that the coexistence of oxidation could have is not well established. The formation of AGE involves oxidative reactions and it has been demonstrated that lipoperoxidation and non-enzymatic glycosylation are mutually potentiated processes (Sobal, 2000). Thus, glycosylation of LDL is not only noxious per se but also because it promotes LDL oxidation.

### 2.2.5 Proteoglycan-bound LDL (PG-LDL)

PG are the main constituents of the arterial intima. It has been hypothesized that subendothelial retention of lipoproteins due to the binding of LDL to PG is the initial event in atherogenesis, even prior to endothelial dysfunction or inflammation (Williams & Tabas, 2005). The retention itself increases the time of LDL in the subendothelial space and, therefore, the possibility that further modifications occur. Furthermore, the binding LDL-PG also has a direct effect on LDL modification because this binding promotes changes in the structure of apoB that facilitate processes such as oxidation or lipolysis mediated by SMase or $sPLA_2$ (Hevonoja, 2000). On the other hand, LDL-PG complexes are taken up by cells through different types of SR, promoting foam cell formation.

## 3. Modified LDL in human plasma

For many years it was considered that LDL modification was a phenomenon occurring mainly in the intima layer of the arterial wall. Oxidative modification was the most studied process, and most researchers accepted that the abundance in plasma of soluble molecules with antioxidant capacity (albumin, uric acid, bilirubin, glutathione, ascorbic acid) would inhibit oxidation of lipoproteins. Moreover, the binding of oxLDL by SR expressed in circulating monocytes is known to promote a rapid clearance of extensively oxidized LDL. However, progress in enzyme immunoassay procedures has provided direct evidence of oxLDL in circulating plasma. Besides oxLDL, similar methods have been used to detect other forms of modified LDL in blood. These include glLDL, AGE-LDL, carbamylated LDL (ca-LDL), desialylated LDL and electronegative LDL (LDL(-)).

### 3.1 Oxidized LDL in plasma

Despite the abundance of antioxidant defences in blood, increased oxidative stress has been described in plasma from patients with atherosclerosis. Early studies reported that increased levels of oxidized lipids in plasma were associated with atherosclerosis development (Avogaro, 1986). In agreement with that, the existence of oxLDL in blood is increased in subjects with high cardiovascular risk (Holvoet, 1999; Holvoet, 1998) or in diseases, such as diabetes, obesity, metabolic syndrome and hyperlipemia (Ishigaki, 2009). Although it cannot be totally ruled out that a part of oxLDL could be formed in blood, it is generally accepted that oxLDL originates primarily in the arterial wall and that the molecules reach the blood from the subendothelial space. For this reason, oxLDL is considered not only a biomarker of atherosclerosis development but also a reflection of the presence of unstable and ruptured atherosclerotic plaques (Fraley & Tsimikas, 2006). The fact that oxLDL increases temporarily during the acute phase of myocardial infarction or stroke supports this notion (Fraley & Tsimikas, 2006; Nishi, 2002; Uno, 2003) and some studies have raised the possibility that plasma oxLDL could predict future cardiovascular events (Meisinger, 2005). The concentration of oxLDL in plasma is very low, and data reported by several authors are disperse, ranging from 0.01% to 0.5% of total LDL. The heterogeneous nature of oxLDL is one reason to explain variation in the reports of oxLDL concentration, but another could be the use of several antibodies that recognize different epitopes (Ishigaki, 2009). The fact that in vitro oxidation does not reproduce the same epitopes generated during in vivo modification makes it difficult to develop a golden standard.

Several studies have shown that besides its utility as a biomarker, oxLDL in plasma acts as a pathogenic factor. It has been reported that oxLDL contributes to increase the systemic inflammatory status by stimulating the activity of the transcription factor NF-kB in peripheral blood mononuclear cells (Cominacini, 2005). More direct demonstration of the implication of oxLDL in blood has been obtained by increasing the expression of SR, such as SRA1 (Whitman, 2002), LOX-1 (Ishigaki, 2008), or the chimerical fusion protein SRA1-growth hormone (Laukkanen, 2000), which favours oxLDL removal from blood. These studies showed an inhibition of atherosclerosis development. It was recently reported that repeated administration of the chimerical fusion protein Fc-CD68 decreases the extent of atherosclerosis in hyperlipemic mice (Zeibig, 2011). However, these studies have been tested to date in animal models only. Regarding humans, several trials have reported that lipid-lowering therapy in atherosclerotic patients lowers oxLDL, although this decrease is parallel to that of LDL cholesterol (Ky, 2008). However, no trial with a therapy specifically focused on oxLDL is yet available. The development of novel therapies for lowering oxLDL itself is a promising strategy for atherosclerosis treatment.

### 3.2 Glycated LDL in plasma

The concentration of glLDL in plasma from patients with diabetes is increased, reflecting the hyperglycemia in these patients. This concentration varies depending on the method used for its quantification (ELISA, affinity chromatography), but it is generally higher than that of oxLDL (Cohen, 1993; Reaven, 1995). The proportion of glLDL in diabetics can reach up to 7-8% of total LDL and approximately half in normoglycemic subjects. It is important to note that glLDL is present in all individuals, and even in normoglycemic subjects the concentration in plasma is higher than that of oxLDL. This suggests glLDL plays a role in the development of atherosclerosis even in absence of hyperglycemia. Interestingly, glLDL is more abundant in the subfractions of LDL that are smallest and have the highest density, probably because these small-dense LDL particles are prone to non-enzymatic glycosylation (Younis, 2009). These particles are also more susceptible to oxidation and have a relatively low affinity to the LDL receptor. These properties are related to the strong association between small-dense LDL and high cardiovascular risk (Krauss, 1995).

Alternative pathways can also result in LDL glycosylation without a direct involvement of glucose. Metabolites of glucose such as glyoxal, methylglyoxal or glycaldehyde have a higher reducing capacity as glycating agents (Rabbani & Thornalley, 2011). Minimal modification by methylglyoxal renders LDL particles with atherogenic properties, including binding to PG and susceptibility to aggregation (Rabbani, 2011). LDL particles with this low level of modification are increased in diabetic patients (Rabbani, 2010).

A more advanced form of glLDL is AGE-LDL, in which AGE are formed due to auto-oxidation of Amadori adducts yielding a number of products, such as carboxymethyl lysine or pentosyl lysine (Brownlee, 2000). AGE-LDL has atherogenic characteristics that are similar to oxLDL, probably because their oxidized lipid content is similar. Although it was generally considered that AGE-LDL was generated in the arterial wall this modified form of LDL has also been detected in blood (Lopes-Virella & Virella, 2010). AGE-LDL, like other AGE-containing proteins, is recognized in circulation by RAGE. RAGE activation stimulates cytokyne and growth factors release (Ramasamy, 2009). An excess of stimulation (i.e. an excess of AGE-LDL) plays an essential role in atherogenic alterations.

### 3.3 Carbamylated LDL (ca-LDL)

Carbamylation of proteins is a post-translational modification in which amine-containing residues react with cyanate, a compound that derives from urea or from thiocyanate. This modification is relatively frequent in patients with chronic uremia or in heavy smokers. Both situations are closely related to increased cardiovascular risk and carbamylated LDL (ca-LDL) is increased in the plasma in both groups of subjects (Basnakian, 2010). Ca-LDL is recognized by SR, promotes monocyte adhesion to endothelium, stimulates cell proliferation and causes cell injury (Apostolov, 2007; Carracedo, 2011).

### 3.4 Desialylated LDL (ds-LDL)

Native LDL has high content of sialic acid in the carbohydrate chains attached to apoB. Tertov and colleagues isolated a fraction of desialylated LDL from plasma (Tertov, 1990). This fraction, which was increased in patients with advanced atherosclerosis, induced foam cell formation in cultured smooth muscle cells and presented inflammatory properties (Orekhov, 1991). They suggested that low sialic acid in LDL was a cardiovascular risk factor (Ruelland, 1993) but this idea was not supported by other authors (Cerne, 2002). Later studies revealed that desialylated LDL was oxidized and that the loss of sialic acid was a consequence of oxidative modification (Tertov, 1995).

## 4. Electronegative LDL, a pool of modified LDL in blood

A common characteristic of most of the previously described modifications is an increase of the negative electric charge. Taking advantage of this property, Avogaro and co-workers fractionated total LDL from human plasma by anion-exchange chromatography, into two subfractions, a major subfraction of native LDL and an electronegatively-charged fraction of LDL (LDL(-)) (Avogaro, 1988). In this first report, LDL(-) accounted for 5-20% of total LDL in normolipemic subjects and presented a number of atherogenic characteristics, including impaired binding to LDLr, high aggregation level, capacity to induce cholesterol accumulation in macrophages and higher conjugated diene (a by-product of lipid peroxidation) content. Since then, a number of studies have tried to elucidate the physico-chemical and biological characteristics of LDL(-) and its relationship with atherosclerosis.

### 4.1 Origin of LDL(-) – Discrepancies regarding the oxidative origin

Early studies focused on the physico-chemical characteristics LDL(-) concluded, in accordance with the high content of oxidized lipids, that LDL(-) was the in vivo counterpart of in vitro oxidized LDL (Cazzolato, 1991). However, as isolation procedures improved and measures to prevent modification increased, the proportion of LDL(-) and the content in lipoperoxides decreased (De Castellarnau, 2000; Demuth, 1996; Sevanian, 1997). Discrepancies regarding the increased content in oxidized lipids in LDL(-), continue; some authors do not find differences compared to native LDL (Benitez, 2007b; Demuth, 1996; Sanchez-Quesada, 2003), and others report increased amounts of oxidized lipids in LDL(-) (Asatryan, 2003; Sevanian, 1997; Ziouzenkova, 2002). But in any case, this level of lipoperoxidation is closer to minimally oxidized LDL than to extensively oxidized LDL suggesting that alternative mechanisms should be involved in LDL(-) formation (Fig. 1).

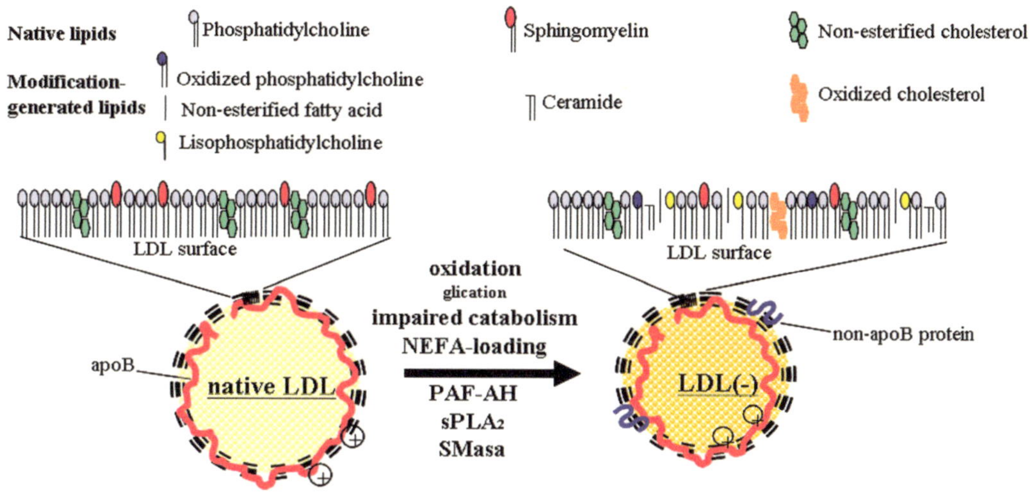


Fig. 1. Formation of LDL(-). The modification of native LDL by one or several mechanisms alters the composition of LDL surface. These alterations include the increase of inflammatory, proliferative and apoptotic lipids and non-apoB proteins in LDL(-), as well as structural abnormalities in apoB.

### 4.1.1 Impaired catabolism of LDL

LDL is a heterogeneous mixture of particles that differ in size (24-28 nm of diameter) and density (1.019-1.063 g/ml). Small-dense particles have fewer lipid molecules while large-buoyant particles have more. It is known that LDL particles at both extremes of the density range have increased electronegative charge compared with mid-density particles (Lund-Katz, 1998). It has been proposed that the origin of LDL(-) could be related with the impairment of the catabolic cascade that transforms VLDL-to-IDL-to-LDL in blood (Sanchez-Quesada, 2004). Such impairment leads to the formation of small-dense or large-buoyant LDL particles. In agreement with this, LDL(-) is most abundant (>80% of LDL(-)) in small-dense particles in normolipemic subjects. Interestingly, in hypercholesterolemic and hypertriglyceridemic patients, LDL(-) are also abundant large-buoyant particles (Sanchez-Quesada, 2002). Another consequence of impaired LDL catabolism is the presence of non-apoB proteins in LDL. Theoretically, the protein moiety of LDL consists of a single copy of a very large protein, apoB. However, it is known that some particles of LDL also contain other proteins. In native LDL, the content of non-apoB proteins is less than 1%. In contrast, LDL(-) contains up to 5% of non-apoB proteins (Bancells, 2010a; Yang, 2003).

### 4.1.2 Lipolysis

Some characteristics of LDL(-), such as high LPC and NEFA content, suggest that a possible mechanism of formation could be mediated by phospholipases. It has been described that in vitro modification of LDL with $sPLA_2$ renders modified particles that mimics some properties of LDL(-) (Asatryan, 2005; Benitez, 2004a; Benitez, 2004b). On the other hand, PAF-AH, which has a 5-10-fold higher activity in LDL(-) than in native LDL, could also play a role in increasing the content of LPC and NEFA and in the generation of LDL(-) (Gaubatz, 2007; Sanchez-Quesada, 2005). Some type of SMase activity could also be involved in LDL(-) generation since a minor subfraction of LDL(-) is aggregated (Bancells, 2010b). It has been reported that LDL(-) has an intrinsic phospholipase C-like (PLC-like) activity that degrades with high affinity both SM and LPC (Bancells, 2008). The origin of such activity is currently unknown, but it could be due to conformational changes in apoB. One or a combination of these phospholipolityc activities could be involved in the formation of LDL(-).

### 4.1.3 Content of non-esterified fatty acids (NEFA)

NEFA are transported in blood mainly associated to albumin. However, in some situations that increase NEFA or decrease albumin there is a partition of NEFA towards other proteins, including lipoproteins. In posprandial lipemia or when high energy is required (such as during heavy exercise) the increase of NEFA in blood increases LDL(-) proportion (Benitez, 2002). NEFA content in LDL(-) is three to four-fold higher than in native LDL (Benitez, 2004a; De Castellarnau, 2000; Demuth, 1996). In this context, it has been reported that the main determinant of the electronegativity of LDL(-) is NEFA (Gaubatz, 2007).

### 4.1.4 Non-enzymatic glycosylation

It would seem reasonable to consider that glLDL contributes in part to the pool of LDL(-), especially in diabetic patients. However, most glycated LDL particles isolable by affinity chromatography do not have a sufficient negative charge to be isolated with LDL(-) and the content of glLDL in LDL(-) is similar to that in native LDL (Benitez, 2007b; Sanchez-Quesada, 2005).

### 4.1.5 Hemoglobin derivatization and carbamylation

Patients with severe renal failure have a high proportion of LDL(-) (Asatryan, 2003). It was reported that LDL from these patients suffered a cross-linking with hemoglobin, rendering a particle with increased negative charge (Ziouzenkova, 2002). Recent studies on carbamylated LDL, however, suggest that carbamylation could underlie the high proportion of LDL(-) in patients with severe renal disease (Apostolov, 2010).

### 4.2 Biological properties of LDL(-)

Whatever the mechanism involved in its formation LDL(-), has several potentially atherogenic properties. These include abnormal binding to receptors, inflammatory and cytotoxic properties, high susceptibility to aggregation and increased affinity to PG (Fig. 2).

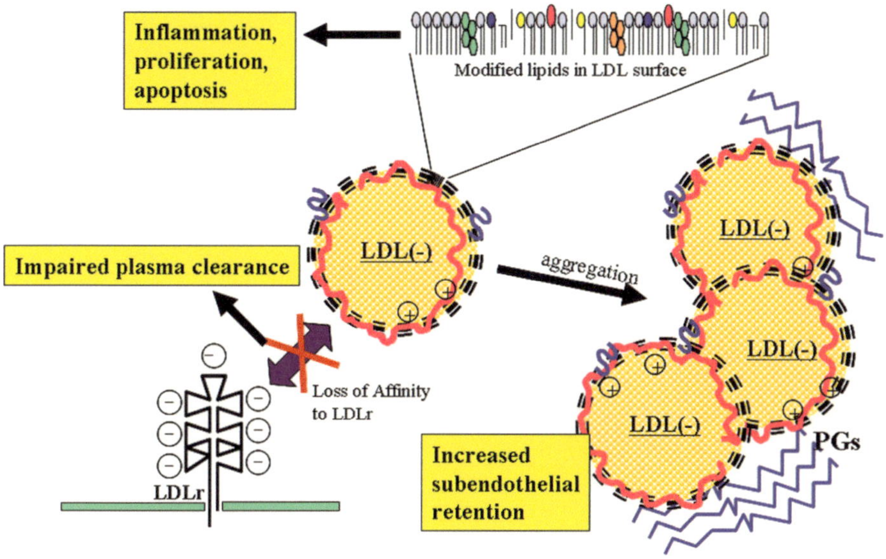


Fig. 2. Atherogenic properties of LDL(-). Modified lipids in LDL(-) surface have inflammatory, proliferative and apoptotic capacity. Aggregation, which is induced by the formation of ceramide, favours the binding to PGs and increases subendothelial retention. The alteration of apoB conformation in LDL(-) induces a partial loss of affinity to the LDLr and impairs its plasma clearance.

#### 4.2.1 Binding to receptors

LDL(-) presents a partial loss of affinity to the LDLr, a property that could lengthen its half-life in blood (Benitez, 2004b). It was initially believed that this was due to the derivatization of lysines in apoB involved in receptor recognition, in a mechanism similar to oxLDL (MDA-Lys) or glLDL (glucose-Lys). However, recent studies have shown that lysines in LDL(-) are not derivatized but have an altered ionization state due to differences in the conformation of apoB (Blanco, 2010). Regarding SR, LDL(-) binds differently to distinct types of SR. The increment of electronegativity in LDL(-) is not sufficient to allow its binding to SRA in macrophages (Benitez, 2004b). However, it has been reported that LDL(-) binds to another SR, LOX-1, in endothelial cells (Lu, 2009). This binding does not promote foam cell formation, but could mediate the signaling of endothelial apoptosis.

#### 4.2.2 Inflammatory activity

LDL(-) has the ability to activate the transcription factors NF-kB, AP-1 and PPAR, inducing the expression of a number of inflammatory molecules in endothelial cells (Abe, 2007; Benitez, 2006; De Castellarnau, 2000; Ziouzenkova, 2003). These molecules include cytokines (IL6) chemokines (IL8, MCP-1, GRO), vascular adhesion molecules (VCAM) and growth factors (GM-CSF, PDGF). Interestingly, LDL(-) also induces the paradoxical expression of the anti-inflammatory cytokine IL10 in lymphocytes and monocytes (Benitez, 2007a). It has been suggested that IL10 production could be a mechanism to control an excessive inflammatory response limiting the extent of injury. LDL(-) could also play a role in angiogenesis modulation since it stimulates vascular endothelial growth factor (VEGF) expression and inhibits the release of the matrix metalloproteinases MMP2 and MMP9 (Lu,

2008; Tai, 2006). The specific molecules that mediate these actions are not well defined; LPC and NEFA probably play a major role, but the action of oxidized lipids remains under discussion (Abe, 2007; Benitez, 2004a; Chen, 2004). If they are present in LDL(-) they could stimulate inflammatory responses, but it is also possible that high PAF-AH activity in LDL (-) degrades readily oxidized phospholipids (Benitez, 2003). Their degradation products, LPC and short-chain NEFA, would therefore be responsible for triggering inflammation.

#### 4.2.3 Cytotoxicity and apoptosis

LDL(-) induces citotoxicity and apoptosis in endothelial cells and macrophages by different signaling pathways. The mechanisms involved are well defined, especially in endothelial cells, where LOX-1 signaling inhibits fibroblast growth factor 2 (FGF2) transcription and Akt phosphorilation (Chen, 2003; Chen, 2007; Lu, 2008; Tang, 2008; Yang, 2007). In contrast, macrophage apoptosis involves the Fas/FasL signaling pathway and the activation of the transcription factor Nrf2 (Pedrosa, 2010).

#### 4.2.4 Binding to proteoglycans

LDL(-) and PG present a high affinity for binding (Bancells, 2009). This could favor the subendothelial retention of LDL(-) and trigger the inflammatory response. Some characteristics in LDL(-) are involved in this higher affinity. Aggregation of lipoproteins favors PG binding, and LDL(-) has a high tendency to aggregate (Bancells, 2010b). In fact, a subfraction of aggregated LDL(-) is responsible for the binding to PG (Bancells, 2009). This subfraction has an abnormal conformation that exposes an epitope in apoB, known as site Ib, that is an alternative binding site to PGs (Bancells, 2011).

### 4.3 Physico-chemical characteristics of LDL(-)

#### 4.3.1 Structure

The earliest physical abnormalities reported in LDL(-) were a great heterogeneity in size and density and a high susceptibility to aggregation (Avogaro, 1988). A subpopulation of aggregated LDL(-) has recently been isolated and characterized. This subpopulation, which accounts for only 0.1-0.5 of total LDL in blood, has high affinity to arterial PG (Bancells, 2009). This increased binding seems to be mediated by abnormal conformation of the amino-terminal extreme of apoB (Bancells, 2011). Further evidence of apoB misfolding, in this case affecting LDLr binding, has been obtained by two dimensional nuclear magnetic resonance analyses (Blanco, 2010). LDL(-) is reported to promote aggregation of non-aggregated LDL particles in a process that fits an amyloidogenic model (Parasassi, 2008). It has been reported that the capacity to induce aggregation could be mediated by the PLC-like activity (Bancells, 2010b), although other authors have suggested that plasma $sPLA_2$ could be involved in apoB misfolding (Greco, 2009). Regarding secondary structure of apoB, some authors have reported loss of secondary $\alpha$-helix structures whereas others did not find differences with native LDL (Asatryan, 2005; Bancells, 2009; Benitez, 2004b; Parasassi, 2001).

#### 4.3.2 Lipids

Although there are contradictory data regarding differences in the lipid content between native LDL and LDL(-) most studies concur in a higher content of triglycerides, NEFA and LPC in LDL(-) (Cazzolato, 1991; De Castellarnau, 2000; Sanchez-Quesada, 2003; Sevanian, 1997; Yang, 2003). The high content of triglycerides reflects impairment of the VLDL-to-IDL-to-LDL cascade. High NEFA could be a consequence of the increase in NEFA concentration in plasma (posprandial lipemia, intense exercise) (Benitez, 2002; Ursini, 1998), or it could come from lipolysis mediated by phospholipases (Benitez, 2004a). This latter possibility would be the same mechanism of increased LPC content in LDL(-).

### 4.3.3 Proteins

The most abundant proteins in LDL(-) are apoA-I (0.15 molecules/particle of LDL(-)), apoE (0.22), apoC-III (0.37) and apoA-II (0.14), with a content 3-5 fold higher in LDL(-) than in native LDL (Bancells, 2010a). The role of these proteins is unclear but their relevance is probably low. However, other proteins whose absolute content in LDL(-) is lower, such as apoF (0.06 molecules/particle), apoJ (0.01) or PAF-AH (0.004) (Bancells, 2010a; Yang, 2007), but their relative content compared with native LDL is 10, 20 and 100-fold higher, respectively, could have a much more relevant role. ApoF is the physiological inhibitor of cholesteryl ester transfer protein (Morton, 2008), a protein that regulates the catabolism of the VLDL-IDL-LDL cascade. It could therefore be one cause of impaired LDL(-) maturation. ApoJ (also known as clusterin) is an extracellular chaperone that binds to hydrophobic unfolded proteins, favoring their extracellular clearance (Oda, 1995). ApoJ binds mainly to aggregated LDL(-), supporting the presence of misfolded apoB in this subfraction. The role of PAF-AH in LDL(-) would be to deactivate oxidized phospholipids, but its undesirable effect would be the formation of LPC and short-chain NEFA. It has been suggested that the PLC-like activity present in LDL(-) could act in cooperation with PAF-AH degrading LPC (Bancells, 2010b). Therefore, this would be a mechanism to limit the deleterious effects exerted by minimal LDL oxidation on vascular cells.

### 4.4 Association of LDL(-) with cardiovascular risk

The proportion of LDL(-) is increased in a number of pathologic situations having a cardiovascular risk. Familial hypercholesterolemia and hypertriglyceridemia present a proportion of LDL(-) 3-5 fold higher than normolipemic healthy subjects (Sanchez-Quesada, 2002; Sanchez-Quesada, 1999). These results were obtained using ultracentrifugation plus anion-exchange chromatography, both being laborious and time-consuming techniques. This limits their use for routine analysis of lipoprotein profiles. However, more reliable techniques for rapid analysis have recently been developed, including capillary electrophoresis and ELISA (Santo Faulin Tdo, 2008; Zhang, 2009; Zhang, 2008). These methods have confirmed previous data obtained by anion-exchange chromatography. Statin therapy decreases the proportion of LDL(-) but the process is not parallel to the lipid-lowering effect. This is because total LDL cholesterol decreases very rapidly (in 2 weeks) whereas LDL(-) decreases more slowly (in up to six months) (Sanchez-Quesada, 1999). This suggests that LDL(-) generation not only depends on lipid metabolism but also on other factors such as chronic inflammation.

Both type 1 and type 2 diabetics have a high proportion of LDL(-) (Moro, 1998; Sanchez-Quesada, 1996; Sanchez-Quesada, 2001; Zhang, 2005). This would suggest that non-enzymatic glycosylation could be involved. However, insulin therapy decreases LDL(-) in type 1 diabetes but not in type 2 diabetes. The different response to insulin treatment has been attributed to differences in the systemic inflammation level, which is higher in type 2 patients. This agrees with the finding that pre-diabetic insulin-resistant subjects with high systemic inflammation also have increased LDL(-) proportion (Zhang, 2005). Therefore, hyperglycemia would not promote the increase of LDL(-) directly but through an increase of systemic inflammation. Another group of subjects with a high proportion of LDL(-) are patients with severe renal disease (Ziouzenkova & Sevanian, 2000). It has been described that α-tocopherol supplementation decreases LDL(-) in hemodialysis patients (Mafra, 2009). Regarding patients with established coronary disease, it has been shown that LDL(-) is increased in patients with angiographically documented coronary artery disease (Tomasik, 2003). Moreover, acute coronary syndromes, such as unstable angina or acute myocardial infarction, have higher levels of LDL(-) than chronic coronary syndromes (Mello, 2011). These observations support the partial subendothelial origin of LDL(-) and open the possibility for LDL(-) to be used as a biomarker of the progression of atherosclerotic lesions.

## 5. Conclusion

LDL is modified by several mechanisms that confer a number of atherogenic properties to these particles. Although it is believed that such modifications are more frequent in the subendothelial space of the artery wall than in blood, different types of modified LDL have been detected in plasma. LDL(-) is a mixture of modified LDL particles that represent the total pool of modified LDL in plasma. The biological and physico-chemical characteristics of LDL(-) and its association with high cardiovascular risk indicate that this lipoprotein plays a direct role in the development of atherosclerosis. However, although statin and insulin treatment decrease the proportion of LDL(-) , the development of a specific therapy for LDL(-) would be of great interest. Another field of research would be the use of LDL(-) as a biomarker. This could be a promising strategy to evaluate the cardiovascular risk and to monitor the success of distinct therapeutic strategies.

## 6. Acknowledgment

JLS-Q and SV are members of the 2009-SGR-1205 and of the 2009-SGR-00761 Research Group from the Generalitat de Catalunya, respectively. JLSQ and SV are funded by PI10/00265, PI10/00975 and CP06/00220 from ISCIII/Spanish Ministry of Health.

## 7. References

Abe, Y., Fornage, M., Yang, C.Y., Bui-Thanh, N.A., Wise, V., Chen, H.H., Rangaraj, G. & Ballantyne, C.M. (2007) L5, the most electronegative subfraction of plasma LDL, induces endothelial vascular cell adhesion molecule 1 and CXC chemokines, which mediate mononuclear leukocyte adhesion. *Atherosclerosis*. 192, 1, 56-66,

Adachi, H. & Tsujimoto, M. (2006) Endothelial scavenger receptors. *Prog Lipid Res*. 45, 5, 379-404, 0163-7827 (Print), 0163-7827 (Linking).

Apostolov, E.O., Ray, D., Savenka, A.V., Shah, S.V. & Basnakian, A.G. (2010) Chronic uremia stimulates LDL carbamylation and atherosclerosis. *J Am Soc Nephrol*. 21, 11, 1852-7, 1533-3450 (Electronic), 1046-6673 (Linking).

Apostolov, E.O., Shah, S.V., Ok, E. & Basnakian, A.G. (2007) Carbamylated low-density lipoprotein induces monocyte adhesion to endothelial cells through intercellular adhesion molecule-1 and vascular cell adhesion molecule-1. *Arterioscler Thromb Vasc Biol*. 27, 4, 826-32, 1524-4636 (Electronic), 1079-5642 (Linking).

Asatryan, L., Hamilton, R.T., Isas, J.M., Hwang, J., Kayed, R. & Sevanian, A. (2005) LDL phospholipid hydrolysis produces modified electronegative particles with an unfolded apoB-100 protein. *J Lipid Res.* 46, 1, 115-22,

Asatryan, L., Ziouzenkova, O., Duncan, R. & Sevanian, A. (2003) Heme and lipid peroxides in hemoglobin-modified low-density lipoprotein mediate cell survival and adaptation to oxidative stress. *Blood.* 102, 5, 1732-9,

Auge, N., Garcia, V., Maupas-Schwalm, F., Levade, T., Salvayre, R. & Negre-Salvayre, A. (2002) Oxidized LDL-induced smooth muscle cell proliferation involves the EGF receptor/PI-3 kinase/Akt and the sphingolipid signaling pathways. *Arterioscler Thromb Vasc Biol.* 22, 12, 1990-5, 1524-4636 (Electronic), 1079-5642 (Linking).

Avogaro, P., Bon, G.B. & Cazzolato, G. (1988) Presence of a modified low density lipoprotein in humans. *Arteriosclerosis.* 8, 1, 79-87,

Avogaro, P., Bon, G.B., Cazzolato, G., Gualandi, G. & Caturelli, G. (1986) Plasma malondialdehyde in coronary patients and in "normal" people at rest and after exercise. *Tex Heart Inst J.* 13, 3, 291-6, 0730-2347 (Print), 0730-2347 (Linking).

Bancells, C., Benitez, S., Jauhiainen, M., Ordonez-Llanos, J., Kovanen, P.T., Villegas, S., Sanchez-Quesada, J.L. & Oorni, K. (2009) High binding affinity of electronegative LDL to human aortic proteoglycans depends on its aggregation level. *J Lipid Res.* 50, 3, 446-55, 0022-2275 (Print), 0022-2275 (Linking).

Bancells, C., Benitez, S., Ordonez-Llanos, J., Oorni, K., Kovanen, P.T., Milne, R.W. & Sanchez-Quesada, J.L. (2011) Immunochemical analysis of the electronegative LDL subfraction shows that abnormal N-terminal apolipoprotein B conformation is involved in increased binding to proteoglycans. *J Biol Chem.* 286, 2, 1125-33, 1083-351X (Electronic), 0021-9258 (Linking).

Bancells, C., Benitez, S., Villegas, S., Jorba, O., Ordonez-Llanos, J. & Sanchez-Quesada, J.L. (2008) Novel phospholipolytic activities associated with electronegative low-density lipoprotein are involved in increased self-aggregation. *Biochemistry.* 47, 31, 8186-94,

Bancells, C., Canals, F., Benitez, S., Colome, N., Julve, J., Ordonez-Llanos, J. & Sanchez-Quesada, J.L. (2010a) Proteomic analysis of electronegative low-density lipoprotein. *J Lipid Res.* 0022-2275 (Electronic), 0022-2275 (Linking).

Bancells, C., Villegas, S., Blanco, F.J., Benitez, S., Gallego, I., Beloki, L., Perez-Cuellar, M., Ordonez-Llanos, J. & Sanchez-Quesada, J.L. (2010b) Aggregated electronegative low-density lipoprotein in human plasma shows high tendency to phospholipolysis and particle fusion. *J Biol Chem.* 1083-351X (Electronic) 0021-9258 (Linking).

Basnakian, A.G., Shah, S.V., Ok, E., Altunel, E. & Apostolov, E.O. (2010) Carbamylated LDL. *Adv Clin Chem.* 51, 25-52, 0065-2423 (Print), 0065-2423 (Linking).

Benitez, S., Bancells, C., Ordonez-Llanos, J. & Sanchez-Quesada, J.L. (2007a) Pro-inflammatory action of LDL(-) on mononuclear cells is counteracted by increased IL10 production. *Biochim Biophys Acta.* 1771, 5, 613-22, 0006-3002 (Print) 0006-3002 (Linking).

Benitez, S., Camacho, M., Arcelus, R., Vila, L., Bancells, C., Ordonez-Llanos, J. & Sanchez-Quesada, J.L. (2004a) Increased lysophosphatidylcholine and non-esterified fatty acid content in LDL induces chemokine release in endothelial cells. Relationship with electronegative LDL. *Atherosclerosis.* 177, 2, 299-305, 0021-9150 (Print), 0021-9150 (Linking).

Benitez, S., Camacho, M., Bancells, C., Vila, L., Sanchez-Quesada, J.L. & Ordonez-Llanos, J. (2006) Wide proinflammatory effect of electronegative low-density lipoprotein on human endothelial cells assayed by a protein array. *Biochim Biophys Acta.* 1761, 9, 1014-21, 0006-3002 (Print), 0006-3002 (Linking).

Benitez, S., Perez, A., Sanchez-Quesada, J.L., Wagner, A.M., Rigla, M., Arcelus, R., Jorba, O. & Ordonez-Llanos, J. (2007b) Electronegative low-density lipoprotein subfraction from type 2 diabetic subjects is proatherogenic and unrelated to glycemic control. *Diabetes Metab Res Rev.* 23, 1, 26-34,

Benitez, S., Sanchez-Quesada, J.L., Lucero, L., Arcelus, R., Ribas, V., Jorba, O., Castellvi, A., Alonso, E., Blanco-Vaca, F. & Ordonez-Llanos, J. (2002) Changes in low-density lipoprotein electronegativity and oxidizability after aerobic exercise are related to the increase in associated non-esterified fatty acids. *Atherosclerosis.* 160, 1, 223-32,

Benitez, S., Sanchez-Quesada, J.L., Ribas, V., Jorba, O., Blanco-Vaca, F., Gonzalez-Sastre, F. & Ordonez-Llanos, J. (2003) Platelet-activating factor acetylhydrolase is mainly associated with electronegative low-density lipoprotein subfraction. *Circulation.* 108, 1, 92-6,

Benitez, S., Villegas, V., Bancells, C., Jorba, O., Gonzalez-Sastre, F., Ordonez-Llanos, J. & Sanchez-Quesada, J.L. (2004b) Impaired binding affinity of electronegative low-density lipoprotein (LDL) to the LDL receptor is related to nonesterified fatty acids and lysophosphatidylcholine content. *Biochemistry.* 43, 50, 15863-72, 0006-2960 (Print), 0006-2960 (Linking).

Berliner, J., Leitinger, N., Watson, A., Huber, J., Fogelman, A. & Navab, M. (1997) Oxidized lipids in atherogenesis: formation, destruction and action. *Thromb Haemost.* 78, 1, 195-9,

Bhakdi, S., Dorweiler, B., Kirchmann, R., Torzewski, J., Weise, E., Tranum-Jensen, J., Walev, I. & Wieland, E. (1995) On the pathogenesis of atherosclerosis: enzymatic transformation of human low density lipoprotein to an atherogenic moiety. *J Exp Med.* 182, 6, 1959-71, 0022-1007 (Print), 0022-1007 (Linking).

Bhakdi, S., Torzewski, M., Paprotka, K., Schmitt, S., Barsoom, H., Suriyaphol, P., Han, S.R., Lackner, K.J. & Husmann, M. (2004) Possible protective role for C-reactive protein in atherogenesis: complement activation by modified lipoproteins halts before detrimental terminal sequence. *Circulation.* 109, 15, 1870-6, 1524-4539 (Electronic), 0009-7322 (Linking).

Blanco, F.J., Villegas, S., Benitez, S., Bancells, C., Diercks, T., Ordonez-Llanos, J. & Sanchez-Quesada, J.L. (2010) 2D-NMR reveals different populations of exposed lysine residues in the apoB-100 protein of electronegative and electropositive fractions of LDL particles. *J Lipid Res.* 51, 6, 1560-5, 0022-2275 (Print), 0022-2275 (Linking).

Boren, J., Lee, I., Zhu, W., Arnold, K., Taylor, S. & Innerarity, T.L. (1998a) Identification of the low density lipoprotein receptor-binding site in apolipoprotein B100 and the modulation of its binding activity by the carboxyl terminus in familial defective apo-B100. *J Clin Invest.* 101, 5, 1084-93, 0021-9738 (Print), 0021-9738 (Linking).

Boren, J., Olin, K., Lee, I., Chait, A., Wight, T.N. & Innerarity, T.L. (1998b) Identification of the principal proteoglycan-binding site in LDL. A single-point mutation in apo-B100 severely affects proteoglycan interaction without affecting LDL receptor binding. *J Clin Invest.* 101, 12, 2658-64, 0021-9738 (Print), 0021-9738 (Linking).

Brown, M.S. & Goldstein, J.L. (1983) Lipoprotein metabolism in the macrophage: implications for cholesterol deposition in atherosclerosis. *Annu Rev Biochem*. 52, 223-61, 0066-4154 (Print), 0066-4154 (Linking).

Brown, M.S. & Goldstein, J.L. (1986) A receptor-mediated pathway for cholesterol homeostasis. *Science*. 232, 4746, 34-47, 0036-8075 (Print), 0036-8075 (Linking).

Brownlee, M. (1992) Glycation products and the pathogenesis of diabetic complications. *Diabetes Care*. 15, 12, 1835-43, 0149-5992 (Print), 0149-5992 (Linking).

Brownlee, M. (2000) Negative consequences of glycation. *Metabolism*. 49, 2 Suppl 1, 9-13, 0026-0495 (Print), 0026-0495 (Linking).

Bucala, R. (1996) Site-specific modification of apolipoprotein B by advanced glycosylation end-products: implications for lipoprotein clearance and atherogenesis. *Nephrol Dial Transplant*. 11 Suppl 5, 17-9, 0931-0509 (Print), 0931-0509 (Linking).

Carracedo, J., Merino, A., Briceno, C., Soriano, S., Buendia, P., Calleros, L., Rodriguez, M., Martin-Malo, A., Aljama, P. & Ramirez, R. (2011) Carbamylated low-density lipoprotein induces oxidative stress and accelerated senescence in human endothelial progenitor cells. *FASEB J*. 25, 4, 1314-22, 1530-6860 (Electronic), 0892-6638 (Linking).

Cazzolato, G., Avogaro, P. & Bittolo-Bon, G. (1991) Characterization of a more electronegatively charged LDL subfraction by ion exchange HPLC. *Free Radic Biol Med*. 11, 3, 247-53,

Cerne, D., Jurgens, G., Ledinski, G., Kager, G., Greilberger, J. & Lukac-Bajalo, J. (2002) Relationship between the sialic acid content of low-density lipoprotein (LDL) and autoantibodies to oxidized LDL in the plasma of healthy subjects and patients with atherosclerosis. *Clin Chem Lab Med*. 40, 1, 15-20, 1434-6621 (Print), 1434-6621 (Linking).

Cohen, M.P., Lautenslager, G. & Shea, E. (1993) Glycated LDL concentrations in non-diabetic and diabetic subjects measured with monoclonal antibodies reactive with glycated apolipoprotein B epitopes. *Eur J Clin Chem Clin Biochem*. 31, 11, 707-13, 0939-4974 (Print), 0939-4974 (Linking).

Cominacini, L., Anselmi, M., Garbin, U., Fratta Pasini, A., Stranieri, C., Fusaro, M., Nava, C., Agostoni, P., Keta, D., Zardini, P., Sawamura, T. & Lo Cascio, V. (2005) Enhanced plasma levels of oxidized low-density lipoprotein increase circulating nuclear factor-kappa B activation in patients with unstable angina. *J Am Coll Cardiol*. 46, 5, 799-806, 0735-1097 (Print), 0735-1097 (Linking).

Curfs, D.M., Ghesquiere, S.A., Vergouwe, M.N., van der Made, I., Gijbels, M.J., Greaves, D.R., Verbeek, J.S., Hofker, M.H. & de Winther, M.P. (2008) Macrophage secretory phospholipase A2 group X enhances anti-inflammatory responses, promotes lipid accumulation, and contributes to aberrant lung pathology. *J Biol Chem*. 283, 31, 21640-8, 0021-9258 (Print), 0021-9258 (Linking).

Chen, C.H. (2004) Platelet-activating factor acetylhydrolase: is it good or bad for you? *Curr Opin Lipidol*. 15, 3, 337-41,

Chen, C.H., Jiang, T., Yang, J.H., Jiang, W., Lu, J., Marathe, G.K., Pownall, H.J., Ballantyne, C.M., McIntyre, T.M., Henry, P.D. & Yang, C.Y. (2003) Low-density lipoprotein in hypercholesterolemic human plasma induces vascular endothelial cell apoptosis by inhibiting fibroblast growth factor 2 transcription. *Circulation*. 107, 16, 2102-8, 1524-4539 (Electronic), 0009-7322 (Linking).

Chen, H.H., Hosken, B.D., Huang, M., Gaubatz, J.W., Myers, C.L., Macfarlane, R.D., Pownall, H.J. & Yang, C.Y. (2007) Electronegative LDLs from familial hypercholesterolemic patients are physicochemically heterogeneous but uniformly proapoptotic. *J Lipid Res*. 48, 1, 177-84, 0022-2275 (Print), 0022-2275 (Linking).

De Castellarnau, C., Sanchez-Quesada, J.L., Benitez, S., Rosa, R., Caveda, L., Vila, L. & Ordonez-Llanos, J. (2000) Electronegative LDL from normolipemic subjects induces IL-8 and monocyte chemotactic protein secretion by human endothelial cells. *Arterioscler Thromb Vasc Biol*. 20, 10, 2281-7,

Demuth, K., Myara, I., Chappey, B., Vedie, B., Pech-Amsellem, M.A., Haberland, M.E. & Moatti, N. (1996) A cytotoxic electronegative LDL subfraction is present in human plasma. *Arterioscler Thromb Vasc Biol*. 16, 6, 773-83,

Dersch, K., Ichijo, H., Bhakdi, S. & Husmann, M. (2005) Fatty acids liberated from low-density lipoprotein trigger endothelial apoptosis via mitogen-activated protein kinases. *Cell Death Differ*. 12, 8, 1107-14, 1350-9047 (Print), 1350-9047 (Linking).

Divchev, D. & Schieffer, B. (2008) The secretory phospholipase A2 group IIA: a missing link between inflammation, activated renin-angiotensin system, and atherogenesis? *Vasc Health Risk Manag*. 4, 3, 597-604, 1176-6344 (Print), 1176-6344 (Linking).

Esterbauer, H., Dieber-Rotheneder, M., Waeg, G., Striegl, G. & Jurgens, G. (1990) Biochemical, structural, and functional properties of oxidized low-density lipoprotein. *Chem Res Toxicol*. 3, 2, 77-92, 0893-228X (Print), 0893-228X (Linking).

Esterbauer, H., Wag, G. & Puhl, H. (1993) Lipid peroxidation and its role in atherosclerosis. *Br Med Bull*. 49, 3, 566-76, 0007-1420 (Print), 0007-1420 (Linking).

Fogelman, A.M., Shechter, I., Seager, J., Hokom, M., Child, J.S. & Edwards, P.A. (1980) Malondialdehyde alteration of low density lipoproteins leads to cholesteryl ester accumulation in human monocyte-macrophages. *Proc Natl Acad Sci U S A*. 77, 4, 2214-8, 0027-8424 (Print), 0027-8424 (Linking).

Fraley, A.E. & Tsimikas, S. (2006) Clinical applications of circulating oxidized low-density lipoprotein biomarkers in cardiovascular disease. *Curr Opin Lipidol*. 17, 5, 502-9, 0957-9672 (Print), 0957-9672 (Linking).

Frostegard, J. (2010) Low level natural antibodies against phosphorylcholine: a novel risk marker and potential mechanism in atherosclerosis and cardiovascular disease. *Clin Immunol*. 134, 1, 47-54, 1521-7035 (Electronic), 1521-6616 (Linking).

Gaubatz, J.W., Gillard, B.K., Massey, J.B., Hoogeveen, R.C., Huang, M., Lloyd, E.E., Raya, J.L., Yang, C.Y. & Pownall, H.J. (2007) Dynamics of dense electronegative low density lipoproteins and their preferential association with lipoprotein phospholipase A(2). *J Lipid Res*. 48, 2, 348-57,

Goldstein, J.L. & Brown, M.S. (1985) The LDL receptor and the regulation of cellular cholesterol metabolism. *J Cell Sci Suppl*. 3, 131-7, 0269-3518 (Print), 0269-3518 (Linking).

Goldstein, J.L., Ho, Y.K., Basu, S.K. & Brown, M.S. (1979) Binding site on macrophages that mediates uptake and degradation of acetylated low density lipoprotein, producing massive cholesterol deposition. *Proc Natl Acad Sci U S A*. 76, 1, 333-7, 0027-8424 (Print), 0027-8424 (Linking).

Greco, G., Balogh, G., Brunelli, R., Costa, G., De Spirito, M., Lenzi, L., Mei, G., Ursini, F. & Parasassi, T. (2009) Generation in human plasma of misfolded, aggregation-prone electronegative low density lipoprotein. *Biophys J*. 97, 2, 628-35,

Hartvigsen, K., Chou, M.Y., Hansen, L.F., Shaw, P.X., Tsimikas, S., Binder, C.J. & Witztum, J.L. (2009) The role of innate immunity in atherogenesis. *J Lipid Res*. 50 Suppl, S388-93,

Henriksen, T., Mahoney, E.M. & Steinberg, D. (1981) Enhanced macrophage degradation of low density lipoprotein previously incubated with cultured endothelial cells: recognition by receptors for acetylated low density lipoproteins. *Proc Natl Acad Sci U S A*. 78, 10, 6499-503, 0027-8424 (Print), 0027-8424 (Linking).

Hessler, J.R., Morel, D.W., Lewis, L.J. & Chisolm, G.M. (1983) Lipoprotein oxidation and lipoprotein-induced cytotoxicity. *Arteriosclerosis*. 3, 3, 215-22, 0276-5047 (Print), 0276-5047 (Linking).

Hessler, J.R., Robertson, A.L., Jr. & Chisolm, G.M., 3rd (1979) LDL-induced cytotoxicity and its inhibition by HDL in human vascular smooth muscle and endothelial cells in culture. *Atherosclerosis*. 32, 3, 213-29, 0021-9150 (Print), 0021-9150 (Linking).

Hevonoja, T., Pentikainen, M.O., Hyvonen, M.T., Kovanen, P.T. & Ala-Korpela, M. (2000) Structure of low density lipoprotein (LDL) particles: basis for understanding molecular changes in modified LDL. *Biochim Biophys Acta*. 1488, 3, 189-210, 0006-3002 (Print), 0006-3002 (Linking).

Holvoet, P., Collen, D. & Van de Werf, F. (1999) Malondialdehyde-modified LDL as a marker of acute coronary syndromes. *JAMA*. 281, 18, 1718-21, 0098-7484 (Print), 0098-7484 (Linking).

Holvoet, P., Vanhaecke, J., Janssens, S., Van de Werf, F. & Collen, D. (1998) Oxidized LDL and malondialdehyde-modified LDL in patients with acute coronary syndromes and stable coronary artery disease. *Circulation*. 98, 15, 1487-94, 0009-7322 (Print), 0009-7322 (Linking).

Ishigaki, Y., Katagiri, H., Gao, J., Yamada, T., Imai, J., Uno, K., Hasegawa, Y., Kaneko, K., Ogihara, T., Ishihara, H., Sato, Y., Takikawa, K., Nishimichi, N., Matsuda, H., Sawamura, T. & Oka, Y. (2008) Impact of plasma oxidized low-density lipoprotein removal on atherosclerosis. *Circulation*. 118, 1, 75-83, 1524-4539 (Electronic), 0009-7322 (Linking).

Ishigaki, Y., Oka, Y. & Katagiri, H. (2009) Circulating oxidized LDL: a biomarker and a pathogenic factor. *Curr Opin Lipidol*. 20, 5, 363-9, 1473-6535 (Electronic), 0957-9672 (Linking).

Klouche, M., Gottschling, S., Gerl, V., Hell, W., Husmann, M., Dorweiler, B., Messner, M. & Bhakdi, S. (1998) Atherogenic properties of enzymatically degraded LDL: selective induction of MCP-1 and cytotoxic effects on human macrophages. *Arterioscler Thromb Vasc Biol*. 18, 9, 1376-85, 1079-5642 (Print), 1079-5642 (Linking).

Klouche, M., May, A.E., Hemmes, M., Messner, M., Kanse, S.M., Preissner, K.T. & Bhakdi, S. (1999) Enzymatically modified, nonoxidized LDL induces selective adhesion and transmigration of monocytes and T-lymphocytes through human endothelial cell monolayers. *Arterioscler Thromb Vasc Biol*. 19, 3, 784-93, 1079-5642 (Print), 1079-5642 (Linking).

Klouche, M., Rose-John, S., Schmiedt, W. & Bhakdi, S. (2000) Enzymatically degraded, nonoxidized LDL induces human vascular smooth muscle cell activation, foam cell transformation, and proliferation. *Circulation*. 101, 15, 1799-805, 1524-4539 (Electronic), 0009-7322 (Linking).

Krauss, R.M. (1995) Dense low density lipoproteins and coronary artery disease. *Am J Cardiol*. 75, 6, 53B-57B, 0002-9149 (Print), 0002-9149 (Linking).

Krieger, M., Abrams, J.M., Lux, A. & Steller, H. (1992) Molecular flypaper, atherosclerosis, and host defense: structure and function of the macrophage scavenger receptor. *Cold Spring Harb Symp Quant Biol*. 57, 605-9, 0091-7451 (Print), 0091-7451 (Linking).

Ky, B., Burke, A., Tsimikas, S., Wolfe, M.L., Tadesse, M.G., Szapary, P.O., Witztum, J.L., FitzGerald, G.A. & Rader, D.J. (2008) The influence of pravastatin and atorvastatin on markers of oxidative stress in hypercholesterolemic humans. *J Am Coll Cardiol*. 51, 17, 1653-62, 1558-3597 (Electronic), 0735-1097 (Linking).

Laukkanen, J., Lehtolainen, P., Gough, P.J., Greaves, D.R., Gordon, S. & Yla-Herttuala, S. (2000) Adenovirus-mediated gene transfer of a secreted form of human macrophage scavenger receptor inhibits modified low-density lipoprotein degradation and foam-cell formation in macrophages. *Circulation*. 101, 10, 1091-6, 1524-4539 (Electronic), 0009-7322 (Linking).

Lopes-Virella, M.F. & Virella, G. (2010) Clinical significance of the humoral immune response to modified LDL. *Clin Immunol*. 134, 1, 55-65, 1521-7035 (Electronic), 1521-6616 (Linking).

Lu, J., Jiang, W., Yang, J.H., Chang, P.Y., Walterscheid, J.P., Chen, H.H., Marcelli, M., Tang, D., Lee, Y.T., Liao, W.S., Yang, C.Y. & Chen, C.H. (2008) Electronegative LDL impairs vascular endothelial cell integrity in diabetes by disrupting fibroblast growth factor 2 (FGF2) autoregulation. *Diabetes*. 57, 1, 158-66,

Lu, J., Yang, J.H., Burns, A.R., Chen, H.H., Tang, D., Walterscheid, J.P., Suzuki, S., Yang, C.Y., Sawamura, T. & Chen, C.H. (2009) Mediation of electronegative low-density lipoprotein signaling by LOX-1: a possible mechanism of endothelial apoptosis. *Circ Res*. 104, 5, 619-27,

Lund-Katz, S., Laplaud, P.M., Phillips, M.C. & Chapman, M.J. (1998) Apolipoprotein B-100 conformation and particle surface charge in human LDL subspecies: implication for LDL receptor interaction. *Biochemistry*. 37, 37, 12867-74, 0006-2960 (Print), 0006-2960 (Linking).

Llorente-Cortes, V. & Badimon, L. (2005) LDL receptor-related protein and the vascular wall: implications for atherothrombosis. *Arterioscler Thromb Vasc Biol* 25, 3, 497-504, 1524-4636 (Electronic), 1079-5642 (Linking).

MacPhee, C.H., Moores, K.E., Boyd, H.F., Dhanak, D., Ife, R.J., Leach, C.A., Leake, D.S., Milliner, K.J., Patterson, R.A., Suckling, K.E., Tew, D.G. & Hickey, D.M. (1999) Lipoprotein-associated phospholipase A2, platelet-activating factor acetylhydrolase, generates two bioactive products during the oxidation of low-density lipoprotein: use of a novel inhibitor. *Biochem J*. 338 ( Pt 2), 479-87, 0264-6021 (Print), 0264-6021 (Linking).

Mafra, D., Santos, F.R., Lobo, J.C., de Mattos Grosso, D., Barreira, A.L., Velarde, L.G., Abdalla, D.S. & Leite, M., Jr. (2009) Alpha-tocopherol supplementation decreases electronegative low-density lipoprotein concentration [LDL(-)] in haemodialysis patients. *Nephrol Dial Transplant*. 24, 5, 1587-92,

Meisinger, C., Baumert, J., Khuseyinova, N., Loewel, H. & Koenig, W. (2005) Plasma oxidized low-density lipoprotein, a strong predictor for acute coronary heart disease events in apparently healthy, middle-aged men from the general population. *Circulation*. 112, 5, 651-7, 1524-4539 (Electronic), 0009-7322 (Linking).

Mello, A.P., da Silva, I.T., Abdalla, D.S. & Damasceno, N.R. (2011) Electronegative low-density lipoprotein: origin and impact on health and disease. *Atherosclerosis*. 215, 2, 257-65, 1879-1484 (Electronic), 0021-9150 (Linking).

Menzel, E.J., Sobal, G. & Staudinger, A. (1997) The role of oxidative stress in the long-term glycation of LDL. *Biofactors*. 6, 2, 111-24, 0951-6433 (Print), 0951-6433 (Linking).

Miller, Y.I., Chang, M.K., Binder, C.J., Shaw, P.X. & Witztum, J.L. (2003) Oxidized low density lipoprotein and innate immune receptors. *Curr Opin Lipidol*. 14, 5, 437-45, 0957-9672 (Print), 0957-9672 (Linking).

Minuz, P., Lechi, C., Gaino, S., Bonapace, S., Fontana, L., Garbin, U., Paluani, F., Cominacini, L., Zatti, M. & Lechi, A. (1995) Oxidized LDL and reduction of the antiaggregating activity of nitric oxide derived from endothelial cells. *Thromb Haemost*. 74, 4, 1175-9, 0340-6245 (Print), 0340-6245 (Linking).

Moro, E., Zambon, C., Pianetti, S., Cazzolato, G., Pais, M. & Bittolo Bon, G. (1998) Electronegative low density lipoprotein subform (LDL-) is increased in type 2 (non-insulin-dependent) microalbuminuric diabetic patients and is closely associated with LDL susceptibility to oxidation. *Acta Diabetol*. 35, 3, 161-4,

Morton, R.E., Gnizak, H.M., Greene, D.J., Cho, K.H. & Paromov, V.M. (2008) Lipid transfer inhibitor protein (apolipoprotein F) concentration in normolipidemic and hyperlipidemic subjects. *J Lipid Res*. 49, 1, 127-35, 0022-2275 (Print), 0022-2275 (Linking).

Naito, M., Yamada, K., Hayashi, T., Asai, K., Yoshimine, N. & Iguchi, A. (1994) Comparative toxicity of oxidatively modified low-density lipoprotein and lysophosphatidylcholine in cultured vascular endothelial cells. *Heart Vessels*. 9, 4, 183-7, 0910-8327 (Print), 0910-8327 (Linking).

Negishi, M., Shimizu, H., Okada, S., Kuwabara, A., Okajima, F. & Mori, M. (2004) 9HODE stimulates cell proliferation and extracellular matrix synthesis in human mesangial cells via PPARgamma. *Exp Biol Med (Maywood)*. 229, 10, 1053-60, 1535-3702 (Print), 1535-3699 (Linking).

Nishi, K., Itabe, H., Uno, M., Kitazato, K.T., Horiguchi, H., Shinno, K. & Nagahiro, S. (2002) Oxidized LDL in carotid plaques and plasma associates with plaque instability. *Arterioscler Thromb Vasc Biol*. 22, 10, 1649-54, 1524-4636 (Electronic), 1079-5642 (Linking).

Oda, T., Wals, P., Osterburg, H.H., Johnson, S.A., Pasinetti, G.M., Morgan, T.E., Rozovsky, I., Stine, W.B., Snyder, S.W., Holzman, T.F. & et al. (1995) Clusterin (apoJ) alters the aggregation of amyloid beta-peptide (A beta 1-42) and forms slowly sedimenting A beta complexes that cause oxidative stress. *Exp Neurol*. 136, 1, 22-31,

Oorni, K., Hakala, J.K., Annila, A., Ala-Korpela, M. & Kovanen, P.T. (1998) Sphingomyelinase induces aggregation and fusion, but phospholipase A2 only aggregation, of low density lipoprotein (LDL) particles. Two distinct mechanisms leading to increased binding strength of LDL to human aortic proteoglycans. *J Biol Chem*. 273, 44, 29127-34,

Oorni, K., Pentikainen, M.O., Ala-Korpela, M. & Kovanen, P.T. (2000) Aggregation, fusion, and vesicle formation of modified low density lipoprotein particles: molecular mechanisms and effects on matrix interactions. *J Lipid Res*. 41, 11, 1703-14,

Orekhov, A.N., Tertov, V.V. & Mukhin, D.N. (1991) Desialylated low density lipoprotein--naturally occurring modified lipoprotein with atherogenic potency. *Atherosclerosis*. 86, 2-3, 153-61, 0021-9150 (Print), 0021-9150 (Linking).

Parasassi, T., Bittolo-Bon, G., Brunelli, R., Cazzolato, G., Krasnowska, E.K., Mei, G., Sevanian, A. & Ursini, F. (2001) Loss of apoB-100 secondary structure and conformation in hydroperoxide rich, electronegative LDL(-). *Free Radic Biol Med*. 31, 1, 82-9,

Parasassi, T., De Spirito, M., Mei, G., Brunelli, R., Greco, G., Lenzi, L., Maulucci, G., Nicolai, E., Papi, M., Arcovito, G., Tosatto, S.C. & Ursini, F. (2008) Low density lipoprotein misfolding and amyloidogenesis. *Faseb J*. 22, 7, 2350-6,

Pedrosa, A.M., Faine, L.A., Grosso, D.M., de Las Heras, B., Bosca, L. & Abdalla, D.S. (2010) Electronegative LDL induction of apoptosis in macrophages: involvement of Nrf2. *Biochim Biophys Acta*. 1801, 4, 430-7, 0006-3002 (Print), 0006-3002 (Linking).

Pentikainen, M.O., Lehtonen, E.M., Oorni, K., Lusa, S., Somerharju, P., Jauhiainen, M. & Kovanen, P.T. (1997) Human arterial proteoglycans increase the rate of proteolytic fusion of low density lipoprotein particles. *J Biol Chem*. 272, 40, 25283-8,

Pentikainen, M.O., Oorni, K., Ala-Korpela, M. & Kovanen, P.T. (2000) Modified LDL - trigger of atherosclerosis and inflammation in the arterial intima. *J Intern Med*. 247, 3, 359-70,

Petit, L., Lesnik, P., Dachet, C., Moreau, M. & Chapman, M.J. (1999) Tissue factor pathway inhibitor is expressed by human monocyte-derived macrophages : relationship to tissue factor induction by cholesterol and oxidized LDL. *Arterioscler Thromb Vasc Biol*. 19, 2, 309-15, 1079-5642 (Print), 1079-5642 (Linking).

Quehenberger, O., Jurgens, G., Zadravec, S. & Esterbauer, H. (1988) Oxidation of human low density lipoprotein initiated by copper (II) chloride. *Basic Life Sci*. 49, 387-90, 0090-5542 (Print), 0090-5542 (Linking).

Rabbani, N., Chittari, M.V., Bodmer, C.W., Zehnder, D., Ceriello, A. & Thornalley, P.J. (2010) Increased glycation and oxidative damage to apolipoprotein B100 of LDL cholesterol in patients with type 2 diabetes and effect of metformin. *Diabetes*. 59, 4, 1038-45, 1939-327X (Electronic), 0012-1797 (Linking).

Rabbani, N., Godfrey, L., Xue, M., Shaheen, F., Geoffrion, M., Milne, R. & Thornalley, P.J. (2011) Glycation of LDL by Methylglyoxal Increases Arterial Atherogenicity: A Possible Contributor to Increased Risk of Cardiovascular Disease in Diabetes. *Diabetes*. 1939-327X (Electronic), 0012-1797 (Linking).

Rabbani, N. & Thornalley, P.J. (2011) Glyoxalase in diabetes, obesity and related disorders. *Semin Cell Dev Biol*. 22, 3, 309-17, 1096-3634 (Electronic), 1084-9521 (Linking).

Ramasamy, R., Yan, S.F. & Schmidt, A.M. (2009) RAGE: therapeutic target and biomarker of the inflammatory response--the evidence mounts. *J Leukoc Biol*. 86, 3, 505-12, 1938-3673 (Electronic), 0741-5400 (Linking).

Reaven, P.D., Herold, D.A., Barnett, J. & Edelman, S. (1995) Effects of Vitamin E on susceptibility of low-density lipoprotein and low-density lipoprotein subfractions to oxidation and on protein glycation in NIDDM. *Diabetes Care*. 18, 6, 807-16, 0149-5992 (Print), 0149-5992 (Linking).

Ross, R. (1999) Atherosclerosis--an inflammatory disease. *N Engl J Med*. 340, 2, 115-26, 0028-4793 (Print), 0028-4793 (Linking).

Ruelland, A., Gallou, G., Legras, B., Paillard, F. & Cloarec, L. (1993) LDL sialic acid content in patients with coronary artery disease. *Clin Chim Acta*. 221, 1-2, 127-33, 0009-8981 (Print), 0009-8981 (Linking).

Sanchez-Quesada, J.L., Benitez, S. & Ordonez-Llanos, J. (2004) Electronegative low-density lipoprotein. *Curr Opin Lipidol*. 15, 3, 329-35,

Sanchez-Quesada, J.L., Benitez, S., Otal, C., Franco, M., Blanco-Vaca, F. & Ordonez-Llanos, J. (2002) Density distribution of electronegative LDL in normolipemic and hyperlipemic subjects. *J Lipid Res*. 43, 5, 699-705,

Sanchez-Quesada, J.L., Benitez, S., Perez, A., Wagner, A.M., Rigla, M., Carreras, G., Vila, L., Camacho, M., Arcelus, R. & Ordonez-Llanos, J. (2005) The inflammatory properties of electronegative low-density lipoprotein from type 1 diabetic patients are related to increased platelet-activating factor acetylhydrolase activity. *Diabetologia*. 48, 10, 2162-9,

Sanchez-Quesada, J.L., Camacho, M., Anton, R., Benitez, S., Vila, L. & Ordonez-Llanos, J. (2003) Electronegative LDL of FH subjects: chemical characterization and induction of chemokine release from human endothelial cells. *Atherosclerosis*. 166, 2, 261-70,

Sanchez-Quesada, J.L., Otal-Entraigas, C., Franco, M., Jorba, O., Gonzalez-Sastre, F., Blanco-Vaca, F. & Ordonez-Llanos, J. (1999) Effect of simvastatin treatment on the electronegative low-density lipoprotein present in patients with heterozygous familial hypercholesterolemia. *Am J Cardiol*. 84, 6, 655-9,

Sanchez-Quesada, J.L., Perez, A., Caixas, A., Ordonmez-Llanos, J., Carreras, G., Payes, A., Gonzalez-Sastre, F. & de Leiva, A. (1996) Electronegative low density lipoprotein subform is increased in patients with short-duration IDDM and is closely related to glycaemic control. *Diabetologia*. 39, 12, 1469-76,

Sanchez-Quesada, J.L., Perez, A., Caixas, A., Rigla, M., Payes, A., Benitez, S. & Ordonez-Llanos, J. (2001) Effect of glycemic optimization on electronegative low-density lipoprotein in diabetes: relation to nonenzymatic glycosylation and oxidative modification. *J Clin Endocrinol Metab*. 86, 7, 3243-9,

Santo Faulin Tdo, E., de Sena, K.C., Rodrigues Telles, A.E., de Mattos Grosso, D., Bernardi Faulin, E.J. & Parra Abdalla, D.S. (2008) Validation of a novel ELISA for measurement of electronegative low-density lipoprotein. *Clin Chem Lab Med*. 46, 12, 1769-75,

Sevanian, A., Bittolo-Bon, G., Cazzolato, G., Hodis, H., Hwang, J., Zamburlini, A., Maiorino, M. & Ursini, F. (1997) LDL- is a lipid hydroperoxide-enriched circulating lipoprotein. *J Lipid Res*. 38, 3, 419-28, 0022-2275 (Print), 0022-2275 (Linking).

Sobal, G., Menzel, J. & Sinzinger, H. (2000) Why is glycated LDL more sensitive to oxidation than native LDL? A comparative study. *Prostaglandins Leukot Essent Fatty Acids*. 63, 4, 177-86, 0952-3278 (Print), 0952-3278 (Linking).

Sonoki, K., Iwase, M., Iino, K., Ichikawa, K., Ohdo, S., Higuchi, S., Yoshinari, M. & Iida, M. (2003) Atherogenic role of lysophosphatidylcholine in low-density lipoprotein modified by phospholipase A2 and in diabetic patients: protection by nitric oxide donor. *Metabolism*. 52, 3, 308-14, 0026-0495 (Print), 0026-0495 (Linking).

Sparrow, C.P., Parthasarathy, S. & Steinberg, D. (1988) Enzymatic modification of low density lipoprotein by purified lipoxygenase plus phospholipase A2 mimics cell-mediated oxidative modification. *J Lipid Res*. 29, 6, 745-53, 0022-2275 (Print), 0022-2275 (Linking).

Stary, H.C. (2000) Natural history and histological classification of atherosclerotic lesions: an update. *Arterioscler Thromb Vasc Biol*. 20, 5, 1177-8, 1079-5642 (Print), 1079-5642 (Linking).

Steinberg, D. (2009) The LDL modification hypothesis of atherogenesis: an update. *J Lipid Res*. 50 Suppl, S376-81, 0022-2275 (Print), 0022-2275 (Linking).

Steinberg, D., Parthasarathy, S., Carew, T.E., Khoo, J.C. & Witztum, J.L. (1989) Beyond cholesterol. Modifications of low-density lipoprotein that increase its atherogenicity. *N Engl J Med*. 320, 14, 915-24, 0028-4793 (Print), 0028-4793 (Linking).

Suriyaphol, P., Fenske, D., Zahringer, U., Han, S.R., Bhakdi, S. & Husmann, M. (2002) Enzymatically modified nonoxidized low-density lipoprotein induces interleukin-8 in human endothelial cells: role of free fatty acids. *Circulation*. 106, 20, 2581-7, 1524-4539 (Electronic), 0009-7322 (Linking).

Tabas, I. (1999) Secretory sphingomyelinase. *Chem Phys Lipids*. 102, 1-2, 123-30, 0009-3084 (Print), 0009-3084 (Linking).

Tai, M.H., Kuo, S.M., Liang, H.T., Chiou, K.R., Lam, H.C., Hsu, C.M., Pownall, H.J., Chen, H.H., Huang, M.T. & Yang, C.Y. (2006) Modulation of angiogenic processes in cultured endothelial cells by low density lipoproteins subfractions from patients with familial hypercholesterolemia. *Atherosclerosis*. 186, 2, 448-57,

Tang, D., Lu, J., Walterscheid, J.P., Chen, H.H., Engler, D.A., Sawamura, T., Chang, P.Y., Safi, H.J., Yang, C.Y. & Chen, C.H. (2008) Electronegative LDL circulating in smokers impairs endothelial progenitor cell differentiation by inhibiting Akt phosphorylation via LOX-1. *J Lipid Res*. 49, 1, 33-47,

Tedgui, A. & Mallat, Z. (2006) Cytokines in atherosclerosis: pathogenic and regulatory pathways. *Physiol Rev*. 86, 2, 515-81, 0031-9333 (Print), 0031-9333 (Linking).

Tellis, C.C. & Tselepis, A.D. (2009) The role of lipoprotein-associated phospholipase A2 in atherosclerosis may depend on its lipoprotein carrier in plasma. *Biochim Biophys Acta*. 1791, 5, 327-38, 0006-3002 (Print), 0006-3002 (Linking).

Tertov, V.V., Bittolo-Bon, G., Sobenin, I.A., Cazzolato, G., Orekhov, A.N. & Avogaro, P. (1995) Naturally occurring modified low density lipoproteins are similar if not identical: more electronegative and desialylated lipoprotein subfractions. *Exp Mol Pathol*. 62, 3, 166-72, 0014-4800 (Print), 0014-4800 (Linking).

Tertov, V.V., Sobenin, I.A., Tonevitsky, A.G., Orekhov, A.N. & Smirnov, V.N. (1990) Isolation of atherogenic modified (desialylated) low density lipoprotein from blood of atherosclerotic patients: separation from native lipoprotein by affinity chromatography. *Biochem Biophys Res Commun*. 167, 3, 1122-7, 0006-291X (Print), 0006-291X (Linking).

Tjoelker, L.W. & Stafforini, D.M. (2000) Platelet-activating factor acetylhydrolases in health and disease. *Biochim Biophys Acta*. 1488, 1-2, 102-23,

Tomasik, A., Jachec, W., Skrzep-Poloczek, B., Widera-Romuk, E., Wodniecki, J. & Wojciechowska, C. (2003) Circulating electronegatively charged low-density lipoprotein in patients with angiographically documented coronary artery disease. *Scand J Clin Lab Invest*. 63, 4, 259-65, 0036-5513 (Print), 0036-5513 (Linking).

Uno, M., Kitazato, K.T., Nishi, K., Itabe, H. & Nagahiro, S. (2003) Raised plasma oxidised LDL in acute cerebral infarction. *J Neurol Neurosurg Psychiatry*. 74, 3, 312-6, 0022-3050 (Print), 0022-3050 (Linking).

Ursini, F., Zamburlini, A., Cazzolato, G., Maiorino, M., Bon, G.B. & Sevanian, A. (1998) Postprandial plasma lipid hydroperoxides: a possible link between diet and atherosclerosis. *Free Radic Biol Med*. 25, 2, 250-2, 0891-5849 (Print), 0891-5849 (Linking).

Van Berkel, T.J., Van Eck, M., Herijgers, N., Fluiter, K. & Nion, S. (2000) Scavenger receptor classes A and B. Their roles in atherogenesis and the metabolism of modified LDL and HDL. *Ann N Y Acad Sci*. 902, 113-26; discussion 126-7, 0077-8923 (Print), 0077-8923 (Linking).

van Blitterswijk, W.J., van der Luit, A.H., Veldman, R.J., Verheij, M. & Borst, J. (2003) Ceramide: second messenger or modulator of membrane structure and dynamics? *Biochem J*. 369, Pt 2, 199-211, 0264-6021 (Print), 0264-6021 (Linking).

Whitman, S.C., Rateri, D.L., Szilvassy, S.J., Cornicelli, J.A. & Daugherty, A. (2002) Macrophage-specific expression of class A scavenger receptors in LDL receptor(-/-) mice decreases atherosclerosis and changes spleen morphology. *J Lipid Res*. 43, 8, 1201-8, 0022-2275 (Print), 0022-2275 (Linking).

Williams, K.J. & Tabas, I. (2005) Lipoprotein retention--and clues for atheroma regression. *Arterioscler Thromb Vasc Biol*. 25, 8, 1536-40, 1524-4636 (Electronic), 1524-4636 (Linking).

Witztum, J.L. (1997) Role of modified lipoproteins in diabetic macroangiopathy. *Diabetes*. 46 Suppl 2, S112-4,

Witztum, J.L., Mahoney, E.M., Branks, M.J., Fisher, M., Elam, R. & Steinberg, D. (1982) Nonenzymatic glucosylation of low-density lipoprotein alters its biologic activity. *Diabetes*. 31, 4 Pt 1, 283-91, 0012-1797 (Print), 0012-1797 (Linking).

Witztum, J.L. & Steinberg, D. (1991) Role of oxidized low density lipoprotein in atherogenesis. *J Clin Invest*. 88, 6, 1785-92, 0021-9738 (Print), 0021-9738 (Linking).

Yang, C.Y., Chen, H.H., Huang, M.T., Raya, J.L., Yang, J.H., Chen, C.H., Gaubatz, J.W., Pownall, H.J., Taylor, A.A., Ballantyne, C.M., Jenniskens, F.A. & Smith, C.V. (2007) Pro-apoptotic low-density lipoprotein subfractions in type II diabetes. *Atherosclerosis*. 193, 2, 283-91, 0021-9150 (Print), 0021-9150 (Linking).

Yang, C.Y., Raya, J.L., Chen, H.H., Chen, C.H., Abe, Y., Pownall, H.J., Taylor, A.A. & Smith, C.V. (2003) Isolation, characterization, and functional assessment of oxidatively modified subfractions of circulating low-density lipoproteins. *Arterioscler Thromb Vasc Biol*. 23, 6, 1083-90, 1524-4636 (Electronic), 1079-5642 (Linking).

Younis, N., Charlton-Menys, V., Sharma, R., Soran, H. & Durrington, P.N. (2009) Glycation of LDL in non-diabetic people: Small dense LDL is preferentially glycated both in vivo and in vitro. *Atherosclerosis*. 202, 1, 162-8, 1879-1484 (Electronic), 0021-9150 (Linking).

Zeibig, S., Li, Z., Wagner, S., Holthoff, H.P., Ungerer, M., Bultmann, A., Uhland, K., Vogelmann, J., Simmet, T., Gawaz, M. & Munch, G. (2011) Effect of the oxLDL binding protein Fc-CD68 on plaque extension and vulnerability in atherosclerosis. *Circ Res*. 108, 6, 695-703, 1524-4571 (Electronic), 0009-7330 (Linking).

Zhang, B., Kaneshi, T., Ohta, T. & Saku, K. (2005) Relation between insulin resistance and fast-migrating LDL subfraction as characterized by capillary isotachophoresis. *J Lipid Res*. 46, 10, 2265-77,

Zhang, B., Matsunaga, A., Rainwater, D.L., Miura, S., Noda, K., Nishikawa, H., Uehara, Y., Shirai, K., Ogawa, M. & Saku, K. (2009) Effects of rosuvastatin on electronegative LDL as characterized by capillary isotachophoresis: the ROSARY Study. *J Lipid Res*. 50, 9, 1832-41,

Zhang, B., Miura, S., Yanagi, D., Noda, K., Nishikawa, H., Matsunaga, A., Shirai, K., Iwata, A., Yoshinaga, K., Adachi, H., Imaizumi, T. & Saku, K. (2008) Reduction of charge-modified LDL by statin therapy in patients with CHD or CHD risk factors and elevated LDL-C levels: the SPECIAL Study. *Atherosclerosis*. 201, 2, 353-9,

Ziouzenkova, O., Asatryan, L., Sahady, D., Orasanu, G., Perrey, S., Cutak, B., Hassell, T., Akiyama, T.E., Berger, J.P., Sevanian, A. & Plutzky, J. (2003) Dual roles for lipolysis and oxidation in peroxisome proliferation-activator receptor responses to electronegative low density lipoprotein. *J Biol Chem*. 278, 41, 39874-81, 0021-9258 (Print), 0021-9258 (Linking).

Ziouzenkova, O., Asatryan, L., Tetta, C., Wratten, M.L., Hwang, J. & Sevanian, A. (2002) Oxidative stress during ex vivo hemodialysis of blood is decreased by a novel hemolipodialysis procedure utilizing antioxidants. *Free Radic Biol Med*. 33, 2, 248-58, 0891-5849 (Print), 0891-5849 (Linking).

Ziouzenkova, O. & Sevanian, A. (2000) Oxidative modification of low-density lipoprotein (LDL) in HD patients: role in electronegative LDL formation. *Blood Purif*. 18, 3, 169-76,

# 22

# Oxidized LDL and NO Synthesis as Biomarkers of Atherogenesis – Correlations with Metabolic Profile in Elderly

Claudia Borsa[1], Cristina Ionescu[1] and Daniela Gradinaru[1,2*]

[1]*Ana Aslan – National Institute of Gerontology and Geriatrics, Bucharest,*
[2]*Carol Davila – University of Medicine and Pharmacy, Faculty of Pharmacy, Bucharest, Romania*

## 1. Introduction

Atherosclerosis is a complex, multifactorial disease, developed in the arterial wall in response to various forms of injurious stimuli, resulting in excessive inflammatory and fibro-proliferative reactions. The endothelial cells are involved in all stages of atherogenesis and their dysfunction is a key initial event in the atherosclerotic plaque formation (Simionescu, 2007). The vascular endothelium, with its broad spectrum of paracrine and autocrine functions, can be regarded as a multifunctional organ and "chief governor" of body homeostasis. Occupying a strategic location between the blood and tissues, the endothelial cells exist in a "high-risk position" and react progressively to aggressive factors, at first by modulation of the constitutive functions - permeability and biosynthesis (Simionescu & Antohe, 2006; Sima et al., 2009). Atherogenesis is an intricate process involving hyperlipidemia, oxidative stress and vascular inflammation. Among the diversity of mechanisms implicated in the pathogenesis of atherosclerotic vascular diseases two of them have been discovered in parallel and studied extensively: the oxidation of low-density lipoprotein (LDL) and the synthesis of endothelium-derived nitric oxide (NO).

### 1.1 Relationship between oxidized LDL and NO as biomarkers of oxidative stress and endothelial dysfunction

Oxidized LDL and NO are recognized to exert contradictory actions within the vascular endothelium microenvironment and to influence the key events in the development of atherosclerosis such as leukocyte adhesion, platelet aggregation and vascular smooth-muscle cell proliferation and migration. While oxidized LDL (oxLDL) - a biomarker of lipoprotein-associated oxidative stress, is identified as a non-traditional pro-atherogenic emerging cardiovascular risk factor, NO is a free radical signal-transducing molecule that maintains the vasodilating tone, modulates *in vitro* lipid peroxidation reactions and alters proinflammatory gene expression (Figure 1).

Endothelial dysfunction - known to precede the development of atherosclerosis, is a systemic pathological state of the endothelium defined as an imbalance between

---

* Corresponding author

vasodilating and vasoconstricting substances produced by (or acting on) the endothelium (Deanfield et al., 2007), leading to a reduced vasodilation, and even a proinflammatory and prothrombotic state (Cottone & Cerasola, 2008).
The most important of the vasodilating substances is nitric oxide, characterized as a non-eicosanoid component of endothelial-derived relaxation factor (EDRF), which is continuously synthesized by the endothelium under the action of different neurohumoral mediators such as acetylcholine, histamine, bradikinine, vasopressine, thrombine and serotonine (Rubbo et al., 1996).

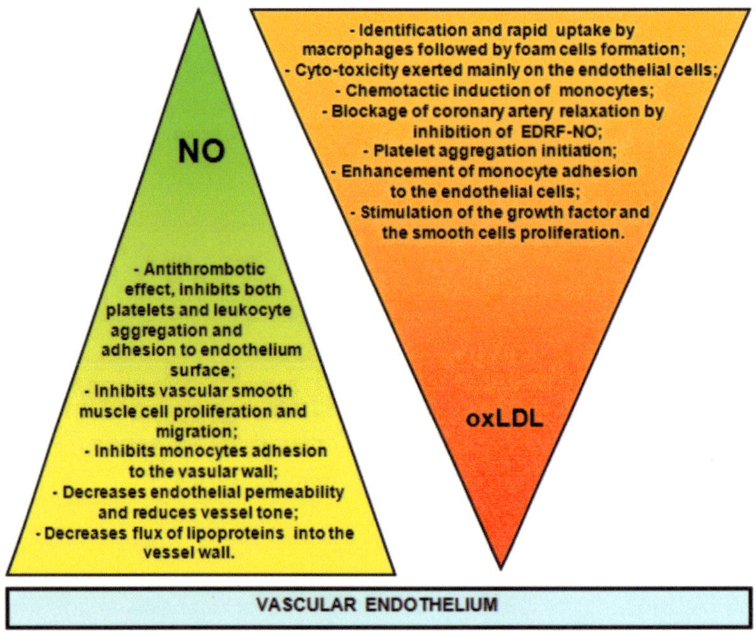


Fig. 1. Antiatherogenic effects and role of nitric oxide (NO) *versus* proatherogenic actions of oxidized LDL (oxLDL) exerted on vascular endothelium.

NO is produced by a variety of mammalian cells including: vascular endothelial cells, neurons, smooth muscle cells, macrophages, neutrophils, platelets, cardiomyocytes and pulmonary epithelium. The family of three enzymes responsible for the synthesis of NO, nitric oxide synthases (NOSs): endothelial (eNOS), neuronal (nNOS), and inducible (iNOS) require calmodulin binding for their activities. The inducible nitric oxide synthases are transcriptionally regulated by cytokines and redox-sensitive transcriptional factors. Bacterial and parasitic antigens, which potently induce the expression of cytokines, also lead to induction of iNOS gene expression (Rubbo et al., 1996; Lundberg & Weitzberg, 2005).
In the endothelial microenvironment, concurrently, a variety of substances that adversely influence endothelial function have been recognized, including free fatty acids, cytokines such as TNF-$\alpha$, and prooxidant molecules - including oxidized low-density lipoprotein (oxLDL). There are strong evidences for the role of oxidative stress in all stages of atherogenesis. Among different molecular targets affected by oxidative stress associated with hyperlipidemia and hyperglycemia, LDL is one of the most significant because is the major cholesterol carrier in the blood and contains also a relevant amount of polyunsaturated fatty acids (PUFAs) - the major substrate for lipid peroxidation.

The initial event in atherogenesis is the increased transcytosis of low-density lipoprotein, and its subsequent deposition, retention and oxidative modification in the subendothelium. It is followed by the infiltration of activated inflammatory cells from the coronary circulation into the arterial wall (Hulsmans & Holvoet, 2010).

The oxLDL is a byproduct of exposure to reactive oxygen species (ROS), and several potential mechanisms have been proposed for LDL oxidation: cell-mediated lipoxygenase and myeloperoxidase activities, non-enzymatic metal ion-mediated oxidation (iron, copper), superoxide generators (xanthine oxidase, NADPH-oxidase), thiol-dependent oxidation, peroxynitrite and other radical generation compounds (Parthasarathy et al., 2008).

Oxidatively modified lipoproteins lead to progression of atherosclerosis through macrophages engulfing oxLDL at the level of scavenger receptors, intracellular depositing of cholesterol esters and at last macrophages transformation into foam cells. Also, oxLDL can induce an immune response leading to anti-oxLDL autoantibodies production, which will determine formation of immune complexes (Steinberg et al., 1989; Tsimikas & Witztum, 2001; Parthasarathy et al., 1999, 2008).

Endothelium relaxant factor is a central molecule in vascular homeostasis as a modulator of endothelial tone and reactivity, exerting pleiotropic positive effects on the cardiovascular system. Important for the cardiovascular biology is the consumption of NO by reactive oxygen species. Oxidative modification of NO not only leads to reduced bioavailability but also produces the toxic oxidant peroxynitrite ($ONOO^-$), which further aggravates the imbalance of protective and aggressive factors (Cai & Harrison, 2000; Schnabel & Blankenberg, 2007). Subsequently, LDL oxidative modifications are made possible through simultaneous NO and superoxide anion radical ($O_2^{\cdot -}$) actions.

A key determinant of the pro-oxidant *versus* oxidant-protective influences of NO is the underlying oxidative status of tissue. When NO is in excess of surrounding oxidants, lipid oxidation and monocyte margination into the vascular wall are attenuated, producing antiatherogenic effects. However, when endogenous tissue rates of oxidant production are accelerated or when tissue oxidant defenses become depleted, NO gives rise to secondary oxidizing species that can increase membrane and lipoprotein lipid oxidation as well as foam cell formation in the vasculature, thus promoting proatherogenic effects (Bloodsworth et al., 2000).

Therefore, targeting particularly upstream targets - substrates for oxidation and inflammation, will be important to better understand interactions of hyperlipidemia, inflammation and oxidation.

Current evidence suggests that endothelial function is an integrative marker of the net effects of damage from traditional and emerging risk factors on the arterial wall and its intrinsic capacity for repair. This endothelial-dependent vascular biology is critical, not only in the initiation and progression of atherosclerosis, but also in the transition from a stable to an unstable disease state with attendant risks. As a result, study of endothelial function has emerged as an important endpoint in clinical research (Deanfield et al., 2007).

### 1.2 Oxidized LDL and NO endothelial synthesis as factors affecting the vascular ageing

Diseases of the vascular system have long been considered to be age-related in terms of their onset and progression. Longevity is a vascular question. More than 50 years ago, a famous anatomist - Rudolf Altschul stated that we have the age of our blood vessels: "a man is as old as his arteries". Senescent cells undergo distinct changes in gene expression that may cause an impairment of cellular function. In endothelial cells these changes result in a phenotype that is pro-inflammatory, pro-atherosclerotic, and prothrombotic. Endothelial cell senescence can be induced by a number of factors implicated in vascular pathologies, particularly by sustained cell replication and oxidative stress (Erusalimski, 2009).

Oxidative stress and inflammation are major determinants of arterial and biological ageing. Recent studies underscore the association between white blood cell (WBC) telomere length, as index of systemic aging, oxidized LDL, and human vascular aging, expressed by the distensibility of the carotid artery. Results showed that higher levels of oxidized LDL are associated with shorter WBC telomeres and increased stiffness of the carotid artery (Nawrot & Staessen, 2008; Nawrot et al., 2010).

Ageing is characterized not only by a reduced arterial compliance and alteration of the contractile properties of the vascular wall, but also by endothelial dysfunction (Alvarez de Sotomayor, et al., 2005; Brandes et al., 2006). At present, there are several reasons to believe that *in vivo* NO synthesis from L-arginine could indeed be impaired in atherosclerosis, hypertension, dyslipidemia, diabetes, obesity, insulin resistance, metabolic syndrome, as well as in ageing (Lind, 2002; Laroia et al., 2003; Hsueh & Quinones, 2003; Holvoet et al., 2003, 2008a; Vickers et al., 2009; Park et al., 2009; Njajou et al., 2009; Huang, 2009; Park et al., 2011; Tabit et al., 2010).

Recent studies support the fact that advancing age increases the LDL susceptibility to oxidation and decreases the nitric oxide availability and bioactivity (Heffernan et al., 2008). Not only LDL but also very low-density lipoprotein (VLDL), beta–VLDL and even HDL undergo oxidative modification that must be taken into consideration in the complex process of atherosclerosis (Parthasarathy et al., 2008). In elderly, higher oxLDL levels were associated with high coronary risk before any clinical manifestation of CHD (Holvoet et al., 2003), and with higher arterial stiffness, independent of cardiovascular disease risk factors (Brinkley et al., 2009). The oxLDL/Apo-B100 ratio and to a lesser extent the oxLDL/LDL-C ratio were significantly negative associated with the flow-mediated-dilation (FMD) of the brachial artery (van der Zwan et al., 2009).

### 1.3 Methods for measuring the circulating oxidized LDL and NO endothelial synthesis

Oxidative biomarkers are now showing strong associations with progression of coronary artery disease (CAD) and predict cardiovascular events, suggesting that they may serve as surrogates and may complement diagnostic investigations. Both *in vitro* and *in vivo*, low-density lipoprotein (LDL) particles are susceptible to oxidation and peroxidation by all of the causes of oxidative stress. Therefore, oxidized LDL are included among the "downstream markers" of oxidative stress. During the last decade, several monoclonal antibodies have been generated, each recognizing at least a substantial subset of the whole spectrum of oxLDL particles, leading to a myriad of new reports on the relation between circulating ox-LDL and cardiovascular pathological processes (Itabe and Ueda, 2007; Tsimikas, 2006).

Currently used assays for oxLDL detect minimally oxidized LDL particles. In addition, concentrations of oxLDL depend on the sensitivity of LDL to oxidation; small dense LDLs contain smaller amounts of antioxidants and are, therefore, more prone to oxidation. The widely applied sensitive immunoassay quantifying the circulating levels of oxLDL uses a monoclonal antibody - 4E6, directed against oxidized apolipoprotein B-100 moiety of LDL (Rietzschel et al., 2008; Holvoet et al., 2008b).

The NO activity is assessed representatively using a variety of clinical invasive and noninvasive methods among which, the use of acetylcholine that induces endothelium-dependent dilation and smooth muscle-mediated constriction. The coronary artery diameter is compared by quantitative angiography before and after infusion of acetylcholine. The functional status of the coronary microvasculature can also be assessed using intracoronary Doppler ultrasound to measure blood flow in resistance vessels in response to substances that produce either endothelial-dependent or endothelial-independent vasodilation. Another noninvasive method of detecting endothelial dysfunction uses high-resolution ultrasound to measure the brachial artery diameter in response to reactive hyperemia, which stimulates NO release and FMD (Davignon & Ganz, 2004).
NO present in the circulation is originating from endothelial, smooth muscle cells, thrombocytes, leukocytes and cardiomiocytes. NO activity is the net result of a balance between its production and its inactivation by oxygen free radicals. NO released "in vivo" by nitric oxide synthase (NOS) activity in endothelial cells and platelets, rapidly autooxidizes to yield nitrite ($NO_2^-$), which interacts with oxyhemoglobin yielding nitrate ($NO_3^-$). Because nitrite plus nitrate are relatively stable compounds in blood, their levels may be a biochemical index of systemic NO production. This is convenient because direct *in vivo* measurements of NO can be very difficult due to the extremely low levels and its short half life. When combined measurements of nitrate and nitrite are conducted, this is usually denoted by the term NOx (Lundberg & Weitzberg, 2005; Hirata et al., 2010).

## 2. Study on correlations of oxLDL and NOx with the metabolic profile in elderly with hyperlipidemia

The LDL oxidation and nitric oxide are the key mediators involved in all stages of atherosclerosis: initiation, progression and complications. Their role is antagonistic: oxLDL have pro-atherogenic and NO antiatherogenic functions on vascular endothelium (Figure 1). A reduction in NO production or activity has been proposed as major mechanisms of endothelial dysfunction and a contributor to atherosclerosis. The endothelial dysfunction is considered an early marker for atherosclerosis and can be detected before structural changes in the vascular wall. An impairment of NO bioactivity or synthesis will reduce its braking effect on processes involved in atherogenesis.

### 2.1 Purpose

In the present study we evaluated the levels of circulating oxidized LDL (oxLDL) and the basal plasma levels of the NO metabolic pathway products, NOx ($NO_2^-$ + $NO_3^-$), and examined their relationships with the global metabolic profile in a group of elderly patients with hyperlipidemia. We explored the determinants of oxLDL and NOx, as well as the relation between oxLDL and NOx in order to investigate whether the oxLDL/NOx and oxLDL/HDL-cholesterol ratios are more informative than the individual variables.

### 2.2 Materials and methods

#### 2.2.1 Study design

The study population included 170 subjects (72 men and 98 women) aged 60 - 70 years, of the patients hospitalized at the Ana Aslan- National Institute of Gerontology and Geriatrics (NIGG), Bucharest, Romania, who were selected according to clinical and biochemical criteria. The subjects did not have diabetes or any liver, kidney, hematological or oncological overt diseases. We selected in a first group 125 subjects with a high cardiovascular risk lipid profile characterized by hypercholesterolemia [serum total cholesterol (TC) > 200 mg/dL and LDL-cholesterol (LDL-C) > 130 mg/dL], associated or not with hypertriglyceridemia [serum triglycerides (TG) < or > 150 mg/dL]. Subjects were not previously diagnosed with cardiovascular disease and were not under treatment with any vasoactive or cardiovascular drugs. None of the patients used lipid-lowering therapy or antioxidants. The second group considered as the control group included 45 apparently healthy subjects with normal lipid profile (TC < 200 mg/dL, LDL-C < 130 mg/dL and TG < 150 mg/dL). Anthropometric and clinical characteristics were collected after a complete clinical examination. All the participants in this study gave their written informed consent, and the study protocol was approved by the Ana Aslan - NIGG ethics committee. All the procedures followed were in accordance with the institutional guidelines. Venous blood samples were drawn after an overnight fast and 24-hours refraining from smoking, caffeinated foods and beverages.

### 2.2.2 Biochemical methods

Total cholesterol (TC), LDL-cholesterol (LDL-C), HDL-cholesterol (HDL-C), triglycerides (TG) and glycemia (G) were determinated by standard enzymatic methods. Results were expressed in mg/dL.

The circulating plasma oxLDL was evaluated by a competitive ELISA kit with the monoclonal antibody 4E6 (kit 10-1158-01, Mercodia, Sweden) directed against an epitope in the apolipoprotein B-100 moiety of oxLDL, formed from substitution of lysine residues of apoB-100 with aldehydes (Holvoet et al., 2008). Results were expressed in U/L plasma.

The total amount of plasma stable metabolic pathway products of NO, [NOx, the sum of nitrites and nitrates ($NO_2^-$ + $NO_3^-$)] was determined using the Griess reagent, following the quantitative conversion of nitrates ($NO_3^-$) to nitrites ($NO_2^-$), with nitrate reductase (kit 23479, SIGMA). Results were expressed in μmols NOx/L plasma. All the biochemical and immunoenzymatic tests were performed on a ChemWell 2190 Analyser (Awareness Technology, USA).

The plasma atherogenic index (Ai) was calculated by the logarithmically transformed ratio of triglycerides on HDL-cholesterol (TG/HDL-C) (1) (Dobiasova, 2006; Dobiasova et al., 2011).

$$Ai = \log(TG/HDL\text{-}C) \qquad (1)$$

### 2.2.3 Statistical analysis

Data are expressed as means±SD. The subjects clinical characteristics were compared using the Mann Whitney Wilcoxon non-parametric test. Differences in means of studied parameters between the groups (hyperlipidemic *vs.* control group) were assessed by Student's paired *t* test. The Pearson's correlation test was used to perform bivariate correlation analysis. Multiple regression analysis was performed to evaluate the independent relation between studied parameters using the Statistical Package for Social Sciences software (SPSS) version 15. Significance was defined at the 0.05 level of confidence.

### 2.3 Results

The study population included 170 subjects aged 60-70 years. In order to establish the link of the traditional markers for the evaluation of the cardiovascular risk (TC, TG and LDL-C) at

systemic level with the oxidative stress and endothelial function parameters, patients were divided into two groups: a group with normal lipid profile (TC<200 mg/dL, LDL<130 mg/dL, TG<150 mg/dL; n=45), and a group with high cardiovascular risk lipid profile (TC>200 mg/dL, LDL>130 mg/dL, TG < or > 150 mg/dL; n = 125).
We firstly collected anthropometric data (body weight, height), clinical parameters, including systolic blood pressure, body mass index (BMI), fasting plasma glucose and the lipid profile in the two groups of our interest.
Both cardiovascular disease risk and healthy control subjects showed not significantly different values of weight and body mass index, but systolic blood pressure, fasting plasma glucose and triglycerides were significantly higher in hyperlipidemic patients. The HDL-cholesterol concentrations of the two groups were comparable. The atherogenic index and the TC /HDL-cholesterol ratio were significantly higher in hyperlipidemic group *versus* control (Table 1).
Also, the increased lipid profile group had a significantly higher circulating levels of oxLDL associated with a significant decrease of the plasma nitric oxide metabolic pathway products (NOx) compared to the normolipidemic group (Table 1).

| Variables | Control Group (n = 45) | Hyperlipidemic Group (n = 125) |
|---|---|---|
| Age (years) | 65±3 | 66±4 |
| Sex (males/females) | 15/30 | 55/70 |
| Systolic blood pressure (mmHg) | 115.6±16.0 | 129.0±21.5** |
| Diastolic blood pressure (mmHg) | 74.6±9.7 | 73.5±12.7 |
| Body mass index (kg/m$^2$) | 22.5±2.9 | 23.2±5.3 |
| Glucose (mg/dL) | 91±12 | 100±12** |
| Total cholesterol (mg/dL) | 182±22 | 285±32** |
| Triglycerides (mg/dL) | 77±22 | 103±48** |
| LDL-cholesterol (mg/dL) | 105±24 | 214±35** |
| HDL-cholesterol (mg/dL) | 56±11 | 54±9 |
| Total cholesterol/HDL-C ratio | 3.40±0.83 | 5.34±1.11** |
| Atherogenic index (Ai) | 0.13±0.15 | 0.24±0.19** |
| Uric acid(mg/dL) | 5.87±2.07 | 6.09±1.94 |
| oxLDL (U/L) | 71.51±13.11 | 85.50±20** |
| NOx (μmol/L) | 32.52±10.63 | 23.52±8.66** |
| oxLDL/HDL cholesterol ratio | 1.35±0.46 | 1.62±0.58* |
| oxLDL/NOx ratio | 2.44±0.92 | 4.13±1.87** |

Values are expressed as means±standard deviation LDL, low-density lipoprotein; HDL-C high-density lipoprotein cholesterol; oxLDL, oxidized low-density lipoprotein; NOx, nitric oxide metabolic pathway products * p values derived from Student *t* test: significantly different *vs.* control group;
* $p < 0.01$; ** $p < 0.001$

Table 1. Clinical characteristics and metabolic variables in control and hyperlipidemic subjects.

To establish which variables other than LDL-C and NO were independent determinants of oxLDL and NO, we explored multiple linear regression models with oxLDL, NOx, oxLDL/HDL-C ratio and oxLDL/NOx ratio, as dependent variables, in control, hyperlipidemia, and whole study population. The results are presented in Table 2 and 3 and Figures 3-6.

In multiple regression analysis for estimating the association between the degree of endothelial dysfunction and metabolic parameters, we found different statistically significant correlations within the two study groups. Tables 2 and 3 show the correlations of oxLDL and NOx with serum metabolic variables, atherogenic markers and indices in normal and hyperlipidemic subjects.

In the control group (table 2) circulating oxLDL level positively correlated with glycemia and triglycerides, as well as the total cholesterol/HDL-cholesterol ratio.

In subjects with high cardio-vascular risk (table 3) significant positive correlations between oxLDL and LDL-cholesterol were pointed out. In both study groups oxLDL was significantly negative correlated with HDL-cholesterol, and significantly positive with the atherogenic index (Ai).

| Variables | oxLDL | oxLDL/HDL-C ratio | NOx | oxLDL/NOx ratio |
|---|---|---|---|---|
| **Control Group (n = 45)** | | | | |
| Glucose (mg/dL) | 0.351* | 0.273 (NS) | 0.164 (NS) | - 0.004 (NS) |
| Total cholesterol (mg/dL) | 0.257 (NS) | - 0.470** | - 0.088 (NS) | 0.097 (NS) |
| Triglycerides (mg/dL) | 0.358* | 0.273 (NS) | - 0.259 (NS) | 0.414** |
| LDL-cholesterol (mg/dL) | 0.257 (NS) | 0.396** | - 0.024 (NS) | 0.031 (NS) |
| HDL-cholesterol (mg/dL) | - 0.471** | - 0.832** | 0.081 (NS) | - 0.291 (NS) |
| Total cholesterol/HDL-C | 0.528** | 0.537** | - 0.075 (NS) | 0.252 (NS) |
| Atherogenic index (Ai) | 0.502** | 0.605** | - 0.267 (NS) | 0.234** |
| Uric acid(mg/dL) | 0.200 (NS) | 0.063 (NS) | 0.184 (NS) | - 0.045 (NS) |
| oxLDL (U/L) | | 0.850** | 0.074 (NS) | 0.404** |
| oxLDL/HDL-C ratio | 0.850** | | 0.045 (NS) | 0.357* |
| NOx (μmol/L) | 0.074 (NS) | 0.045 (NS) | | - 0.826** |
| oxLDL/NOx ratio | 0.404** | 0.357* | - 0.826** | |

LDL, low-density lipoprotein; HDL-C, high-density lipoprotein cholesterol; oxLDL, oxidized low-density lipoprotein; NOx, nitric oxide metabolic pathway products

* $p < 0.05$; ** $p < 0.01$; NS, non-significant

Table 2. Interrelationships between studied markers of lipoxidative stress, endothelial function, and metabolic profile parameters, in control subjects, determined as Pearson's correlation coefficients (r).

As regards the nitric oxide metabolic pathway products, the statistical analysis of the data pointed out a significant negative correlation, between NOx and the total cholesterol/HDL-cholesterol ratio, but only in the hyperlipidemic group (Table 2 and 3).

| Variables | oxLDL | oxLDL/HDL-C ratio | NOx | oxLDL/NOx ratio |
|---|---|---|---|---|
| **Hyperlipidemic Group (n = 125)** | | | | |
| Glucose (mg/dL) | 0.275** | 0.329** | - 0.096 (NS) | 0.245** |
| Total cholesterol (mg/dL) | 0.390** | 0.298** | - 0.340** | 0.437** |
| Triglycerides (mg/dL) | 0.320** | 0.293** | 0.037 (NS) | 0.128 (NS) |
| LDL-cholesterol (mg/dL) | 0.377** | 0.391** | - 0.315** | 0.411** |
| HDL-cholesterol (mg/dL) | - 0.445** | - 0.762** | 0.011 (NS) | - 0.223* |
| Total cholesterol/HDL-C ratio | 0.578** | 0.796** | - 0.191* | 0.416** |
| Atherogenic index (Ai) | 0.549** | 0.637** | 0.054 (NS) | 0.220* |
| Uric acid(mg/dL) | 0.270** | 0.201* | 0.158 (NS) | - 0.006 (NS) |
| oxLDL(U/L) | | 0.895** | - 0.143 (NS) | 0.641** |
| oxLDL/HDL-C ratio | 0.895** | | - 0.111 (NS) | 0.546** |
| NOx (μmol/L) | - 0.143 (NS) | - 0.111 (NS) | | - 0.729** |
| oxLDL/NOx ratio | 0.641** | 0.546** | - 0.729** | |

LDL, low-density lipoprotein; HDL-C, high-density lipoprotein cholesterol; oxLDL, oxidized low-density lipoprotein; NOx, nitric oxide metabolic pathway products
* $p < 0.05$; ** $p < 0.01$; NS, non-significant

Table 3. Interrelationships between studied markers of lipoxidative stress, endothelial function, and metabolic profile parameters, in hyperlipidemic subjects, determined as Pearson's correlation coefficients (r)

To further estimate the extent of oxLDL involvement in endothelial dysfunction, the ratio of oxLDL to HDL-cholesterol and the newly introduced ratio of oxLDL to NOx, were calculated.

Significant differences as regards oxLDL/HDL-cholesterol ratio as well as oxLDL/NOx ratio were found out between the study groups; both ratios were higher in the hyperlipidemic subjects (Table 1).

Moreover, in the group of subjects with cardiovascular risk, oxLDL/NOx ratio correlated significantly with almost each of the traditional parameters of the metabolic profile, namely: glycemia, total cholesterol, LDL-cholesterol and HDL-cholesterol, as well as the Ai and cardiovascular risk markers (TC/HDL-C and oxLDL/HDL-C ratios) (Table 3).

We explored the metabolic determinants of oxLDL and NOx by performing the statistical multiple correlation test in the whole study population (n=170). Regarding the oxLDL we identified significant ($p < 0.01$) positive correlations with each studied parameters of the metabolic profile, such as glycemia ($r = 0.351$), total cholesterol ($r = 0.457$), LDL-cholesterol ($r = 0.456$), triglycerides ($r = 0.414$) and uric acid ($r = 0.253$). A strong significant negative association between oxLDL and HDL-C ($r= -0.425$, $p <0.01$) was pointed out.

In all 170 subjects we pointed out significantly negative correlations ($p < 0.01$) of NOx levels and lipid profile: total cholesterol ($r = - 0.470$), LDL-C ($r = - 0.451$), and the atherogenic risk marker TC/HDL ratio ($r= -0.365$) (Figure 2).

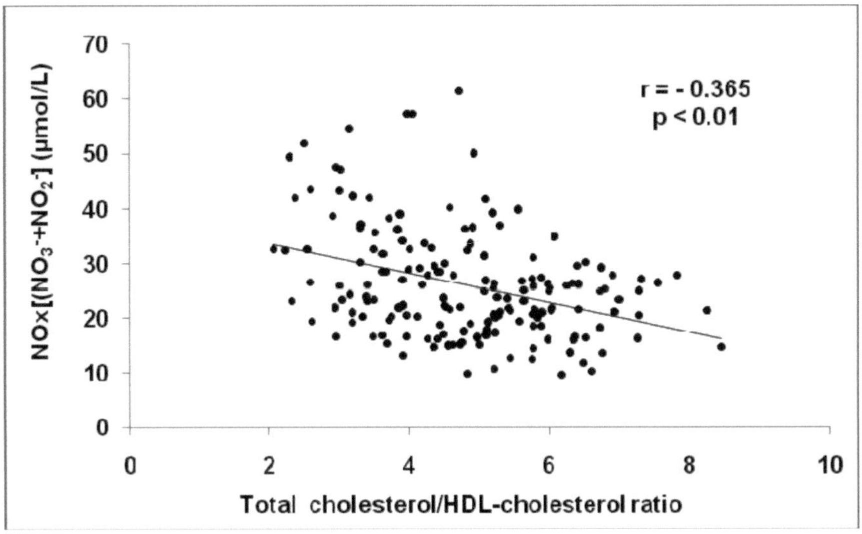


Fig. 2. Plasma nitric oxide metabolic pathway products (NOx) is inversely correlated with total cholesterol/HDL-cholesterol ratio in all the study subjects (n=170)

Finally, it is important to underscore the most interesting significant, negative, correlation, identified between oxLDL and NOx ($r = -0.205$, $p < 0.01$; $n = 170$) in all study population (Figure 3). In the hyperlipidemic group this association was negative but not significant.

The newly introduced ratio oxLDL/NOx was significantly related to the ratio oxLDL/HDL ($r = 0.547$, $p < 0.01$, n=170), the atherogenic index (Ai) and also the total cholesterol/HDL-ratio ($r = 0.478$, $p < 0.01$ and $r = 0.537$, $p < 0.01$) (Figure 4 - A, B, C).

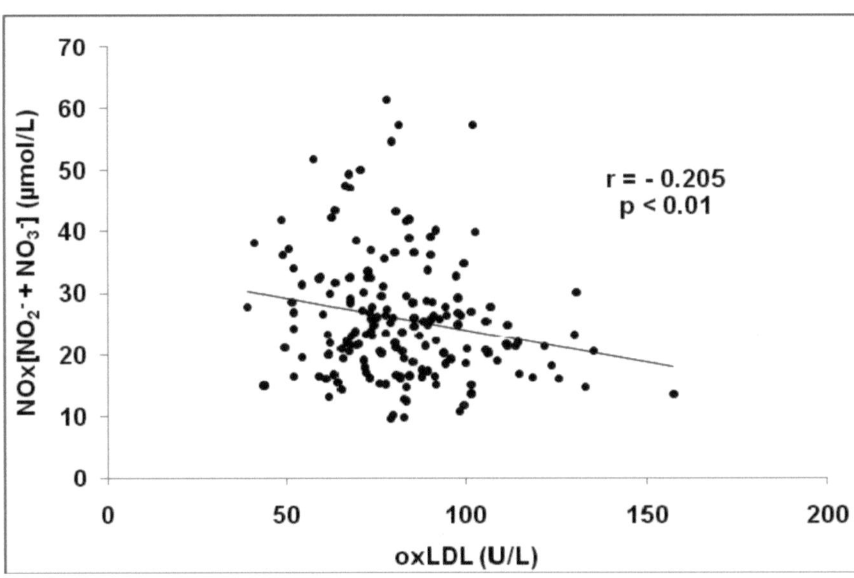


Fig. 3. Oxidized LDL (oxLDL) levels are inversely associated with plasma nitric oxide metabolic pathway products (NOx) in all the study subjects (n = 170).

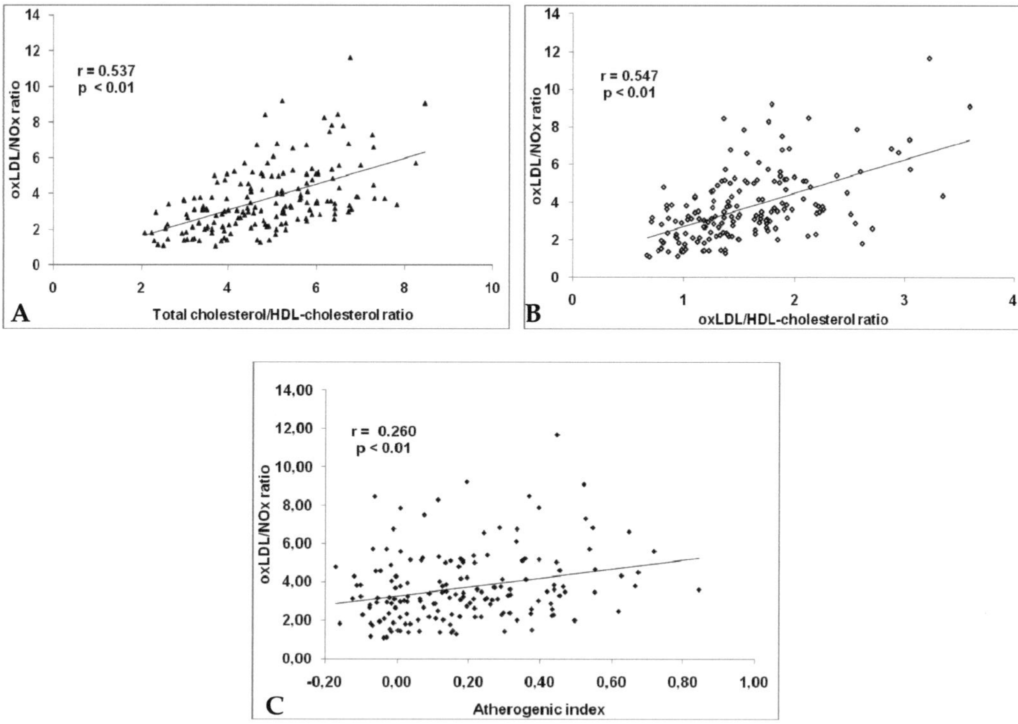


Fig. 4. oxLDL/NOx ratio is directly correlated with total cholesterol/HDL-cholesterol ratio (A), with oxLDL/HDL-cholesterol ratio (B), and with the Atherogenic index (C) in all the study subjects (n=170)

## 2.4 Discussion

The purpose of this work was to point to the interrelationships of oxLDL and NO as biomarkers of oxidative stress and endothelial function and the metabolic profile in elderly. We explored the literature on molecular mechanisms involved in the biochemical and metabolic links of NO and oxLDL. We investigated the metabolic determinants of oxLDL and NOx in 170 elderly subjects. Our research results focused mainly on the correlations between lipid and lipoprotein parameters as indices of atherogenic risk, and lipoxidative stress and endothelial dysfunction biomarkers, namely the nitric oxide metabolic pathway products (NOx) and the circulating oxidized LDL.

Impairment in NO, a common feature in patients with endothelial dysfunction, is considered to predict atherosclerosis and cardiovascular events. On the other hand, elevated levels of oxidized LDL, formed within the arterial wall, are commonly related to the atherogenic profile (Steinberg, 2009; Steinberg & Witzum, 2010). Therefore, in the present study, we evaluated the relationships of oxLDL and NOx as oxidative stress and endothelial dysfunction biomarkers with the metabolic profile and the cardiovascular high-risk profile markers, in 170 elderly patients.

Plasma NOx levels were significantly lower in patients with hyperlipidemia, further suggesting that physiologic levels of NO are necessary to maintain the normal, vasodilatatory and noninflammatory phenotype of the vascular wall. A major finding of this study is that NO release levels measured by its metabolic pathway products significantly negatively correlated with circulating oxLDL concentrations. Overall, this work pointed out the link between the vascular endothelium vasodilating/vasoconstricting imbalance and the metabolic profile in hyperlipidemic elderly patients.

The evaluations of LDL-cholesterol, high-density lipoprotein-cholesterol, and triglycerides are the traditionally recommended lipid screening tests for coronary heart disease (CHD). Several studies do suggest that total cholesterol/HDL-cholesterol ratio, a major lipid index, is better than the individual total cholesterol, LDL-cholesterol, HDL-cholesterol, and triglycerides parameters (Lemieux et al., 2001). This ratio is easily obtained and one of the most powerful important risk factors for CHD. Both oxLDL and NOx significantly correlated with all markers and calculated atherogenic indices (TC/HDL-C, oxLDL/HDL-C and Ai). Hence, our data support the fact that measurements of the oxLDL and NOx levels at different times may help to monitor the state and severity of endothelial dysfunction.

Based on the multiple correlations analysis in both study groups and all subjects we found that TC, TC/HDL-C, and oxLDL/HDL-C ratios are major determinants of oxLDL and NO. These associations are stronger for the newly introduced oxLDL/NOx ratio. As well, the oxLDL/NOx ratio is strongly correlated with the atherogenic index and more importantly, with the oxLDL/HDL-C ratio, the best lipid biomarker used for discriminating between coronary artery disease patients and healthy control subjects, and also the best blood biomarker that reflects atherosclerotic disease activity in the arterial wall (Huang et al., 2008; Lankin et al., 2011)

Our results are in accordance with literature with regard to the damaging effects of hyperlipidemia, mediated or stimulated by oxidative stress. Numerous studies have supported the role of hyperlipidemia in atherosclerosis, endothelial dysfunction and progression of coronary heart diseases (Wallace et al., 2010; Deanfield et al., 2007; Highashino et al., 2010; Van den Oever et al., 2010). The hypothesised mechanisms for this effect are via hyperlipemia-induced oxidative stress, especially LDL oxidation and subsequent reduced NO bioavailibility. The strong significant association of oxidized LDL with plasma lipid profile (TC, LDL-C, TG), atherogenic risk markers (TC/HDL-c, oxLDL/HDL) and atherogenic index (Ai) found out in the hyperlipidemic group as well as the whole population studied, underscore the validity of the observation that hyperlipemia induces LDL oxidation and oxidative stress. The oxidative stress generates the superoxide radicals ($O_2^{.-}$), which are scavenged by nitric oxide to form peroxynitrite ($ONOO^-$), a powerful oxidant. The overproduction of $O_2^{.-}$ has direct and indirect effects on vascular NO bioavailability. Moreover, $O_2^{.-}$ and $ONOO^-$ can oxidize tetrahydrobiopterin ($BH_4$), the cofactor necessary for NO production by eNOS enzyme, leading to eNOS uncoupling, and thus to more $O_2^{.-}$ generation and reduced NO production. Also, the significant negative correlation found out in this study between oxLDL and NOx shows that the excess of LDL oxidation itself may contribute to reduce NO level. Taken toghether, hyperlipidemia, oxidative stress and LDL oxidation result in reduced NO bioavailability via combinatory effects of direct elimination and decreased production of NO. This NO reduced bioavailability compromises all the antiatherogenic functions of the endothelium. This hypothesised mechanism shown above could be a target for interventions to protect against hyperlipidemia-induced atherogenesis and cardiovascular disease.

Based on the strong interrelationships pointed out in this clinical study and the numerous experimental and clinical research in the field of atherosclerosis we summarize in figure 5 the important relationships among hyperlipidemia, oxidative stress, LDL oxidation, nitric oxide and endothelial dysfunction. Hyperlipidemia, oxidative stress and LDL oxidation are harmful at multiple steps in atherogenesis, including direct contributions to endothelial functions. As shown in figure 5, hyperlipidemia induces enhanced oxidative stress, superoxide ($O_2^{\cdot-}$) excessive generation and LDL oxidation. Increased $O_2^{\cdot-}$ generation as a result of excess mitochondrial lipid oxidation, LDL oxidation and other sources, is critically involved in reduced NO bioactivity and endothelial dysfunction, by direct elimination of NO.

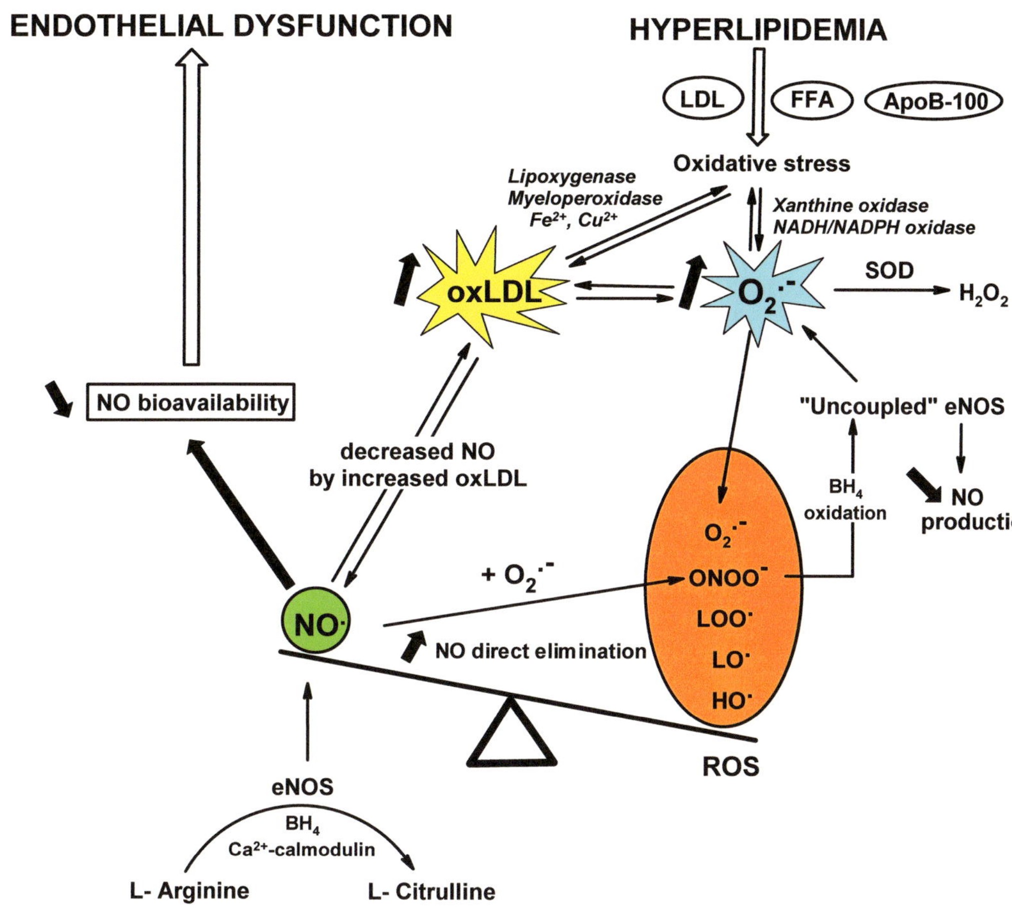


LDL, low-density lipoprotein; oxLDL, oxidized low-density lipoprotein; FFA, free fatty acids; ApoB-100, apolipoprotein B-100; $H_2O_2$, hydrogen peroxide; SOD, superoxide dismutase, ROS, reactive oxygen species; HO·, hydroxyl radical; LO·, alkoxyl radical; LOO·, peroxyl radical; $ONOO^-$, peroxynitrite; eNOS, endothelial nitric oxide synthase; $BH_4$, tetrahydrobiopterin.

Fig. 5. Simplified scheme of the interrelationships between oxidative stress, LDL oxidation and NO in the hyperlipidemic state leading to endothelial dysfunction.

There is abundant experimental evidence indicating the role of NO oxidative inactivation as a mediator of endothelial dysfunction and a pre-pathogenic vascular phenotype (Harrison, 1997; Bermudez et al., 2008). The NO is the kinetically preferred scavenger for $O_2^{\cdot-}$, because their reaction to generate $ONOO^-$ occurs three times faster than the $O_2^{\cdot-}$ elimination by superoxide dismutase (SOD) (Beckman & Koppenol, 1996; Cai & Harrison, 2000). Both excess generation of reactive oxygen species (ROS) including $O_2^{.-}$ and oxidized LDL, and decreased antioxidant defence mechanisms contribute to enhanced degradation of NO. Many studies support the role of the $O_2^{.-}$ as an essential element in the decrease of NO bioavailability in oxidative stress conditions. Thus, studies on rabbbits with aortic atherosclerosis, demonstrated a remarkable decrease in endothelium-related relaxation, which was corrected by SOD treatment (Dulak et al., 1997).

Also, peroxynitrite is itself a powerful oxidant which contributes to enhance oxidative stress and turn the balance NO - ROS in the favour of ROS. Both radicals, $O_2^{.-}$ and $ONOO^-$ can oxidize tetrahydrobiopterin ($BH_4$) leads to eNOS uncoupling, which in turn will produce $O_2^{.-}$ instead of NO, and activate this vicious cycle (Fostermann, 2006). Uncoupling eNOS directly leading to decreased NO production. Not only $BH_4$ oxidation, but also decreases in $BH_4$ concentrations may reduce the NO production. Thus, many studies have shown a significant decrease in $BH_4$ activity in various pathological states, such as: hyperlipidemia, hypercholesterolemia, insulin resistance, probably through the oxLDL increase, as well as increased expression in some proinflammatory cytokine (TNF-alpha, interleukin-1 beta) (Bowers et al., 2011; Wever et al., 1997; Stroes et al., 1997). Furthermore, clinical and experimental studies have confirmed these mechanisms, showing that acute administration of $BH_4$ improve the endothelial dysfunctions related to hyperlipidemia, atherosclerosis and hypertension (Setoguchi et al., 2001). Also, a decrease in arginine and consequently a lack in eNOS substrate bioavailability leads to a failure in NO synthesis (Bermudez et al, 2005).

Recent *in vitro* studies (Bowers et al., 2011) demonstrated that tetrahydrobiopterin (BH4) could reduce oxLDL-induced $O_2^{.-}$ production by NADPH oxidase, increasing NO synthesis in endothelial cells. The superoxide anion production was increased by pretreatment of cells with an inhibitor of $BH_4$ synthesis, and decreased following pretreatment with a $BH_4$ precursor. Thus, $BH_4$ concentrations can modulate the NADPH oxidase-induced imbalance of endothelial NO and $O_2^{.-}$ production. $BH_4$ may be critical in combating oxidative stress, restoring proper redox state and reducing risk for cardiovascular disease including atherosclerosis.

Other mechanisms are also involved in the interrelations of LDL oxidation, nitric oxide and endothelial dysfunction. The oxidized LDL may reduce eNOS levels by inhibiting eNOS gene expression (Dulak et al., 1997) and also can displace eNOS from caveolae by binding to endothelial cell CD36 receptors and by depleting caveolae cholesterol content and therefore disrupt eNOS activity (Barbato et al., 2004). These adverse effects of oxLDL are prevented by HDL via binding to scavenger receptor BI (SR-BI), colocalized with eNOS in endothelial caveolae. This occurs through the maintenance of caveolae cholesterol content by cholesterol ester uptake from HDL. Moreover, HDL binding to SR-BI may stimulate eNOS activity in endothelial cells, and enhance endothelium- and NO-dependent relaxation. Thus, lipoproteins have potent effects on eNOS function in caveolae via actions on both membrane cholesterol homeostasis and the level of activation of the enzyme, processes that may be critically involved in the earliest phases of atherogenesis (Rigotti et al., 1997; Uittenbogaraard et al., 2000; Yuhanna et al., 2001; Schaul, 2003). The significant negative correlations between HDL and oxLDL, oxLDL/HDL ratio, atherogenic index and more important oxLDL/NO ratio pointed out in hyperlipidemic group and all subjects, underscore the beneficial effect of HDL on the endothelium.

Recent studies demonstrated that oxLDL causes impairment of endothelium-dependent, nitric oxide-mediated vasodilation involving L-arginine deficiency. The oxLDL may reduce L-arginine availability to eNOS for NO production, by up-regulating arginase. The experimental studies indicated that oxLDL increased arginase expression in the vascular wall without altering eNOS expression (Wang et al., 2011).

Experimental studies underscore the dual role of oxLDL on endothelial cells causing either proliferation or apoptosis, depending on its concentration and exposure time (Galle et al., 2001). Thus, oxLDL induced proliferation at low (5 to 10 microg/mL) and apoptosis at higher concentrations (50 to 300 microg/mL). Both effects are mediated by $O_2^{.-}$ formation via NADPH oxidase as it major source. Thus, oxLDL contributes importantly to vascular cellular turnover through the induction of oxidative stress. More recently, was demonstrated that oxLDL at low concentrations (5 microg/mL) promotes *in vitro* angiogenesis and activate nitric oxide synthase through PI3K/Akt/eNOS pathway in human coronary artery endothelial cells (Yu et al., 2011).

On the whole, the decline in nitric oxide bioavailability is caused by the cummulative effects of many factors and processes discussed above: the decreased expression of the endothelial NO synthase, a reduction of substrate or cofactors for eNOS, alterations of cellular signaling, eNOS inhibition by asymmetric demethyl arginine, reduced NO production and accelerated NO degradation by hyperlipidemia, oxidative stress and LDL oxidation.

Taking into account overall the atherogenic properties of oxidized LDL, involved in all stages of atherosclerosis (Steinberg et al., 1989; Steinberg, 2009), and the vasoprotective and antioxidant functions of NO (Bermudez et al., 2008; Yasa & Turkseven, 2005), we introduced for the first time the ratio oxLDL to NOx for quantifying their possible cumulative effect on vascular endothelium. The strong positive associations of this ratio with the atherogenic index and the atherogenic risk markers: TC/HDL and oxLDL/HDL ratios, supported us to propose this newly introduced ratio (oxLDL/NOx) as a potential marker of endothelial dysfunction. The future in depth studies, will take into consideration the association with clinical parameters of vascular endothelial functions using acethylcholine to induce endothelium dependent dilation, quantitative angiography, and high resolution ultrasound to measure brachial artery diameter, to further support this new candidate marker.

Wu et al., (2006) suggested in a prospective cohort study that circulating oxLDL as an individual parameter, measured with antibody 4E6, was not an independent overall predictor of coronary heart disease (CHD), after adjustment of lipid markers and less predictive in development of CHD than apoB and total cholesterol/HDL-cholesterol ratio (Wu et al., 2006). Therefore, based on the results obtained in our study it is important to examine in future research whether the ratio oxLDL to NOx correlates with endothelial function and predicts CHD independently of the lipid markers.

Data of this study support the relevance of oxLDL and NOx as biomarkers reflecting, at systemic level, the progressive damage at cellular level under the action of prooxidant pathogenic factors. These biomarkers could be valuable in the complex evaluation of oxidative stress in the endothelium.

Despite numerous evidences of oxidative processes involved in atherosclerosis and the multiple experimental research on their inhibition by traditional antioxidants, and the success in several animal trials, the human clinical trials using antioxidants have failed (Parthasarathy et al., 2008; da Luz et al., 2006). There were not taken into consideration all the factors, aspects, processes, steps and stages involved in early or advanced atherosclerotic lesions, their interrelations, and the most important the pro-oxidant properties and actions of antioxidants in different oxidative process steps and disease stages.

These interrelatioships pointed out in our study could be very important in the management of new effective therapeutic strategies for atherosclerosis and cardiovascular disease. Because oxidative stress, LDL oxidation and endothelial dysfunction centrally contributes to cardiovascular disease, further sustained efforts must be undertaken to translate this knowledge into the characterization and identification of biomarkers that enable preventive or early detection of injuries and allow improved risk stratification by integration into cardiovascular risk stratification models.

### 2.5 Limitations of our study

The study population included only elderly and therefore the results may be different in other age-groups subjects, in order to have identified the early onset of hyperlipidemia-induced vascular impairment. Another important limitation was that we did not evaluate the endothelial function using the flow-mediated dilation (FMD) and ultrasound examination of the right brachial artery.

## 3. Conclusion

The results of this correlations study pointed out that in hyperlipidemic elderly patients the endothelial NO synthesis could indeed be impaired and associated with a higher oxidative stress exerted on circulating LDL particles. Oxidized LDL has a large range of biological effects that contribute to atherogenesis, but NO also has many biological effects that prevent atherogenesis. In this context, the interrelations pointed out between hyperlipidemia, oxidative stress, LDL oxidation and nitric oxide leading to endothelial dysfunctions, emphasized their implications in molecular mechanisms of endothelial dysfunction.

It is important to distinguish between the effect of oxidized LDL and the effect of a deficiency in the release of NO and to draw a link between these two biomarkers. According to the results obtained in this study, we propose the use of a new marker of endothelial dysfunction, the ratio of oxLDL to NOx, which could be a more accurate estimation of the *in vivo* cumulative implications of oxLDL and NO in atherogenesis. Future studies taking into account the association of this newly introduced marker with other markers of endothelial function will be undertaken to support the marker validity.

The strong interrelations pointed out in our study underscore the molecular mechanisms implicated in endothelial dysfunctions and atherosclerosis presented in this chapter. Future research is needed to translate this knowledge into the identification, characterization and validation of new and known biomarkers of lipoxidative stress-induced endothelial dysfunctions and atherosclerosis, and their integration into cardiovascular risk stratifications models.

These findings suggest the importance of understanding the senescent specific changes occurring in endothelium associated with age-related disease. Such an understanding may not only provide answers regarding mechanisms of disease development, but may also provide biomarkers of endothelium specific ageing.

As perspectives, the nutritional and therapeutic strategies should attempt to correct the lipid profile and lipoxidative stress in order to prevent the amplification of redox and inflammatory phenomena that lead to increased cardiovascular risk. As well, therapeutic approaches in the prevention and treatment of atherosclerosis based on improving NO bioactivity and reducing LDL oxidation may become a challenge for future studies.

## 4. Acknowledgements

The authors thank Professor Sampath Parthasarathy for comments that greatly improved the manuscript.
The authors are grateful for the support provided by the 7th Framework Program (FP7) European Study "MARK-AGE, European Study to Establish Biomarkers of Human Ageing".

## 5. References

Alvarez de Sotomayor, M., Perez-Guerrero, C., Herrrera, M.D, Jimenez, L., Marin, R., Marhuenda, E. & Andriantsitohaina, R. (2005). Improvement of Age-related Endothelial Dysfunction by Simvastatin: Effect on NO and COX Pathways. *British Journal of Pharmacology*, Vol.146, No.8, (December 2005), pp. 1130–1138, ISSN 0007-1188

Barbato, J.E. & Tzeng, E. (2004). Nitric Oxide and Arterial Disease. *Journal of Vascular Surgery*, Vol.40, No.1, (July 2004), 187-193. ISSN 0741-5214

Beckman, J.S. & Koppenol, W.H. (1996). Nitric Oxide, Superoxide, and Peroxynitrite: the Good, the Bad and the Ugly. *American Journal of Physiology. Endocrinolgy and metabolism*, Vol.271, No.5Pt1, (November 1996), pp. C1424-C1437, ISSN 0193-1849

Bermudez, V., Bermudez, F., Acosta, G., Acosta, A., Afiez, J., Andara, C., Leal, E., Cano, C., Hernandez, R. & Israili, Z. (2008). Molecular Mechanisms of Endothelial Dysfunction: From Nitric Oxide Synthesis to ADMA Inhibition. *American Journal of Therapeutics*, Vol.15, No.4, (July 2008), pp. 326-333, ISSN 1075-2765

Bloodsworth, A., O'Donnell, V.B. & Freeman, B.A. (2000). Nitric Oxide Regulation of Free Radical- and Enzyme-Mediated Lipid and Lipoprotein Oxidation. *Arteriosclerosis, Thrombosis and Vascular Biology*, Vol.20, No.7, (July 2000), pp. 1707- ISSN 1524-4636

Bowers, M.C., Hargrove, L.A., Kelly, K.A., Wu, G. & Meininger, C.J. (2011). Tetrahydrobiopterin Attenuates Superoxide-Induced Reduction in Nitric Oxide. *Frontiers in Bioscience*, Vol.16, No.3, (June 2011), pp. 1263-1272, ISSN 1945-0516

Brandes, R.P., Fleming, I. & Busse R. (2005). Endothelial Aging. *Cardiovascular Research*, Vol.66, No.2, (May 2005), pp. 286 - 294, ISSN 1755-4715

Brinkley, T.E., Nicklas, B.J., Kanaya, A.M., Satterfield, S., Lakatta, E.G., Simonsick, E.M., Sutton-Tyrrell, K. & Kritchevsky, S.B. (2009). Plasma Oxidized Low-Density Lipoprotein Levels and Arterial Stiffness in Older Adults: the Health, Aging, and Body Composition Study. *Hypertension*, Vol.53, No.5, (May 2009), pp. 846-852, ISSN 0194911X

Cai, H. & Harrison, D.G. (2000). Endothelial Dysfunction in Cardiovascular Diseases: The Role of Oxidant Stress. *Circulation Research*, Vol.87, No.10, (November 2000), pp. 840-844, ISSN 0009-7300

Cottone, S. & Giovanni, C. (2008). Oxidative Stress, Inflammation and Endothelial Biomarkers in Arterial Hypertension. *Current Hypertension Reviews*, Vol.4, No.2, (May 2008), pp. 86-99, ISSN 1573-4021

Da Luz, P. L., Favarato, D. & Laurindo, F.R.M. (2006). Oxidative Theory of Atherosclerosis. Why Did Large Trials Not Show Benefit? *International Journal of Atherosclerosis,* Vol.1, No.2, (August, 2006), pp. 124-136

Davignon, J. & Ganz, P. (2004). Role of Endothelial Dysfunction in Atherosclerosis. *Circulation,* Vol.109, No.23., (suppl III), (June 2004), pp. III-27-III-32, ISSN 0009-7300

Deanfield, J.E., Halcox & J.P., Rabelink, T.J. (2007). Endothelial Function and Dysfunction. Testing and Clinical relevance. *Circulation,* Vol.115, No.10, (March 2007), pp. 1285-1295, ISSN 0009-7322

Dobiasova, M. (2006). AIP- Atherogenic Index of Plasma as a Significant Predictor of Cardiovascular Risk from Research to Practice. *Vnitrni Lekarstvi,* Vol.52, No.1, (January 2006), pp. 64-71, ISSN 0042-773X

Dobiasova, M., Frohlich, J., Sedova, M., Cheung, M.S. & Brown, B. G. (2011). Cholesterol Esterification and Atherogenic Index of Plasma Correlate with Lipoprotein Size and Findings on Coronary Angiography. *Journal of Lipid Research,*Vol.52, No.3 (March 2011), pp. 566-571, ISSN 1539-7262

Dulak, J., Polus, M., Guevara, I., Polus, A., Hartwich, J. & Dembinska-Kiec, A. (1997). Regulation of Inducible Nitric Oxide Synthase (iNOS) and GTP Cyclohydrolase I Gene Expression by oxLDL in Rat Vascular Smooth Muscle Cells. *Journal of Physiology and Pharmacology,* Vol.48, No.4, (December 1997), pp. 689-697, ISSN 0008-4212

Erusalimski, J.D. (2009). Vascular Endothelial Senescence: From Mechanisms to Pathophysiology. *Journal of Applied Physiology,* Vol.106, No.1, (January 2009), pp. 326–332, ISSN 8750-7587

Forstermann, U. (2006). Endothelial NO Synthase as a Source of NO and Superoxide. *European Journal of Clinical Pharmacology,* Vol.62, Suppl.1, (February 2006), pp. 5-12, ISSN 1432-1041

Galle, J., Heinloth, A., Wanner, C. & Heermeier, K. (2001). Dual Effect of Oxidized LDL on Cell Cycle in Human Endothelial Cells Through Oxidative Stress. *Kidney International. Supplement,* Vol. 59, No.78, (February 2001), pp. S120-123, ISSN 0085-2538

Harrison, D. (1997). Perspective Series: Nitric Oxide and Nitric Oxide Synthases. *Journal of Clinical Investigation,* Vol.100, No.10, (November 1997), pp. 2153-2157, ISSN 0021-9738

Heffernan, K.S., Vieira, V.J. & Valentine, R.J. (2008). Microvascular Function and Ageing: L-Arginine, Tetrahydrobiopterin and the Search for the Fountain of Vascular Youth. *Journal of Physiology,* Vol.586, No.Pt 8, (April 2008), pp. 2041–2042, ISSN 0022-3751

Higashino, H., Tabuchi, M., Yamagata, S., Kurita, T. Miya, H., Mukai, H. & Miya, Y. (2010). Serum Nitric Oxide Metabolite Levels in Groups of Patients with Various Diseases in Comparison of Healthy Control Subjects. *Journal of Medical Sciences,* Vol.10, No.1, (January 2010), pp. 1-11, ISSN 1863-4362

Hirata, Y., Nagata, D., Suzuki, E., Nishimatsu, H., Suzuki, J. & Nagai, R. (2010). Diagnosis and Treatment of Endothelial Dysfunction in Cardiovascular Disease. *International Heart Journal,* Vol.51, No.1, (January 2010), pp. 1-6, ISSN 1349-2365

Holvoet, P., Harris, T.B., Tracy, R.P., Verhamme, P., Newman, A.B., Rubin, S.M., Simonsick, E.M., Colbert, L.H. & Kritchevsky, S.B. (2003). Association of High Coronary Heart Disease Risk Status with Circulating Oxidized LDL in the Well-Functioning

Elderly: Findings from the Health, Aging, and Body Composition Study. *Arteriosclerosis, Thrombosis and Vascular Biology,* Vol. 23, No.8, (August 2003), pp. 1444–1448, ISSN 1524-4636

Holvoet, P., Lee, D.H., Steffes, M., Gross, M. & Jacobs, D.R. Jr. (2008). Association Between Circulating Oxidized Low-Density Lipoprotein and Incidence of the Metabolic Syndrome. The *Journal of the American Medical Association,* Vol.299, No.19, (May 2008), pp. 2287-2293, ISSN 0098-7484

Holvoet, P., De Keyzer, D. & Jacobs, D.R. Jr. (2008). Oxidized LDL and the Metabolic Syndrome. *Future Lipidology,* Vol.3, No.6, (December 2008), pp. 637 - 649, ISSN 1746-0875

Hsueh, W.A. & Quinones, M.J. (2003). Role of Endothelial Dysfunction in Insulin Resistance. *American Journal of Cardiology.* Vol.92, No.4A, (August 2003), pp. 10J-17J, ISSN 0002-9149.

Huang, H., Mai, W., Dan, L., Hao, Y., Tao, J. & Dong, Y. (2008). The Oxidation Ratio of LDL: A Predictor for Coronary Artery Disease. *Disease Markers,* Vol.24, No.6, (August 2008), pp.341-349, ISSN 1875-8630

Huang, P.L. (2009). eNOS, Metabolic Syndrome and Cardiovascular Disease. *Trends in Endocrinology and Metabolism,* Vol.20, No.6, (August 2009), pp. 295-302, ISSN 1043-2760

Hulsmans, M. & Holvoet, P. (2010). The Vicious Circle Between Oxidative Stress and Inflammation in Atherosclerosis. *Journal of Cellular and Molecular Medicine,* Vol.14, No.1-2, (January 2010), pp. 70-77, ISSN 1582-1838

Heffernan, K.S., Vieira, V.J. & Valentine, R.J. (2008). Microvascular Function and Ageing: L-Arginine, Tetrahydrobiopterin and the Search for the Fountain of Vascular Youth. *Journal of Physiology,* Vol.586, No.Pt 8, (April 2008), pp. 2041–2042, ISSN 0022-3751

Itabe, H. & Ueda, M. (2007). Measurement of Plasma Oxidized Low-Density Lipoprotein and its Clinical Implications. *Journal of Atherosclerosis and Thrombosis,* Vol.14, No.1, ( February 2007), pp. 1-11, ISSN 1340-3478

Lankin, V., Viigimaa, M., Tikhaze, A., Kumskova, E., Konovalova, G., Abina, J., Zemtsovskaya, G., Kotkina, T., & Yanushevs, V.T. (2011) Cholesterol-Rich Low Density Lipoproteins are Also More Oxidized. *Molecular and Cellular Biochemistry,* online publication, (June 2011), ISSN 1573-4919

Laroia, S.T., Ganti, A.K., Laroia, A.T. & Tendulkar, K.K. (2003). Endothelium and the Lipid Metabolism: the Current Understanding. *International Journal of Cardiology,* Vol.88, No.1, (March 2003), pp. 1–9, ISSN 0167-5273

Lemieux, I., Lamarche, B., Couillard, C., Pascot, A., Cantin, B., Bergeron, J., Dagenais, G.R. & Despres, J.P. (2001). Total Cholesterol/HDL Cholesterol Ratio vs LDL Cholesterol/HDL Cholesterol Ratio as Indices of Ischemic Heart Disease Risk in Men. *Archives of Internal Medicine,* Vol.161, No.24, (December 2001), pp. 2685-2692, ISSN 1538-3679

Liao, J.K., Shin, W.S., Lee, W.Y. & Clark, S.L. (1995). Oxidized Low-Density Lipoprotein Decreases the Expression of Endothelial Nitric Oxide Synthase. *Journal of Biological Chemistry,* Vol.270, No.1, (January 1995), pp. 319-24, ISSN 1083-351X

Lind, L. (2002). Lipids and Endothelium-Dependent Vasodilation - A Review. *Lipids,* Vol.37, No.1, (January 2002), pp. 1-15, ISSN 2090-3049

Lundberg, J.O. & Weitzberg, E. (2005). NO Generation from Nitrite and its Role in Vascular Control. *Arteriosclerosis, Thrombosis and Vascular Biology*, Vol.25, No.5, (March 2005), pp. 915-922, ISSN 1524-4636

Nawrot, T.S. & Staessen, J.A. (2008). Genetic Variation and Environmental Factors in Biological and Arterial Ageing. *Verhandelingen Koninklijke Academie. Geneeskunde van Belgie*, Vol.70, No.5-6, (May 2008), pp. 323-338, ISSN 0300-9017

Nawrot, T.S., Staessen, J.A., Holvoet, P., Struijker-Boudier, H.A., Schiffers, P., Van Bortel, L.M., Fagard, R.H., Gardner, J.P., Kimura, M. & Aviv, A. (2010). Telomere Length and its Associations with Oxidized-LDL, Carotid Artery Distensibility and Smoking. *Frontiers in Biosciences,* Vol.1, No.2, (June 2010), pp. 1164-1168, ISSN 1093-4715

Njajou, O.T., Kanaya, A.M., Holvoet, P., Connelly, S., Strotmeyer, E.S., Harris, T.B., Cummings, S.R. & Hsueh, W.C. (2009). Association Between Oxidized LDL, Obesity and Type 2 Diabetes in a Population-Based Cohort, the Health, Aging and Body Composition Study. *Diabetes Metabolism Research and Reviews*, Vol.25, No.8, (September 2009), pp. 733-739, ISSN 1520-7560

Park, K., Gross, M., Lee, D.H., Holvoet, P., Himes, J.H., Shikany, J.M. & Jacobs, D.R. Jr. (2009). Oxidative Stress and Insulin Resistance: the Coronary Artery Risk Development in Young Adults Study. *Diabetes Care*, Vol.32, No.7,(July 2009), pp. 1302-1307, ISSN 1935-5548

Park, S.H., Kim, J.Y., Lee, J.H. & Park, H.Y. (2010). Elevated Oxidized Low-Density Lipoprotein Concentrations in Postmenopausal Women with the Metabolic Syndrome. *Clinica Chemica Acta*, Vol.412, No.5-6, (November 2010), pp. 435-440, ISSN 0009-8981

Parthasarathy, S., Litvinov, D., Selvarajan, K. & Garelnabi, M. (2008). Lipid Peroxidation and Decomposition- Conflicting Roles in Plaque Vulnerability and Stability. *Biochimica Biophysica Acta*, Vol.1781, No.5, (May 2008), pp. 221–231, ISSN 0006-3002

Parthasarathy, S., Santanam, N., Ramachandran, S. & Meilhac, O. (1999). Oxidants and Antioxidants in Atherogenesis: an Appraisal. *Journal of Lipid Research*, Vol.40, No.12, (December 1999), pp. 2143–2157, ISSN 1539-7262

Rietzschel, E.R., Langlois, M., De Buyzere, M.L., Segers, P., De Bacquer, D., Bekaert, S., Cooman, L., Van Oostveldt, P., Verdonck, P., De Backer, G.G. & Gillebert T.G. (2008). Oxidized Low-Density Lipoprotein Cholesterol Is Associated With Decreases in Cardiac Function Independent of Vascular Alterations. *Hypertension,* Vol.52, No.3, (September 2008), pp. 535-541, ISSN 0194911X

Rigotti, A., Trigatti, B.L., Penman, M., Rayburn, H., Herz, J. & Krieger, M. (1997). A Targeted Mutation in the Murine Gene Encoding the High Density Lipoprotein (HDL) Receptor Scavenger Receptor Class B Type I Reveals its Key Role in HDL Metabolism. *Proceedings of the National Academy of Sciences U S A*, Vol.94, No.23, (November 1997), pp. 12610–12615, ISSN 0027-8424

Rubbo, H., Darley-Usmar, V. & Freeman, B.A. (1996). Nitric Oxide Regulation of Tissue Free Radical Injury. *Chemical Research in Toxicology*, Vol.9, No.5, (July-August 1996), pp. 809–820, ISSN 1520-5010

Schnabel, R. & Blankenberg, S. (2007). Oxidative Stress in Cardiovascular Disease-Successful Translation From Bench to Bedside? *Circulation,* Vol.116, No.12, (September 2007), pp. 1338-1340, ISSN 0009-7322

Setoguchi, S., Mohri, M., Shimokava, H., & Takeshita, A. (2001).Tetrahydrobiopterin Improves Endothelial Dysfunction in Coronary Microcirculation in Patients Without Epicardial Coronary Artery Disease. *Journal of the American College of Cardiology*, Vol.38, No.2, (August 2001), pp. 493-98, ISSN 0735-1097

Shaul, P.W. (2003). Endothelial Nitric Oxide Synthase, Caveolae and the Development of Atherosclerosis. Journal of Physiology, Vol.547, No.1, (February 2003), pp. 21-33, ISSN 1469-7793

Sima, A., Stancu, C. & Simionescu, M. (2009). Vascular Endothelium in Atherosclerosis, *Cell and Tissue Research*, Vol.335, No.1, (January 2009), pp. 191-203, ISSN 0302-766X

Simionescu, M. & Antohe, F. (2006). Functional Ultrastructure of the Vascular Endothelium: Changes in Various Pathologies. *Handbook of Experimental Pharmacology*, 2006, Vol.176, No.1, pp. 41-69, ISSN 0171-2004

Simionescu, M. (2007). Implications of Early Structural-Functional Changes in the Endothelium for Vascular Disease. *Arteriosclerosis, Thrombosis and Vascular Biology*, Vol.27, No.2, (February 2007), pp. 266-274, ISSN 1079-5642

Steinberg, D., Parthasarathy, S., Carew, T.E., Khoo, J.C. & Witztum, J.L. (1989). Beyond Cholesterol: Modifications of Low Density Lipoprotein that Increase its Atherogenicity. *New England Journal of Medicine*, Vol.320, No.14, (April 1989), pp. 915-24, ISSN 1533-4406

Steinberg, D. (2009). The LDL Modification Hypothesis of Atherogenesis: an Update. *Journal of Lipid Research*, Vol.50, Supplement, (April 2009), pp. S376 - S381, ISSN 1539-7262

Steinberg, D. & Witzum, J.L. (2010). Oxidized Low-Density Lipoprotein and Atherosclerosis. History of Discovery. *Arteriosclerosis, Thrombosis and Vascular Biology*, Vol.30, No.12, (November 2010), pp. 2311 - 2316, ISSN 1524-4636

Stroes, E., Kastelein, J., Cosentino, F., Erkelens, W., Wever, R., Koomans, H., Lüscher, T. & Rabelink, T. (1997). Tetrahydrobiopterin Restores Endothelial Function in Hypercholesterolemia. *Journal of Clinical Investigation*, Vol.99, No. 1, (January1997), pp. 41-46, ISSN 1365-2362.

Tabit, C.E., Chung, W.B., Hamburg, N.M. & Vita, J.A. (2010). Endothelial Dysfunction in Diabetes Mellitus: Molecular Mechanisms and Clinical Implications. *Reviews in Endocrine & Metabolic Disorders*, Vol.11, No.1, (March 2010), pp. 61-74, ISSN 1573-2606

Tsimikas, S. (2006). Oxidative Biomarkers in the Diagnosis and Prognosis of Cardiovascular Disease. *American Journal of Cardiology*, Vol.98, No.11A, (December 2006), pp. 9P-17P, ISSN 0002-914

Tsimikas, S. & Witztum, J.L. (2001). Measuring Circulating Oxidized Low-Density Lipoprotein to Evaluate Coronary Risk. *Circulation*, Vol.103, No.15, (April 2001), pp. 1930-1932, ISSN 0009-7322

Uittenbogaard, A., Shaul, P.W., Yuhanna, I.S., Blair, A. & Smart, E.J. (2000). High Density Lipoprotein Prevents Oxidized Low Density Lipoprotein-Induced Inhibition of Endothelial Nitric-Oxide Synthase Localization and Activation in Caveolae. *Journal of Biological Chemistry*, Vol.275, No.15, (April 2000), pp. 11278–11283, ISSN1083-351X

Van den Oever, I.A., Raterman, H.G., Nurmohamed, M.T. & Simsek, S. (2010). Endothelial Dysfunction, Inflammation and Apoptosis in Diabetes Mellitus. *Mediators of Inflammation*, (June 2010), pp. 1-15, ISSN 1466-1861

Van der Zwan, L. P., Teerlink, T., Dekker, J.M., Henry, R.M.A., Stehouwer, C.D.A., Jakobs, C., Heine, R.J. & Scheffe,r P.G. (2009). Circulating Oxidized LDL: Determinants and Association with Brachial Flow-Mediated Dilation. *Journal of Lipid Research*, Vol.50, No.2, (February 2009), pp. 342–349, ISSN 1539-7262

Vickers, K.C., Maguire, C.T., Wolfert, R., Burns, A.R., Reardon, M., Geis, R., Holvoet, P. & Morrisett, J.D. (2009). Relationship of Lipoprotein-Associated Phospholipase A2 and Oxidized Low Density Lipoprotein in Carotid Atherosclerosis. *Journal of Lipid Research*, Vol.50, No.9, (September 2009), pp. 1735-1743, ISSN1539-7262

Wallace, J.P., Johnson, B., Padilla, J. & Mather, K. (2010). Postprandial Lipaemia, Oxidative Stress and Endothelial Function: a Review. *International Journal of Clinical Practice*, Vol.64, No.3, (January 2010), pp. 389-403, ISSN 1368-5031

Wang, W., Hein, T.W., Zhang, D.C., Zawieja, D.C., Liao, J.C. & Kuo, L. (2011). Oxidized Low-Density Lipoprotein Inhibits Nitric Oxide Mediated Coronary Arteriolar Dilation by Up-Regulating Endothelial Arginase I. *Microcirculation*, Vol.18, No.1, (January 2011), pp. 36-45, ISSN 1549-8719.

Wever, R.M.F., Dam, T., van Rijn, H.J., Groot, F & Rabelink, T. (1997). Tetrahydrobiopterin Regulates Superoxide and Nitric Oxide Generation by Recombinant Endothelial Nitric Oxide Synthase. *Biochemical and Biophysical Research Communications*, Vol.37, No.2 (August 1997), pp. 340-344, ISSN 0006-291X

Wu, T., Willett, W.C., Rifai, N., Shai, I., Manson, J.E & Rimm, E.B. (2006). Is Plasma Oxidized Low-Density Lipoprotein, Measured with the Widely Used Antibody 4E6, an Independent Predictor of Coronary Heart Disease Among U.S. Men and Women? *Journal of the American College of Cardiology*, Vol.48, No.5, (August 2006), pp. 973-979, ISSN 0735-1097

Yasa, M. & Turkseven, S. (2005). Vasoprotective Effects of Nitric Oxide in Atherosclerosis. *FABAD Journal of Pharmaceutical Sciences*, Vol.30, No.1, (March 2005), pp. 41-53, ISSN 1300-4182

Yu, S., Wong, S.L., Lau, C.W., Huang, Y. & Yu, C.M. (2011). Oxidized LDL at Low Concentration Promotes In-vitro Angiogenesis and Activate Nitric Oxide Synthase Through PI3K/Akt/eNOS Pathway in Human Coronary Artery Endothelial Cells. *Biochemical and Biophysical Research Communications*, Vol.407, No.1, (April 2011), pp. 44-48, ISSN 0006-291X

Yuhanna, I.S., Zhu, Y., Cox, B.E., Hahner, L.D., Osborne-Lawrence, S., Lu, P., Marcel, Y.L., Anderson, R.G., Mendelsohn, M.E., Hobbs, H.H. & Shaul, P.W. (2001). High-Density Lipoprotein Binding to Scavenger Receptor-BI Activates Endothelial Nitric Oxide Synthase, *Nature Medicine*, Vol.7, No.7, (July 2001), pp. 853–857, ISSN 1078-8956

# 23

# Are Hemochromatosis Mutations Protective Against Iron-Mediated Atherogenesis?

Jerome L. Sullivan
*University of Central Florida College of Medicine, Orlando, USA*

## 1. Introduction

Modest levels of stored iron, far less than conventional iron overload, may promote cardiovascular disease, i.e. sustained iron depletion may be protective [1-6]. This so-called "iron hypothesis" was initially presented to explain for the sex difference in cardiovascular disease and the increase in disease following menopause. The idea, although continually debated for more than 25 years, has achieved standing as a plausible and testable hypothesis [7-18] [19].

The hypothesis has not yet been definitively tested. A first randomized clinical trial (FeAST) to address aspects of the hypothesis was recently reported [7]. The FeAST trial [7] had significant limitations as a general test of the idea: 1) it was a trial of secondary prevention, and 2) the iron reduction protocol fell far short of achieving full iron depletion. Zacharski et al [7] reported that reducing iron stores significantly improves survival for patients with symptomatic but stable peripheral arterial disease (PAD), if iron reduction begins at a young age. The FeAST trial provides compelling support for a new trial designed to test the original hypothesis.

Controversial results from multiple epidemiological studies investigating a variety of atherosclerotic events using all kinds of variable parameters of body iron load have presented a confusing picture of the iron hypothesis [20]. Confusion became complete when it appeared that patients with homozygous hemochromatosis who were afflicted with serious, life long iron overload had no increased atherosclerosis and might even be protected against atherosclerosis. In the debate on the hypothesis, the disease pattern in homozygous hemochromatosis has been intrepreted as perhaps the most persuasive evidence against the hypothesis [21]. This "hemochromatosis paradox" is seen as a anomaly that makes the hypothesis untenable for some investigators. How can normal stored iron levels be bad for the vascular system, when massive amounts of stored iron in genetic iron overload are not associated with increased atherosclerosis?

## 2. Hemochromatosis and atherosclerosis: More to it than iron load alone

An early corollary to the iron hypothesis was the proposal that heterozygous hemochromatosis might be a significant risk factor for premature myocardial infarction [22]. This was proposed despite the general impression at the time that homozygous hemochromatosis was not prominently associated with increased atherosclerosis. In the absence of definitive data, this was not seen as necessarily incompatible with the iron hypothesis [22-24]. An impact on cardiovascular event rates in hemochromatosis was not excluded based on available data. In addition, even without promotion of atherosclerosis by genetic iron overload, relevant issues that continue to be unresolved include roles of hemochromatosis mutation-associated iron overload in myocardial reperfusion injury [2;24-26] and endothelial dysfunction [27;28]. Future investigations are needed, as long term exposure to non-transferrin bound iron (NTBI) in genetic iron overload may contribute to life-long progression of atherosclerosis as it promotes monocyte-endothelium interaction and inflammatory pathways.

Mutational effects other than promotion of an increase in total body iron were not considered in the 1990 hypothesis relating heterozygosity to early onset of myocardial infarction [22]. The idea that total body iron load was the only factor that might influence cardiovascular disease expression in hemochromatosis was restated as recently as 2007 in a JAMA editorial on the status of the iron hypothesis by Hu [8]:

*"The 1996 discovery of HFE gene mutations responsible for most cases of hereditary hemochromatosis [[29]] has led to the use of genetic markers of iron stores (ie, heterozygosity for the C282Y mutation in the HFE gene as a marker of lifelong moderate iron overload) in epidemiologic studies. In contrast to biomarkers, genetic markers of iron overload can be measured exactly and are not influenced by such factors as inflammation, recent blood loss, diet, and use of medications (eg, aspirin)."*

The corollary hypothesis that heterozygosity might be associated with myocardial infarction [22] led to a number of investigations, especially after the identification of the disease-causing mutation in most cases of hemochromatosis in 1996 [29]. Early findings appeared to support some increase in cardiovascular events among heterozygotes [23;30;31]. However, these studies taken together with subsequent investigations [32-36] do not support an increase in myocardial infarction, stroke or atherosclerosis in patients who are heterozygous for hemochromatosis. In fact, the body of relevant work, including some older studies [37;38] does not exclude protection against atherosclerosis in hemochromatosis. In an autopsy series that examined coronary artery disease in heavily iron overloaded individuals, Miller and Hutchins [37] reported an odds ratio of coronary artery disease with iron overload of 0.18. This is suggestive of a significant protective effect in patients presumptively homozygous for hemochromatosis who comprised 80% of the autopsy cases reviewed by Miller and Hutchins [37]. Could some poorly understood feature of homozygous hemochromatosis confound the relationship between iron load and atherosclerosis?

## 3. Hepcidin and a resolution of the hemochromatosis paradox

An iron loading mutation is not just "a marker of lifelong moderate iron overload" as indicated by Hu [8]. Hemochromatosis mutations also radically alter the distribution of body iron [39]. Iron-poor Kupffer cells adjacent to iron-loaded hepatocytes are a classic finding in hereditary hemochromatosis [39]. Another classic finding in homozygotes is a relative scarcity of coronary artery iron deposition despite extensive iron deposits in myocardial tissue [39;40].

In 1998, Moura et al [41] reported that monocytes from hereditary hemochromatosis patients released twice as much iron in the low molecular weight form as normal human monocytes after erythrocyte phagocytosis. Thus, even before the discovery and understanding of the iron regulatory hormone, hepcidin [42-44], there was an understanding of *"a macrophage defect in hemochromatosis leading to a constriction. of the macrophage/reticuloendothelial iron pool" [24]. This macrophage defect [41] in hereditary hemochromatosis was suggested as a factor that might "protect homozygotes from foam cell formation and thus, to a degree, gives some specific protection against atherosclerosis,"* [24] with a partial protective effect in heterozygotes.

The discovery of hepcidin [42-44] and the details of its influence on iron metabolism [45-49] illuminated patterns of macrophage iron retention and led to a conceptual *volte-face* on the possibility of diminished atherosclerosis in homozygotes [4;6].

Hepcidin is the major regulator for the amount of iron retained within macrophages. Production of hepcidin is regulated by iron intake and a number of interrelated factors. Elevated levels, favoring macrophage iron retention, are seen with increased iron intake, infection and inflammation. Iron loading in secondary iron overload in wild type individuals is associated with increased hepcidin expression. Reduced hepcidin levels and iron-poor macrophages accompany iron deficiency, hypoxia, anemia and hereditary hemochromatosis. Hepcidin binds to the iron exporter protein ferroportin, leading to the internalization, and intracellular degradation of ferroportin. Loss of the iron exporter function of ferroportin from macrophages leads to intracellular retention of iron and to reduced serum iron levels. In intestinal epithelial cells, hepcidin-induced loss of ferroportin results in reduced iron internalization into the systemic circulation.

Remarkably, the most extreme reductions in hepcidin level are associated with the opposite extremes of total body iron load, i.e. in iron deficiency anemia and in homozygous hemochromatosis [50]. Loss of hepcidin expression can be produced by mutations in hepcidin, hemojuvelin, *TFR2*, and *HFE* [51]. Mutations at these sites leads to hereditary iron overload. In this discussion, the term "hemochromatosis" indicates hereditary iron overload associated with one of the mutations causing lower hepcidin expression. The homozygous *HFE* C282Y mutation is the most common cause of hereditary iron overload and is associated with lower liver expression of hepcidin mRNA [51].

The very low hepcidin levels seen in homozygous hemochromatosis are associated with systemic iron loading because reduced hepcidin levels permit unregulated ferroportin-mediated transfer of iron from intestinal epithelial cells into the systemic iron pool. The more extreme the degree of hepcidin deficiency, the more severe the level of parenchymal iron load, but also the more extreme the macrophage iron retention deficit. These patterns offer a potential resolution of the paradox of the proposed protection by iron depletion in wild type subjects against cardiovascular disease despite of the lack of increased atherosclerosis in genetic iron overload [4;6]. Hepcidin may act as an iron-dependent risk factor for atherosclerosis by causing iron loading of plaque macrophages with promotion of foam cell formation. According to this proposal, hepcidin amplifies the plaque iron loading effects of an increased iron load as iron itself upregulates hepcidin concentration. At the other end of the iron status spectrum, iron deficiency downregulates hepcidin and promotes removal of iron from plaque macrophages. In hemochromatosis, the associated hepcidin deficiency is hypothesized to reduce progressive iron accumulation within arterial walls and foam cell formation. Hemochromatosis patients may thus enjoy a specific protection against plaque progression in proportion to the severity of hepcidin deficiency. Hepcidin deficiency would not protect these patients from direct iron-mediated injury to heart muscle from parenchymal iron accumulation in myocardial tissue. The corollary hypothesis that identifies hepcidin as a risk factor for atherogenesis [4] may explain the conundrum of decreased atherosclerosis in the face of massive iron loading and provide additional justification for the contention that the macrophage has a key role in atherogenesis.

Previous studies, especially the work of Miller and Hutchins [37] and Pirart and Barbier [38], raised the possibility of a protective effect of hereditary hemochromatosis against atherosclerosis. An unknown *"facteur constitutionnel"* [38] linked to hemochromatosis that enhances resistance to vascular lesions was proposed. A mechanistic hypothesis to explain the findings [37;38] was not proposed as the studies were done prior to identification of either the principal iron overloading genotypes or the iron regulatory hormone hepcidin. More recent evidence supporting the hypothesis that hemochromatosis-associated hepcidin deficiency is protective against atherosclerosis has been reported [52]. Valenti et al [52] studied vascular disease, iron status, hepcidin levels and *HFE* mutations in 506 consecutive patients with nonalcholic fatty liver disease (NAFLD). None were homozygous for hereditary hemochromatosis. Serum ferritin was associated with common carotid intima-media thickness (CC-IMT) ($p = 0.048$) and with prevalence of atherosclerotic carotid plaques ($p = 0.0004$), except in patients whose heterozygous *HFE* mutations lower hepcidin levels. Hyperferritinemia was associated with vascular damage only in patients with wild type *HFE* genotypes ($p<0.0001$). Hepcidin was elevated in those without such an *HFE* mutation and was found to be an independent predictor of the presence of carotid atherosclerosis.

## 4. Iron, hepcidin, inflammation and vascular disease

Inflammation accelerates atherogenesis [53]. The mechanism may involve iron- and hepcidin-mediated mechanisms [4;6]. Hepcidin is upregulated by interleukin-6 (IL-6), a cytokine induced by inflammatory processes. IL-6 has also been found to be a cardiovascular disease risk factor [54]. An important end result of any process that induces IL-6 is increased deposition of iron within reticuloendothelial cells, including atherosclerotic plaque macrophages, because of hepcidin upregulation. Continued inflammation-mediated hepcidin synthesis maintains iron in storage sites even in the face of a low hematocrit as in the anemia of inflammation (i.e. the "anemia of chronic disorders").

Hepatic hepcidin may be normally upregulated in inflammation even in hemochromatosis homozygotes who usually have markedly low hepcidin levels [55]. The effects of inflammatory processes in hemochromatosis patients on possible redistribution of iron from parenchymal cells to the reticuloendothelial compartment, including arterial plaque macrophages, are not currently known. Interactions between mutational effects and inflammation-induced effects on hepcidin level may result in complex epidemiological patterns in studies of cardiovascular disease expression in hemochromatosis patients.

## 5. Blunted inflammatory responses in macrophages in hemochromatosis or induced iron depletion

A recent study of macrophages in the *Hfe* knockout (*Hfe* -/-) mouse [56] is pertinent to the present discussion of iron, inflammation and atherosclerosis. Wang et al [56] found attenuated inflammatory responses in a mouse model of human hemochromatosis and reduced translation of cytokine mRNAs in *Hfe* -/- macrophages in response to Salmonella and LPS exposure. Intramacrophage iron levels were decreased in the *Hfe* -/- mice in association with upregulation of macrophage iron exporter ferroportin (FPN). Salmonella- and LPS-induced inflammatory responses were diminished in the *Hfe* knockout animals. Less severe enterocolitis was observed in vivo and reduced macrophage TNF- and IL-6 secretion was observed in vitro.

Of special significance in the present discussion, the reduced translation of cytokine mRNAs of the mutant macrophages could be reproduced in wild-type cells by reducing the intracellular iron concentration with chelation. Atherosclerotic plaque macrophages in patients with hemochromatosis mutations associated with diminished hepcidin may display similar attenuated inflammatory responses such as those from *Hfe* -/- mice [56], and thereby a diminished tendency to form atherosclerotic foam cells.

## 6. Iron, hemochromatosis and other cell types in vascular disease

Iron plays a role in vascular disease in other cell types than the macrophage, e.g. endothelial cells [3;9;14;18;57-59] and vascular smooth muscle cells [60-62]. Patients with hemochromatosis have endothelial dysfunction that is improved by iron reduction therapy [63]. This suggests that iron overload itself rather than mutational effects of iron overload genes influences endothelial function. Proliferaton of vascular smooth muscle cells [60-62] also requires iron. How hemochromatosis mutations might modifies iron-mediated atherogenic processes in these cell types will require additional studies.

## 7. Serum cholesterol level, hemochromatosis, macrophage iron loss, and cardiovascular disease

Adams et al [64] reported that hemochromatosis patients homzygous for C282Y have diminished serum cholesterol and low-density lipoprotein (LDL) levels. Systemically lower cholesterol and LDL could represent an additional mechanism by which hemochromatosis patients are relatively protected from atherosclerosis. This could be associated with the iron retention deficit in mutant macrophages. A role for macrophage iron metabolism in regulation of cellular lipid level has been proposed [65]. As noted above, the most extreme reductions in hepcidin level are seen at the opposite extremes of total body iron load, i.e. in both iron deficiency anemia and in homozygous hemochromatosis. Consistent with a hepcidin level similar to that in hemochromatosis, iron deficiency is also associated with lower systemic levels of serum cholesterol and LDL [12;66;67]. Future studies are needed to determine if lower macrophage iron level in iron deficiency or inherited iron overload negatively regulates systemic cholesterol level.

## 8. Mutational protection against atherogenesis: Epidemiological implications

The literature on the role of iron in cardiovascular disease in the general population is contradictory and inconsistent, as has often been noted [8]. There have been misconceptions regarding the hypothesis leading to inadequate study designs [20;68]. Another key limitation of previous studies that has not been addressed is the possibility of a protective effect of hemochromatosis mutations against iron-mediated atherogenesis. If hemochromatosis mutations confer protection against atherogenesis, previous epidemiological studies of iron and atherosclerosis may be critically flawed. The highest serum ferritin levels in population groups whose hemochromatosis gene status has not been ascertained will select a disproportionate share of subjects who are heterozygous or homozygous for hemochromatosis. These high serum ferritin individuals may have less disease because of mutational protection against atherosclerosis and may confound underlying associations of iron load and atherosclerosis in normal subjects.

## 9. Penetrance and testing the hepcidin hypothesis

This problem of clinical penetrance of the hemochromatosis mutations needs to be considered in the design of a study to test the hepcidin hypothesis. There is undoubtedy a variable impact of genotype on hepcidin expression. Genotype of subjects in a study to test the hypothesis shouldbe determined; however, testing the hypothesis would not rely directly on showing an association of genotype with disease. The hypothesis suggests that protection against atherogenesis is inversely proportional to hepcidin expression. In an epidemiological study, the hypothesis suggests that, among those with any one of a number of iron overloading genotypes, protection against atherogenesis would be seen in proportion to the degree of life long hepcidin downregulation.

It would be inappropriate to simply look at a group of all subjects with hepcidin expression below some prespecified level. It would be necessary to exclude the iron deficient subjects from a group defined by such a criterion, as iron deficiency is associated with quite low hepcidin levels. A future interventional study of the effect of long term iron deficiency-induced reduction in hepcidin expression on atherogenesis would be of interest.

## 10. Conclusions and future directions

The hypothesis that iron depletion protects against atherosclerosis may apply even in hemochromatosis homozygotes because of the mutational effect of selective iron depletion of the macrophage, a key cell type in atherogenesis. In homozygotes, a sea of tissue iron deposition surrounds islands of iron depleted cells of the reticuloendothelial system. Low hepcidin expression is a mutational feature of hemochromatosis and also of systemic iron deficiency that may protect against iron-mediated atherogenesis in both conditions. What is known at present about disease patterns in genetic iron overload is compatible with the hypothesis that iron depletion protects against atherosclerosis. Hereditary hemochromatosis may be a special case of selective cellular iron depletion that inhibits atherogenesis.

More detailed investigations are needed on hepcidin as a risk factor for atherosclerosis including more studies of atherosclerotic disease in patients with hemochromatosis mutations. Work is also needed on the effects of the inflammatory response on iron metabolism, especially the impact of inflammatory processes on hepcidin and macrophage iron in patients with hemochromatosis mutations.

It would be of interest to replicate the low hepcidin levels of those with hemochromatosis mutations in normal subjects and to assess the effects of low hepcidin levels on atherogenesis. A well established and safe method that would have the effect of reducing hepcidin production in normal subjects is induced iron depletion. Long-term modest reduction in storage iron can be achieved in patients with established vascular disease and is associated with decreased cancer mortality [69] and, among younger participants, decreased cardiovascular mortality [7].

In humans with intact hepcidin responses, atherosclerotic plaque has a substantially higher iron concentration than that in healthy arterial wall [15]. Increased lesional iron is also seen in cholesterol fed animals. In a series of studies with rabbits fed a 1% cholesterol diet, Watt and colleagues [70-74] used nuclear microscopy to show a 7-fold increase in iron concentration within newly formed atherosclerotic lesions compared to healthy arteries. Iron accumulation was seen at the onset of lesion formation.

A role for iron in foam cell formation and lesion progression has been implicated by numerous observations and experiments [4-6;75-83]. Recent work shows that iron can be mobilized out of atherosclerotic plaque by manipulation of body iron status, and that this process may be associated with reduction in lesion size. Animal experiments suggest that systemic lowering of stored iron levels reduces intralesional iron content and also the size of atherosclerotic plaques [70;84]. It is well known that iron-deficient erythropoiesis can mobilize and relocate almost all stored iron in the body to maturing erythroid precursors. In iron deficiency, mobilization is facilitated by extreme downregulation of hepcidin. Key questions in future human studies include the following: What duration and degree of iron reduction therapy is needed for restoring iron levels in atherosclerotic vessel segments to the much lower level seen in healthy vascular tissue? How much reduction in the level of hepcidin is required to facilitate the relocation of stored iron from intralesional macrophages to erythroid precursors? And, is it possible in normal subjects to inhibit the formation of atherosclerotic foam cells by rendering their macrophages as iron poor as in those with hemochromatosis mutations?

## 11. Conflict of interest disclosures

None.

## 12. References

[1] Sullivan JL. Iron and the sex difference in heart disease risk. Lancet 1981; 1(8233):1293-1294.

[2] Sullivan JL. The iron paradigm of ischemic heart disease. Am Heart J 1989; 117(5):1177-1188.

[3] Sullivan JL. Stored Iron and Vascular Reactivity. Arterioscler Thromb Vasc Biol 2005; 25(8):1532-1535.

[4] Sullivan J. Macrophage Iron, Hepcidin, and Atherosclerotic Plaque Stability. Exp Biol Med 2007; 232(8):1014-1020.

[5] Li W, XU LH, Forssell C, Sullivan JL, YUAN XM. Overexpression of Transferrin Receptor and Ferritin Related to Clinical Symptoms and Destabilization of Human Carotid Plaques. Proc Soc Exp Biol Med 2008; 233(7):818-826.

[6] Sullivan JL. Iron in arterial plaque: A modifiable risk factor for atherosclerosis. Biochimica et Biophysica Acta (BBA) - General Subjects 2009; 1790(7):718-723.

[7] Zacharski LR, Chow BK, Howes PS, Shamayeva G, Baron JA, Dalman RL, Malenka DJ, Ozaki CK, Lavori PW. Reduction of Iron Stores and Cardiovascular Outcomes in Patients With Peripheral Arterial Disease: A Randomized Controlled Trial. JAMA 2007; 297(6):603-610.

[8] Hu FB. The Iron-Heart Hypothesis: Search for the Ironclad Evidence. JAMA 2007; 297(6):639-641.

[9] Zheng H, Cable R, Spencer B, Votto N, Katz SD. Iron stores and vascular function in voluntary blood donors. Arterioscler Thromb Vasc Biol 2005; 25(8):1577-1583.

[10] Salonen JT, Nyyssonen K, Korpela H, Tuomilehto J, Seppanen R, Salonen R. High stored iron levels are associated with excess risk of myocardial infarction in eastern Finnish men [see comments]. Circulation 1992; 86(3):803-811.

[11] Yuan XM, Li W. The iron hypothesis of atherosclerosis and its clinical impact. Ann Med 2003; 35(8):578-591.
[12] Facchini FS, Saylor KL. Effect of iron depletion on cardiovascular risk factors: studies in carbohydrate-intolerant patients. Ann N Y Acad Sci 2002; 967:342-351.
[13] Kell DB. Iron behaving badly: inappropriate Iron chelation as a major contributor to the aetiology of vascular and other progressive inflammatory and degenerative diseases. BMC Med Genomics 2009; 2(1):2.
[14] Kartikasari AE, Georgiou NA, Visseren FL, Kats-Renaud H, van Asbeck BS, Marx JJ. Intracellular labile iron modulates adhesion of human monocytes to human endothelial cells. Arterioscler Thromb Vasc Biol 2004; 24(12):2257-2262.
[15] Stadler N, Lindner RA, Davies MJ. Direct Detection and Quantification of Transition Metal Ions in Human Atherosclerotic Plaques: Evidence for the Presence of Elevated Levels of Iron and Copper. Arterioscler Thromb Vasc Biol 2004; 24(5):949-954.
[16] Raman SV, Winner MW, III, Tran T, Velayutham M, Simonetti OP, Baker PB, Olesik J, McCarthy B, Ferketich AK, Zweier JL. In Vivo Atherosclerotic Plaque Characterization Using Magnetic Susceptibility Distinguishes Symptom-Producing Plaques. J Am Coll Cardiol Img 2008; 1(1):49-57.
[17] You SA, Archacki SR, Angheloiu G, Moravec CS, Rao S, Kinter M, Topol EJ, Wang Q. Proteomic approach to coronary atherosclerosis shows ferritin light chain as a significant marker: evidence consistent with iron hypothesis in atherosclerosis. Physiol Genomics 2003; 13(1):25-30.
[18] Duffy SJ, Biegelsen ES, Holbrook M, Russell JD, Gokce N, Keaney JF, Jr., Vita JA. Iron chelation improves endothelial function in patients with coronary artery disease. Circulation 2001; 103(23):2799-2804.
[19] Valenti L, Dongiovanni P, Motta BM, Swinkels DW, Bonara P, Rametta R, Burdick L, Frugoni C, Fracanzani AL, Fargion S. Serum hepcidin and macrophage iron correlate with MCP-1 release and vascular damage in patients with metabolic syndrome alterations. Arterioscler Thromb Vasc Biol 2011; 31(3):683-690.
[20] Sullivan JL. Misconceptions in the debate on the iron hypothesis. Journal of Nutritional Biochemistry 2001; 12:33-37.
[21] Burt MJ, Halliday JW, Powell LW. Iron and coronary heart disease [editorial] [see comments]. BMJ 1993; 307(6904):575-576.
[22] Sullivan JL. Heterozygous hemochromatosis as a risk factor for premature myocardial infarction. Medical Hypotheses 1990; 31:1-5.
[23] Sullivan JL. Iron and the Genetics of Cardiovascular Disease. Circulation 1999; 100(12):1260-1263.
[24] Sullivan JL, Zacharski LR. Hereditary haemochromatosis and the hypothesis that iron depletion protects against ischemic heart disease. Eur J Clin Invest 2001; 31(5):375-377.
[25] Kramer JH, Lightfoot FG, Weglicki WB. Cardiac tissue iron: effects on post-ischemic function and free radical production, and its possible role during preconditioning. Cell Mol Biol (Noisy -Le-Grand) 2000; 46(8):1313-1327.
[26] Turoczi T, Jun L, Cordis G, Morris JE, Maulik N, Stevens RG, Das DK. HFE Mutation and Dietary Iron Content Interact to Increase Ischemia/Reperfusion Injury of the Heart in Mice. Circ Res 2003; 92(11):1240-1246.

[27] Kartikasari AER, Georgiou NA, Visseren FLJ, Kats-Renaud H, Sweder van Asbeck B, Marx JJM. Endothelial activation and induction of monocyte adhesion by nontransferrin-bound iron present in human sera. FASEB J 2005;05-4700fje.

[28] Lekakis J, Papamicheal C, Stamatelopoulos K, Cimponeriu A, Voutsas A, Vemmos K, Mavrikakis M, Stamatelopoulos S. Hemochromatosis associated with endothelial dysfunction: evidence for the role of iron stores in early atherogenesis. Vasc Med 1999; 4(3):147-148.

[29] Feder JN, Gnirke A, Thomas W, Tsuchihashi Z, Ruddy DA, Basava A, Dormishian F, Domingo R, Jr., Ellis MC, Fullan A, Hinton LM, Jones NL, Kimmel BE, Kronmal GS, Lauer P, Lee VK, Loeb DB, Mapa FA, McClelland E, Meyer NC, Mintier GA, Moeller N, Moore T, Morikang E, Prass CE, Quintana L, Starnes SM, Schatzman RC, Brunke KJ, Drayna DT, Risch NJ, Bacon BR, Wolff RK. A novel MHC class I-like gene is mutated in patients with hereditary haemochromatosis. Nat Genet 1996; 13(4):399-408.

[30] Roest M, van der Schouw YT, de Valk B, Marx JJ, Tempelman MJ, de Groot PG, Sixma JJ, Banga JD. Heterozygosity for a hereditary hemochromatosis gene is associated with cardiovascular death in women [see comments]. Circulation 1999; 100(12):1268-1273.

[31] Tuomainen TP, Kontula K, Nyyssonen K, Lakka TA, Helio T, Salonen JT. Increased risk of acute myocardial infarction in carriers of the hemochromatosis gene Cys282Tyr mutation : a prospective cohort study in men in eastern Finland [see comments]. Circulation 1999; 100(12):1274-1279.

[32] Franco RF, Zago MA, Trip MD, ten Cate H, van den EA, Prins MH, Kastelein JJ, Reitsma PH. Prevalence of hereditary haemochromatosis in premature atherosclerotic vascular disease. Br J Haematol 1998; 102(5):1172-1175.

[33] Ellervik C, Tybjaerg-Hansen A, Grande P, Appleyard M, Nordestgaard BG. Hereditary hemochromatosis and risk of ischemic heart disease: a prospective study and a case-control study. Circulation 2005; 112(2):185-193.

[34] van der A, Peeters PHM, Grobbee DE, Roest M, Marx JJM, Voorbij HM, van der Schouw YT. HFE mutations and risk of coronary heart disease in middle-aged women. European Journal of Clinical Investigation 2006; 36(10):682-690.

[35] van der A, Rovers MM, Grobbee DE, Marx JJM, Waalen J, Ellervik C, Nordestgaard BG, Olynyk JK, Mills PR, Shepherd J, Grandchamp B, Boer JMA, Caruso C, Arca M, Meyer BJ, van der Schouw YT. Mutations in the HFE Gene and Cardiovascular Disease Risk: An Individual Patient Data Meta-Analysis of 53 880 Subjects. Circ Cardiovasc Genet 2008; 1(1):43-50.

[36] Njajou OT, Hollander M, Koudstaal PJ, Hofman A, Witteman JC, Breteler MM, van Duijn CM. Mutations in the hemochromatosis gene (HFE) and stroke. Stroke 2002; 33(10):2363-2366.

[37] Miller M, Hutchins GM. Hemochromatosis, multiorgan hemosiderosis, and coronary artery disease. JAMA 1994; 272(3):231-233.

[38] Pirart J, Barbier P. [Protective effects of hemochromatosis against senile and diabetic angiopathies]. Diabetologia 1971; 7(4):227-236.

[39] Sheldon JH. Haemochromatosis. London, United Kingdom: Oxford University Press, 1935.

[40] JAMES TN. Pathology of the cardiac conduction system in hemochromatosis. N Engl J Med 1964; 271:92-94.
[41] Moura E, Noordermeer MA, Verhoeven N, Verheul AFM, Marx JJM. Iron Release From Human Monocytes After Erythrophagocytosis In Vitro: An Investigation in Normal Subjects and Hereditary Hemochromatosis Patients. Blood 1998; 92(7):2511-2519.
[42] Pigeon C, Ilyin G, Courselaud B, Leroyer P, Turlin B, Brissot P, Loreal O. A new mouse liver-specific gene, encoding a protein homologous to human antimicrobial peptide hepcidin, is overexpressed during iron overload. J Biol Chem 2001; 276(11):7811-7819.
[43] Park CH, Valore EV, Waring AJ, Ganz T. Hepcidin, a Urinary Antimicrobial Peptide Synthesized in the Liver. J Biol Chem 2001; 276(11):7806-7810.
[44] Nicolas G, Bennoun M, Devaux I, Beaumont C, Grandchamp B, Kahn A, Vaulont S. Lack of hepcidin gene expression and severe tissue iron overload in upstream stimulatory factor 2 (USF2) knockout mice. Proceedings of the National Academy of Sciences of the United States of America 2001; 98(15):8780-8785.
[45] Nemeth E, Valore EV, Territo M, Schiller G, Lichtenstein A, Ganz T. Hepcidin, a putative mediator of anemia of inflammation, is a type II acute-phase protein. Blood 2003; 101(7):2461-2463.
[46] Nemeth E, Ganz T. Regulation of Iron Metabolism by Hepcidin. Annual Review of Nutrition 2006; 26(1):323-342.
[47] Nemeth E, Rivera S, Gabayan V, Keller C, Taudorf S, Pedersen BK, Ganz T. IL-6 mediates hypoferremia of inflammation by inducing the synthesis of the iron regulatory hormone hepcidin. J Clin Invest 2004; 113(9):1271-1276.
[48] Nguyen NB, Callaghan KD, Ghio AJ, Haile DJ, Yang F. Hepcidin expression and iron transport in alveolar macrophages. Am J Physiol Lung Cell Mol Physiol 2006; 291(3):L417-L425.
[49] Ganz T, Nemeth E. Iron imports. IV. Hepcidin and regulation of body iron metabolism. Am J Physiol Gastrointest Liver Physiol 2006; 290(2):G199-G203.
[50] Kemna E, Tjalsma H, Laarakkers C, Nemeth E, Willems H, Swinkels D. Novel urine hepcidin assay by mass spectrometry. Blood 2005; 106(9):3268-3270.
[51] Lee PL, Beutler E. Regulation of Hepcidin and Iron-Overload Disease. Annual Review of Pathology: Mechanisms of Disease 2009; 4(1):489-515.
[52] Valenti L, Swinkels DW, Burdick L, Tjalsma H, Bertelli C, Fatta C, Bignamini D, DONGIOVANNI P, Rametta R, Motta BM, Fargion S, Fracanzani AL. Serum ferritin and hepcidin levels predict vascular damage in patients with nonalcoholic fatty liver disease. Poster session presented at: International BioIron Society 2009 Meeting; 2009 Jun 7-11; Porto, Portugal. 2009. Ref Type: Abstract
[53] Paoletti R, Gotto AM, Jr., Hajjar DP. Inflammation in Atherosclerosis and Implications for Therapy. Circulation 2004; 109(23_suppl_1):III-20.
[54] Ridker PM, Rifai N, Stampfer MJ, Hennekens CH. Plasma Concentration of Interleukin-6 and the Risk of Future Myocardial Infarction Among Apparently Healthy Men. Circulation 2000; 101(15):1767-1772.
[55] van Deuren M, Kroot JJ, Swinkels DW. Time-course analysis of serum hepcidin, iron and cytokines in a C282Y homozygous patient with Schnitzler's syndrome treated with IL-1 receptor antagonist. Haematologica 2009.

[56] Wang L, Johnson EE, Shi HN, Walker WA, Wessling-Resnick M, Cherayil BJ. Attenuated Inflammatory Responses in Hemochromatosis Reveal a Role for Iron in the Regulation of Macrophage Cytokine Translation. J Immunol 2008; 181(4):2723-2731.
[57] Zheng H, Dimayuga C, Hudaihed A, Katz SD. Effect of dexrazoxane on homocysteine-induced endothelial dysfunction in normal subjects. Arterioscler Thromb Vasc Biol 2002; 22(7):E15-E18.
[58] Li L, Frei B. Prolonged Exposure to LPS Increases Iron, Heme, and p22phox Levels and NADPH Oxidase Activity in Human Aortic Endothelial Cells: Inhibition by Desferrioxamine. Arterioscler Thromb Vasc Biol 2009; 29(5):732-738.
[59] Kartikasari AE, Georgiou NA, de Geest M, Kats-Renaud JH, Bouwman JJ, van Asbeck BS, Marx JJ, Visseren FL. Iron enhances endothelial cell activation in response to Cytomegalovirus or Chlamydia pneumoniae infection. Eur J Clin Invest 2006; 36(10):743-752.
[60] Porreca E, Ucchino S, Di Febbo C, Di Bartolomeo N, Angelucci D, Napolitano AM, Mezzetti A, Cuccurullo F. Antiproliferative effect of desferrioxamine on vascular smooth muscle cells in vitro and in vivo. Arterioscler Thromb 1994; 14(2):299-304.
[61] Pahl PM, Yan XD, Hodges YK, Rosenthal EA, Horwitz MA, Horwitz LD. An exochelin of Mycobacterium tuberculosis reversibly arrests growth of human vascular smooth muscle cells in vitro. J Biol Chem 2000; 275(23):17821-17826.
[62] Pang JH, Jiang MJ, Chen YL, Wang FW, Wang DL, Chu SH, Chau LY. Increased ferritin gene expression in atherosclerotic lesions. J Clin Invest 1996; 97(10):2204-2212.
[63] Gaenzer H, Marschang P, Sturm W, Neumayr Gu, Vogel W, Patsch J, Weiss Gu. Association between increased iron stores and impaired endothelial function in patients with hereditary hemochromatosis*1. Journal of the American College of Cardiology 2002; 40(12):2189-2194.
[64] Adams PC, Pankow JS, Barton JC, Acton RT, Leiendecker-Foster C, McLaren GD, Speechley M, Eckfeldt JH. HFE C282Y Homozygosity Is Associated With Lower Total and Low-Density Lipoprotein Cholesterol: The Hemochromatosis and Iron Overload Screening Study. Circ Cardiovasc Genet 2009; 2(1):34-37.
[65] Kraml PJ, Klein RL, Huang Y, Nareika A, Lopes-Virella MF. Iron loading increases cholesterol accumulation and macrophage scavenger receptor I expression in THP-1 mononuclear phagocytes. Metabolism 2005; 54(4):453-459.
[66] Choi JW, Kim SK, Pai SH. Changes in Serum Lipid Concentrations during Iron Depletion and after Iron Supplementation. Ann Clin Lab Sci 2001; 31(2):151-156.
[67] Ozdemir A, Sevinc C, Selamet U, Turkmen F. The relationship between iron deficiency anemia and lipid metabolism in premenopausal women. Am J Med Sci 2007; 334(5):331-333.
[68] Sullivan JL. Iron versus cholesterol--perspectives on the iron and heart disease debate. J Clin Epidemiol 1996; 49(12):1345-1352.
[69] Zacharski LR, Chow BK, Howes PS, Shamayeva G, Baron JA, Dalman RL, Malenka DJ, Ozaki CK, Lavori PW. Decreased Cancer Risk After Iron Reduction in Patients With Peripheral Arterial Disease: Results From a Randomized Trial. J Natl Cancer Inst 2008;djn209.
[70] Minqin R, Rajendran R, Pan N, Kwong-Huat TB, Ong WY, Watt F, Halliwell B. The iron chelator desferrioxamine inhibits atherosclerotic lesion development and

decreases lesion iron concentrations in the cholesterol-fed rabbit. Free Radic Biol Med 2005; 38(9):1206-1211.

[71] Ponraj D, Makjanic J, Thong PS, Tan BK, Watt F. The onset of atherosclerotic lesion formation in hypercholesterolemic rabbits is delayed by iron depletion. FEBS Lett 1999; 459(2):218-222.

[72] Minqin R, Watt F, Huat BT, Halliwell B. Correlation of iron and zinc levels with lesion depth in newly formed atherosclerotic lesions. Free Radic Biol Med 2003; 34(6):746-752.

[73] Ren M, Rajendran R, Ning P, Tan Kwong Huat B, Choon Nam O, Watt F, Jenner A, Halliwell B. Zinc supplementation decreases the development of atherosclerosis in rabbits. Free Radical Biology and Medicine 2006; 41(2):222-225.

[74] Watt F, Rajendran R, Ren MQ, Tan BKH, Halliwell B. A nuclear microscopy study of trace elements Ca, Fe, Zn and Cu in atherosclerosis. Nuclear Instruments and Methods in Physics Research Section B: Beam Interactions with Materials and Atoms 2006; 249(1-2):646-652.

[75] Yuan XM, Anders WL, Olsson AG, Brunk UT. Iron in human atheroma and LDL oxidation by macrophages following erythrophagocytosis. Atherosclerosis 1996; 124(1):61-73.

[76] Lee FY, Lee TS, Pan CC, Huang AL, Chau LY. Colocalization of iron and ceroid in human atherosclerotic lesions. Atherosclerosis 1998; 138(2):281-288.

[77] Lee TS, Lee FY, Pang JH, Chau LY. Erythrophagocytosis and iron deposition in atherosclerotic lesions. Chin J Physiol 1999; 42(1):17-23.

[78] Li W, Hellsten A, XU LH, Zhuang DM, Jansson K, Brunk UT, YUAN XM. Foam cell death induced by 7[beta]-hydroxycholesterol is mediated by labile iron-driven oxidative injury: Mechanisms underlying induction of ferritin in human atheroma. Free Radical Biology and Medicine 2005; 39(7):864-875.

[79] Tavora F, Ripple M, Li L, Burke A. Monocytes and neutrophils expressing myeloperoxidase occur in fibrous caps and thrombi in unstable coronary plaques. BMC Cardiovascular Disorders 2009; 9(1):27.

[80] Yuan XM, Li W, Baird SK, Carlsson M, Melefors O. Secretion of ferritin by iron-laden macrophages and influence of lipoproteins. Free Radic Res 2004; 38(10):1133-1142.

[81] Li W, Xu LH, Yuan XM. Macrophage hemoglobin scavenger receptor and ferritin accumulation in human atherosclerotic lesions. Ann N Y Acad Sci 2004; 1030:196-201.

[82] Li W, Hellsten A, Nyhalah JD, Yuan XM. Enhanced expression of natural resistance-associated macrophage protein 1 in atherosclerotic lesions may be associated with oxidized lipid-induced apoptosis. Ann N Y Acad Sci 2004; 1030:202-207.

[83] Li W, Ostblom M, XU LH, Hellsten A, Leanderson P, Liedberg B, Brunk UT, Eaton JW, YUAN XM. Cytocidal effects of atheromatous plaque components: the death zone revisited. FASEB J 2006; 20(13):2281-2290.

[84] Lee TS, Shiao MS, Pan CC, Chau LY. Iron-deficient diet reduces atherosclerotic lesions in apoE-deficient mice. Circulation 1999; 99(9):1222-1229

# 24

# Paraoxonase Polymorphisms and Platelet Activating Factor Acetylhydrolase Activity as a Genetic Risk Factors in Cerebral Atherosclerosis

Zlata Flegar-Meštrić[1], Mirjana Mariana Kardum Paro[1], Sonja Perkov[1], Vinko Vidjak[2] and Marija Grdić Rajković[3]
*[1]Institute of Clinical Chemistry and Laboratory Medicine,*
*[2]Clinical Department for Diagnostic and Clinical Radiology,*
*Merkur University Hospital, Zagreb*
*[3]Department of Medical Biochemistry and Hematology, Faculty of Pharmacy and Biochemistry, University of Zagreb, Zagreb,*
*Croatia*

## 1. Introduction

Atherosclerosis is a progressive disease characterized by the accumulation of lipids and fibrous elements in the large arteries (Lusis, JA. 2000). Investigations into the genetics of atherosclerosis, along with biochemical approaches, have greatly advanced today knowledge of the mechanisms of this complex multifactorial disease (Lusis et al., 2004a, 2004b; Lusis &Weiss , 2010). According to the oxidation hypothesis, oxidative stress is a key mechanism through which atherosclerosis as a chronic inflammatory disease develops. It is mediated by reactive oxygen species that alter the fundamental properties of cholesterol, cholesterol esters, and phospholipids on lipoproteins, as well as other proteins, to make them dysfunctional, immunogenic, and pro-atherogenic (Tsimikas et. al., 2009). Oxidative stress can be enhanced by non-enzymatic pathways, such as by copper and iron cations, as well as by enzymatic pathways, such as by lipoxygenases, myeloperoxidase, and NADPH oxidase. These pro-oxidant pathways are balanced by anti-oxidant mechanisms, such as anti-oxidant vitamins (alpha-tocopherol and carotenoids) present within lipoproteins, and anti-oxidant enzymes, such as superoxide dismutase and glutathione peroxidase. Many of these enzymes and products of oxidation can be measured in the circulation, including oxidized low-density lipoprotein, oxidized phospholipids, isoprostanes, and myeloperoxidase, and have been shown to predict the presence of cardiovascular disease (CVD) and incident cardiovascular events (Tsimikas et al., 2007, 2009).

Human serum paraoxonase [(PON1); aryldialkylphosphatase (EC 3.1.8.1)] is associated with high density lipoprotein particles (HDL) responsible in part for the ability of HDL to prevent lipid peroxidation. The decreased serum paraoxonase (PON1) activity in patients with atherosclerosis disease may cause decreased HDL antioxidant capacity and therefore significantly influence the risk of the development of atherosclerosis (Aviram, M. 2004;

Nieminen et al., 2006; Shih DM. & Lusis AJ. 2009). The enormous between-individual biological variability in serum PON1 activity seems to be regulated mainly by genetic determinants. The paraoxonase gene family includes *pon1*, *pon2* and *pon3* genes which produce three enzyme paraoxonase 1 (PON1), paraoxonase 2 (PON2) and paraoxonase 3 (PON3). These genes are located on the long arm of chromosome 7 and they are structurally similar. They share about 70% of identity in nucleotide sequences and about 60% of identity in amino acid sequences. PON1 mRNA is expressed in the liver, and PON3 mRNA is expressed primarily in the liver but also in the kidneys. On the other hand PON2 mRNA is ubiquitously expressed in different kinds of tissues like kidneys, liver, lungs, small intestine, placenta, spleen, stomach and testicles and in the cells of the artery wall (including endothelial cell, smooth muscle cell and macrophages) (Draganov, DI. & La Du, BN. 2004; Ng et al., 2005).

PON1 is a 354 amino acid long glycosylated protein and has an apparent mass of 43-47 kDa. The enzyme is synthesized in the liver and is secreted into plasma. In the plasma, PON1 is mainly bounded to high density lipoproteins (HDL) but also small amount of this enzyme was detected in very low-density lipoprotein (VLDL), and postprandial chylomicrons. PON1 has hydrophobic signal sequence on the N-terminal region, from which only the initiator methionine residue is removed, and this region is for the association of PON1 with HDL (Draganov, DI. & La Du, BN. 2004; Fuhrman et al., 2005.) PON1 possesses organophosphatase, arylesterase and lactonase activities and hydrolyzes different kinds of substrates (like paraoxon, chlorpyrifos oxon, diazoxon, sarin, soman, phenylacetate, tiophenylacetate homogentisic acid lactone, dihydrocoumarin, γ-butyrolactone and homocysteine thiolactone) (Draganov, DI. & La Du, BN. 2004; Ng et al., 2005). PON1 is also well known to possess antioxidative and antiatherogenic activity, to protect HDL and low-density lipoprotein (LDL) from oxidation, and to destroy biologically active oxidized lipids on lipoproteins and in arterial cells (Draganov, DI. & La Du, BN. 2004; Aviram, M. 2004).

More than 160 polymorphisms of *pon1* gene are known, and some of them have been recognized to affect PON1 concentration and activity (Deakin, SP. & James, RW. 2004; Costa et al., 2005). Two polymorphisms in the coding region of *pon1* gene result in the substitution of amino acid glutamine with arginine at the position 192 (Q192R polymorphism, the exchange of codon CAA to CGA in exon 6) and in the substitution of amino acid leucine to methionine at the position 55 (L55M polymorphism, the exchange of codon TTG to ATG in exon 3) (Adkins et al., 1993). Q192 and R192 alloenzymes have a different affinity and catalytic activity towards numerous substrates, the R192 alloenzyme hydrolyzes paraoxon six times faster than Q192 alloenzyme while Q192 alloenzyme hydrolyzes sarin, soman and diazoxon faster than R192 alloenzyme (Deakin, SP. & James, RW. 2004). These two alloenzymes are also different in their ability to protect LDL from oxidation *in vitro*, Q192 alloenzyme is more efficient than R192 alloenzyme (Deakin, SP. & James, RW. 2004; Mackness et al., 1999). L55M polymorphism affects PON1 mRNA levels, concentration and enzyme activity. M55 alloenzyme is associated with a lower level of PON1 mRNA, concentration and activity (Deakin, SP. & James, RW. 2004). These two alloenzymes are also different in protection of LDL against oxidation, where M55 alloenzyme shows to be more protective (Mackness et al., 1999). In the promoter region of *pon1* gene at least five polymorphisms were detected and -108C>T polymorphism is one of them. This polymorphism affects *pon1* gene expression, and enzyme concentration and activity. It is believed that -108C>T polymorphism is the main contributor to serum PON1 variation (accounting for 23-24% of total variation), while other polymorphisms in *pon1* promoter region made little or no difference to serum PON1 levels (Deakin, SP. & James, RW. 2004; Leviev, I. & James, RW. 2000; Suehiro et al., 2000).

As it was mentioned earlier, PON2 is a ubiquitously expressed intracellular protein with a relative molecular mass of approximately 44 kDa (Ng et al., 2005; Li et al., 2003). PON2 has antioxidant properties, lowers the intracellular oxidative stress and prevents the cell-mediated oxidation of LDL (Ng at al., 2005; Li et al., 2003). In the *pon2* gene two common polymorphisms were identified. Alanine or glycine could be at the position 148 (A148G), and serine or cysteine could be at the position 311 (S311C). S311C polymorphism has been related with eg. coronary artery disease, ischemic stroke in patients with type 2 diabetes mellitus, Alzheimer's disease and reduced bone mass in postmenopausal women (Ng at al., 2005; Li et al., 2003). The mechanisms by which PON2 exerts its atheroprotective effects remain to be clarified. Large-scale epidemiologic studies are needed to further examine the relationship between PON2 genetic polymorphisms and risk for CVD (Shih, DM. & Lusius, AJ. 2009).

Human PON3 is a '40-kDa protein primarily synthesized in the liver with biological activity similar to PON1. PON3 is a secreted protein associated with HDL in the plasma and can participate in the prevention of LDL oxidation. The PON3 protein may play a role, distinct from that of PON1, in the lipoprotein metabolism of the kidney. These characteristics link PON3 with a group of enzymes, such as PON1, platelet-activating factor–acetylhydrolase, and lecithin-cholesterol acyltransferase, which together may contribute to the antiatherogenic properties of HDL, but the role of PON3 in atherosclerosis needs further investigation (Reddy et al., 2001; Getz, GS. & Resardon, CA. 2004).

Another lipoprotein-associated enzyme, the platelet-activating factor acetylhydrolase (PAF-AH), also referred to as lipoprotein-associated phospholipase $A_2$ (Lp-$PLA_2$), is an enzyme (EC 3.1.1.47) recently described as a potentially useful plasma biomarker associated with cardiovascular disease (Srinivasan, B. & Bahson, BJ. 2010; Koenig et al., 2004; Yamada et al., 2000; Karasawa, K. 2006; Mallat et al., 2010). The biological role of Lp-$PLA_2$ (PAF-AH) has been controversial, with contradictory antiatherogenic and proatherogenic functions. The antiatherogenic properties of Lp-PLA2 were first suggested because plasma PAF-AH might play an anti-inflammatory role in human diseases by preventing the accumulation of PAF (1-O-alkyl-2-acetyl-sn-glycero-3-phosphocholine) and PAF-like oxidized phospholipids (Karasawa, K. 2006; Mallat et al., 2010; Mitsios et al., 2006). PAF is a biologically active phospholipid involved in diverse pathologies such as inflammation and atherosclerosis. PAF can activate various cell types including platelets. In the presence of PAF, platelets aggregate and degranulate, releasing biologically potent agents. PAF is hydrolyzed and converted to lysoPAF by the catalytic reaction of PAF-AH (Mitsios et al., 2006). The atherogenic role of Lp-$PLA_2$ comes from the observation that this enzyme can also produce lysophosphatidylcholine and oxidatively modified nonesterified fatty acids which could promote the pathogenesis of atherosclerosis (Karasawa, K. 2006; Mallat et al., 2010). Lysophosphatidylcholine is an important chemoattractant for macrophages and T cells, it induces migration of vascular smooth muscle cells, affects endothelial function, and increases the expression of adhesion molecules and cytokines (Garza et al., 2007; Tsimikas et al., 2009).

Phospholipases $A_2$ ($PLA_2$s) comprise distinct sets of enzymes with different localizations:
the intracellular (cytosolic) enzymes that are $Ca^{2+}$ dependent (c$PLA_2$), $Ca^{2+}$ independent (i$PLA_2$), or specific for PAF (intracellular PAF acetylhydrolase) and extracellular (plasma) enzymes, either associated with lipoproteins (Lp-$PLA_2$) or secreted $PLA_2$s (s$PLA_2$) (Mallat et al., 2010). Extracellular (plasma) PAF-AH shares 41% sequence identity with intracellular (cytosolic) Type II PAFAH, whereas both enzymes show less structural similarity to Type I PAF-AH (Karasawa, K. 2006; Mitsios et al., 2006). Secreted $PLA_2$s (s$PLA_2$) represent a

diverse family of structurally related, disulfide-rich calcium-dependent secreted enzymes that hydrolyze the sn-2 position of glycerophospholipids generating potent lipid mediators: lysophospholipids and free fatty acids, including the precursor of eicosanoids, arachidonic acid. Extracellular levels of secreted $PLA_2$s are increased in both plasma and inflammatory fluids in various inflammatory diseases ( Karabina et al., 2010; Mallat et al., 2010 ).
The extracellular (plasma) enzyme Lp-$PLA_2$ is a single polypeptide that originates mostly from cells of the hematopoietic lineage, primarily from monocytes/macrophages (Karabina et al., 2010; Stafforini, DM. 2009). Lp-$PLA_2$ (PAF-AH) exhibits unique substrate specificity toward PAF and oxidized phospholipids. In human plasma, PAF-AH activity is associated mainly with the apolipoprotein B (apoB)-containing lipoproteins and primarily with low-density lipoprotein (LDL). A small proportion of the circulating enzyme activity is also associated with high density lipoprotein and lipoprotein(a), an atherogenic lipoprotein particle that appears to be a preferential carrier of oxidized phospholipids in human plasma (Mallat et al., 2010; Wolfert et al., 2004; Karasawa, K. 2006). In plasma, approximately 80% of Lp-$PLA_2$ is attached to low-density lipoproteins (LDLs), and the remaining 20% is linked to high-density lipoproteins (HDLs) and lipoprotein (a) (Garza et al., 2007). HDL protects LDL from oxidation and HDL-associated PAF-AH might be involved in this effect together with other HDL-associated enzymes, including PON1 and lecithin-cholesterol acyltransferase (LCAT) . Dyslipidemia-induced decrease in the ratio of HDL-associated PAF-AH to the plasma PAF-AH levels might thus lead to the promotion of atherosclerosis (Karasawa, K. 2006 ; Garza et al., 2007). Many studies appeared on the role of lipoprotein–associated $PLA_2$ and secreted $PLA_2$s in atherosclerosis at the level of biology and epidemiology. It is still unclear whether these PLA2s act as true biological effectors of cardiovascular diseases in humans and whether they have proven utility as biomarkers of disease severity (Mallat et al., 2010).
We explored relations between serum PON1 and PAF-AH activities as well as the distribution of polymorphisms of *pon1* and *pon2* genes and cerebral atherosclerosis in well-characterized groups of patients with angiografically assessed severe stenosis of cerebral arteries and matched control no-stenosis group.

## 2. Patients and methods

### 2.1 Patients

The study comprised 119 patients, 35 women and 84 men with symptoms of cerebrovascular insufficiency and stenosis of carotid artery more than 50% of the lumen. Among them, 87 (73.1%) had transitory ischemic attacks, 19 (16.0%) had suffered a cerebrovascular insult with motor deficit 5-9 months previously, and 13 patients (10.9%) had headache and vertigo with carotid bruit. All patients were examined by neurologists and referred to Doppler examination. At the Doppler examination, all of them had stenosis of one or both carotid arteries more than 50% of the arterial lumen and were preceded to digital subtraction angiography (DSA) and possible endovascular carotid PTA/stent treatment. Based on the angiographic findings, for the purpose of present investigation they were divided in two groups. The first group consisted of 73 patients, 25 female, median age 67 years (range, 41-79 years) and 48 male, median age 65 years (range, 46-83 years) with a moderate degree of carotid extra cranial stenosis between 50% and 69% of the arterial lumen. In this group there was no intracranial stenosis of cerebral arteries. The second group consisted of 46 patients, 10 female, median age 67 years (range, 46-78 years) and 36 male, median age 68 years (range, 54-78 years) in whom stenosis between 70-99% or obliteration of the carotid artery was angiographically determined. In this group, intracranial stenosis less than 50% of the lumen of carotid arteries in three patients were found.

The control no-stenosis group consisted of 90 patients, 46 female, median age 60 years (range, 44-76 years) and 44 male, median age 63 years (range, 46-82 years) with suspected cerebrovascular symptoms, but with normal Doppler examination of the carotid arteries. Vertigo, headache and transitory vision problems were indications for Doppler examination for 72 patients (80%). Twelve out of 90 (13.3%) patients had had nonischemic cerebrovascular insult a few months or years priorly with new symptoms like headache, suspected motor deficit or vertigo. The remaining six patients (6.7%) had the same symptoms combined with the carotid bruit. All of them had normal appearance and normal hemodynamic results at Doppler examination of carotid arteries. The third group of patients, with Doppler established carotid stenosis between 1-49% of cerebral arteries, was not included in the present investigation. They were proceeded to other non-invasive carotid investigations like MR angiography or multislice CT angiography.

All Doppler and DSA procedures were performed at the Institute for Diagnostic and Interventional Radiology of the Merkur University Hospital. Doppler examinations were performed at the center of excellence with more than 3,000 examinations per year. DSA was performed by the interventional radiologists skilled in neurovascular interventions.

Smokers were defined as those reporting daily smoking. Obesity was defined in terms of the patient's body mass index (BMI) calculated as weight in kg/height in $m^2$.

The patients with the BMI ≥ 25 were considered overweight. Written informed consent was obtained from all subjects according to the guidelines of our Ethics Committee.

This study was approved by the Ethics Committee of the Merkur University Hospital, Zagreb, Croatia.

### 2.2 Samples

Blood samples were collected by venopuncture after overnight fasting and under controlled pre-analytical conditions. Serum was prepared 30 min after blood collection into vacutainer tubes (Becton Dickinson) without additives by centrifugation at 3000 rpm for 15 minutes. Blood collected in EDTA-coated tubes was used for determination of *pon1 and pon2* genotypes while sera were analyzed for triacylglycerol, total cholesterol, LDL and HDL-cholesterol concentrations and PON1 and PAF-AH activities.

### 2.3 Methods

#### 2.3.1 Serum triacylglycerol, total cholesterol, LDL and HDL cholesterol assays

Serum triacylglycerol and total cholesterol were measured by enzymatic PAP- method. HDL-cholesterol was measured with direct method based on selective inhibition of the non-HDL fractions by means of polyanions. A homogeneous assay for the selective measurement of LDL-cholesterol in serum was used. All measurements were performed on fresh sera on the day of blood collection using standard commercial kits (Olympus Diagnostic GmbH, Hamburg, Germany) on the Olympus AU 600 analyzer (Olympus Mishima Co., Ltd., Shizuoka, Japan).

#### 2.3.2 Paraoxonase activity measurement

PON1 paraoxonase activity was assessed by using paraoxon as the substrate in the presence of NaCl (NaCl stimulated activity) (Juretić et al., 2006). The assay was performed on Olympus AU 600 biochemical analyzer (Olympus Mishima Co., Ltd., Shizuoka, Japan) at

37°C, as previously described, with a minor modification (Grdić et al., 2008). Briefly, 15 µL of serum was added to 300 µL of reaction mixture containing 2.5 mmol/L paraoxon of ~90% purity, 2.2 mmol/L $CaCl_2$ and 1.0 mol/L NaCl in 0.1 mol/L Tris- HCl buffer, pH 8.0. The release of p-nitrophenol from paraoxon was measured at 410/480 nm (ε410/480=17900 L/ mol cm) and the enzyme activity is expressed in international units per 1 L of serum and standardized against concentration of HDL-cholesterol . Serum samples were kept frozen at -80°C until the day of analysis.

### 2.3.3 Paraoxonase polymorphisms determinations

Polymorphisms of *pon1* and *pon2* genes were determined by the polymerase chain reaction (PCR) followed by restriction fragment length polymorphism analysis (PCR-RFLP) (Table 1). The PCR reaction was performed in a Gene Amp PCR System 2720 (Applied Biosystems) PCR machine. *Pon1* gene polymorphisms (Q192R, L55M and -108C>T) were determined by the method described by Campo et al., (Campo et al., 2004). with some modifications concerning the sequence of 1CT primer, annealing temperature and restriction enzyme for -108C>T polymorphism (Grdić et al., 2008; Grdić Rajković et al., 2011).

*Pon2* gene polymorphism (S311C) was determined by the method described by Sanghera et al. (Sangera et al., 1998) with a few modifications including the sequence of 2SC primer and annealing temperature (Grdić et al., 2011). Briefly, the amplification mixture (total volume 25 µL) for each *pon1* gene polymorphism and for *pon2* gene polymorphism contained 250 ng of genomic DNA, 0.4 µmol/L of each primer, 0.2 mmol/L of each dNTP, 2mmol/LMgCl2, 0.5 units of PlatinumTaqDNA Polymerase and 2.5 µL of reaction buffer (200mmol/L Tris-HCl, pH 8.4 and 500mmol/L KCl). PCR reaction was carried out using the following procedure: the first step of predenaturation at 95 °C for 12 min, 35 cycles of amplification (30 seconds at 94 °C followed by 30 seconds at specific primers annealing temperature and 60 seconds at 72 °C), and the last cycle of final extension at 72 °C for 7 min. PCR was attenuated by lowering the temperature to 4 °C for at least 6 min. The primers, annealing temperatures and lengths of PCR fragments are given in Table 1. Endonuclease mixture for each polymorphism explored in this study (total volume 15 µL) contained 9 µL of amplified fragment, an appropriate buffer for each restriction enzyme and 4 units of BspPI (for *pon1* Q192R), 5 units of Hin1II (for *pon1* L55M), 3 units of BsrBI (for *pon1* -108C>T) and 3 units of DdeI (for *pon2* S311C). For separation of restriction products electrophoresis on 4% agarose gel in TAE buffer (0.04 mol/L Tris-HCl, 5 mmol/L Na-acetate, 0.04 mmol/L EDTA, pH 7.9) and stained with ethidium bromide (final concentration was 0.5 µg/mL) were used. The length of RFLP fragments is given in Table 1.

Determination of *pon1* Q192R, *pon1* L55M and *pon1* -108C>T polymorphisms by the PCR-RFLP procedure using specific restriction enzymes were described in details previously (Grdić et al., 2008, 2011). Briefly, for *pon1* Q192R polymorphism undigested fragment (238 bp) was detected in genotype QQ, digested fragments (175 and 63 bp) were detected in genotype RR, and both digested and undigested fragments (238, 175 and 63 bp) were detected in genotype QR. For *pon1* L55M polymorphism undigested fragment (172 bp) was detected in genotype LL, digested fragments (103 and 69 bp) were detected in genotype MM, and digested and undigested fragments (172, 103 and 69 bp) were detected in genotype LM. For *pon1*-108C>T polymorphism undigested fragment (240 bp) was detected in genotype TT, digested fragment (212 bp) was detected in genotype CC, and both undigested and digested fragments (240 and 212 bp) were detected in genotype CT .

| Poly-morphism | Primer | °C | Restriction enzyme | PCR fragment | RFLP fragments |
|---|---|---|---|---|---|
| *pon1* Q192R | $1_{QR}$: 5′ TATTGTTGCTGTGGGACCTGAG 3′ | 60 | BspPI | 238 bp | Q allele: 238 bp |
| | $2_{QR}$: 5′ CCTGAGAATCTGAGTAAATCCACT 3′ | | | | R allele: 175+63 bp |
| *pon1* L55M | $1_{LM}$: 5′ CCTGCAATAATATGAAACAACCTG 3′ | 63 | Hin1II | 172 bp | L allele: 172 bp |
| | $2_{LM}$: 5′ TGAAAGACTTAAACTGCCAGTC 3′ | | | | M allele: 103+69 bp |
| *pon1* -108C>T | $1_{CT}$: 5′ AGCTAGCTGCCGACCCGGCGGGGAGGaG 3′ | 68 | BsrBI | 240 bp | C allele: 212+28 bp |
| | $2_{CT}$: 5′ GGCTGCAGCCCTCACCACAACCC 3′ | | | | T allele: 240 bp |
| *pon2* S311C | $1_{SC}$: 5′ ACATGCATGTACGGTGGTCTTATA 3′ | 55 | DdeI | 265 bp | S allele: 123+75+67 bp |
| | $2_{SC}$: 5′ AGCAATTCATAGAAAATTAATTGTTA 3′ | | | | C allele: 142+123 bp |

Table 1. Conditions for PCR-RFLP method. The lower case base "a" in *pon1* -108CNT 1CT primer indicates a mismatch, introducing a restriction site for restriction enzyme BsrBI.

Determination of *pon2* S311C polymorphism by PCR-RFLP procedure using DdeI restriction enzyme was carried out as follows. The exchange of the nucleotide C with G results in substitution of codon TCT to TGT (exon 9 of *pon2* gene), and with substitution of serine to cystein at position 311 (S311C, SNP ID rs7493). S and C alleles have a restriction site for DdeI restriction enzyme but the presence of codon TCT in S allele introduces an additional restriction site for this enzyme. The amplified fragment of 265 bp was digested in two fragments (142 and 123 bp) in both S and C allele. In the case of S allele 142 bp fragment is additionally digested in two fragments (75 and 67 bp). Fragments of 123, 75 and 67 bp were detected in genotype SS, fragments of 142 and 123 bp were detected in genotype CC, and fragments of 142, 123, 75 and 67 bp were detected in genotype SC.

### 2.3.4 PAF-AH activity assay

Platelet-activating factor acetylhydrolase (PAF-AH) activity was measured in plain serum with the new automated spectrophotometric assay (Azwell Inc., Auto PAF-AH, Osaka, Japan) at 37°C (Kosaka et al., 2000). In the first phase, 2μL of serum was added to 240 μL of 200 mmol/L HEPES (*N*-2-hydroxyethylpiperazine-*N*′-2-ethanesulfonic acid) buffer (Reagent 1), pH 7.6 and pre-incubated at 37°C for 5 min. The reaction was started by adding 80 μL of 20 mmol/L citric acid monohydrate buffer, pH 4.5 containing 90 mmol/L 1-myristoyl-2-(4-nitrophenylsuccinyl)phosphatidylcholine (Reagent 2). The liberation of *p*-nitrophenol was monitored at 405 and 505 nm at 1 and 3 min after the addition of Reagent 2 using the automatic biochemical analyzer OlympusAU600 (Olympus Mishima Co., Ltd., Shizuoka, Japan). Enzyme activities are expressed in international units per liter of serum and standardized against concentration of LDL-cholesterol. Serum samples were kept frozen at -80°C until the day of analysis.

### 2.3.5 Quality control of measurements

The Institute of Clinical Chemistry and Laboratory Medicine of the Merkur University Hospital has been accredited to ISO 15189, Medical laboratories - Particular requirements for quality and competence since 2007 (ISO 15189, 2008). Analytical methods for measurement of serum triacylglycerol, total cholesterol, LDL and HDL-cholesterol concentrations as well as for paraoxonase polymorphisms determinations used in this study have been accredited according to this norm (Flegar- Meštrić et al., 2010a). Traceability of analytical methods is achieved through a manufacturer's reference materials (calibrators) or reference methods for enzyme activities. Analyzer-based calibrations are routinely performed for compensation of systematic effects. Estimates of within-laboratory precision are provided by internal quality control data using commercial control sera (Olympus Diagnostic) for triacylglycerol, total cholesterol, LDL and HDL-cholesterol concentrations and pool serum samples for the paraoxonase and PAF-AH activities. Trueness estimates are based on the long-term results of external quality assessment (EQA) obtained by the participation of the Institute of Clinical Chemistry and Laboratory Medicine of the Merkur University Hospital in the National External Quality Assessment Scheme organized by the Croatian Society of Medical Biochemists and international EQA schemes for general and special medical biochemistry organized by Labquality - WHO Collaborating Centre for Education and Training in Laboratory Quality Assurance, FIN-00520 Helsinki, Finland (Flegar-Meštrić, Z. et al., 2010b). According to the requirements of the international standard ISO 15189, interlaboratory comparisons were performed for the paraoxonase polymorphisms determinations between the Institute of Clinical Chemistry and Laboratory Medicine of the Merkur University Hospital and Faculty of Pharmacy and Biochemistry, University of Zagreb, Croatia. Estimation of measurement uncertainties is done on the basis of the "Guide to the Expression of Uncertainty in Measurement" (GUM, 2005). The uncertainty components that we use are uncertainties related to calibrator, within-laboratory precision and trueness estimates based on the results of external quality assessment (EQA). The expanded measurement uncertainties (k=2) obtained for triacylglycerol, total cholesterol, LDL and HDL-cholesterol concentrations and pool serum samples for the paraoxonase and PAF-AH activities in the normal concentration range were 4.8, 4.0, 8.0, 11.1, 4.2 and 3.8%, respectively.

### 2.4 Statistical analysis

The Mann-Whitney U-test was applied to evaluate the differences between the groups, with $p< 0.05$ considered statistically significant. The correlations between serum PAF-AH activity and concentrations of total and LDL cholesterol were estimated using Pearson's correlation. Chi-square test was used for comparisons of allele and genotype proportions. MedCalc statistical program (MedCalc Software Version 8.1.0.0, 2005 Frank Schoonjans for Windows, available at the website:www.medcalc.be/) was used.

## 3. Results

### 3.1 Patients

The results of the Mann-Whitney U-test showed that, according to the demographic and lifestyle characteristics (age, body mass index), the control no-stenosis group matched the groups of patients with different degrees of cerebrovascular stenosis (Table 2). The chi-squared test showed no significant differences between sex and cerebrovascular stenosis subgroups (Yates corrected $\chi^2$ =0.003, p=0.338 in the group with <70% of stenosis; Yates corrected $\chi^2$ =0.023, p=0.638 in the group with >70% of stenosis) or smoking habits and cerebrovascular stenosis subgroups (Yates corrected $\chi^2$ =0.001, p=0.478 in the group with <70% of stenosis; Yates corrected $\chi^2$ =0.012, p=0.962 in the group with >70% of stenosis). The proportion of daily smokers in the group of patients with <70% of stenosis was 33.3% and 32.6% in the group of patients with >70% of stenosis versus 25.8 % in control no-stenosis group. The mean values of the body mass index in all groups examined were more than 25 kg/m$^2$, indicating overweight.

### 3.2 Serum triacylglycerol, total cholesterol, LDL and HDL cholesterol concentrations

Comparing the results obtained for the traditional risk factors (triacylglycerol, total cholesterol, HDL-cholesterol, LDL-cholesterol) between the groups of patients with cerebrovascular stenosis and control no-stenosis group using the Mann-Whitney univariate statistic method, significant differences were found for all serum lipid parameters (p<0.05) (Table 2).

| Parameter | Control no-stenosis group (N=90) | Patients with cerebrovascular stenosis | | | |
|---|---|---|---|---|---|
| | | <70% of stenosis (N=73) | *P* | >70% of stenosis (N=46) | *P* |
| Age (years) | 61 (44-82) | 66 (41 - 83) | 0.068 | 68 (46 - 83) | 0.160 |
| Body mass index (kg/m$^2$) | 26.3 (20.2 - 35.7) | 25.7 (19.1 - 34.1) | 0.143 | 26.5 (19.0 - 35.1) | 0.944 |
| Total cholesterol (mmol/L) | 6.3 (4.2 - 8.4) | 5.4 (3.4 - 11.5) | 0.001 | 5.7 (3.5 - 9.6) | 0.000 |
| Triacylglicerol (mmol/L) | 1.39 (0.34 - 4.14) | 1.75 (0.43 - 8.18) | 0.003 | 1.66 (0.71 - 5.09) | 0.026 |
| HDL- cholesterol (mmol/L) | 1.6 (1.0 - 3.1) | 1.3 (0.7 - 2.3) | 0.000 | 1.1 (0.8 - 1.8) | 0.000 |
| LDL- cholesterol (mmol/L) | 3.9 (2.6 - 5.9) | 3.6 (1.8 - 6.3) | 0.021 | 3.5 (1.2 - 8.4) | 0.001 |

Table 2. Demographic and biochemical parameters for control no-stenosis group and patients with <70% and >70% of cerebrovascular stenosis. Results are given as medians, with ranges in parentheses. p values: significance level for difference between the group of patients with cerebrovascular stenosis and the control no-stenosis group tested by Mann-Whitney test; p <0.05 was considered as statistically significant.

### 3.3 Paraoxonase activity measurement

Basal and stimulated PON1 activities differ significantly between patients group with stenosis and the control no-stenosis group, and HDL standardized basal and stimulated PON1 activity did not show statistical difference. Kolmogorov –Smirnov test for normal distribution reject normality for all examined data (Table 3) . There were no statistically significant relationships between basal and stimulated PON1 activity and examined lipid and lipoprotein parameters (tryacylglicerol, total cholesterol, HDL cholesterol, LDL cholesterol) (Table 4).

| Paraoxonase (unit) | Control no-stenosis group (N=90) | Patients with cerebrovascular stenosis (N=119) | p |
|---|---|---|---|
| | Median (IQR) | Median (IQR) | |
| Basal PON1 activity (U/L) | 187 (137) | 103 (180) | 0.0056 |
| NaCl -stimulated PON1 activity (U/L) | 379 (326) | 213 (339) | 0.0079 |
| HDL standardized basal PON1 activity (U/mmol) | 110 (125) | 93 (142) | 0.9390 |
| HDL standardized NaCl -stimulated PON1 activity (U/mmol) | 228 (238) | 189 (310) | 0.9605 |

Table 3. Serum paraoxonase (PON1) activity and HDL standardized paraoxonase activity in control no-stenosis group and patients with cerebrovascular stenosis. Abbreviation: IQR, Interquartile range; p values: significance level for difference between the group of patients with cerebrovascular stenosis and the control no-stenosis group tested by Mann-Whitney test; p <0.05 was considered as statistically significant.

| | Correlation coefficient | | | |
|---|---|---|---|---|
| | Control no-stenosis group (N=90) | | Patients with cerebrovascular stenosis (N=119) | |
| | Basal PON1 activity | | | |
| | r | p | r | p |
| Tryacylglicerol | 0.1638 | 0.1229 | 0.0754 | 0.4211 |
| Total cholesterol | 0.0105 | 0.9219 | 0.1534 | 0.1003 |
| HDL cholesterol | 0.1278 | 0.2301 | 0.1146 | 0.2205 |
| LDL cholesterol | -0.3067 | 0.3182 | 0.1201 | 0.1992 |
| | NaCl stimulated PON1 activity | | | |
| Tryacylglicerol | 0.1587 | 0.1358 | 0.0691 | 0.4606 |
| Total cholesterol | -0.0140 | 0.8956 | 0.1589 | 0.0844 |
| HDL cholesterol | 0.1283 | 0.2281 | 0.1154 | 0.2173 |
| LDL cholesterol | -0.1262 | 0.2359 | 0.1306 | 0.1623 |

Table 4. Relationships between paraoxonase activity and serum lipids and lipoproteins levels. p <0.05 was considered as statistically significant.

### 3.4 Paraoxonase polymorphisms determinations

Genotype frequencies of *pon1* and *pon2* polymorphisms found in the group of patients with angiografically assessed stenosis of cerebral arteries vs. control no-stenosis group are presented in Table 5 and Figures 1-4. Observed and expected genotype frequencies of all examined *pon1* and *pon2* genes polymorphisms were in Hardy-Weinberg equilibrium. There were no statistically significant differences between genotype frequencies of *pon1* and *pon2* (Table 5) as well as for the alleles frequencies in patients group vs. control no-stenosis group (p>0,05) (Table 6).

| Genotype | Control no-stenosis group (N=81) | | Patients with cerebrovascular stenosis (N=71) | | p |
|---|---|---|---|---|---|
| | n | % | n | % | |
| *pon1* L55M | | | | | |
| LL | 33 | 40 | 32 | 45 | *P = 0,910* |
| LM | 41 | 51 | 25 | 35 | |
| MM | 7 | 9 | 14 | 20 | |
| *pon1* Q192R | | | | | |
| QQ | 38 | 47 | 33 | 47 | *P = 0,995* |
| QR | 39 | 48 | 32 | 45 | |
| RR | 4 | 5 | 6 | 8 | |
| *pon1* -108C>T | | | | | |
| CC | 22 | 27 | 18 | 25 | *P = 0,912* |
| CT | 47 | 58 | 32 | 45 | |
| TT | 12 | 15 | 21 | 30 | |
| *pon2* S311C | | | | | |
| SS | 44 | 54 | 45 | 63 | *P = 0,981* |
| CS | 37 | 46 | 24 | 34 | |
| CC | 0 | 0 | 2 | 3 | |

Table 5. Genotype frequencies of *pon1* and *pon2* polymorphisms in control no-stenosis group and patients with cerebrovascular stenosis. Data are shown as number (n) and percentage (%) of individuals having a certain genotype; checked by Chi-square test.

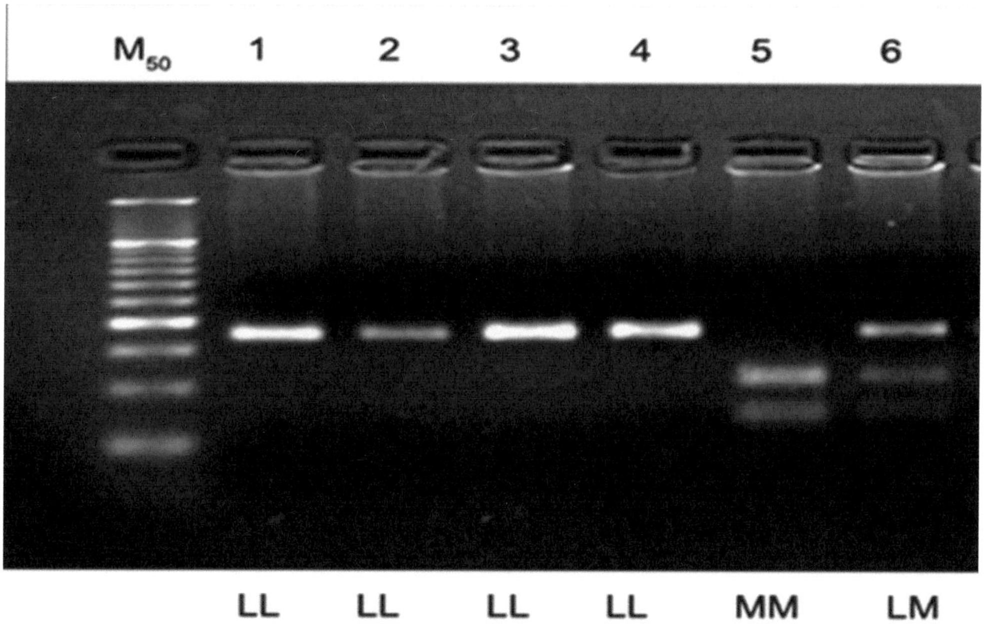


Fig. 1. Determination of L55M *pon1* gene polymorphism by the PCR-RFLP procedure using *Hin*1II restriction enzyme. Lines 1- 4 LL, line 5 MM, and line 6 LM genotype.

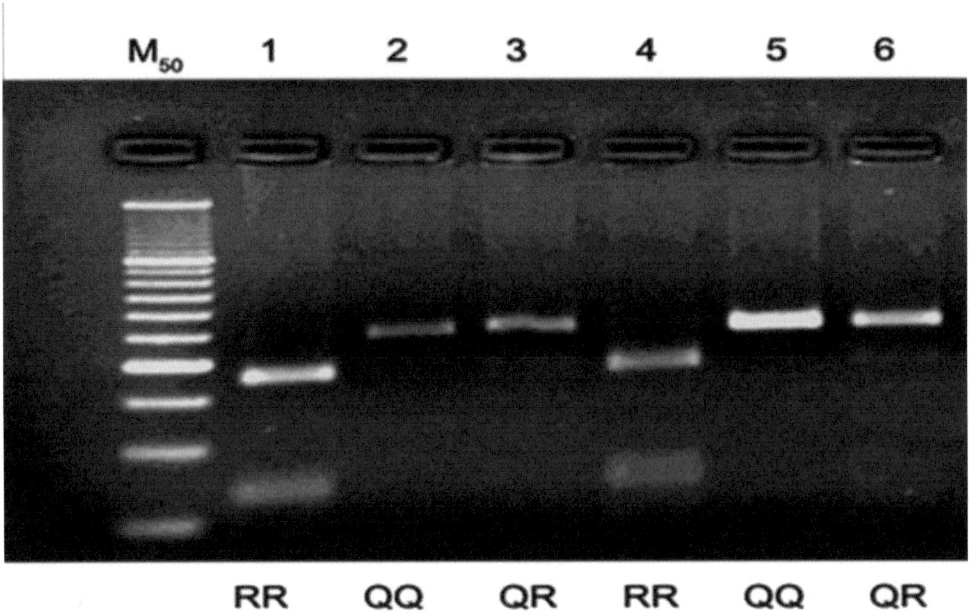


Fig. 2. Determination of Q192R *pon1* gene polymorphism by the PCR-RFLP procedure using *Bsp*PI restriction enzyme. Line 1 RR, line 2 QQ, line 3 QR, line 4 RR, line 5 QQ, and line 6 QR genotype.

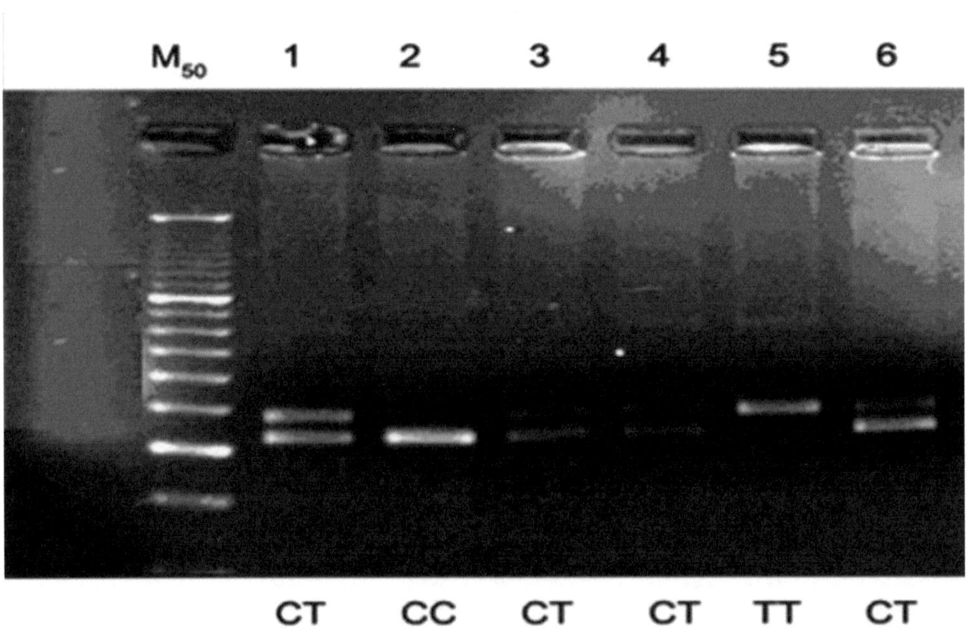


Fig. 3. Determination of -108C>T *pon1* gene polymorphism by the PCR-RFLP procedure using *Bsr*BI restriction enzyme. Line 1 CT, line 2 CC, lines 3, 4 CT, line 5 TT and line 6 CT genotype.

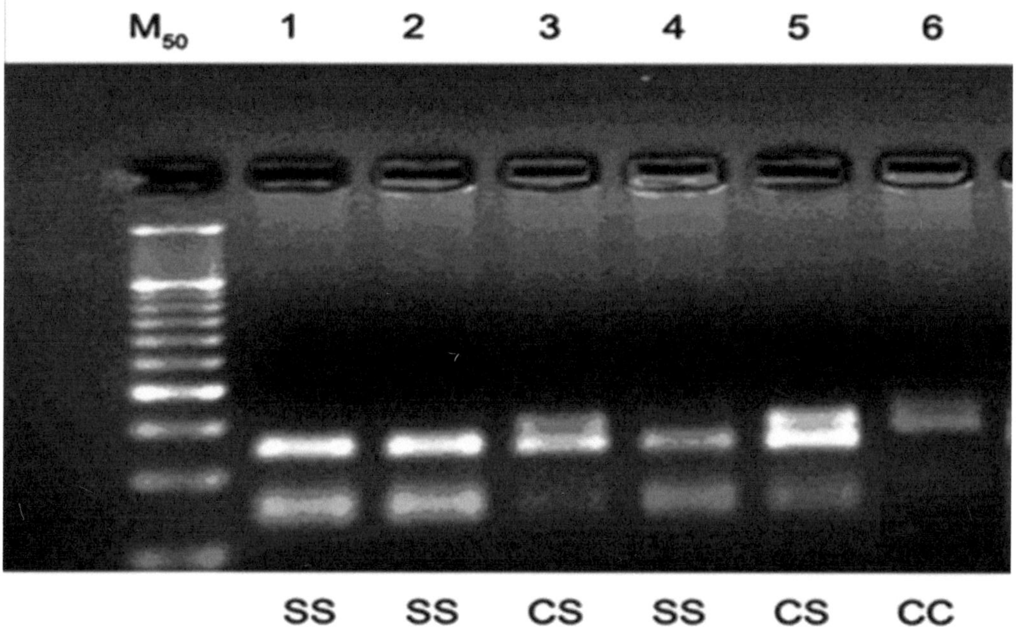


Fig. 4. Determination of S311C *pon2* gene polymorphism by the PCR-RFLP procedure using *Dde*I restriction enzyme. Lines 1- 2 SS, line 3 CS, line 4 SS, line 5 CS, and line 6 CC genotype.

| **Allele** | **Control no-stenosis group** | | **Patients with cerebrovascular stenosis** | | **p** |
|---|---|---|---|---|---|
| | n | % | n | % | |
| *pon1* L55M | | | | | |
| L | 107 | 62 | 89 | 63 | *P = 0,9744* |
| M | 65 | 38 | 53 | 37 | |
| *pon1* Q192R | | | | | |
| Q | 115 | 66 | 139 | 70 | *P = 0,8477* |
| R | 47 | 34 | 61 | 30 | |
| *pon1* -108C>T | | | | | |
| C | 91 | 56 | 95 | 48 | *P = 0,1246* |
| T | 71 | 44 | 105 | 52 | |
| *pon2* S311C | | | | | |
| S | 125 | 77 | 160 | 80 | *P = 0,5980* |
| C | 37 | 23 | 40 | 20 | |

Table 6. Allele frequencies of *pon1* and *pon2* polymorphisms in control no-stenosis group and patients with cerebrovascular stenosis. Data are shown as number (n) and percentage (%) of individuals having a certain allele; checked by Chi-square test.

### 3.5 PAF-AH activity assay

The values of PAF-AH activity did not differ significantly between control no-stenosis group and group of patients with cerebrovascular stenosis (Table 7) while LDL standardized PAF-AH activity (U/mmol) showed significant difference. The PAF-AH activity showed significant relationship with total and LDL cholesterol in both groups studied (Table 8).

| | Control no-stenosis group | Patients with cerebrovascular stenosis | |
|---|---|---|---|
| | Median (IQR) | Median (IQR) | p |
| PAF-AH activity (U/L) | 405 (134) | 414 (171) | 0.769 |
| LDL standardized PAF-AH activity (U/mmol) | 99 (30) | 119 (41) | <0.0001 |

Table 7. Serum Platelet-activating factor acetylhydrolase (PAF-AH) activity in groups studied. p values: significance level for difference between the group of patients with cerebrovascular stenosis and the control no-stenosis group tested by Mann-Whitney test; p <0.05 was considered as statistically significant.

| | Correlation coefficient | | | |
|---|---|---|---|---|
| | Control no-stenosis group | | Patients with cerebrovascular stenosis | |
| | r | p | r | p |
| Tryacylglicerol | 0.353 | 0.0006 | 0.153 | 0.1018 |
| Total cholesterol | 0.417 | <0.0001 | 0.591 | <0.0001 |
| HDL cholesterol | -0.360 | 0.0005 | -0.006 | 0.9495 |
| LDL cholesterol | 0.459 | <0.0001 | 0.5879 | <0.0001 |

Table 8. Relationships between platelet-activating factor acetylhydrolase (PAF-AH) activity and serum lipids and lipoproteins levels. p <0.05 was considered as statistically significant.

## 4. Discussion

Atherosclerosis, a disease of large arteries, is the primary cause of heart disease and stroke (Lusis, JA. 2000). Epidemiological studies over the past 50 years have revealed various risk factors for atherosclerosis and cardiovascular disease, which can be grouped into factors with an important genetic component and those that are largely environmental (Gupta et al., 2009; Lusis, JA. 2000). The results of our study indicated that significant changes associated with cerebrovascular stenosis could be the result of the environmental factors and demographic characteristics of the examined population, which is in accordance with previous studies that have investigated the atherosclerosis and the severity and extent of cardiovascular disease (Mallat et al., 2010; Costa et al., 2005; Granér et al., 2006). All groups examined in our study were characterized by a high frequency of cigarette smoking and overweight, which is consistent with the results of a previous large cross-sectional epidemiological study of Croatian population (Turek et al., 2001), and could be considered as the possible risk factors that contribute to the increased risk of cerebrovascular stenosis (Flegar-Meštrić et al., 2007; Vrhovski-Hebrang et al., 2002).

It has been reported that raised levels of atherogenic lipoproteins are a prerequisite for most forms of atherosclerotic disease (Mallat et al., 2010; Tsimikas et al., 2009; Lusis, JA. 2000).

In our study, the median values obtained in the groups of patients with different degrees of cerebrovascular stenosis were for total cholesterol, LDL-cholesterol and tryacilglycerols higher and for HDL-cholesterol lower than the recommended values for prevention of atherosclerotic disease (De Backer et al., 2004), indicating a possible contribution of dyslipidemia to the risk of developing future stenosis of cerebral arteries.

Today, the aim of cardiovascular risk prevention is to determine atherosclerotic disease activity and shift the present focus from identification of stenosis, which is a focal disease, to identification of patients with inflamed and rupture-prone plaque (Karabina et al., 2010). Numerous biomarkers have been proposed to better discern the vulnerability of plaque rupture, pathogenesis, or cardiovascular risk. Epidemiologic, genetic, and biochemical studies support an antiatherogenic role for paraoxonase (PON) 1. The two other members of the PON gene family, namely, PON2 and PON3, have also been reported to possess antioxidant properties and may exhibit antiatherogenic capacities as well (Shih, DM & Lusis, AJ. 2009). Previous studies have demonstrated that PON1 expression is down regulated by oxidative stress. In contrast, more recent studies have shown that PON2 expression is up regulated in response to oxidative stress-inducing agents, while PON3 expression remains unchanged (Ng et al., 2005). Although PON1 activity is determined genetically, various factors, such as diet, lifestyle and environmental factors, can influence PON1 activity (Ng et al., 2005; Gupta et al., 2009). Between individuals, there is an approximately 10- to 40-fold variation in PON1 activity (Gupta et al., 2009).

Only a few studies have examined the relationship between PON1 activity and angiographically proven cardiovascular disease (Graner et al., 2006; Mackness et al., 2001). Our results indicated that basal and stimulated PON1 activities were significantly decreased in patients group with angiographically proven cerebrovascular stenosis (>50%) versus control no-stenosis group ($p<0.05$), and there were no statistically significant relationships between basal and stimulated PON1 activity and examined lipid parameters (total cholesterol, LDL-cholesterol, HDL-cholesterol and tryacilglycerols), $p>0.05$. Those results are in line with previous studies, indicating that PON1 activities toward paraoxon are lower in subjects with cardiovascular disease than in control subjects regardless of the PON1 genotype. This would suggest that the quality of the PON1 enzyme is a more important factor in cardiovascular disease than the PON1 gene (Mackness et al., 2001).

Polymorphisms in *pon1* and *pon2* genes (L55M and Q192R in *pon1*, and S311C in *pon2*) have been reported to be associated with the risk for the development of atherosclerosis as well as polymorphism in *pon1* promoter region (-108C>T) (Pasdar et al., 2006; Granér et al., 2006).

Paraoxonase-1 has several genetic polymorphisms that modify its activity and mass concentration. Hypothesized differences in the ability of the polymorphic forms to protect oxidation of LDL have led to numerous studies attempting to determine the relationship between *PON1* polymorphisms and cardiovascular disease. The results of meta-analysis of 88 studies on 4 *PON* polymorphisms [Q192R, L55M, and T(−107)C in the *PON1* and the S311C in the *PON2*] suggested an overall weak association between the R192 polymorphism and CHD risk. Despite these limitations, this meta-analysis suggests that Q192R polymorphisms may increase the risk of CHD, but no significant effect for L55M, T(−107)C and S311C polymorphisms (Wang et al., 2011). Additionally, it has been reported that no significant genotypic or allelic frequency differences between stroke cases and controls for any of the structural polymorphisms of the *PON* genes tested were found (Pasdar et al., 2006).

In our study, there were no significant differences in genotype or allele frequencies of *pon1* and *pon2* genes between patients with stenosis of cerebral arteries and controls, indicating that there is no relationship between examined polymorphisms and reduced paraoxonase activity in patients group with angiographically proven cerebrovascular stenosis.

The platelet-activating factor acetylhydrolase (PAF-AH) or lipoprotein-associated phospholipase $A_2$ (Lp-PL$A_2$) is among the multiple biomarkers that have been associated with an increased CHD risk (Karabina et al., 2010; Garza et al., 2007; Tsimikas et al., 2009; Reddy et al., 2009; Wolfert et al., 2004). A recent meta-analysis of 14 prospective epidemiologic studies involving more than 20,000 patients established a high relative risk for cardiovascular events with high Lp-PLA2.( Garza et. al., 2007; Ballantyne et al., 2007). The LDL-associated PAF-AH activity increases in parallel with the severity of hypercholesterolemia, thus one of the major factors that determines plasma levels of PAF-AH is the rate of removal of LDL from the circulation (Karabina et al., 2010; Tsimikas et al., 2009). In our study, the PAF-AH activity shows the most significant linear relationship with total cholesterol and LDL cholesterol in the control no-stenosis group and the group of patients with cerebrovascular stenosis. It has been reported that increased Lp-PL$A_2$ activity is significantly related to incident cardiovascular disease (cardiovascular death, myocardial infarction, stroke, and transient ischemic attack) (Tsimikas et al., 2009; Mallat et al., 2010). In our study, the median serum PAF-AH activity did not differ significantly between patients with cerebrovascular stenosis and control no-stenosis group (median values 414 U/L versus 405 U/L, p>0,05), which is consistent with results of our previous study (Flegar-Meštrić et al., 2003), while LDL standardized PAF-AH activity a showed significant difference between the patients with cerebrovascular stenosis and control group (median values 119 U/mmol versus 99 U/mmol, p<0,0001).

Previous studies show that Lp-PL$A_2$ is a unique inflammatory biomarker that plays a critical role in the development of atherosclerosis and may be involved in the causal pathway of plaque inflammation and plaque rupture (Munzel, T. & Gori, T. 2009; Cariquist et al., 2007). The association of Lp-PL$A_2$ with cardiovascular risk among different population studies independent of classical risk factors makes the premise even stronger that Lp-PL$A_2$ is involved in progression of atherosclerosis to advanced rupture-prone unstable plaques (Reddy et al., 2009) . As Lp-PL$A_2$ is produced by macrophages and foam cells of atherosclerotic plaques that are numerous in unstable plaque, the differentiation between stable versus unstable plaque could be established by the presence of elevated Lp-PL$A_2$ (Reddy et al., 2009; Munzel, T. & Gori, T. 2009; Hiramoto et al., 1997; Zalewski, A. & Macphee, C. 2005). However, the clinical utility of Lp-PL$A_2$ activity for prediction of cardiovascular risk has to be explored in future studies.

## 5. Conclusion

The results of the present study show that basal and stimulated PON1 activities were significantly decreased in the patients group with cerebrovascular stenosis (group of patients with symptoms of cerebrovascular insufficiency and stenosis of carotid artery more than 50% of the lumen) versus control no-stenosis group (p<0.05). There were no statistically significant relationships between PON1 activity and lipid parameters (total cholesterol, LDL-cholesterol, HDL-cholesterol and tryacilglycerols), p>0.05. According to the results obtained, we assume that decreased PON1 activities in patients with cerebrovascular stenosis may cause a decreased HDL antioxidant capacity and therefore contribute to the increased risk of the development of cerebrovascular atherosclerosis. However, there were no significant differences in genotype or allele frequencies of *pon1* and *pon2* genes between patients with stenosis of cerebral arteries and no-stenosis control group, indicating that changes in paraoxonase activity are determined by both genetic and environmental factors. Our results show the most significant linear relationship between PAF-AH activity and total cholesterol and LDL-cholesterol ( p<0.001) in the control no-stenosis group, as well as in the group of patients with cerebrovascular stenosis. The median serum PAF-AH activity did not differ significantly between the patients with cerebrovascular stenosis and control no-stenosis group (p>0,05), while LDL standardized PAF-AH activity showed significant difference between both examined groups (p<0.0001). According to our results, the LDL-standardized PAF-AH activity could be used as an additional discriminating biochemical indicator of cerebrovascular stenosis.

## 6. Acknowledgement

This work was supported by a grant of the Ministry of Science, Education and Sports of the Republic of Croatia (No. 044-0061245-0551).

## 7. References

Adkins, S.; Gan, KN.; Mody, M. & La Du, BN. (1993). Molecular basis for the polymorphic forms of human serum paraoxonase/arylesterase: glutamine or arginine at position 191, for the respective A or B allozymes. *American Journal of Human Genetics*, Vol.52, No.3, pp. 598-608, ISSN

Aviram M. (2004). Introduction to the serial review on paraoxonases, oxidative stress, and cardiovascular diseases. *Free Radical Biology and Medicine,* Vol.37, No.9, (November 2004), pp. 1301-1303, ISSN 0891-5849

Ballantyne, C., Cushman, M., Psaty, B., et al. (2007). Collaborative meta-analysis of individual participant data from observational studies of Lp-PLA2 and cardiovascular diseases. *European Journal of Cardiovascular Prevention & Rehabilitation,* Vol. 14, No.1, (February 2007), pp. 3–11, ISSN 1741-8267

Carlquist, JF.; Muhlestein, JB. & Anderson, JL. (2007). Lipoprotein-associated phospholipase $A_2$: a new biomarker for cardiovascular risk assessment and potential therapeutic target. *Expert Review of Molecular Diagnostics,* Vol.7, No.5, (September 2007), pp. 511-517 , ISSN

Costa, LC.; Vitalone, A.; Cole, TB.& Furlong, CE. (2005). Modulation of paraoxonase (PON1) activity. *Biochemical Pharmacoloy,* Vol.69, No.4, (February 2005), pp. 541-550, ISSN 0006-2952

Deakin, SP.& James, RW. (2004). Genetic and environmental factors modulating serum concentrations and activities of the antioxidant enzyme paraoxonase-1. *Clinical Science,* Vol.107, No. 5, (November 2004), pp. 435-47, ISSN 0143-5221

De Backer, G.; Ambrosioni, E.; Borch-Johnsen, K.; Brotons, C.; Cifkova, R.; Dallongeville, J.; Ebrahim, S.; Faergeman, O.; Graham, I.; Mancia, G.; Manger, CV.; Orth-Gomér, K.; Perk, J.; Pyörälä, K.; Rodicio, JL.; Sans, S.; Sansoy, V.; Sechtem, U.; Silber, S.; Thomsen, T. & Wood, D. (2004). European guidelines on cardiovascular disease prevention in clinical practice. Third Joint Task Force of European and other societies on cardiovascular disease prevention in clinical practice (constituted by representatives of eight societies and by invited experts). *Atherosclerosis*, Vol. 173, No. 1, (November 2003), pp. 381-391, ISSN 1523-3804

Draganov, DI. & La Du, BN. (2004). Pharmacogenetics of paraoxonases: a brief review. *Naunyn Schmidebergs Archives of Pharmacology* , Vol. 369, No.1, (January 2004), pp. 78-88, ISSN 1432-1912

Flegar-Meštrić, Z.; Nazor, A.; Perkov, S.; Šurina, B.; Kardum-Paro, MM.; Šiftar, Z.; Sikirica, M.; Sokolić, I.; Ožvald, I. & Vidas Ž. (2010a). Accreditation of medical laboratories in Croatia - experiences of the Institute of clinical chemistry, University Hospital Merkur, Zagreb. *Collegium Antropologicum*, Vol. 34, No.1, (Mart 2010), pp. 181-186, ISSN 0350-6134

Flegar-Meštrić, Z.; Perkov, S.; Nazor, A.; Sikirica, M.& Juretić, D. (2010b). Long-term evaluation of EQA data in Croatia, *EQAnews* No.1, pp.16-17, EQALM Symposium 2010, Lisbon, October, 2010.

Flegar-Meštrić, Z.; Vrhovski-Hebrang, D.; Preden-Kereković, V.; Perkov, S.; Hebrang, A.; Grga, A.; Januš, D. & Vidjak, V. (2007). C-Reactive protein level in severe stenosis of cerebral arteries. *Cerebrovascular Disease*, Vol. 23, No.5-6 (April 2007), pp. 430-434, ISSN 1015-9770

Flegar-Meštrić, Z.; Vrhovski-Hebrang, D.; Juretić, D.; Perkov, S.; Preden-Kereković, V.; Hebrang, A.; Vidjak, V.; Odak, D.; Grga, A. & Kosaka, T. (2003). Serum platelet-activating factor acetyl-hydrolase activity in patients with angiographically established cerebrovascular stenosis. *Proceedings of 15th IFCC - FESCC European Congress of Clinical Chemistry, EUROMEDLAB*, Barcelona 2003; Monduzzi Editore; International Proceedings Division, pp. 369-372

Fuhrman, B.; Volkova, N. & Aviram, M. (2005). Paraoxonase 1 (PO N1) is present in postprandial chylomicrons. *Atherosclerosis,* Vol.180, No.1, (May 2005), pp. 55-61, ISSN 1523-3804

Garza, CA.; Montori, VM.; McConnell JP,Somers VK., Kullo IJ. & Lopez-Jimenez, F. (2007). Association between lipoprotein-associated phospholipase A2 and cardiovascular disease: a systematic review. *Mayo Clinic Proceedings,* Vol.82, No.2, (February 2007), pp. 159–65, ISSN 0025-6196

Getz , GS. & Reardon, CA. (2004). Paraoxonase, a cardioprotective enzyme: continuing issues. *Current Opinion in Lipidology* , Vol.15, No.3, (June 2004), pp. 261-267, ISSN 0957-9672

Granér,M., James, RW., Kahri, J., Nieminen, MS., Syvänne, M. & Taskinen, MR. (2006). Association of Paraoxonase-1 Activity and Concentration With Angiographic Severity and Extent of Coronary Artery Disease. *Journal of the American College of Cardiology,* Vol. 47, No.12 , (Jun 2006), pp. 2429-2435, ISSN 0735-1097

Grdić, M.; Barišić, K.; Rumora, L.; Salamunić, I.; Tadijanović, M.; Žanić Grubišić, T.; Pšikalová, R., Flegar-Meštrić, Z.& Juretić, D. (2008). Genetic frequencies of paraoxonase 1 gene polymorphisms in Croatian population. *Croatica Chemica Acta,* Vol. 81, No.1, pp. 105-11, ISSN 0011-1643

Grdić Rajković, M.; Barišić, K.; Juretić, D.; Žanić Grubišić, T.; Flegar-Meštrić, Z. & Rumora, L. (2011). Polymorphisms of *pon1* and *pon2* genes in hemodialyzed patients. *Clinical Biochemistry, doi:10.1016/j.clinbiochem.2011.05.012,* ISSN 0009-9120

Guide to the expression of uncertainty in measurement (GUM), (1995). second ed. BIPM/IEC/IFCC/ISO/IUPAC/IUPAP/OIML, Geneva. Switzerland

Gupta, N., Gill, K. & Singh, S. (2009). Paraoxonase: Structure, gene polymorphism & role in coronary artery disease. *The Indian Journal of Medical Research,* Vol. 130, No.4, (October 2009), pp. 361-368, ISSN 0971-5916

Hiramoto, M.; Yoshida, H.; Imaizumi, T.; Yoshimizu, N.& Satoh, K. (1997). A mutation in plasma platelet-activating factor acetylhydrolase (Val279 --> Phe) is a genetic risk factor for stroke. *Stroke,* Vol. 28, No.12 , (December 1997), pp. 2417–2420, ISSN 00392499

International Organization for Standardization. Medical laboratories - Particular requirements for quality and competence, HRN EN ISO 15189:2008. second ed.

Juretić, D.; Motejlkova, A.; Kunović, B.; Rekić, B.; Flegar-Meštrić, Z.; Vujić, L.; Mesić, R.; Lukač-Bajalo, J.& Simeon-Rudolf, V. (2006). Paraoxonase/arylesterase in serum of patients with type II diabetes mellitus. *Acta Pharmaceutica,* Vol.56, No.1, (Mart 2006), pp. 59-68, ISSN 846-9558

Karabina, SA.; Gora, S.; Atout, R. & Ninio, E. (2010). Extracellular phospholipases in atherosclerosis. *Biochimie,* Vol.92, No. 6, (Jun 2010), pp. 594-600, ISSN 0300-9084

Karasawa, K. (2006). Clinical aspects of plasma platelet-activating factor-acetylhydrolase. *Biochimica et Biophysica Acta,*. Vol.1761, (May 2006), pp. 1359–1372, ISSN

Koenig, W.; Khuseyinova, N.; Löwel, H.; Trishler, G. & Meisinger, C. (2004).Lipoprotein-associated phospholipase A2 adds to risk prediction of incident coronary events by C-reactive protein in apparently healthy middle-aged men from the general population: results from the 14–year follow-up of a large cohort from southern Germany. *Circulation,* Vol. 110, No. 14, (October 2004) pp. 1903-1908, ISSN 0009-7322

Kosaka, T.; Yamaguchi, M.; Soda, Y.; Kishimoto, T.; Tago, A.; Toyosato, M.& Mizuno, K. (2000). Spectrophotometric assay for serum platelet-activating factor acetylhydrolase activity. *Clinica Chimica Acta,* Vol.296, No.1-2, (Jun 2000), pp. 151–161, ISSN 009-8981

Leviev, I. & James, RW. (2000). Promoter polymorphisms of human paraoxonase *PON1* gene and serum paraoxonase activities and concentrations. *Arteriosclerosis, Thrombosis and Vascular Biology,* Vol.20, No.2, (February 2000), pp. 516 -521, ISSN 1079-5642

Li, HL.; Liu, DP. & Liang, CC. (2003). Paraoxonase gene polymorphisms, oxidative stress, and diseases. *Journal of Molecular Medicine,* Vol.81, No.12, (December 2003), pp. 766-779, ISSN 0946-2716

Lusis, JA. (2000). Atherosclerosis. *Nature,* Vol.407, No.6801, (September 2000), pp. 233-241, ISSN 0028-0836

Lusis, JA.; Fogelman, AM. & Fonarow, GC. (2004b). Genetic Basis of Atherosclerosis: Part II: Clinical Implications. *Circulation,* Vol.110, No. 14, ( October 2004), pp. 2066-2071, ISSN 009-7322

Lusis, JA.; Fogelman, AM. & Fonarow, GC. (2004a). Genetic Basis of Atherosclerosis: Part I: New Genes and Pathways. *Circulation,* Vol.110, No.13, (September 2004), pp. 1868-1873, ISSN 009-7322

Lusis, JA. & Weis JN. (2010). Cardiovascular Networks: Systems-Based Approaches to Cardiovascular Disease. *Circulation,* Vol.121, No.1, (Januar 2010), pp. 157-170, ISSN 009-7322

Mackness, B.; Durrington, PN. & Mackness,MI. (1999). Polymorphisms of paraoxonase genes and low-density lipoprotein lipid peroxidation. *Lancet,* Vol.353, No.9151, (February 1999), pp. 468-469, ISSN 0140-6736

Mackness,B., Gershan K. Davies, GK., Wajdi Turkie, W., Lee, E., David H. Roberts, DH et al. (2001). Paraoxonase Status in Coronary Heart Disease: Are Activity and Concentration More Important Than Genotype?. *Arteriosclerosis Thrombosis and Vascular Biology,* Vol. 21, No.9, (September 2001), pp. 1451-1457, ISSN 1049-8834

Mallat, Z.; Lambeau, G & Tedgui, A. (2010). Lipoprotein-Associated and Secreted Phospholipases A2 in Cardiovascular Disease. Roles as Biological Effectors and Biomarkers. *Circulation,* Vol.122, No.21, (November 2010), pp. 2183-2200, ISSN 0009-7322

Mitsios, JV.; Vini, MP.; Stengel, D.; Ninio E.& and Tselepis, AD. (2006). Human Platelets Secrete the Plasma Type of Platelet-Activating Factor Acetylhydrolase Primarily Associated With Microparticles. *Arteriosclerosis, Thrombosis and Vascular Biology,* Vol.26, (May 2006), pp. 1907-1913, ISSN 1049-8834

Munzel, T. & Gori, T. Lipoprotein-associated phospholipase A2, a marker of vascular inflammation and systemic vulnerability. *European Heart Journal,* Vol.30, No.23, (December 2009), pp. 2829-2831, ISSN 1520-765X

Ng, CJ.; Shiha, DM.; Hamaa ,SY.; Villaa, N.; Navaba, M. & Reddy, ST. (2005). The paraoxonase gene family and atherosclerosis. *Free Radical Biology & Medicine,* Vol.38, No.2, (January 2005), pp. 153–163, ISSN 0891-5849

Nieminen, M.; Syvänne,M. & Taskinen, MR. (2006). Association of Paraoxonase-1 Activity and Concentration With Angiographic Severity and Extent of Coronary Artery Disease. *Journal of the American College of Cardiology,* Vol. 47, No.12 , (Jun 2006), pp. 2429-2435, ISSN 0735-1097

Pasdar, A.; Helen Ross-Adams, H.; Cumming, A.; Cheung, J.; Whalley, L.; St Clair, D. & MacLeod, MJ.(2006). Paraoxonase gene polymorphisms and haplotype analysis in a stroke population. *BMC Medical Genetics,* Vol. 7, (Mart 2006), pp. 28, ISSN 1471-2350

Reddy, KJ.; Singh, M.; Bangit, JR. & Batsell, RR. (2009). The role of lipoprotein-associated phospholipase A2 on cardiovascular disease risk assessment and plaque rupture: a clinical review. *Journal of Clinical Lipidology,* Vol.3, No.2, (April 2009), pp. 85–93, ISSN 19333-2874

Reddy, TS.; Wadleigh, DJ.; Grijalva, V.; Carey Ng, C.; Hama, S.;Gangopadhyay, A.; Shih, DM.; Lusis, AJ.; Navab, M. & Fogelman, AM. (2001). Human Paraoxonase-3 Is an HDL-Associated Enzyme With Biological Activity Similar to Paraoxonase-1 Protein but Is Not Regulated by Oxidized Lipids. *Arteriosclerosis, Thrombosis and Vascular Biology,* Vol.21, No.4, (April 2001), pp. 542-547, ISSN 1049-8834

Shih, DM. & Lusis, AJ. (2009). The roles of PON1 and PON2 in cardiovascular disease and innate immunity. *Current Opinion in Lipidology*, Vol.20, No.4, (August 2009), pp. 288-292, ISSN 0957-9672

Srinivasan, P. & Bahnson, BJ. (2010) Molecular Model of Plasma PAF Acetylhydrolase-Lipoprotein Association: Insights from the Structure. *Pharmaceuticals,* Vol. 3, pp. 541-557, ISSN 1424-8247

Stafforini, DM.; Satoh, K.; Atkinson, DL.; Tjoelker, LW.; Eberhardt, C.; Yoshida, H.; Imaizumi, T.; Takamatsu, S.; Zimmerman, GA.; McIntyre, TM.; Gray, PW. & Prescott, SM.(1996). Platelet-activating factor acetylhydrolase deficiency. A missense mutation near the active site of an anti-inflammatory phospholipase. *Journal of Clinical Investigation,* Vol.97, No.12, (June 1996), pp. 2784-2791, ISSN 0021-9738

Stafforini, DM. (2009). Biology of platelet-activating factor acetylhydrolase (PAF-AH, lipoprotein associated phospholipase A2). *Cardiovascular Drugs Therapy.* Vol. 23, No. 1, (February 2008), p.p. 73-83, ISSN 1473-7159

Suehiro, T.; Nakamura, T.; Inoue, M.; Shiinoki, T.; Ikeda, Y. & Kumon, Y. (2000). A polymorphism upstream from the human paraoxonase (*PON1*) gene and its association with *PON1* expression. *Atherosclerosis,* Vol.150, No.2, (Jun 2000), pp. 295-298, ISSN 1523-3804

Tsimikas, S.; Willeit, J.; Knoflach, M.; Mayr , M.; Egger, G.; Notdurfter, M.; Witztum, JL.; Wiedermann, CJ.; Xu, Q & Kiechl, S. (2009). Lipoprotein associated phospholipase A2 activity, ferritin levels, metabolic syndrome, and 10-year cardiovascular and non-cardiovascular mortality: results from the Bruneck study. *European Heart Journal,* Vol.30, No.1, pp. 107–115, ISSN 0195-668X

Tsimikas, S.; Tsironis, LD. & Tselepsis, AD. (2007). New Insights Into the Role of Lipoprotein(a)-Associated Lipoprotein-Associated Phospholipase A2 in Atherosclerosis and Cardiovascular Disease. *Arteriosclerosis Thrombosis and Vascular Biology,* Vol.27, No.10, (October 2007), pp. 2094-2099, ISSN 1079-5642

Turek, S.; Rudan. I.; Smolej-Narančić, N.; Szirovica, L.; Ćubrilo-Turek, M.; Žerjavić-Hrabak, V.; Rak-Kaić, A.; Vrhovski-Hebrang, D.; Prebeg, Z.; Ljubičić, M.; Janičijević, B. & Rudan, P. (2001). A large cross-sectional study of health attitudes, knowledge, behavior and risks in the post-war Croatian population (the First Croatian Health Project). *Collegium Antropologicum,* Vol. 25, No.1, (Jun 2001), pp. 77-96, ISSN 0350-6134

Vrhovski-Hebrang, D.; Flegar-Meštrić, Z.; Preden-Kereković, V.; Perkov, S.; Hebrang, A.; Januš, D. & Grga, A. (2002). Biochemical risk factors in angiographically established stenosis of cerebral arteries. *Croatian Medical Journal,* Vol. 43, No.6, (December 2002), pp. 696-701, ISSN 1332-8166

Wang, M.; Lang, X.; Zou, L.; Huang, Sh. & Xu, Z. (2011). Four genetic polymorphism of paraoxonase gene and risk of coronary heart disease: A meta-analysis based on 88 case-control studies. *Atherosclerosis,* Vol. 214, No.2, (February 2011), pp. 377-385, ISSN 1523-3804

Wolfert, RL., Kim, NW., Selby, RG., Sarno, MJ., Warnick, RG. & Sudhir, K. (2004). Biological variability and specificity of lipoprotein-associated phospholipase A2 (Lp-PLA2), a novel marker of cardiovascular risk. *Circulation,* Vol. 110, No. 14, (November 2004) pp. 309, ISSN 0009-7322

Yamada, Y.; Yoshida, H.; Ichihara, S.; Imaizumi, T.; Satoh, K. & Yokota, M. (2000). Correlations between plasma platelet-activating factor acetylhydrolase (PAF-AH) activity and PAF-AH genotype, age, and atherosclerosis in a Japanese population. *Atherosclerosis*, Vol. 150, No.1, (May 2000), pp. 209–216, ISSN 1523-3804

Zalewski, A. & Macphee, C. (2005). Role of Lipoprotein-Associated Phospholipase A2 in Atherosclerosis Biology, Epidemiology, and Possible Therapeutic Target. *Arteriosclerosis, Thrombosis and Vascular Biology*, Vol.25, No.5, (May 2005), pp. 923-931, ISSN 1049-8834

# 25

# G Protein-Coupled Receptor Dependent NF-κB Signaling in Atherogenesis

Phillip C. Delekta[1], Robert L. Panek[1], Linda M. McAllister-Lucas[2] and Peter C. Lucas[1]
[1]*Department of Pathology, University of Michigan Medical School,*
[2]*Department of Pediatrics, University of Michigan Medical School,*
*USA*

## 1. Introduction

Over the past decade we have witnessed an explosion of information regarding the molecular mechanisms underlying atherogenesis. While at one time atherosclerosis was viewed as a passive process of lipid deposition within muscular arteries, resulting in progressive luminal stenosis, we now understand that the process is much more complex. In particular, there is a growing appreciation for the role of both adaptive and innate immunity in atherogenesis, and for the contribution of other, non-traditional inflammatory stimuli. Indeed, atherogenesis is now understood primarily as an inflammatory disorder and much of the therapeutic focus has turned to devising approaches for reducing systemic levels of pro-inflammatory mediators and/or preventing these mediators from altering the biochemistry and physiology of the cells that make up the vessel wall. The inflammatory component of atherogenesis is particularly important from a clinical standpoint since it appears that atherosclerotic lesions characterized by on-going inflammation are those that are most unstable and susceptible to rupture, possibly leading to luminal thrombosis and acute myocardial infarction.

In this chapter, we provide a brief overview of the mechanisms underlying atherogenesis, highlighting known pro-inflammatory influences. We then focus on activation of the NF-κB family of transcription factors as a major molecular mediator of inflammation and summarize recent work that has provided new insights into how a diverse set of G protein-coupled receptors (GPCRs) may use a common mechanism to communicate NF-κB activation in cells native to the vessel wall, particularly endothelial cells. These discoveries may provide novel avenues for therapeutic intervention as we refine our approach to treating patients at risk for atherosclerosis.

## 2. Basic concepts and mechanisms in atherogenesis

Atherosclerosis is a chronic, progressive process through which lipid deposition, extracellular matrix production, immune cell infiltration, and smooth muscle cell proliferation all conspire to produce arterial obstruction and to disrupt normal arterial vasoreactivity (Hansson, 2005). Atherosclerosis and its related diseases account for nearly a third of all deaths, making it the most common cause of disease-related death in the world (Hansson, 2005; Murray and Lopez, 1997). Although the process is gradual, often taking decades to proceed to a life-threatening stage, it is useful to think of atherogenesis as a series of distinct stages (Fig. 1). We will review these only briefly, as they are discussed in more detail elsewhere in this book.

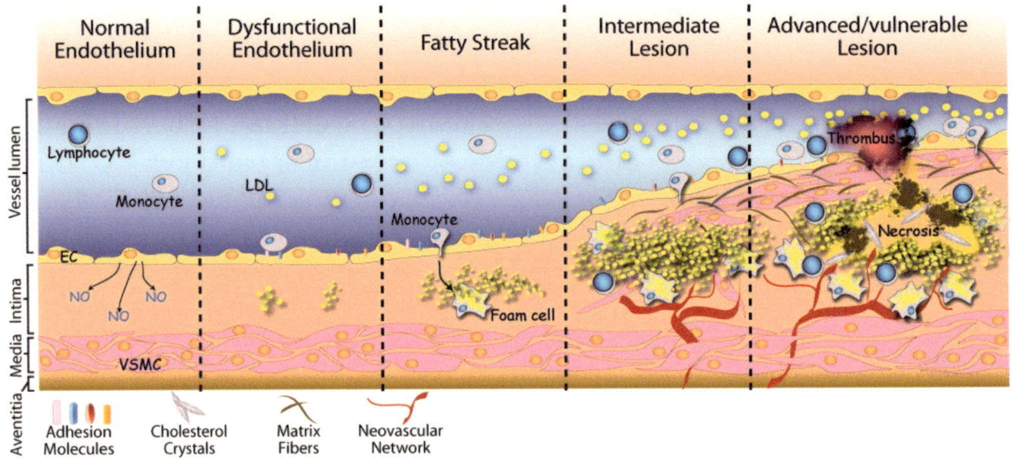


Fig. 1. The role of the endothelium through the stages of plaque formation. It should be noted that while endothelial dysfunction represents the first stage of plaque formation, it continues through all other stages as well. See text for a detailed description of each stage.

### 2.1 Endothelial dysfunction

The earliest recognizable stage in the development of atherosclerosis is characterized by changes in the cellular physiology of endothelial cells, referred to as endothelial dysfunction (Sitia et al., 2010). Endothelial cells form a single cell-thick, selectively permeable barrier, separating circulating blood components from the vessel wall. Aside from their barrier function, these cells also influence overall vessel function, in particular by regulating levels of nitric oxide (NO) which influences vascular contractility and tone (Jin and Loscalzo, 2010). Endothelial dysfunction ensues when these cells are exposed to injurious stimuli, resulting in a disruption in their ability to maintain a proper barrier and to promote vascular relaxation. As will be discussed, many features of endothelial dysfunction can be linked to the stimulation of signal transduction pathways culminating in NF-κB activation (de Winther et al., 2005). In particular, NF-κB activation induces expression of chemokines such as monocyte chemotactic factor (MCP-1), and adhesion molecules such as vascular and intercellular adhesion molecules (VCAM-1 and ICAM-1), which serve to recruit circulating monocytes and facilitate their process of transmigration through the endothelial barrier into the subendothelial space (de Winther et al., 2005) (Fig. 1). In addition, NF-κB activation plays a role in reorganizing tight and adherens junctions, which represent the glue connecting one endothelial cell to the next (Aveleira et al., 2010). Alteration in tight junctions can then influence the permeability of the endothelial layer to serum proteins and lipids. Finally, NF-κB activation has a complex role in controlling various aspects of NO production, and vice versa (Csiszar et al., 2008; Farmer and Kennedy, 2009; Laroux et al., 2001). As such, factors that act on endothelial cells to induce NF-κB represent important players in the initiation of atherogenesis.

### 2.2 Fatty streak

The fatty streak is a waxy yellow deposit in the subendothelial space that represents the first grossly visual evidence of atherogenesis (Packard and Libby, 2008). The fatty streak is formed by the accumulation of lipid and lipid-laden macrophages, also known as foam cells, which are recruited during endothelial dysfunction to the intimal space. While these streaks typically develop into more advanced lesions, they do have the potential to involute and resolve, so that at least at this stage, the process of atherogenesis is a reversible one. Lipid residing in the intima, particularly when in an oxidized form (Ox-LDL), can act to further endothelial dysfunction, initiating a vicious cycle that perpetuates fatty streak formation and can lead to more advanced lesions (Packard and Libby, 2008). This occurs in part through activation of scavenger receptors on the basolateral surface of endothelial cells, including the lectin-like oxidized LDL receptor-1 (LOX-1) (Mitra et al., 2011). Among other effects, LOX-1 activation upregulates VCAM-1 and ICAM-1 leading to further monocyte recruitment, upregulates the receptor for Angiotensin II (AGTR1), and increases release of reactive oxygen species (ROS) which cause further oxidation of LDL particles (Mitra et al., 2011).

### 2.3 Intermediate lesion

As the plaque progresses, there is further expansion of the intimal space with lipid and macrophages. Other leukocytes, including lymphocytes and mast cells, begin to accumulate and play key regulatory roles (Hansson, 2005; Packard and Libby, 2008). In this stage, vascular smooth muscle cells (VSMCs) begin to proliferate and some migrate into the superficial intima, leaving their usual position in the media. This occurs in response to increasing concentrations of growth factors released from endothelial cells and inflammatory cells in the developing lesion. The VSMCs in turn contribute to plaque size through their proliferation and through production of extracellular matrix proteins (collagen, elastin, proteoglycans). However, it is these matrix proteins and VSMCs that together form a protective fibrous cap separating the inflammatory core of the plaque from the endothelial layer (Libby et al., 2011). Thus, the integrity of the fibrous cap is essential for maintaining a stable lesion. Also during this stage, the vessel undergoes compensatory remodelling in an effort to maintain luminal patency, although there is invariably a progressive stenosis (Rader and Daugherty, 2008). Part of the remodelling process includes the ingrowth of a neovascular network, extending from the vasa vasorum of the outer adventitial layer of the vessel into the central portion of plaque (Libby et al., 2011) (Fig. 1). While this neovascularization serves a stabilizing function by providing for adequate blood supply to the plaque, and preventing cellular hypoxia in this region, these newly formed vessels are also leaky, delicate, and prone to rupture. In this way, neovascularization represents a double-edged sword, simultaneously promoting and risking lesion stability.

### 2.4 Advanced/vulnerable lesion

With increasing cycles of lipid deposition and inflammation, the plaque becomes progressively unstable and prone to rupture due to a multitude of factors. The lipid core may become necrotic, leading to release of cytotoxic substances and cellular debris. Hemorrhage of the lipid core microvasculature may occur, leading to intra-lesional thrombosis and production of pro-inflammatory molecules including thrombin. These effects attract more leukocytes to further weaken the plaque (Libby et al., 2011).

Ultimately, it is the integrity of the surface endothelial lining of the plaque that represents the greatest clinical concern. Any damage to these endothelial cells may then lead to exposure of the extracellular matrix to circulating blood. This includes the exposure of tissue factor (TF), which triggers the coagulation cascade and can lead to life-threatening local thrombosis. Damage to the endothelium may occur via processes occurring in the vessel lumen, for example as a consequence of shear stresses induced by hypertension and plasma turbulence. Alternatively, damage may come from below, as a consequence of inflammation in the plaque. Ongoing inflammation within the lipid core weakens the fibrous cap, in part because inflammatory cells release proteases that degrade the extracellular matrix. For example, macrophages release matrix metalloproteinase 9 (MMP-9), which alone is sufficient to induce rupture of advanced lesions in mice (Gough et al., 2006). T lymphocytes uniquely contribute to plaque instability via the production of IFN-γ which then downregulates VSMC matrix production (Packard and Libby, 2008). Thus, lesions that are most susceptible to rupture are those that have been weakened over time by the action of matrix-degrading proteases and have a paucity of VSMCs to provide a protective barrier separating the lipid core from surface endothelial cells (Libby et al., 2011).

## 3. Specific GPCR agonists as contributors to vascular inflammation

The GPCR family represents the largest family of cell surface receptors, and includes over 800 known members (Dorsam and Gutkind, 2007; Lappano and Maggiolini, 2011). GPCRs are structurally defined by an extracellular N-terminal tail, seven trans-membrane domains linked together by 6 alternating intracellular and extracellular loops, and a C-terminal tail (Strader et al., 1994). Members of this receptor family respond to a diverse array of ligands including peptides, amines, glycoproteins and enzymes. The receptors relay extracellular signals by activating multiple intracellular signaling pathways which include those for ERK, Akt, JNK, p38MAPK, STAT, and NF-κB activation, to name only a few (Dorsam and Gutkind, 2007; Lappano and Maggiolini, 2011). Several GPCR agonists have been identified as key regulators of both endothelial cell function and atherogenesis. Below we discuss three such agonists that play particularly prominent roles in the pathophysiologic stages of atherogenesis.

### 3.1 Angiotensin II

Angiotensin II (Ang II) is a GPCR agonist, long known for its classic role in controlling blood pressure through regulating vascular smooth muscle tension, influencing renal reabsorption of sodium and water, and through stimulating aldosterone release from the adrenal. However, in recent years our understanding of this peptide hormone has broadened, and it is now appreciated that Ang II exerts a much wider spectrum of responses (Luft, 2001). In particular, Ang II is now appreciated for its profound pro-inflammatory effects, exerted on both endothelial and smooth muscle cells of the vasculature (Phillips and Kagiyama, 2002). Through this role, Ang II is thought to promote atherogenesis via mechanisms that are independent from its impact on blood pressure. Consistent with this notion, animal models of Ang II-dependent atherosclerosis, as well as large clinical trials investigating angiotensin converting enzyme (ACE) inhibitors or AGTR1 blockers (eg, HOPE, EUROPA, and LIFE), have demonstrated that the contribution of Ang II to atherogenesis cannot be explained solely by its ability to promote hypertension (Bertrand, 2004; Ferrario and Strawn, 2006; Kintscher et al., 2004). Instead, there is emerging evidence that perhaps the greatest impact of Ang II lies in its ability to directly induce pro-inflammatory signal transduction.

AGTR1 is expressed on both endothelial cells and VSMCs (Brasier et al., 2002). In addition, all the components of a local renin-angiotensin system (RAS) exist within the vasculature, so that Ang II can be locally produced and act in an autocrine or paracrine fashion, supplementing the effects of systemically circulating Ang II (Sata and Fukuda, 2010). Although Ang II influences numerous aspects of endothelial cell physiology, at least four categories of genes are induced that contribute to atherogenesis (Fig. 2). These include **1)** genes whose products promote recruitment and activation of monocytes and other inflammatory cells (eg, chemokines, cytokines, and adhesion molecules such as MCP-1, IL-6, IL-8, ICAM-1, VCAM-1, and E-selectin), **2)** genes whose products destabilize plaque and promote both proliferation and migration of underlying VSMCs (eg, MMP-9, PAI-1, and IGF-1R), **3)** genes whose products mediate endothelial dysfunction, particularly in the presence of oxidized LDL (eg, LOX-1), and **4)** genes encoding secondary cytokines that can feed back to ECs and VSMCs, further enhancing the pro-inflammatory milieu (eg, TNFα, Il-1β) (Fig. 2) (Brasier et al., 2002; de Winther et al., 2005; Pober and Sessa, 2007). Importantly, activation of LOX-1 sets in motion a destructive feed-forward cycle, whereby it enhances the expression of both AGTR1 and angiotensin converting enzyme (ACE) (Li et al., 2000; Li et al., 2003). This in turn results in enhanced local production of Ang II (Fig. 2). As will be discussed, all the above are NF-κB regulated genes, highlighting NF-κB activation as a key pro-atherogenic signaling event.

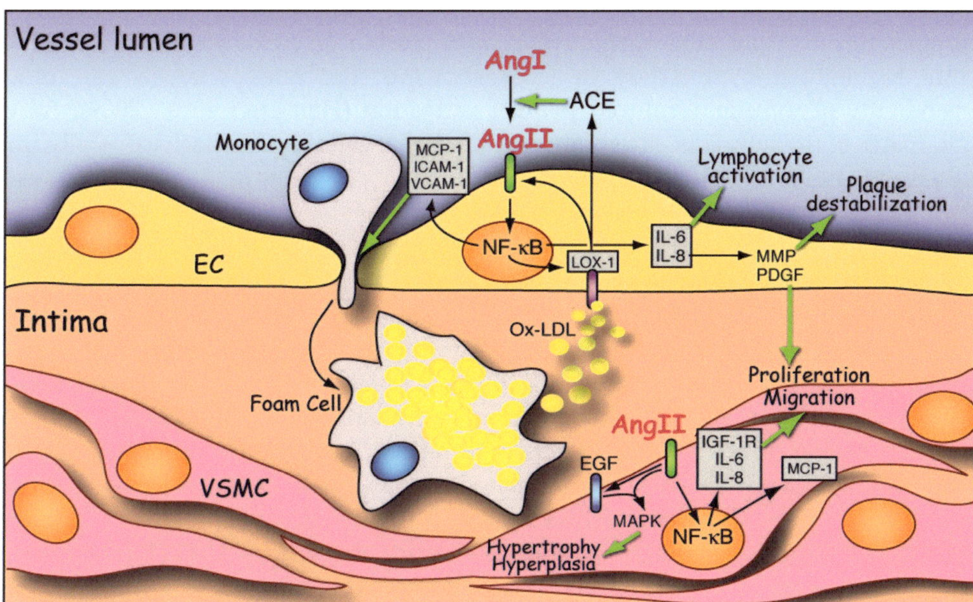


Fig. 2. Pleiotropic effects of Ang II on vascular pathophysiology.

Ang II, either made locally within the vessel wall or present following diffusion from the vessel lumen, can also act on VSMCs. Here, AGTR1 activation results in many of the same pro-inflammatory responses that are seen in endothelial cells. Additionally, MAPK pathways are activated, partly through transactivation of EGF receptors, thereby promoting the hypertrophy and hyperplasia of VSMCs that is characteristic of atherosclerotic lesions (Fig. 2) (Eguchi et al., 1998; Ohtsu et al., 2006; Saito and Berk, 2001).

### 3.2 Thrombin

Thrombin is known historically for its role in the clotting cascade. Active thrombin is generated from the inactive precursor, prothrombin, via cleavage by a complex consisting of factor Xa and factor Va, assembled through the actions of tissue factor (TF) (Borissoff et al., 2011). Thrombin then plays a role in generating a stable clot, in part through cleaving fibrinogen to produce fibrin, and through its actions on platelets. However, as is the case for Ang II, there is increasing appreciation for the receptor-mediated, pro-inflammatory effects of thrombin. Unlike most GPCR agonists, thrombin is a serine protease and acts on its cognate receptors through an unusual mechanism. The best studied thrombin receptor on endothelial cells is perhaps the protease activated receptor-1 (PAR-1) (Borissoff et al., 2009). In this case, thrombin binds to an extracellular hirudin-like domain on PAR-1 and cleaves the receptor at a specific site, exposing a cryptic ligand, SFLLRN, present near the N-terminal tail of the receptor. The newly exposed amino acid sequence acts as a tethered ligand by binding to a pocket on extracellular loop 2 and permanently activating the receptor (Borissoff et al., 2009). A synthetic peptide with the same SFLLRN sequence, also known as TRAP-6, can be used to induce the same response from PAR-1 as thrombin (Coughlin, 2005).

Both PAR-1 and its agonist thrombin are major participants in the regulation of endothelial cell biology and atherogenesis, affecting cell signaling, gene expression, endothelial permeability, angiogenesis, and vascular tone (Hirano, 2007). Indeed, the importance of direct pro-atherogenic effects of thrombin on cells of the vessel wall were recently highlighted by a study in mice showing that atherosclerosis can proceed independently of thrombin-induced platelet activation (Hamilton et al., 2009). As with Ang II, many of the effects of thrombin on endothelial cells can be mechanistically linked to NF-κB activation.

### 3.3 IL-8

A vast array of chemokines and associated GPCRs exist that influence vascular biology (Rosenkilde and Schwartz, 2004). For the purposes of this review, we highlight only one, IL-8 (CXCL8), because of the recent work demonstrating parallels between the molecular signaling pathways activated by IL-8 and those activated by both Ang II and thrombin (Martin et al., 2009). IL-8 is a CXC chemokine with many immunomodulatory functions and a broad range of biological effects. The effects of IL-8 are mediated primarily through CXCR2, a GPCR that is expressed on a broad range of cells, including endothelial cells (Rosenkilde and Schwartz, 2004). IL-8 is upregulated within developing atherosclerotic lesions, in part due to the stimulatory effect of Ox-LDL (Braunersreuther et al., 2007). Among its many effects, IL-8 induces expression of vascular endothelial growth factor (VEGF), which is synthesized and released by endothelial cells and can act in an autocrine/paracrine fashion to induce angiogenesis within the lipid core and to increase vascular permeability (Gavard et al., 2009). As with Ang II and thrombin, many of the pro-inflammatory effects of IL-8 can be attributed to the activation of NF-κB. In particular, IL-8 induction of the *VEGF* gene occurs through NF-κB binding sites in its promoter (Martin et al., 2009). See Table 1 for a summary of several pro-atherogenic effects of IL-8, and other GPCR agonists, that have been ascribed to NF-κB activation.

| GPCR | Affected cell type in plaque | NF-κB related pro-atherogenic effects |
|---|---|---|
| Angiotensin II Type 1 receptor | Endothelial cells | • Release of pro-inflammatory cytokines<br>• Recruitment and activation of inflammatory cells<br>• Destabilization of plaque |
| | VSMCs | • Proliferation and migration into plaque |
| CXCR2 (IL-8 receptor) | Endothelial cells | • Expression of VEGF<br>• Promotion of plaque neovascularization<br>• Enhancement of vascular permeability |
| Protease Activated Receptor-1 (thrombin receptor) | Endothelial cells | • Recruitment of inflammatory cells<br>• Enhancement of vascular permeability<br>• Promotion of plaque neovascularization<br>• Stimulation of vasoconstriction |

Table 1. Selected effects of three GPCRs and their ligands on atherogenesis.

## 4. GPCR connectivity to NF-κB

For ligand activated GPCRs, many, but not all, signaling events are initiated through the activation of heterotrimeric G proteins (Dorsam and Gutkind, 2007; Lappano and Maggiolini, 2011). The cytoplasmic loops within GPCRs serve to recruit these G proteins, consisting of α, β, and γ subunits. Upon agonist binding, the receptors promote exchange of GDP for GTP on the Gα subunit, leading to its dissociation from the Gβγ subunits. Both GTP-bound Gα and Gβγ subunits are then able to stimulate a range of downstream effectors. At least part of the specificity in receptor signaling stems from the fact that there are numerous Gα subtypes, broadly grouped into four classes ($G\alpha_s$, $G\alpha_i$, $G\alpha_{q/11}$, and $G\alpha_{12/13}$), and GPCRs will preferentially couple to certain subtypes (Dorsam and Gutkind, 2007; Lappano and Maggiolini, 2011).

Receptors that couple to $G\alpha_{q/11}$ are known to activate protein kinase C (PKC) isoforms through G protein-dependent stimulation of phospholipase C, $Ca^{2+}$ mobilization, and DAG generation. These include receptors for agonists described above (Ang II, thrombin, IL-8) as well as others that potentially influence endothelial biology in the context of atherogenesis, including endothelin-1, lysophosphatidic acid (LPA), and SDF-1/CXCL12 . For some time, it has been clear that PKC activation by select GPCRs is a prerequisite for subsequent NF-κB activation, but we are only now beginning to unravel the specific mechanistic links between PKC and the NF-κB machinery. In order to discuss these links, we will first briefly review the salient features of the NF-κB family of transcription factors, and their regulation. For a more nuanced treatment, the reader is referred to one of the more complete reviews of the topic (Hayden and Ghosh, 2008; Oeckinghaus and Ghosh, 2009; Vallabhapurapu and Karin, 2009).

### 4.1 The NF-κB family

The NF-κB family denotes a group of five transcription factors and includes the proteins RelA (p65), RelB, c-Rel, NF-κB1 (p105/50), and NF-κB2 (p100/52) (Oeckinghaus and Ghosh, 2009). All share a highly conserved Rel homology domain (RHD) which directs their dimerization, nuclear localization, and DNA binding activities (Oeckinghaus and Ghosh, 2009). Upon entering the nucleus, NF-κB subunits bind to the NF-κB consensus sequence, GGPuNNPyPyCC, present within the regulatory regions of target genes. Along with an array of co-factors, NF-κB transcription factors are able to induce or repress transcription of a wide variety of genes. Several pathways exist for activating NF-κB, depending upon the specific cellular stimulus, and this affects which NF-κB subunits are recruited into action.

### 4.2 The canonical NF-κB signaling pathway

In the unstimulated cell, the canonical NF-κB subunits, RelA and p50, stand at the ready in the cytoplasm, retained there by a family of regulatory proteins termed inhibitors of κB (IκBs). These IκB proteins conceal the nuclear localization sequences on RelA and p50, preventing their nuclear translocation. Various stimuli, including ligands for the TNF, interleukin, Toll-like, and antigen receptor families, act to induce intracellular signaling pathways that culminate in activation of the chief canonical regulatory complex, termed the IκB kinase (IKK) complex (Fig. 3A). The IKK complex is composed of three principal subunits, one regulatory subunit (NEMO/IKKγ), and two catalytic subunits (IKKα and IKKβ) (Oeckinghaus and Ghosh, 2009). Once activated, the catalytic subunits, particularly IKKβ, phosphorylate IκBs, leading to their ubiquitination and proteosomal degradation. This frees the RelA/p50 complex for nuclear translocation and transcriptional regulation.

While the steps leading from IKK activation to IκB phosphorylation and degradation are well-conserved, no matter what the stimulus, specificity is built into the system in that different receptors use vastly different signaling mechanisms for communicating with the IKK complex (dotted lines in Fig. 3A). It is in dissecting these "private pathways" for IKK activation that much of the recent progress in NF-κB research has been made. This is a crucial area of discovery, since identifying molecules that specifically mediate IKK activation in response to selected receptor ligands may allow for development of pharmaceuticals that interrupt (or enhance) the response to those ligands and not others. This could be a critically important area of discovery since general inhibition of NF-κB can have substantial negative side-effects including the initiation of a generalized state of immunodeficiency, or impairment of growth/development.

### 4.3 The non-canonical (alternative) NF-κB signaling pathway

A distinct set of stimuli, including CD40 ligand, BAFF, and lymphotoxin-β, work to activate a second set of NF-κB subunits (Oeckinghaus and Ghosh, 2009). Activation of their cognate receptors causes phosphorylation of p100, in complex with its partner, RelB (Fig. 3B). This occurs through the kinase activity of IKKα, but does not require the other components of the IKK complex. Instead, IKKα activation requires the upstream activation of NF-κB inducing kinase (NIK), which serves not only to phosphorylate and activate IKKα, but also appears to assist in recruiting p100. Once phosphorylated, p100 undergoes partial proteolysis, producing p52, and it is the RelB/p52 complex that is active as a regulator of transcription. Thus, in essence the p100 precursor acts much the same as an IκB, preventing non-canonical NF-κB activity. An area of intense interest relates to the question of whether the non-canonical NF-κB complex of RelB/p52 regulates a distinct set of genes from those regulated by RelA/p50. Importantly, while GPCRs are known to stimulate the canonical pathway, their potential for activating non-canonical signaling remains to be elucidated.

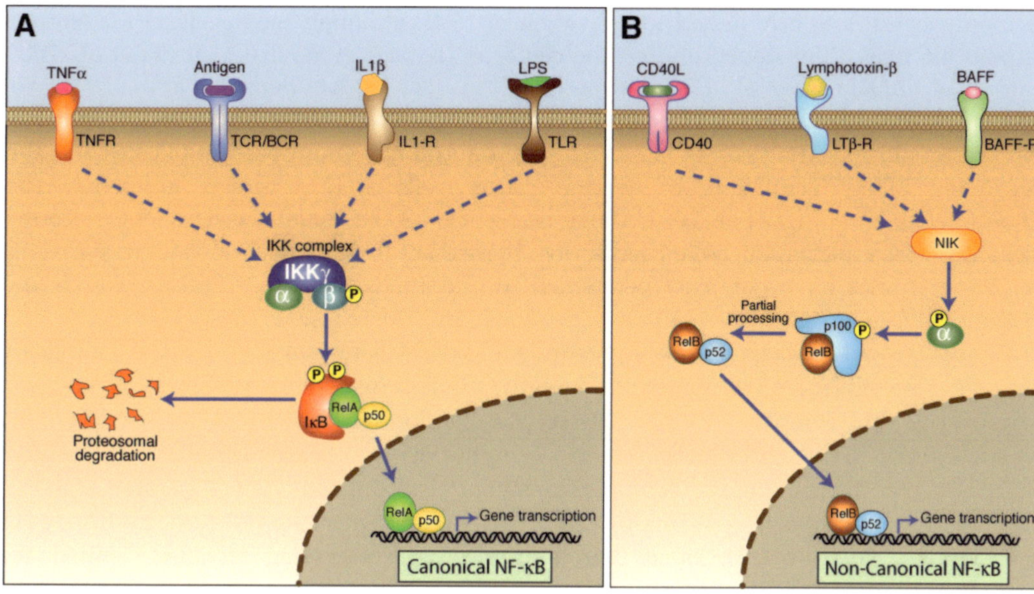


Fig. 3. Distinct pathways for canonical and non-canonical NF-κB activation.

### 4.4 Unique/emerging NF-κB signaling pathways

Although the canonical and non-canonical pathways for NF-κB activation have historically received the most attention, it is clear that several other mechanisms are in place for activating NF-κB subunits. Bearing in mind that several different NF-κB heterodimer complexes have been identified, it is likely that our understanding of alternative routes for NF-κB activation will only grow as the regulation of these complexes is explored in more detail. For example, recent work in B cells has demonstrated that c-Rel/p50 heterodimers can be regulated by a unique, non-proteosome dependent pathway for IκB degradation (O'Connor et al., 2004). Further, kinases other than IKKβ have been identified that can act to phosphorylate IκB proteins, leading to their degradation (McElhinny et al., 1996; Schwarz et al., 1996). Finally, other levels of control exist beyond the simple degradation of IκB proteins. Several groups have shown that NF-κB subunits are targets of secondary modification, including phosphorylation and acetylation, alterations that can affect their ability to interact with both DNA consensus sites and transcriptional co-regulators. Thus, as the body of experimental data grows, it will no doubt become obvious that the concepts of canonical and non-canonical activation, outlined above and in Fig. 3, represent only a framework for a much more complicated system of regulation.

### 4.5 GPCR dependent NF-κB signaling

Activation of certain GPCRs expressed on vascular cells, including the receptors for Ang II, thrombin, and IL-8, leads to all the hallmarks of canonical NF-κB activation. Although the precise mechanisms underlying this response have been unclear, it has long been appreciated that canonical activation requires proximal stimulation of PKC (Fraser, 2008). For example, Ang II induction of NF-κB in both endothelial cells, VSMCs, and cardiomyocytes is tightly linked to activation of PKC, although the specific PKC isoform responsible may differ depending on the cell type (Brasier et al., 2000; Hiroki et al., 2004; Kalra et al., 2002; Liao et al., 1997; Parmentier et al., 2006; Rouet-Benzineb et al., 2000). For PAR-1, PKCδ is known as the primary PKC mediating NF-κB activation in endothelial cells (Minami et al., 2004; Rahman et al., 2001). PKCα and δ have both been implicated in LPA-dependent NF-κB activation, in ovarian cancer cells and in airway epithelial cells, respectively (Cummings et al., 2004; Mahanivong et al., 2008). Finally, several PKC isoforms, including PKCα and PKCβ, have been shown to mediate IL-8/CXCR2-dependent signaling, but these studies have not been performed in endothelial cells or VSMCs (Waugh and Wilson, 2008).

In that upstream PKC activation is a prerequisite for GPCR-responsive NF-κB signaling, we and others recognized a parallel theme with the antigen-responsive activation of NF-κB in lymphocytes. In B lymphocytes, antigen receptor ligation induces PKCβ, and this is critical for subsequent NF-κB activation, while in T lymphocytes it is PKCθ that is crucial (Lucas et al., 2004). Over the past decade, a tremendous volume of data has been generated to define the precise molecular steps linking PKC activation with the NF-κB machinery in lymphocytes. This work revealed that a multi-protein signaling complex, termed the CARMA1/Bcl10/MALT1 (CBM) signalosome serves as a molecular bridge between the two, and is necessary for lymphocytes to mount a normal, NF-κB-dependent immune response to antigenic challenge (Lucas et al., 2004; Thome, 2004; Wegener and Krappmann, 2007). Taking cues from the lymphocyte field, we and others worked to define a novel molecular pathway that explains how GPCR-dependent PKC activation can result in NF-κB signaling. This pathway utilizes an analogous CBM signalosome, present in cells outside of the immune system, and is detailed in the next section.

It is important to note, however, that the discovery of a GPCR-responsive CBM signalosome must be viewed in the larger context of GPCR signaling, with the realization that other signaling pathways are active, some of which may influence NF-κB through independent mechanisms. For example, Brasier and colleagues have uncovered a distinct mechanism by which ligand-activated AGTR1 induces RelA in VSMCs (Brasier, 2010). In these cells, substantial levels of RelA are found inactive in the nucleus under resting conditions. Ang II stimulation induces a pathway of RhoA and NIK activation, culminating in NIK-dependent phosphorylation of the nuclear RelA species on serine 536 (Choudhary et al., 2007; Cui et al., 2006). This phosphorylated pool of RelA is free from IκB regulation and dynamically cycles through the nucleus, interacting with target genes (Bosisio et al., 2006; Sasaki et al., 2005). This mechanism of regulation has been shown to impact the NF-κB responsive, *IL-6* gene. Consistent with this observation, we have seen only a partial effect of blocking the CBM signalosome on Ang II-dependent IL-6 induction, underscoring the concept that different NF-κB responsive genes may respond to different NF-κB transcription factor complexes and/or different modes of NF-κB regulation.

## 5. The CARMA3/Bcl10/MALT1 signalosome; missing link for GPCR activity

### 5.1 Lessons learned from lymphocytes

CARMA1 (also known as Bimp3/CARD11) is a member of the membrane-associated guanylate kinase (MAGUK) superfamily of molecular scaffolds that each utilize multiple discrete protein interaction domains to cluster receptors and cytosolic signaling molecules at the cell membrane (Dimitratos et al., 1999; Fanning and Anderson, 1999). As such, all MAGUKS contain three defining interactions domains: the PSD-95/Dlg/ZO-1 homologous (PDZ) domain, the Src-homology (SH3) domain, and the guanylate kinase (GUK)-like domain (Fig. 4A). CARMA1 is expressed exclusively in lymphocytes, and a few related cells of the immune system, and is one of three known members of the CARMA subfamily. This subfamily is distinguished from members of other MAGUK subfamilies by the presence of additional coiled-coil and caspase recruitment (CARD) domains.

Numerous biochemical and genetic studies have now definitively established that CARMA1 is an essential component of the antigen-induced NF-κB signaling pathway in T cells. Data indicate that CARMA1 acts as a molecular bridge, linking PKC activation with stimulation of the downstream signaling proteins, Bcl10 and MALT1 (Fig. 4B) (Lucas et al., 2004). Together, CARMA1, Bcl10, and MALT1 form a complex (referred to as the CBM signalosome) that is recruited to the lymphocyte immunological synapse following receptor engagement. In this complex, the small Bcl10 protein appears to function as an adaptor, capable of oligomerizing MALT1. Finally, MALT1 acts as an effector subunit by stimulating IKKγ, the IKK regulatory subunit, in part through promoting its K63-linked ubiquitination (Sun et al., 2004; Zhou et al., 2004). This subsequently leads to activation of the catalytic subunits, IKKα and IKKβ, thereby allowing them to phosphorylate IκB and free NF-κB for nuclear transport. The details as to how MALT1 achieves regulation of the IKK complex are still unfolding, with the current dogma suggesting that the process includes a coordinated series of K63-linked ubiquitination events, not only of IKKγ but of several other proteins in the complex, as well as IKKβ phosphorylation, probably via the kinase TAK1.

A second mechanism of action for MALT1 has recently emerged and gained considerable attention. This relates to the discovery that MALT1 is a substrate-specific protease (McAllister-Lucas and Lucas, 2008). Although such enzymatic activity has long been postulated, based on recognition of a "caspase-like" active site in the C-terminus of MALT1 (Uren et al., 2000), it wasn't until only recently that substrates for MALT1 cleavage were identified. So far, three have been identified, and their cleavage sites mapped (Coornaert et al., 2008; Rebeaud et al., 2008; Staal et al., 2011). Two of the substrates, A20 and CYLD, are deubiquitinases, known for their ability to dampen NF-κB signaling through their ubiquitin editing functions, affecting various players in the NF-κB machinery. Thus, by targeting these two proteins for cleavage, it is thought that MALT1 proteolytic activity serves to maximize the level of NF-κB activation, following antigen stimulation of lymphocytes. Indeed, cleavage of A20 leads to loss of its inhibitory effect and magnified antigen-dependent NF-κB activation (Coornaert et al., 2008). In theory, the same could occur with cleavage of CYLD, although initial work has only shown an impact on the related JNK pathway (Staal et al., 2011).

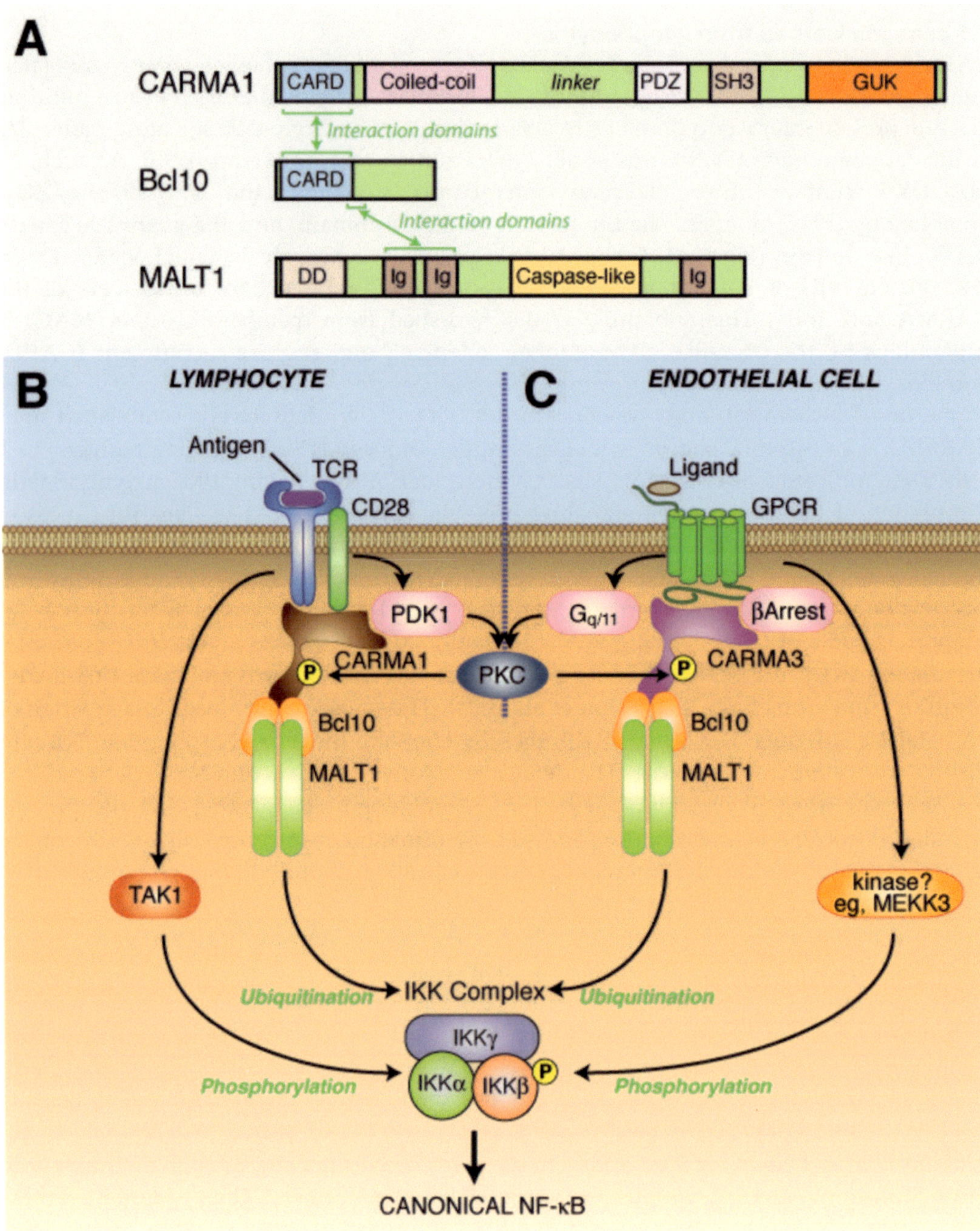


Fig. 4. A, Schematic diagram of proteins that make up the CBM signalosome. B and C, Similarities and differences exist between the mechanisms through which the CARMA1- and CARMA3-containing signalosomes act to stimulate the IKK complex; see text for description.

Many of the details concerning how the CBM complex is recruited and activated at the T cell immunological synapse have become clear only recently. First, Ghosh and co-workers demonstrated that, following T cell receptor stimulation, the enzyme 3-phosphoinositide-dependent kinase 1 (PDK1) serves to anchor both activated PKCθ and CARMA1 within close proximity to one another, at the immunological synapse (Fig. 4B) (Lee et al., 2005). PDK1 is a kinase known to phosphorylate PKC at a specific site within its "activation loop" (Belham et al., 1999; Mora et al., 2004; Newton, 2001, 2003). This phosphorylation appears to serve as a priming reaction, allowing PKC to then respond to activating signals, such as $Ca^{2+}$ or DAG, depending on the specific isoform. However, the ability of PDK1 to interact with CARMA1 represents a newly defined role for this kinase. Although PDK1 plays a key role in recruiting the CBM signalosome to the T cell receptor, it may not represent the only molecular link; for example, recent work has demonstrated that the protein ADAP is also crucial in this regard (Medeiros et al., 2007).

A second major finding was that PKC acts to phosphorylate specific sites within the linker region of CARMA1, which resides between the CARD/coiled-coil domains and the domains present in all MAGUK proteins (PDZ/SH3/GUK) (Matsumoto et al., 2005; Sommer et al., 2005). This appears to result in a conformational change in CARMA1, allowing for exposure of the CARD domain (Sommer et al., 2005). Consequently, Bcl10 and MALT1 can then be effectively recruited to the immunological synapse because their recruitment depends primarily on a CARD-CARD interaction between CARMA1 and Bcl10. Finally, the IKK complex is recruited and can thereby be activated by the fully assembled CBM complex (Shinohara et al., 2005; Stilo et al., 2004; Weil et al., 2003). It should be noted that the majority of the work defining the mechanism of action of the CBM signalosome has been carried out using T cell models. Interestingly, not all of the concepts are likely to hold true for B cells. In particular, based on phenotypic differences between *MALT1*$^{-/-}$ mice and *BCL10*$^{-/-}$ or *CARMA1*$^{-/-}$ mice, there is some debate as to whether MALT1 is an obligate player in B cell receptor-dependent NF-κB activation.

### 5.2 CARMA3, a CARMA homologue expressed in cells outside the immune system

Except for CARMA1, the key molecules mediating antigen-dependent NF-κB activation in lymphocytes are ubiquitously expressed in a diverse array of cells. However, we and others had noted that a highly related protein, CARMA3 (Bimp1/CARD10), is expressed more broadly than the immune cell-specific CARMA1 (McAllister-Lucas et al., 2001; Wang et al., 2001b). The *CARMA1* and *CARMA3* genes encode proteins that are highly similar; the CARDS and coiled-coil domains share approximately 60% and 50% sequence identity with one another, respectively, while the PDZ, SH3 and GUK domains share approximately 20-30% identity. The functional similarities between CARMA3 and CARMA1 are illustrated by the fact that CARMA3 can rescue antigen-induced NF-κB activation in CARMA1-deficient T cells (Matsumoto et al., 2005). Of potential importance to cardiovascular pathophysiology, all three proteins of a putative CARMA3-containing CBM complex are abundant in heart and aorta, and western blotting confirms their presence in those tissues at the protein level (McAllister-Lucas et al., 2010; McAllister-Lucas et al., 2007). As a result, we wondered if CARMA3 might scaffold an analogous CBM signalosome in cells outside the immune system. The known dependence on PKC activation for GPCR-responsive NF-κB stimulation led to the hypothesis that specific GPCRs might represent candidates for receptors that could communicate with CARMA3 and it associated signaling molecules.

Using distinct systems and approaches, we and two other groups simultaneously demonstrated that two GPCRs could harness a CARMA3-containing CBM signalosome for the purposes of NF-κB activation (Klemm et al., 2007; McAllister-Lucas et al., 2007; Wang et al., 2007) (Fig. 4C). Our group demonstrated the essential role of CARMA3, Bcl10, and MALT1 in the Ang II-dependent activation of canonical NF-κB (McAllister-Lucas et al., 2007). This initial work focused on hepatocytes as a model, but subsequent work demonstrated that the same CBM machinery is active in endothelial cells following Ang II stimulation (McAllister-Lucas et al., 2010). Individually knocking down each component of the putative CARMA3/Bcl10/MALT1 complex completely blocked Ang II-dependent IκB phosphorylation, a marker of canonical NF-κB activation, or induction of an NF-κB responsive reporter gene. In addition, expression of a dominant negative mutant of CARMA3 was sufficient to impair Ang II-dependent K63-linked IKKγ polyubiquitination.

The other two studies focused on mouse embryonic fibroblasts (MEFs) from *BCL10*$^{-/-}$ and *MALT1*$^{-/-}$ mouse strains. In contrast to wild-type MEFs, these knockout cells showed a complete lack of NF-κB activation when stimulated with lysophosphatidic acid (LPA) (Klemm et al., 2007; Wang et al., 2007). Follow-up work revealed the same phenomenon with *CARMA3*$^{-/-}$ MEFs (Grabiner et al., 2007). Like the receptor for Ang II (AGTR1), receptors for LPA ($LPA_{1-4}$) are prototypical GPCRs, coupled primarily with $G\alpha_{q/11}$ subunits. With regard to pathophysiology, LPA receptor-induced NF-κB activation has been linked to a variety of consequences, depending upon the cell type affected, which include the promotion of carcinoma cell survival and spread, as well as endothelial dysfunction. However, despite the potential importance of the CBM complex in mediating LPA-dependent effects in endothelial cells or VSMCs, studies have yet to be published that specifically link LPA receptors to the CBM components in the vasculature.

Following these initial studies, several groups have added to the list of GPCRs capable of harnessing the CARMA3-containing CBM signalosome. To date, however, the only receptors that have been specifically shown to utilize the signalosome in endothelial cells are those for Ang II (AGTR1), thrombin (PAR-1) and IL-8 (CXCR2) (Delekta et al., 2010; Martin et al., 2009; McAllister-Lucas et al., 2010).

### 5.3 Distinct mechanisms for recruiting CARMA1- and CARMA3-containing signalosomes

Although there are strong parallels between the mechanisms underlying recruitment and activation of the CARMA1-containing CBM signalosome of lymphocytes and the CARMA3-containing CBM signalosome of endothelial cells, there are also notable differences. Most striking are the differences in how the signalosomes communicate with their cognate receptors. We have already described work demonstrating a crucial role for PDK1 in scaffolding an interaction with antigen receptors in the T cell. In contrast, PDK1 may have no role in coordinating GPCR-dependent CBM assembly; at least for PAR-1, knockdown of PDK1 in endothelial cells has no effect on thrombin-dependent NF-κB activation (Delekta et al., 2010). Instead, we and others have implicated β-arrestin 2 as a protein that could serve the function of scaffolding CARMA3 to select GPCRs (Delekta et al., 2010; Sun and Lin, 2008).

Traditionally, the β-arrestin proteins have been known for their role in down-regulating activated GPCRs through receptor endocytosis, leading to their recycling or degradation. Activated GPCRs are phosphorylated by various G protein receptor kinases (GRKs), which then allows recruitment of arrestins to the receptors. This helps to uncouple G proteins from the receptors and assists in receptor internalization through clathrin-coated pits. But more recently, arrestins have become known as scaffold proteins that facilitate the recruitment and activation of a number of distinct secondary signaling molecules (DeFea, 2011). In this way, arrestins are now appreciated not just for their ability to terminate GPCR signaling, but also for their ability to promote a second layer of GPCR-dependent responses.

Lin and colleagues originally showed that β-arrestin 2 deficient MEFs were unable to respond to LPA treatment with an NF-κB signal (Sun and Lin, 2008). They then determined that β-arrestin 2 bound to CARMA3. Further, co-immunoprecipitation experiments demonstrated that CARMA3 could interact with the LPA receptor only when β-arrestin 2 was present to act as a bridge. Subsequent work showed that β-arrestin 2 deficient MEFs are also defective in thrombin-dependent NF-κB activation (Delekta et al., 2010). Thus, it is likely that for GPCR signaling, β-arrestin 2 serves a scaffolding role, analogous to what has been shown for PDK1 in the lymphocyte system (Fig. 4C).

Despite the progress that has been made in understanding the regulation of CARMA3-containing CBM signalosomes, much remains to be learned. The CARMA1-containing complex has been studied for a much longer period of time, and many of the finer details have been explored in more detail. For example, the sites of PKC-dependent CARMA1 phosphorylation, which allow for unfolding of CARMA1 and exposure of the CARD domain, have been mapped (Matsumoto et al., 2005; Sommer et al., 2005). In addition, other kinases have been identified that can positively or negatively regulate CARMA1 (Bidere et al., 2009; Brenner et al., 2009; Ishiguro et al., 2006; Shinohara et al., 2007). In contrast, mechanisms for regulation of CARMA3 remain mostly speculative at this time.

### 5.4 Distinct mechanisms for CARMA1- and CARMA3-dependent IKK activation

Another area of potential distinction, differentiating CARMA1- and CARMA3-containing signalosomes, relates to their ability to facilitate IKK complex phosphorylation, a necessary step for full IKK activation. As described previously, MALT1 is thought to play a major role as an "effector" protein in the CBM complex, coordinating the activation of the IKK complex. This occurs at least in part through the ability of MALT1 to direct multiple K63-linked ubiquitin modifications, targeting IKKγ, Bcl10, and even MALT1 itself. In the lymphocyte, these ubiquitin chains may then serve as a scaffold to recruit the kinase, TAK1, which completes the activation of the IKK complex through phosphorylation of IKKβ at specific residues within its activation loop (Shinohara et al., 2005; Wang et al., 2001a). As for the activation of TAK1, this appears to occur through a parallel pathway, initiated by the antigen receptor, that does not depend upon the CBM complex (Shambharkar et al., 2007) (Fig. 4B).

Interestingly, recent work has shown that TAK1 is dispensable for LPA-dependent NF-κB activation. Instead, another mitogen-activated protein kinase, MEKK3, takes its place (Sun et al., 2009). Thus, the ligand-activated LPA receptor induces a parallel pathway, independent of the CARMA3-containing CBM complex, that causes MEKK3 activation, subsequently leading to IKKβ phosphorylation (Fig. 4C). It remains an open question as to whether MEKK3 will be involved in IKK complex activation downstream of all GPCRs, or whether distinct kinases will act in concert with the CARMA3-containing CBM complex, depending on the specific GPCR being induced.

## 6. The CARMA3/Bcl10/MALT1 signalosome and endothelial phenotype

### 6.1 Role for endothelial NF-κB activation in atherogenesis

As discussed earlier, many pieces of evidence implicate endothelial cell NF-κB activation as an important GPCR-mediated signaling event favoring atherogenesis. Recently, this concept was reinforced by elegant studies using two related mouse models (Gareus et al., 2008). These researchers first generated an endothelial-specific *IKKγ*$^{-/-}$ mouse, to disrupt any NF-κB signaling in this cell type. These *IKKγ*$^{-/-}$ mice were crossed with a mouse model of atherosclerosis (*ApoE*$^{-/-}$) and fed a cholesterol-rich diet. After ten weeks, these mice showed a 30% reduction in plaque size, 40% reduction of T cells in plaques, and an overall retardation in the progression to advanced plaques as compared to *IKKγ*$^{+/+}$/*ApoE*$^{-/-}$ mice under the same diet. To further demonstrate the specific role of endothelial NF-κB in atherogenesis, an additional transgenic mouse model was created, expressing dominant negative IκBα (IκB-SR) under control of the Tie2 promoter. This effectively targeted expression of the dominant negative mutant to endothelial cells. Since the dominant negative mutant lacks phosphorylation acceptor sites for IKKβ, its expression effectively keeps NF-κB subunits sequestered in an inactive state, regardless of whether or not the cell is being stimulated by any of the classic NF-κB inducers. These mice were once again backcrossed with *ApoE*$^{-/-}$ mice and placed on a high cholesterol diet for ten weeks, after which they showed a 60% reduction in plaque size and a significant reduction in plaque progression as compared to *ApoE*$^{-/-}$ mice with normally functioning NF-κB (Gareus et al., 2008). The endothelium of IκB-SR/*ApoE*$^{-/-}$ mice was almost completely free from expression of most cytokines, chemokines and adhesion molecules. Taken together, this study provides exceptionally strong evidence that NF-κB activation within the endothelium alone is necessary to drive a significant atherogenesis response.

### 6.2 The GPCR-CBM-NF-κB axis in endothelial dysfunction and atherogenesis

To date, three GPCRs have been linked to the CBM signalosome and NF-κB activation, specifically in endothelial cells. These are the receptors for Ang II, thrombin, and IL-8. Others are sure to follow; for example, clear evidence exists for an important role for LPA receptor-dependent NF-κB activation in endothelial biology, but to date the connections between this receptor and the CBM signalosome have been explored only in cell models outside vascular biology. In the following sections, we describe the specific work that has been done to investigate the GPCR-CBM-NF-κB signaling axis in endothelial cells, focusing on the cellular and pathophysiologic consequences of activating this signaling axis.

#### 6.2.1 IL-8 and VEGF induction

Vascular endothelial growth factor (VEGF) is a key endothelial-specific growth factor that is induced in response to tissue damage. VEGF modulates endothelial cell phenotypes by inducing cell proliferation, promoting cell migration, and inhibiting apoptosis, and is regarded as a key regulator of angiogenesis (Ferrara et al., 2003). In atherogenesis, VEGF may play a role in promoting the pathologic ingrowth of the neovascular network from the vasa vasorum, into plaque developing in the subintimal space. These effects are mediated through VEGF binding to its own receptors, VEGFR-1/2 (Ferrara et al., 2003).

Under certain conditions such as tissue hypoxia, VEGF synthesis and secretion is regulated via activation of the transcription factor, hypoxia inducible factor-1 (HIF-1) (Semenza, 2007). Although hypoxia is a potent stimulus for VEGF expression, inflammatory cytokines have also been reported to stimulate VEGF expression through mechanisms that have not been fully delineated. One recent study, however, revealed that regulation of VEGF expression in endothelial cells can occur via CBM signalosome-mediated activation of NF-κB (Martin et al., 2009). These investigators showed that the pro-inflammatory cytokine IL-8 (CXCL8) stimulated VEGF production and secretion through activation of its cognate GPCR, CXCR2. This receptor, in turn, was linked to the CBM signaling complex and NF-κB activation. Importantly, the effect of IL-8 on VEGF induction was independent of HIF-1 but entirely dependent on NF-κB. Inhibition of any of the CBM components by siRNA was effective at reducing NF-κB activation and resulted in a marked inhibition of VEGF mRNA expression and protein secretion. Further, this was accompanied by decreased autocrine VEGFR2 activation. These results suggest that the CBM signalosome is necessary for regulating VEGF production in endothelial cells in response to certain inflammatory cytokines, and might indirectly contribute to the VEGF-dependent transition of the endothelium into a pro-angiogenic phenotype.

#### 6.2.2 Thrombin and endothelial cell/monocyte adhesion

As discussed earlier, thrombin and its receptor, PAR-1, are thought to induce a variety of pro-inflammatory responses that may also contribute to endothelial phenotype changes (Hirano, 2007). Thrombin levels are increased at sites of vascular injury and thrombosis, where the persistent stimulation of its receptor leads to endothelial dysfunction, thereby increasing inflammatory responses leading to further vessel wall damage and atherosclerotic lesion progression. One of the key responses to local thrombin production is the increase in endothelial cell expression of adhesion molecules, allowing for firm adhesion of circulating monocytes and other leukocytes (Minami et al., 2004). Our lab has specifically shown that thrombin-dependent activation of the CBM-NF-κB signaling axis in endothelial cells results in upregulation of two such adhesion molecules, VCAM-1 and ICAM-1, at both the mRNA and protein levels (Delekta et al., 2010). Further, we showed that thrombin-induced adhesion of monocytes to endothelial cells requires the intact CBM signalosome; siRNA-mediated knockdown of Bcl10 in endothelial cells altered their phenotype to completely abolish thrombin-dependent monocyte adherence. Further work will be required to test the role of the CBM proteins in modulating other aspects of thrombin-dependent endothelial dysfunction.

#### 6.2.3 Ang II and *in vivo* atherogenesis

Similar to thrombin, Ang II produced locally in the vasculature has been reported to induce a number of inflammatory responses, including the expression of NF-κB-sensitive adhesion molecules and cytokines in endothelial cells, and the recruitment of inflammatory cells to the vessel wall (Daugherty and Cassis, 2004). Our group recently showed that Ang II activation of its receptor, present on endothelial cells and on VSMCs, stimulates NF-κB through the CBM signalosome (McAllister-Lucas et al., 2010).

Further, we tested the effects of manipulating the signalosome *in vivo*. In these studies, we utilized the *ApoE*$^{-/-}$ mouse strain described earlier, which is hyperlipidemic and prone to developing atherosclerosis. The development of lesions, however, can be dramatically accelerated through infusion with Ang II, even at subpressor doses. When infusions are carried out for as little as 4 weeks, the mice develop prominent and premature atherosclerotic lesions, even in the absence of a high-fat diet; these can be visualized grossly by staining the intimal surfaces of the aorta with Oil-red-O, a stain that reacts to lipid-laden lesions (Fig. 5). This effect of Ang II infusion is generally accepted to be the result of its direct pro-inflammatory effects on the vessel wall, which conspires with hyperlipidemia to cause accelerated atherogenesis. We tested the role of the CBM signalosome by crossing *ApoE*$^{-/-}$ and *Bcl10*$^{-/-}$ mice to generate a double knock-out line (McAllister-Lucas et al., 2010). The absence of Bcl10 in the ApoE-deficient strain revealed a dramatic phenotype in which the mice were protected from developing Ang II-induced atherosclerosis and aortic aneurysms (Fig. 5). Additionally, the reduction in atherosclerotic lesions in aortas from *ApoE*$^{-/-}$/*Bcl10*$^{-/-}$ mice was associated with reduced aortic gene expression of several pro-inflammatory molecules, as compared to *ApoE*$^{-/-}$ mice infused with Ang II in the same way.

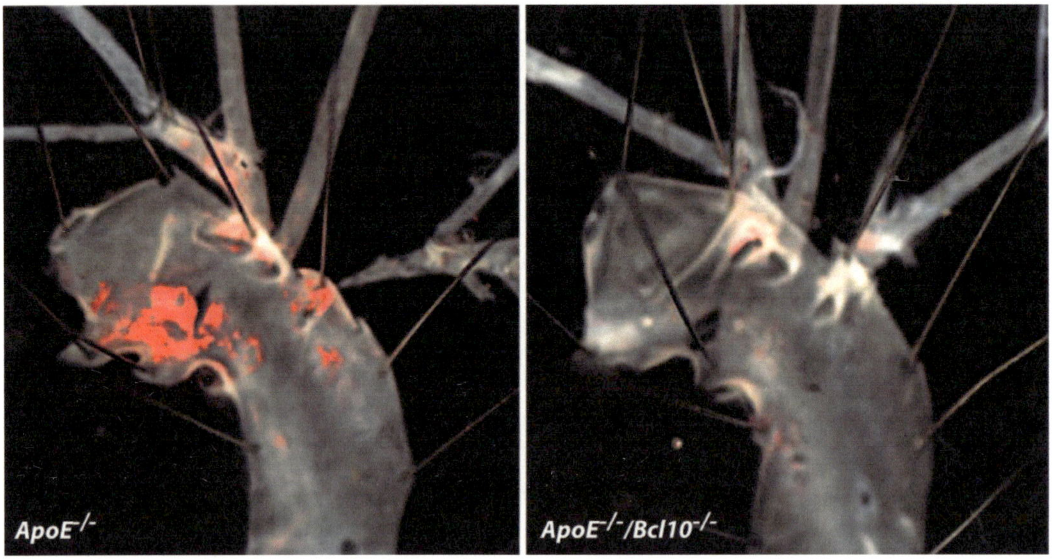


Fig. 5. Representative aortic arches from mice infused with Ang II for 4 weeks. Genotypes are as indicated. Aortas are stained with Oil-red-O to highlight lipid-laden intimal lesions (fatty streaks-advanced lesions). See text and McAllister-Lucas et al., 2010 for details.

### 6.2.4 LPA and the CBM signalosome in atherogenesis?

As mentioned, it is likely that other GPCRs will be linked to the CBM-NF-κB signaling axis in endothelial cells, since several have already been linked in this way through work on other cell types. In particular, the receptors for LPA are likely to harness the CBM proteins in endothelial cells, considering their prominent role in affecting endothelial cell biology. A new study by Schober and colleagues demonstrates that LPA, produced via oxidation of LDL particles, enhances atherosclerotic lesion formation in *ApoE*$^{-/-}$ mice (Zhou et al., 2011). This effect is mediated largely via LPA receptor-dependent elaboration of CXCL1 (GRO-α) on the surface of endothelial cells. CXCL1 is a chemokine that acts to promote monocyte recruitment to the endothelial wall, and thus plays a role in promoting atherogenesis. The authors showed that CXCL1 expression was in part NF-κB dependent. Thus, since LPA-stimulated NF-κB activation has been shown to require the CBM complex in MEFs and in ovarian cancer cells (Grabiner et al., 2007; Klemm et al., 2007; Mahanivong et al., 2008; Wang et al., 2007), it is likely that the same will hold true for endothelial cells.

## 7. Therapeutic opportunities

Identification of the CBM signalosome as a critical mediator of GPCR-dependent pro-inflammatory effects suggests that pharmaceutical targeting of the CBM proteins could represent a new strategy for preventing or treating atherosclerosis. Since disruption of the CBM signalosome blocks NF-κB activation and inflammatory signaling downstream of AGTR1, PAR-1, CXCR2 and probably other GPCRs within the vessel wall that contribute to endothelial dysfunction and atherogenesis, inhibiting vascular CBM activity may prove beneficial. Potential pharmaceutical approaches include: **1)** preventing specific upstream events that link GPCR stimulation to CBM activation, **2)** blocking key post-translational modifications of CBM components, and **3)** directly targeting the activity of CBM components themselves.

### 7.1 Upstream targets

The specific upstream molecular mechanisms by which GPCR stimulation promotes assembly and activation of the CBM have not yet been extensively investigated, and these mechanisms likely vary significantly depending on ligand, GPCR and cell type. However, there are some clues to potential therapeutic targets that could be critical for GPCR-induced CBM activation in the vasculature. For example, β–arrestin 2 associates with CARMA3, and studies thus far demonstrate that β–arrestin 2 is required for both LPA and thrombin to induce GPCR-dependent NF-κB activation (Delekta et al., 2010; Sun and Lin, 2008). Intriguingly, recent studies demonstrate that in VSMCs, β–arrestin 2 mediates AGTR1-dependent prevention of apoptosis and is required for both LPA and thrombin-induced vascular smooth muscle cell proliferation (Ahn et al., 2009; Kim et al., 2008). Furthermore, deficiency of β–arrestin 2 protects LDL receptor knockout (*ldlr*$^{-/-}$) mice from aortic atherosclerosis (Kim et al., 2008). Together, these studies suggest that somehow targeting β–arrestin 2 could represent a rational therapeutic strategy for preventing GPCR-dependent CBM activation and combating atherosclerosis. Precisely how to inhibit β–arrestin 2-dependent CBM activation remains to be investigated, but one potential approach would be to block GRK-mediated phosphorylation of GPCRs, thus preventing phosphorylation-dependent recruitment of β–arrestin 2 to the GPCR (DeFea, 2011). In addition, "G-protein-biased ligands" which selectively activate G-protein-mediated signaling downstream of specific GPCRs, while inhibiting β–arrestin-mediated signaling, are currently under development, and such agents may prove to be useful in modulating β–arrestin 2/CBM-dependent vascular inflammatory disease (Whalen et al., 2011).

### 7.2 Targets involved in CBM modification

In addition to β–arrestin 2-mediated recruitment of CARMA3, another critical step in GPCR-induced CBM activation that represents a potential therapeutic target is the PKC-mediated phosphorylation of CARMA3. As discussed above, T-cell receptor (TCR) or B-cell receptor (BCR) stimulation induces PKC-dependent phosphorylation of CARMA1, thus causing a conformational change that allows CARMA1 to recruit Bcl10/MALT1 to the receptor and form the CARMA1-Bcl10-MALT1 (CBM) complex (Matsumoto et al., 2005; Sommer et al., 2005). It is not yet known if a similar mechanism of PKC-induced CARMA3 phosphorylation occurs downstream of GPCRs, although it is well established that GPCR stimulation leads to phosphorylation and activation of various PKC isoforms and treatment with broad-spectrum PKC inhibitors can block GPCR-dependent NF-κB activation. However, a pharmaceutical approach targeting PKC in atherogenesis is likely to be complex (Ding et al., 2011), since as we described earlier, each GPCR may utilize distinct PKC isoforms to communicate with the CBM complex. Nevertheless, progress is being made on this front; a recent report demonstrated that treatment with the DAG/calcium-dependent PKC inhibitor, Go6976, and siRNA-mediated silencing of PKCα both blocked AGTR1-dependent NF-κB signaling in VSMCs (Doyon and Servant, 2010). Likewise, PKC inhibitors RO318220 and GF109203X have been shown to abrogate thrombin-dependent pro-inflammatory signaling in human aortic VSMCs (Chung et al., 2010). Perhaps the PKCβ isoform has been most thoroughly studied in the context of atherosclerosis. For example, genetic knockdown of PKCβ or treatment with the PKCβ inhibitor, ruboxistaurin, results in decreased atherosclerosis in ApoE-deficient mice (Harja et al., 2009), and this same PKC inhibitor has also been shown to reduce endothelial dysfunction in human patients (Mehta et al., 2009). Because there is much evidence supporting a critical role for PKCs in atherogenesis and there are multiple isoform-specific PKC inhibitors already available, it will be of great interest to determine whether inhibition of particular PKCs blocks CBM activation by specific GPCRs within the vasculature and whether these effects are associated with a pharmaceutical benefit in the setting of atherosclerosis.

Like PKC-mediated phosphorylation of CARMA3, other post-translational modifications of CBM components may be critical to GPCR-induced CBM activity and could therefore represent potential targets for pharmaceutical intervention in GPCR-driven atherosclerosis. In lymphocytes, several kinases and phosphatases have been implicated in regulating the phosphorylation status of CARMA1 and Bcl10, and similarly, several ubiquitin ligases and deubiquitinases have been implicated in regulating the ubiquitination status of all three components of the CBM complex. In contrast to antigen receptor-dependent CBM activation in lymphocytes, GPCR-dependent regulation of the phosphorylation and ubiquitination of CARMA3, Bcl10 and MALT1 has not yet been investigated, although it seems likely that at least some of the same processes that regulate CBM activity in response to antigen receptor stimulation will also play a role in GPCR-dependent CBM regulation. Future studies may identify specific kinases, phosphatases, ubiquitin ligases and/or deubiquitinases that could be targeted in an effort to treat atherosclerosis by inhibiting GPCR/CBM pro-inflammatory activity in the vasculature.

### 7.3 Targeting the enzymatic activity of the CBM signalosome itself

MALT1, recently discovered to be a protease, is the only component of the CBM complex that is known to possess intrinsic enzymatic activity, and inhibition of MALT1 proteolytic activity may indeed represent a promising new therapeutic target for the treatment of atherosclerosis. As described in section 5.1, three proteolytic substrates for MALT1 have been identified so far: the MALT1 binding partner Bcl10, and the NF-κB-inhibiting deubiquitinases A20 and CYLD (Coornaert et al., 2008; Rebeaud et al., 2008; Staal et al., 2011). In T-cells, MALT1-dependent cleavage of Bcl10 is induced by TCR stimulation and may play a role in integrin-mediated T-cell adhesion (Rebeaud et al., 2008). Whether

GPCR stimulation can induce MALT1-dependent cleavage of Bcl10 has not yet been investigated, and how Bcl10 cleavage might impact endothelial or VSMC function is totally unknown. TCR stimulation also induces the cleavage of A20 by MALT1, and this results in loss of A20's ability to inhibit TCR-dependent NF-κB activation. It is speculated that A20 cleavage, which separates the N-terminal deubiquitination domain from the C-terminal substrate interaction domain, prevents the removal of activating K63-linked polyubiquitin from A20's substrates, which include TRAFs 2 and 6, Bcl10, IKKγ and MALT1 itself, and that preserving these activating ubiquitination events promotes NF-κB activity. In this way, MALT1-dependent A20 cleavage can amplify the degree of NF-κB dependent gene expression (Coornaert et al., 2008). Whether GPCRs within the vasculature such as AGTR1, PAR-1, CXCR2 or LPA receptors induce MALT1-dependent A20 cleavage is not known. Intriguingly, A20 appears to have a protective effect against atherosclerosis in both mice and humans. In *ApoE$^{-/-}$* mice, A20 haploinsufficiency results in a significant increase in atherosclerosis compared to normal A20 controls, whereas transgenic overexpression of A20 results in decreased atherosclerosis (Wolfrum et al., 2007). Moreover, in human diabetic patients, polymorphisms at the *A20* locus leading to reduced levels of A20 expression are associated with increased coronary artery disease (Boonyasrisawat et al., 2007). Whether inhibition of MALT1-mediated cleavage of A20 might impact GPCR-driven atherogenesis remains to be investigated, but based on these studies, one might predict that preventing A20 cleavage could be protective. Initial studies suggest that MALT1-induced cleavage of CYLD is required for TCR-induced JNK activation (Staal et al., 2011), but MALT1-dependent CYLD cleavage has not been studied in the vasculature. Interestingly, CYLD overexpression attenuates neointimal formation in a rat model of carotid artery injury (Takami et al., 2008). How these studies of CYLD relate to GPCR/CBM-mediated atherogenesis remain to be investigated. Clearly much remains to be learned about the role of MALT1 proteolytic activity and its biologic affects. Future studies will hopefully elucidate whether MALT1 proteolytic activity contributes to vascular pathobiology and whether inhibiting this activity represents a rational therapeutic approach to atherogenesis.

## 8. Conclusion

There is a pressing need to understand the molecular mechanisms underlying cardiovascular disease, as it is the leading cause of disease-related deaths worldwide. Atherosclerosis is a chronic inflammatory disease of the vasculature in which the pro-inflammatory transcription factor, NF-κB, is a chief driving force. NF-κB-dependent plaque formation is mediated via the expression of cytokines, chemokines, and adhesion molecules, and via changes in endothelial biology including a reduction in NO production. While many inducers of NF-κB have been identified that act on endothelial cells, selective GPCR ligands clearly represent major players in the process of atherogenesis. Up until recently, little was known about the precise molecular mechanisms through which GPCRs communicate NF-κB activation in endothelial cells. However, dramatic progress has now been made in understanding this process, and we have outlined much of this work here in this chapter. It is hoped that delineating the molecules mediating GPCR-dependent NF-κB activation will provide new avenues for pharmaceutical development, adding a new layer of therapeutic opportunity in our efforts to combat atherogenesis.

## 9. Acknowledgments

This work was supported by grants from the National Institutes of Health (NIH), U.S.A., R01HL082914 and R01DK079973.

## 10. References

Ahn, S., Kim, J., Hara, M.R., Ren, X.R., & Lefkowitz, R.J. (2009). {beta}-Arrestin-2 Mediates Anti-apoptotic Signaling through Regulation of BAD Phosphorylation. *J Biol Chem.* 284, 8855-8865

Aveleira, C.A., Lin, C.M., Abcouwer, S.F., Ambrosio, A.F., & Antonetti, D.A. (2010). TNF-alpha signals through PKCzeta/NF-kappaB to alter the tight junction complex and increase retinal endothelial cell permeability. *Diabetes.* 59, 2872-2882

Belham, C., Wu, S., & Avruch, J. (1999). Intracellular signalling: PDK1--a kinase at the hub of things. *Curr Biol.* 9, R93-96

Bertrand, M.E. (2004). Provision of cardiovascular protection by ACE inhibitors: a review of recent trials. *Curr Med Res Opin.* 20, 1559-1569

Bidere, N., et al. (2009). Casein kinase 1alpha governs antigen-receptor-induced NF-kappaB activation and human lymphoma cell survival. *Nature.* 458, 92-96

Boonyasrisawat, W., Eberle, D., Bacci, S., Zhang, Y.Y., Nolan, D., Gervino, E.V., Johnstone, M.T., Trischitta, V., Shoelson, S.E., & Doria, A. (2007). Tag polymorphisms at the A20 (TNFAIP3) locus are associated with lower gene expression and increased risk of coronary artery disease in type 2 diabetes. *Diabetes.* 56, 499-505

Borissoff, J.I., Spronk, H.M., Heeneman, S., & ten Cate, H. (2009). Is thrombin a key player in the 'coagulation-atherogenesis' maze? *Cardiovasc Res.* 82, 392-403

Borissoff, J.I., Spronk, H.M., & ten Cate, H. (2011). The hemostatic system as a modulator of atherosclerosis. *N Engl J Med.* 364, 1746-1760

Bosisio, D., Marazzi, I., Agresti, A., Shimizu, N., Bianchi, M.E., & Natoli, G. (2006). A hyper-dynamic equilibrium between promoter-bound and nucleoplasmic dimers controls NF-kappaB-dependent gene activity. *Embo J.* 25, 798-810

Brasier, A.R. (2010). The nuclear factor-kappaB-interleukin-6 signalling pathway mediating vascular inflammation. *Cardiovasc Res.* 86, 211-218

Brasier, A.R., Jamaluddin, M., Han, Y., Patterson, C., & Runge, M.S. (2000). Angiotensin II induces gene transcription through cell-type-dependent effects on the nuclear factor-kappaB (NF-kappaB) transcription factor. *Mol Cell Biochem.* 212, 155-169

Brasier, A.R., Recinos, A., 3rd, & Eledrisi, M.S. (2002). Vascular inflammation and the renin-angiotensin system. *Arterioscler Thromb Vasc Biol.* 22, 1257-1266

Braunersreuther, V., Mach, F., & Steffens, S. (2007). The specific role of chemokines in atherosclerosis. *Thromb Haemost.* 97, 714-721

Brenner, D., et al. (2009). Phosphorylation of CARMA1 by HPK1 is critical for NF-kappaB activation in T cells. *Proc Natl Acad Sci U S A.* 106, 14508-14513

Choudhary, S., Lu, M., Cui, R., & Brasier, A.R. (2007). Involvement of a novel Rac/RhoA guanosine triphosphatase-nuclear factor-kappaB inducing kinase signaling pathway mediating angiotensin II-induced RelA transactivation. *Mol Endocrinol.* 21, 2203-2217

Chung, S.W., Park, J.W., Lee, S.A., Eo, S.K., & Kim, K. (2010). Thrombin promotes proinflammatory phenotype in human vascular smooth muscle cell. *Biochem Biophys Res Commun.* 396, 748-754

Coornaert, B., Baens, M., Heyninck, K., Bekaert, T., Haegman, M., Staal, J., Sun, L., Chen, Z.J., Marynen, P., & Beyaert, R. (2008). T cell antigen receptor stimulation induces MALT1 paracaspase-mediated cleavage of the NF-kappaB inhibitor A20. *Nat Immunol.*

Coughlin, S.R. (2005). Protease-activated receptors in hemostasis, thrombosis and vascular biology. *J Thromb Haemost.* 3, 1800-1814

Csiszar, A., Wang, M., Lakatta, E.G., & Ungvari, Z. (2008). Inflammation and endothelial dysfunction during aging: role of NF-kappaB. *J Appl Physiol.* 105, 1333-1341

Cui, R., Tieu, B., Recinos, A., Tilton, R.G., & Brasier, A.R. (2006). RhoA mediates angiotensin II-induced phospho-Ser536 nuclear factor kappaB/RelA subunit exchange on the interleukin-6 promoter in VSMCs. *Circ Res.* 99, 723-730

Cummings, R., Zhao, Y., Jacoby, D., Spannhake, E.W., Ohba, M., Garcia, J.G., Watkins, T., He, D., Saatian, B., & Natarajan, V. (2004). Protein kinase Cdelta mediates lysophosphatidic acid-induced NF-kappaB activation and interleukin-8 secretion in human bronchial epithelial cells. *J Biol Chem.* 279, 41085-41094

Daugherty, A., & Cassis, L. (2004). Angiotensin II-mediated development of vascular diseases. *Trends Cardiovasc Med.* 14, 117-120

de Winther, M.P., Kanters, E., Kraal, G., & Hofker, M.H. (2005). Nuclear factor kappaB signaling in atherogenesis. *Arterioscler Thromb Vasc Biol.* 25, 904-914

DeFea, K.A. (2011). Beta-arrestins as regulators of signal termination and transduction: how do they determine what to scaffold? *Cell Signal.* 23, 621-629

Delekta, P.C., Apel, I.J., Gu, S., Siu, K., Hattori, Y., McAllister-Lucas, L.M., & Lucas, P.C. (2010). Thrombin-dependent NF-{kappa}B activation and monocyte/endothelial adhesion are mediated by the CARMA3.Bcl10.MALT1 signalosome. *J Biol Chem.* 285, 41432-41442

Dimitratos, S.D., Woods, D.F., Stathakis, D.G., & Bryant, P.J. (1999). Signaling pathways are focused at specialized regions of the plasma membrane by scaffolding proteins of the MAGUK family. *Bioessays.* 21, 912-921

Ding, R.Q., Tsao, J., Chai, H., Mochly-Rosen, D., & Zhou, W. (2011). Therapeutic potential for protein kinase C inhibitor in vascular restenosis. *J Cardiovasc Pharmacol Ther.* 16, 160-167

Dorsam, R.T., & Gutkind, J.S. (2007). G-protein-coupled receptors and cancer. *Nat Rev Cancer.* 7, 79-94

Doyon, P., & Servant, M.J. (2010). Tumor necrosis factor receptor-associated factor-6 and ribosomal S6 kinase intracellular pathways link the angiotensin II AT1 receptor to the phosphorylation and activation of the IkappaB kinase complex in vascular smooth muscle cells. *J Biol Chem.* 285, 30708-30718

Eguchi, S., et al. (1998). Calcium-dependent epidermal growth factor receptor transactivation mediates the angiotensin II-induced mitogen-activated protein kinase activation in vascular smooth muscle cells. *J Biol Chem.* 273, 8890-8896

Fanning, A.S., & Anderson, J.M. (1999). Protein modules as organizers of membrane structure. *Curr Opin Cell Biol.* 11, 432-439

Farmer, D.G., & Kennedy, S. (2009). RAGE, vascular tone and vascular disease. *Pharmacol Ther.* 124, 185-194

Ferrara, N., Gerber, H.P., & LeCouter, J. (2003). The biology of VEGF and its receptors. *Nat Med.* 9, 669-676

Ferrario, C.M., & Strawn, W.B. (2006). Role of the renin-angiotensin-aldosterone system and proinflammatory mediators in cardiovascular disease. *Am J Cardiol.* 98, 121-128

Fraser, C.C. (2008). G protein-coupled receptor connectivity to NF-kappaB in inflammation and cancer. *Int Rev Immunol.* 27, 320-350

Gareus, R., Kotsaki, E., Xanthoulea, S., van der Made, I., Gijbels, M.J., Kardakaris, R., Polykratis, A., Kollias, G., de Winther, M.P., & Pasparakis, M. (2008). Endothelial cell-specific NF-kappaB inhibition protects mice from atherosclerosis. *Cell Metab.* 8, 372-383

Gavard, J., Hou, X., Qu, Y., Masedunskas, A., Martin, D., Weigert, R., Li, X., & Gutkind, J.S. (2009). A role for a CXCR2/phosphatidylinositol 3-kinase gamma signaling axis in acute and chronic vascular permeability. *Mol Cell Biol.* 29, 2469-2480

Gough, P.J., Gomez, I.G., Wille, P.T., & Raines, E.W. (2006). Macrophage expression of active MMP-9 induces acute plaque disruption in apoE-deficient mice. *J Clin Invest.* 116, 59-69

Grabiner, B.C., Blonska, M., Lin, P.C., You, Y., Wang, D., Sun, J., Darnay, B.G., Dong, C., & Lin, X. (2007). CARMA3 deficiency abrogates G protein-coupled receptor-induced NF-{kappa}B activation. *Genes Dev.* 21, 984-996

Hamilton, J.R., Cornelissen, I., Mountford, J.K., & Coughlin, S.R. (2009). Atherosclerosis proceeds independently of thrombin-induced platelet activation in ApoE-/- mice. *Atherosclerosis.* 205, 427-432

Hansson, G.K. (2005). Inflammation, atherosclerosis, and coronary artery disease. *N Engl J Med.* 352, 1685-1695

Harja, E., Chang, J.S., Lu, Y., Leitges, M., Zou, Y.S., Schmidt, A.M., & Yan, S.F. (2009). Mice deficient in PKCbeta and apolipoprotein E display decreased atherosclerosis. *Faseb J.* 23, 1081-1091

Hayden, M.S., & Ghosh, S. (2008). Shared principles in NF-kappaB signaling. *Cell.* 132, 344-362

Hirano, K. (2007). The roles of proteinase-activated receptors in the vascular physiology and pathophysiology. *Arterioscler Thromb Vasc Biol.* 27, 27-36

Hiroki, J., et al. (2004). Inflammatory stimuli upregulate Rho-kinase in human coronary vascular smooth muscle cells. *J Mol Cell Cardiol.* 37, 537-546

Ishiguro, K., et al. (2006). Ca2+/calmodulin-dependent protein kinase II is a modulator of CARMA1-mediated NF-kappaB activation. *Mol Cell Biol.* 26, 5497-5508

Jin, R.C., & Loscalzo, J. (2010). Vascular Nitric Oxide: Formation and Function. *J Blood Med.* 2010, 147-162

Kalra, D., Sivasubramanian, N., & Mann, D.L. (2002). Angiotensin II induces tumor necrosis factor biosynthesis in the adult mammalian heart through a protein kinase C-dependent pathway. *Circulation.* 105, 2198-2205

Kim, J., Zhang, L., Peppel, K., Wu, J.H., Zidar, D.A., Brian, L., DeWire, S.M., Exum, S.T., Lefkowitz, R.J., & Freedman, N.J. (2008). Beta-arrestins regulate atherosclerosis and neointimal hyperplasia by controlling smooth muscle cell proliferation and migration. *Circ Res.* 103, 70-79

Kintscher, U., Lyon, C.J., & Law, R.E. (2004). Angiotensin II, PPAR-gamma and atherosclerosis. *Front Biosci.* 9, 359-369

Klemm, S., Zimmermann, S., Peschel, C., Mak, T.W., & Ruland, J. (2007). Bcl10 and Malt1 control lysophosphatidic acid-induced NF-kappaB activation and cytokine production. *Proc Natl Acad Sci U S A.* 104, 134-138

Lappano, R., & Maggiolini, M. (2011). G protein-coupled receptors: novel targets for drug discovery in cancer. *Nat Rev Drug Discov.* 10, 47-60

Laroux, F.S., Pavlick, K.P., Hines, I.N., Kawachi, S., Harada, H., Bharwani, S., Hoffman, J.M., & Grisham, M.B. (2001). Role of nitric oxide in inflammation. *Acta Physiol Scand.* 173, 113-118

Lee, K.Y., D'Acquisto, F., Hayden, M.S., Shim, J.H., & Ghosh, S. (2005). PDK1 nucleates T cell receptor-induced signaling complex for NF-kappaB activation. *Science.* 308, 114-118

Li, D., Saldeen, T., Romeo, F., & Mehta, J.L. (2000). Oxidized LDL upregulates angiotensin II type 1 receptor expression in cultured human coronary artery endothelial cells: the potential role of transcription factor NF-kappaB. *Circulation.* 102, 1970-1976

Li, D., Singh, R.M., Liu, L., Chen, H., Singh, B.M., Kazzaz, N., & Mehta, J.L. (2003). Oxidized-LDL through LOX-1 increases the expression of angiotensin converting enzyme in human coronary artery endothelial cells. *Cardiovasc Res.* 57, 238-243

Liao, D.F., Monia, B., Dean, N., & Berk, B.C. (1997). Protein kinase C-zeta mediates angiotensin II activation of ERK1/2 in vascular smooth muscle cells. *J Biol Chem.* 272, 6146-6150

Libby, P., Ridker, P.M., & Hansson, G.K. (2011). Progress and challenges in translating the biology of atherosclerosis. *Nature.* 473, 317-325

Lucas, P.C., McAllister-Lucas, L.M., & Nunez, G. (2004). NF-kappaB signaling in lymphocytes: a new cast of characters. *J Cell Sci.* 117, 31-39

Luft, F.C. (2001). Angiotensin, inflammation, hypertension, and cardiovascular disease. *Curr Hypertens Rep.* 3, 61-67

Mahanivong, C., Chen, H.M., Yee, S.W., Pan, Z.K., Dong, Z., & Huang, S. (2008). Protein kinase C alpha-CARMA3 signaling axis links Ras to NF-kappa B for lysophosphatidic acid-induced urokinase plasminogen activator expression in ovarian cancer cells. *Oncogene.* 27, 1273-1280

Martin, D., Galisteo, R., & Gutkind, J.S. (2009). CXCL8/IL8 stimulates vascular endothelial growth factor (VEGF) expression and the autocrine activation of VEGFR2 in endothelial cells by activating NFkappaB through the CBM (Carma3/Bcl10/Malt1) complex. *J Biol Chem.* 284, 6038-6042

Matsumoto, R., Wang, D., Blonska, M., Li, H., Kobayashi, M., Pappu, B., Chen, Y., Wang, D., & Lin, X. (2005). Phosphorylation of CARMA1 Plays a Critical Role in T Cell Receptor-Mediated NF-kappaB Activation. *Immunity.* 23, 575-585

McAllister-Lucas, L.M., et al. (2001). Bimp1, a MAGUK family member linking protein kinase C activation to Bcl10-mediated NF-kappaB induction. *J Biol Chem.* 276, 30589-30597

McAllister-Lucas, L.M., Jin, X., Gu, S., Siu, K., McDonnell, S., Ruland, J., Delekta, P.C., Van Beek, M., & Lucas, P.C. (2010). The CARMA3-Bcl10-MALT1 signalosome promotes angiotensin II-dependent vascular inflammation and atherogenesis. *J Biol Chem.* 285, 25880-25884

McAllister-Lucas, L.M., & Lucas, P.C. (2008). Finally, MALT1 is a protease! *Nat Immunol.* 9, 231-233

McAllister-Lucas, L.M., et al. (2007). CARMA3/Bcl10/MALT1-dependent NF-kappaB activation mediates angiotensin II-responsive inflammatory signaling in nonimmune cells. *Proc Natl Acad Sci USA.* 104, 139-144

McElhinny, J.A., Trushin, S.A., Bren, G.D., Chester, N., & Paya, C.V. (1996). Casein kinase II phosphorylates I kappa B alpha at S-283, S-289, S-293, and T-291 and is required for its degradation. *Mol Cell Biol.* 16, 899-906

Medeiros, R.B., Burbach, B.J., Mueller, K.L., Srivastava, R., Moon, J.J., Highfill, S., Peterson, E.J., & Shimizu, Y. (2007). Regulation of NF-kappaB activation in T cells via association of the adapter proteins ADAP and CARMA1. *Science.* 316, 754-758

Mehta, N.N., Sheetz, M., Price, K., Comiskey, L., Amrutia, S., Iqbal, N., Mohler, E.R., & Reilly, M.P. (2009). Selective PKC beta inhibition with ruboxistaurin and endothelial function in type-2 diabetes mellitus. *Cardiovasc Drugs Ther.* 23, 17-24

Minami, T., Sugiyama, A., Wu, S.Q., Abid, R., Kodama, T., & Aird, W.C. (2004). Thrombin and phenotypic modulation of the endothelium. *Arterioscler Thromb Vasc Biol.* 24, 41-53

Mitra, S., Deshmukh, A., Sachdeva, R., Lu, J., & Mehta, J.L. (2011). Oxidized Low-Density Lipoprotein and Atherosclerosis Implications in Antioxidant Therapy. *Am J Med Sci.*

Mora, A., Komander, D., van Aalten, D.M., & Alessi, D.R. (2004). PDK1, the master regulator of AGC kinase signal transduction. *Semin Cell Dev Biol.* 15, 161-170

Murray, C.J., & Lopez, A.D. (1997). Global mortality, disability, and the contribution of risk factors: Global Burden of Disease Study. *Lancet.* 349, 1436-1442

Newton, A.C. (2001). Protein kinase C: structural and spatial regulation by phosphorylation, cofactors, and macromolecular interactions. *Chem Rev.* 101, 2353-2364

Newton, A.C. (2003). Regulation of the ABC kinases by phosphorylation: protein kinase C as a paradigm. *Biochem J.* 370, 361-371

O'Connor, S., Shumway, S.D., Amanna, I.J., Hayes, C.E., & Miyamoto, S. (2004). Regulation of constitutive p50/c-Rel activity via proteasome inhibitor-resistant IkappaBalpha degradation in B cells. *Mol Cell Biol.* 24, 4895-4908

Oeckinghaus, A., & Ghosh, S. (2009). The NF-kappaB family of transcription factors and its regulation. *Cold Spring Harb Perspect Biol.* 1, a000034

Ohtsu, H., Dempsey, P.J., Frank, G.D., Brailoiu, E., Higuchi, S., Suzuki, H., Nakashima, H., Eguchi, K., & Eguchi, S. (2006). ADAM17 mediates epidermal growth factor receptor transactivation and vascular smooth muscle cell hypertrophy induced by angiotensin II. *Arterioscler Thromb Vasc Biol.* 26, e133-137

Packard, R.R., & Libby, P. (2008). Inflammation in atherosclerosis: from vascular biology to biomarker discovery and risk prediction. *Clin Chem.* 54, 24-38

Parmentier, J.H., Pavicevic, Z., & Malik, K.U. (2006). ANG II stimulates phospholipase D through PKCzeta activation in VSMC: implications in adhesion, spreading, and hypertrophy. *Am J Physiol Heart Circ Physiol.* 290, H46-54

Phillips, M.I., & Kagiyama, S. (2002). Angiotensin II as a pro-inflammatory mediator. *Curr Opin Investig Drugs.* 3, 569-577

Pober, J.S., & Sessa, W.C. (2007). Evolving functions of endothelial cells in inflammation. *Nat Rev Immunol.* 7, 803-815

Rader, D.J., & Daugherty, A. (2008). Translating molecular discoveries into new therapies for atherosclerosis. *Nature.* 451, 904-913

Rahman, A., Anwar, K.N., Uddin, S., Xu, N., Ye, R.D., Platanias, L.C., & Malik, A.B. (2001). Protein kinase C-delta regulates thrombin-induced ICAM-1 gene expression in endothelial cells via activation of p38 mitogen-activated protein kinase. *Mol Cell Biol.* 21, 5554-5565

Rebeaud, F., et al. (2008). The proteolytic activity of the paracaspase MALT1 is key in T cell activation. *Nat Immunol.* 9, 272-281

Rosenkilde, M.M., & Schwartz, T.W. (2004). The chemokine system -- a major regulator of angiogenesis in health and disease. *Apmis.* 112, 481-495

Rouet-Benzineb, P., Gontero, B., Dreyfus, P., & Lafuma, C. (2000). Angiotensin II induces nuclear factor- kappa B activation in cultured neonatal rat cardiomyocytes through protein kinase C signaling pathway. *J Mol Cell Cardiol.* 32, 1767-1778

Saito, Y., & Berk, B.C. (2001). Transactivation: a novel signaling pathway from angiotensin II to tyrosine kinase receptors. *J Mol Cell Cardiol.* 33, 3-7

Sasaki, C.Y., Barberi, T.J., Ghosh, P., & Longo, D.L. (2005). Phosphorylation of RelA/p65 on serine 536 defines an I{kappa}B{alpha}-independent NF-{kappa}B pathway. *J Biol Chem.* 280, 34538-34547

Sata, M., & Fukuda, D. (2010). Crucial role of renin-angiotensin system in the pathogenesis of atherosclerosis. *J Med Invest.* 57, 12-25

Schwarz, E.M., Van Antwerp, D., & Verma, I.M. (1996). Constitutive phosphorylation of IkappaBalpha by casein kinase II occurs preferentially at serine 293: requirement for degradation of free IkappaBalpha. *Mol Cell Biol.* 16, 3554-3559

Semenza, G.L. (2007). Vasculogenesis, angiogenesis, and arteriogenesis: mechanisms of blood vessel formation and remodeling. *J Cell Biochem.* 102, 840-847

Shambharkar, P.B., Blonska, M., Pappu, B.P., Li, H., You, Y., Sakurai, H., Darnay, B.G., Hara, H., Penninger, J., & Lin, X. (2007). Phosphorylation and ubiquitination of the IkappaB kinase complex by two distinct signaling pathways. *Embo J.* 26, 1794-1805

Shinohara, H., Maeda, S., Watarai, H., & Kurosaki, T. (2007). IkappaB kinase beta-induced phosphorylation of CARMA1 contributes to CARMA1 Bcl10 MALT1 complex formation in B cells. *J Exp Med.* 204, 3285-3293

Shinohara, H., Yasuda, T., Aiba, Y., Sanjo, H., Hamadate, M., Watarai, H., Sakurai, H., & Kurosaki, T. (2005). PKC beta regulates BCR-mediated IKK activation by facilitating the interaction between TAK1 and CARMA1. 202, 1423-1431

Sitia, S., et al. (2010). From endothelial dysfunction to atherosclerosis. *Autoimmun Rev.* 9, 830-834

Sommer, K., Guo, B., Pomerantz, J.L., Bandaranayake, A.D., Moreno-Garcia, M.E., Ovechkina, Y.L., & Rawlings, D.J. (2005). Phosphorylation of the CARMA1 Linker Controls NF-kappaB Activation. *Immunity.* 23, 561-574

Staal, J., Driege, Y., Bekaert, T., Demeyer, A., Muyllaert, D., Van Damme, P., Gevaert, K., & Beyaert, R. (2011). T-cell receptor-induced JNK activation requires proteolytic inactivation of CYLD by MALT1. *Embo J.* 30, 1742-1752

Stilo, R., Liguoro, D., Di Jeso, B., Formisano, S., Consiglio, E., Leonardi, A., & Vito, P. (2004). Physical and functional interaction of CARMA1 and CARMA3 with Ikappa kinase gamma-NFkappaB essential modulator. *J Biol Chem.* 279, 34323-34331

Strader, C.D., Fong, T.M., Tota, M.R., Underwood, D., & Dixon, R.A. (1994). Structure and function of G protein-coupled receptors. *Annu Rev Biochem.* 63, 101-132

Sun, J., & Lin, X. (2008). Beta-arrestin 2 is required for lysophosphatidic acid-induced NF-kappaB activation. *Proc Natl Acad Sci U S A.* 105, 17085-17090

Sun, L., Deng, L., Ea, C.K., Xia, Z.P., & Chen, Z.J. (2004). The TRAF6 ubiquitin ligase and TAK1 kinase mediate IKK activation by BCL10 and MALT1 in T lymphocytes. *Mol Cell.* 14, 289-301

Sun, W., et al. (2009). MEKK3 is required for lysophosphatidic acid-induced NF-kappaB activation. *Cell Signal.* 21, 1488-1494

Takami, Y., et al. (2008). Potential role of CYLD (Cylindromatosis) as a deubiquitinating enzyme in vascular cells. *Am J Pathol.* 172, 818-829

Thome, M. (2004). CARMA1, BCL-10 and MALT1 in lymphocyte development and activation. *Nat Rev Immunol.* 4, 348-359

Uren, A.G., O'Rourke, K., Aravind, L.A., Pisabarro, M.T., Seshagiri, S., Koonin, E.V., & Dixit, V.M. (2000). Identification of paracaspases and metacaspases: two ancient families of caspase-like proteins, one of which plays a key role in MALT lymphoma. *Mol Cell.* 6, 961-967

Vallabhapurapu, S., & Karin, M. (2009). Regulation and function of NF-kappaB transcription factors in the immune system. *Annu Rev Immunol.* 27, 693-733

Wang, C., Deng, L., Hong, M., Akkaraju, G.R., Inoue, J., & Chen, Z.J. (2001a). TAK1 is a ubiquitin-dependent kinase of MKK and IKK. *Nature.* 412, 346-351

Wang, D., You, Y., Lin, P.C., Xue, L., Morris, S.W., Zeng, H., Wen, R., & Lin, X. (2007). Bcl10 plays a critical role in NF-kappaB activation induced by G protein-coupled receptors. *Proc Natl Acad Sci U S A.* 104, 145-150

Wang, L., et al. (2001b). Card10 is a novel caspase recruitment domain/membrane-associated guanylate kinase family member that interacts with BCL10 and activates NF-kappa B. *J Biol Chem.* 276, 21405-21409

Waugh, D.J., & Wilson, C. (2008). The interleukin-8 pathway in cancer. *Clin Cancer Res.* 14, 6735-6741

Wegener, E., & Krappmann, D. (2007). CARD-Bcl10-Malt1 signalosomes: missing link to NF-kappaB. *Sci STKE.* 2007, pe21

Weil, R., Schwamborn, K., Alcover, A., Bessia, C., Di Bartolo, V., & Israel, A. (2003). Induction of the NF-kappaB cascade by recruitment of the scaffold molecule NEMO to the T cell receptor. *Immunity.* 18, 13-26

Whalen, E.J., Rajagopal, S., & Lefkowitz, R.J. (2011). Therapeutic potential of beta-arrestin- and G protein-biased agonists. *Trends Mol Med.* 17, 126-139

Wolfrum, S., Teupser, D., Tan, M., Chen, K.Y., & Breslow, J.L. (2007). The protective effect of A20 on atherosclerosis in apolipoprotein E-deficient mice is associated with reduced expression of NF-kappaB target genes. *Proc Natl Acad Sci U S A.* 104, 18601-18606

Zhou, H., Wertz, I., O'Rourke, K., Ultsch, M., Seshagiri, S., Eby, M., Xiao, W., & Dixit, V.M. (2004). Bcl10 activates the NF-kappaB pathway through ubiquitination of NEMO. *Nature.* 427, 167-171

Zhou, Z., et al. (2011). Lipoprotein-derived lysophosphatidic acid promotes atherosclerosis by releasing CXCL1 from the endothelium. *Cell Metab.* 13, 592-600

# 26

# Vasoprotective Effect of Foods as Treatments: Chicken Collagen Hydrolysate

Tomomi Kouguchi, Youzuo Zhang,
Mikako Sato, Yoshihisa Takahata and Fumiki Morimatsu
*Nippon Meat Packers, Inc., R & D Center*
*Japan*

## 1. Introduction

Collagen is a major protein in living organisms and accounts for about one-third of all protein in mammalian bodies, including the human body. Recently, collagen peptides have been used as foods that take advantage of their tertiary functions. We have been focusing on the vasoprotective effect of collagen peptides.

Chicken collagen hydrolysate (CCH) is obtained by treating chicken feet with enzymes to produce an angiotensin-converting enzyme (ACE) inhibitory peptide. Administration of this CCH for 12 weeks reduces blood pressure in humans. We therefore investigated the mechanism of the vasoprotective effect of CCH. We tested whether prolonged CCH treatment of rats or mice would restore endothelial cell function and improve proinflammatory cytokine levels. We found that CCH treatment improved the vasorelaxation of rat aorta damaged with L-NG-nitroarginine methyl ester , an NO synthesis inhibitor. CCH treatment also reduced the serum levels of IL-6, sICAM-1, and TNF-α in an atherosclerotic mouse model, C57BL/6.KOR-ApoE$^{sh1}$.

These findings indicate the usefulness of collagen peptides as foods promoting anti-atherogenesis via a vasoprotective effect.

Years have passed since functional foods and their tertiary function first attracted attention. The primary function of foods is to supply the nutrients required to sustain life, and the secondary function is to satisfy taste preferences. The tertiary function of foods is to exert biological regulatory effects, such as biophylaxis, homeostatic maintenance, and disease prevention, which are activated upon food intake. Purified food ingredients that have tertiary functions are widely consumed as supplements. Multitudes of supplements are available on today's market: besides common vitamins, minerals, and amino acids, there are catechins, which are antioxidant constituents of tea (Katiyar, 2003), soy isoflavones, which have female hormone–like actions (Weijer, 2002), and docosahexaenoic acids and eicosapentaenoic acids, which decrease triglyceride levels (Tamai, 2004). Collagen is being used widely, not only in supplements but also as an ingredient of common food products such as beverages, yogurts, and breads.

Collagen is a major protein in living organisms and accounts for about one-third of all protein in mammalian bodies, including the human body. It forms an extracellular matrix that plays a role in the formation of connective tissues and acts as a scaffold for cells, but its accumulation declines with age. The majority of the collagen in the body exhibits a triple helix structure; with heating, this structure is lost and the collagen becomes gelatin like. Moreover, as a result of enzymatic degradation that eliminates its gelation ability, the gelatin increases in solubility and becomes collagen peptides (Fig. 1), which are frequently consumed by women, in particular. Collagen peptides are consumed as a food product to supply the collagen lost from the body with age, and a substantial number of reports have shown that treatment with collagen peptides increases well-being.

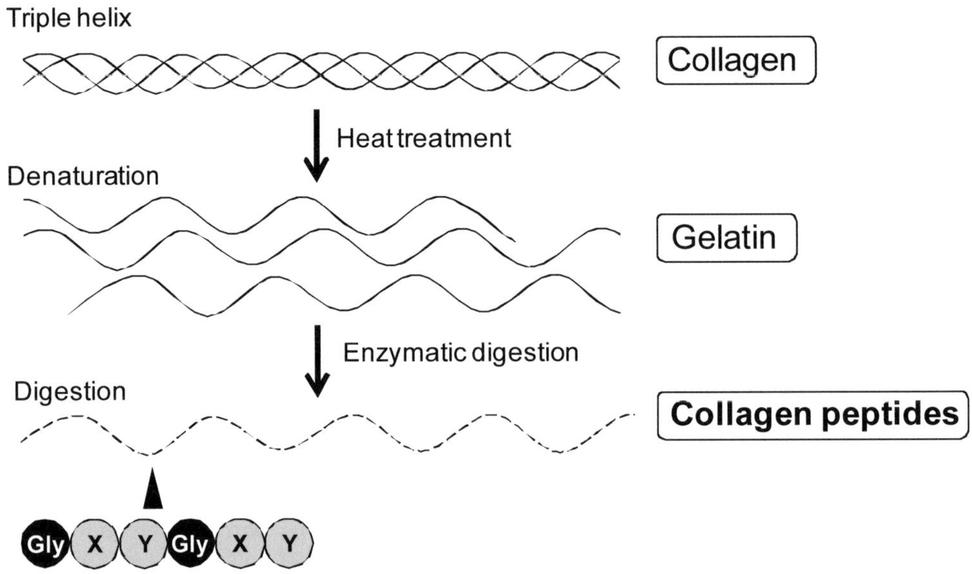


Fig. 1. Collagen in the body exhibits a triple helix structure but is denatured and becomes gelatin-like if heated. Enzyme treatment of denatured collagen produces collagen peptides, which are composed of atypical repetitions of -Gly-X-Y-Gly-X-Y- and are consumed as functional foods.

### 1.1 The tertiary function of collagen peptides

In recent years, vigorous research has been conducted to elucidate both the mechanism by which collagen peptides are absorbed from food into the body and the tertiary functions of this protein. Orally administered collagen peptides are transferred to the blood in the form of dipeptides or tripeptides, without being completely degraded to amino acids (Iwai, 2009 and Shigemura,2009). A double-blind placebo-controlled trial has confirmed that collagen peptide treatment increases the skin's moisture content (Ohara, 2009). The primary structure of collagen consists of atypical repetitions of -Gly-X-Y- and characteristically includes hydroxyproline, which is produced by posttranslational modification. Many studies have suggested that this particular sequence enables collagen to exert multiple bioactivities, not only in skin and bones, but also in blood vessels, which contain large amounts of collagen (Arborelius, 1999). Accordingly, collagen peptides are expected to have tertiary functions additional to those already known.

### 1.2 Targeting blood vessels

The blood vessels are referred to as the largest organ in the body, because the vascular endothelial cells, which line the vessel lumens, cover an area as large as six tennis courts and weigh 1.5 kg; they are therefore as heavy as the liver. Although blood vessels were once seen as simply the "pipes" that circulate blood, it has become increasingly clear that the vascular endothelial cells receive signals from organs and control blood supply and the secretion of various cytokines on demand (Kato, 2004).

There are many diseases caused by vascular abnormalities, especially in Japan. According to the cause-specific death rates reported by the Ministry of Health, Labor, and Welfare of Japan in 2006, death rates due to circulatory system diseases are extremely high: after malignant neoplasms (30.4%), cardiovascular diseases account for 15.9% of all deaths and cerebrovascular diseases account for 11.8%. From this perspective, protecting the blood vessels from disease should increase the quality of life of many people. We therefore took advantage of the absorbability of collagen peptides and aimed to develop ones targeting the protection of blood vessels.

### 1.3 Development of a low-molecular-weight chicken collagen hydrolysate

Collagen peptides are generally extracted from pig skin or fish scales. However, here we used chicken legs as sources of the new collagen peptides. This was because, although gelatin is known to be allergenic, our previous study showed that the allergenicity of chicken-derived gelatin is the lowest among a number of types (Taguchi, 2002).

Chicken legs were solubilized by acid treatment and the extracted collagen was processed by proteases. The resulting low-molecular-weight collagen peptides were then dried and powdered for subsequent use as low-molecular-weight chicken collagen hydrolysate (CCH) (Saiga, 2008) (Fig. 2). Our preliminary *in vitro* experiments showed that CCH strongly inhibits angiotensin-converting enzyme (ACE). Production of angiotensin II, a vasopressor, is suppressed by the inhibition of ACE in the blood and organs, thereby resulting in a hypotensive effect (Gupta, 2010). Because hypertension is closely related to arteriosclerosis, the inhibition of blood pressure elevation is expected to have a protective effect on the blood vessels. In addition, ACE serves as a kininase II (Sharma, 2009). Because kininase II degrades bradykinin, a vasodilator, inhibition of ACE (or kininase II) by CCH causes bradykinin accumulation in the body. Bradykinin activates endothelial nitric oxide synthase (eNOS) and increases the production of nitric oxide (NO), a vasodilator. In this manner, CCH was expected to have a vasoprotective function—a novel tertiary function of foods—through its ACE inhibitory activity.

## 2. Hypotensive effects of chicken collagen hydrolysate in subjects with hypertension

Arteriosclerosis and hypertension are closely associated with each other. If strong pressure is applied continuously to an artery because of hypertension, the arterial walls are damaged and blood cholesterols infiltrate the walls through the damaged areas and cause arteriosclerosis. In addition, advanced arteriosclerosis narrows the blood vessels and causes blood flow to deteriorate. The heartbeat is then enhanced to improve blood flow, and this causes the blood pressure to increase. In this manner, hypertension accelerates arteriosclerosis and produces a vicious cycle. If we could alleviate hypertension, we would thus also be able to ameliorate arteriosclerosis. We therefore initially conducted a clinical trial to verify the hypotensive effect of CCH in humans (Kouguchi, 2008).

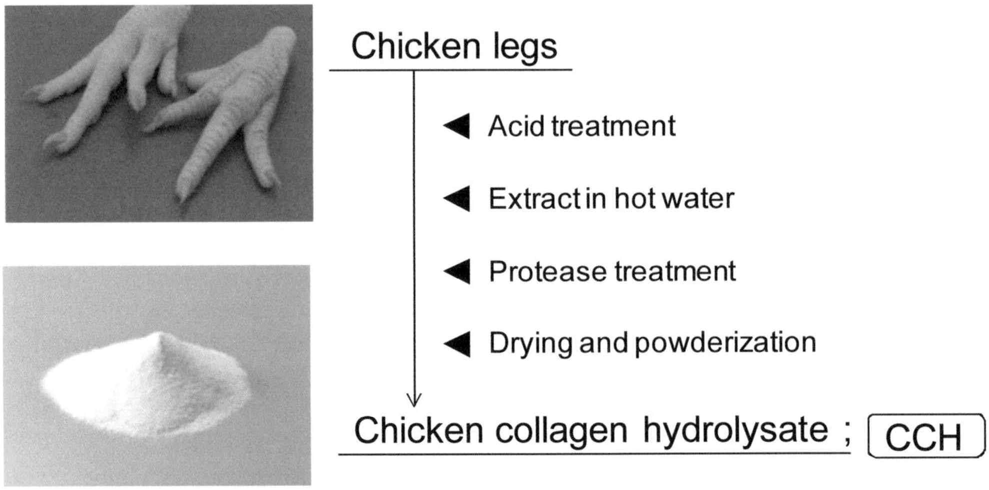


Fig. 2. Process of production of chicken collagen hydrolysate (CCH). Chicken legs are used as the basic ingredient and are treated with acid and then hot water to extract collagen, which was then processed with proteases. The resulting low-molecular-weight collagen peptides are then dried and powered for subsequent use as CCH.

### 2.1 Subjects

Subjects for the test were 120 healthy, antihypertensive drug-free, adult males and females with mild hypertension or high-normal blood pressure. The subjects (males, 59; females, 61) were randomly assigned to two groups. No significant differences in subject characteristics, including sex, age, height, body weight, body mass index, systolic blood pressure, diastolic blood pressure, and pulse rate, were observed between the two groups ($P > 0.2$).

The study was approved by the institutional review board and was performed under the close supervision of the study investigators. The subjects were well informed about the test contents and methods by the study investigators, and they provided written informed consent to protect their rights in accordance with the spirit of the Declaration of Helsinki.

### 2.2 Experimental diets

A drink containing CCH (hereafter, referred to as the test food) or its counterpart without CCH (hereafter, referred to as the placebo) was used in the experiment. The test food contained 2.9 g of CCH; for the placebo, the raw material composition was the same as that of the test food, but without the CCH.

### 2.3 Trial design

The trial was designed as a placebo-controlled, double-blind, parallel-group comparison study. The study ran for a total of 18 weeks: 2 observational weeks before the treatment (pre-treatment observation period), a 12-week treatment period, and 4 weeks for post-treatment observation (post-treatment observation period). All subjects were given a bottle of drink daily during the treatment period. All subjects were directed not to change their daily diets and exercise regimens (Fig.3). They were advised strongly not to overeat, over-drink, or over-exercise.

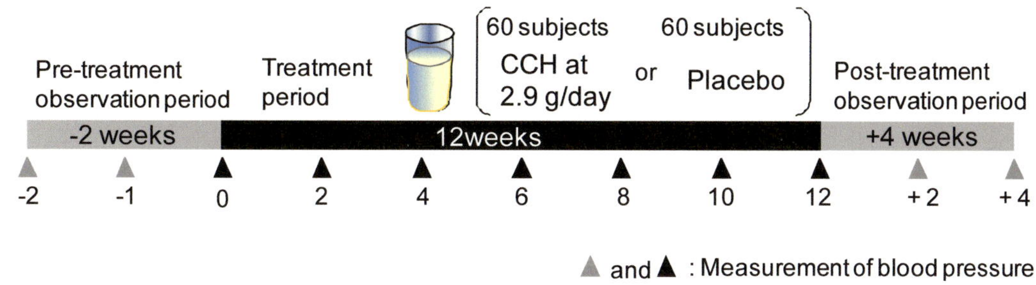


Fig. 3. Clinical trial schedule for CCH administration. The 120 subjects were assigned to two groups and given the experimental or placebo diet for 12 weeks. Blood pressure was measured a total of 11 times in the course of the experiment: twice in the pre-treatment observation period, 7 times in the treatment period, and twice in the post-treatment observation period.

### 2.4 Measurement of blood pressure

Blood pressure was measured a total of 11 times in the course of the experiment: twice in the pre-treatment observation period, 7 times in the treatment period, and twice in the post-treatment observation period. The subjects were kept at rest for at least 10 min before the measurement. Blood pressure in the left cubital fossa was measured while the subjects were seated. Blood pressure was measured more than once with a mercury manometer. The average value of 2 stable measurements (i.e. when the difference of the values was less than 5 mmHg) was recorded as the value recorded. Pulse rate was measured once at each visit. The subjects' condition was also interviewed by a doctor at the time of measurement of blood pressure.

### 2.5 Results

Systolic blood pressures in the test food group were non-significantly lower ($P < 0.1$) than those of the placebo group after 2 weeks of treatment and were significantly lower ($P < 0.05$) than in the placebo group after 12 weeks of treatment (Fig. 4). In the test food group, in comparison with the mean pre-treatment blood pressure (139.7 mm Hg), the blood pressure was significantly lower after 2 weeks (133.9 mm Hg; $P < 0.001$), 4 weeks (135.7 mm Hg; $P < 0.01$), 6 weeks (134.6 mm Hg; $P < 0.001$), 8 weeks (134.4 mm Hg; $P < 0.01$), 10 weeks (134.6 mm Hg; $P < 0.001$), and 12 weeks (133.5 mm Hg; $P < 0.001$). After 2 weeks of treatment, the blood pressure in the test food group was 135.5 mm Hg; this was non-significantly lower than the pre-treatment blood pressure ($P < 0.1$). In the placebo group, blood pressure after 6 weeks of treatment (135.9 mm Hg) was significantly lower than the pre-treatment blood pressure (139.8 mm Hg) ($P < 0.05$).

### 2.6 Discussion

Blood pressures in the test food group decreased continuously during the treatment period. Because the compositional difference between the test food and placebo in this experiment was only the presence or the absence of CCH, the observed antihypertensive effect was considered to be due to CCH treatment. We had previously confirmed that CCH exhibits ACE inhibitory activity and antihypertensive effects in rats (Saiga, 2008). The results of this study indicated that CCH had a similar antihypertensive effect in humans. Moreover, on medical examination some subjects reported a dry cough. Dry cough is typically observed with ACE inhibitor administration and is attributed to bradykinin accumulation in the body. This raises the possibility that the CCH inhibited kininase II and thus caused accumulation of bradykinin, a vasoprotector, which then induced NO production via the stimulation of eNOS. The results suggest that CCH exerts vasoprotective effects by ameliorating blood pressure in humans.

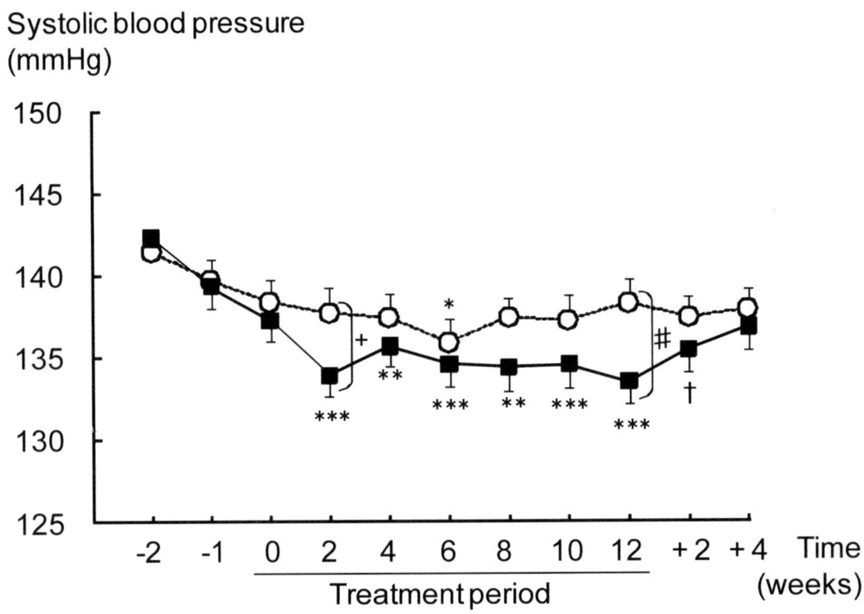


Fig. 4. Time-course of changes in systolic blood pressure in the subjects. Systolic blood pressures in the test food group were non-significantly lower than those in the placebo group after 2 weeks of treatment and were significantly lower than in the placebo group after 12 weeks of treatment. In comparison with the pre-treatment blood pressure (mean of the values at −2, −1, and 0 weeks), the blood pressure in the test food group was consistently and significantly lower throughout the treatment period. Data are mean ± SE values . + $P< 0.1$, # $P< 0.05$ versus placebo group. † $P< 0.1$, ∗ $P< 0.05$, ∗ ∗ $P< 0.01$, ∗ ∗ ∗ $P< 0.001$ versus pre-treatment blood pressure.

In our previous *in vitro* studies, we found that CCH treatment of human umbilical vein endothelial cells directly increased eNOS activation (data not shown). When eNOS expressed in vascular endothelial cells is activated, the cells produce NO. The NO functions as a signal to relax adjacent vascular smooth muscle cells; consequently, this dilates arteries and increases blood flow. Other than NO, vascular endothelial cells excrete vasoactive substances such as endothelin, a vasopressor, and maintain the balance of constriction and dilation of blood vessels. NO production via eNOS is particularly important in maintaining the homeostasis of blood vessels. Taken together, these findings indicate that oral administration of CCH improves blood pressure by inhibiting ACE and protects blood vessels by inducing NO production, thereby inhibiting the development of arteriosclerosis.

## 3. CCH treatment improves vascular endothelial function in rats and thus exerts protective effects on organs

The clinical trial described in the preceding section suggested that CCH protects the blood vessels by inducing NO production. Therefore, we next directly investigated the vasodilatory effect of CCH *ex vivo* by using rat blood vessels. We administered L-N$^{G}$-nitroarginine methyl ester (L-NAME), an NO synthesis inhibitor, to rats to trigger vascular endothelial dysfunction. We then tested whether prolonged CCH treatment of the rats would restore their endothelial function (Zhang, 2010).

### 3.1 Experimental animals

Thirty-six male WKY rats (10 weeks old) were randomly allocated to three groups. The first group (control group) received untreated chow and drinking water. The second group (L-NAME group) received L-NAME in their drinking water (0.5 g/L) for 8 weeks. The third group (L-NAME+CCH group) received L-NAME in their drinking water and CCH (2.0 g/kg daily) via a metal oral Zonde needle. All animal procedures were performed in accordance with the Animal Experimentation Guidelines of the Japanese Association for Laboratory Animal Science and were approved by the Animal Use and Care Committee of Nippon Meat Packers, Inc.

### 3.2 Vasorelaxation assay

A vasorelaxation assay was performed on the tissue of eight or nine rats from each group after 8 weeks of treatment. The rats were anesthetized with diethyl ether and the thoracic aorta was removed. The surrounding connective tissue and fat were carefully removed from the thoracic aorta, which was then cut into 2- to 3-mm-wide rings. Segments of thoracic aorta were mounted between two steel hooks in isolated tissue chambers containing Krebs-Henseleit solution at 37 °C. The isometric tension was recorded with an isometric force-displacement transducer. After an equilibration period, L-norepinephrine bitartrate was added to cause contraction. This was followed by the addition of cumulative doses of acetylcholine chloride to the bath solution to produce relaxation. Vascular relaxation was expressed as a percentage of tension development (Fig.5).

### 3.3 Results

After 8 weeks of treatment, the survival rate of the L-NAME group rats, which had received L-NAME in their drinking water, was 66.7% of that of the control rats. However, rats that had ingested CCH (L-NAME+CCH group) had a significantly better survival rate (91.7% of that of the control group) than the L-NAME rats ($P < 0.05$) (Fig.6). During all of the experiments, monitoring revealed that the rats drank 17 to 30 mL of water and ate 16 to 30 g of chow every day, confirming that their drinking and eating patterns were unaffected by the treatment protocols. Body weight gains did not differ among groups (data not shown).

We measured the vasorelaxant effects of CCH treatment after 8 weeks of treatment (Fig. 7). Treatment with acetylcholine chloride caused concentration-dependent relaxation of the thoracic aorta preparations from all groups after the preparations had been caused to contract by the addition of L-norepinephrine bitartrate. The acetylcholine chloride induced a relaxation response in the thoracic aortas from the L-NAME group (12.7% vasorelaxation); this was significantly less than that in preparations from the control group (69.5%).

Compared with that of the L-NAME group, vasorelaxation of the thoracic aortas from the L-NAME+CCH group (36.0%) was significantly improved by long-term administration of CCH ($P < 0.05$).

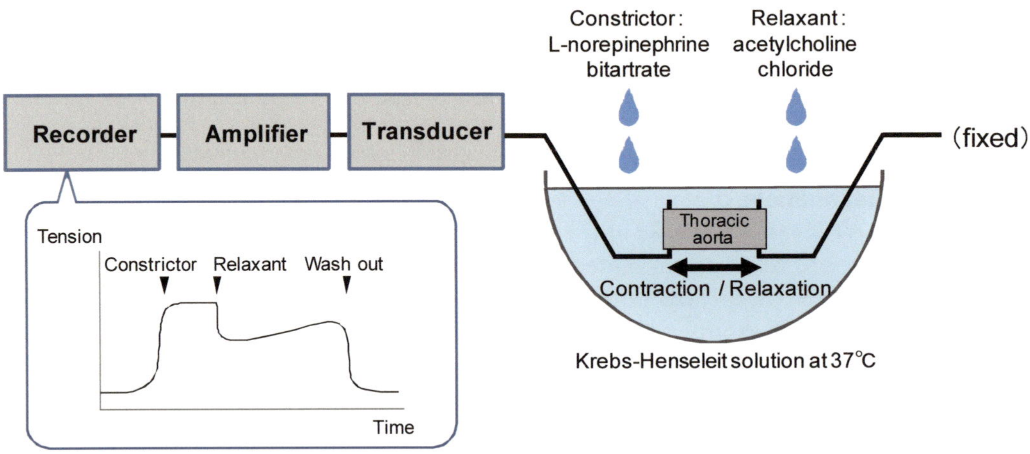


Fig. 5. Schematic of the Magnus apparatus. The excised rat thoracic aorta was cut into 2- to 3-mm-wide rings and the segments were mounted between two steel hooks in isolated tissue chambers containing Krebs-Henseleit solution at 37°C. Drops of L-norepinephrine bitartrate were then added to the tissue chamber to cause the aorta to contract. This was followed by the addition of various doses of acetylcholine chloride to trigger aortic relaxation. The electrical signals for this contraction–relaxation reaction were amplified via a transducer and recorded.

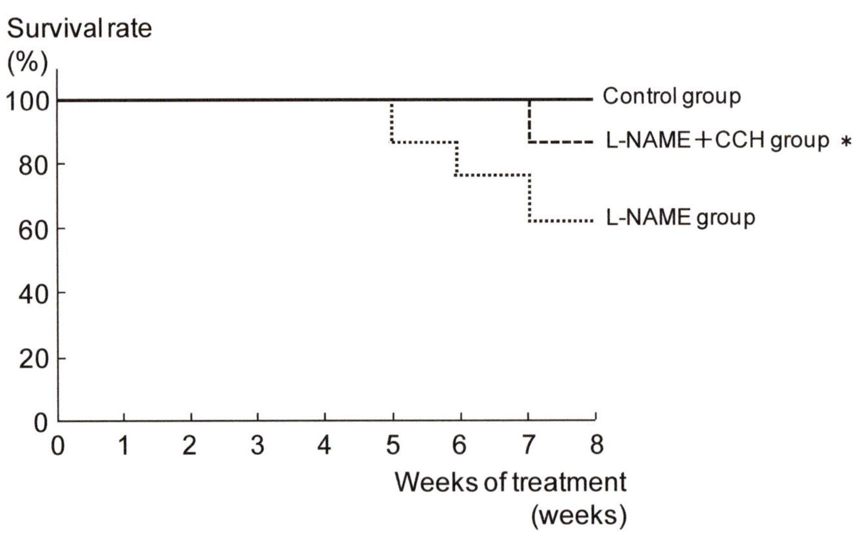


Fig. 6. Survival rates of rats during the test period. Eight weeks into the test period, the survival rate of the L-NAME + CCH group was significantly higher than that of the L-NAME group. Data are mean ± SE values (n=12 rats). * $P< 0.05$ versus L-NAME group.

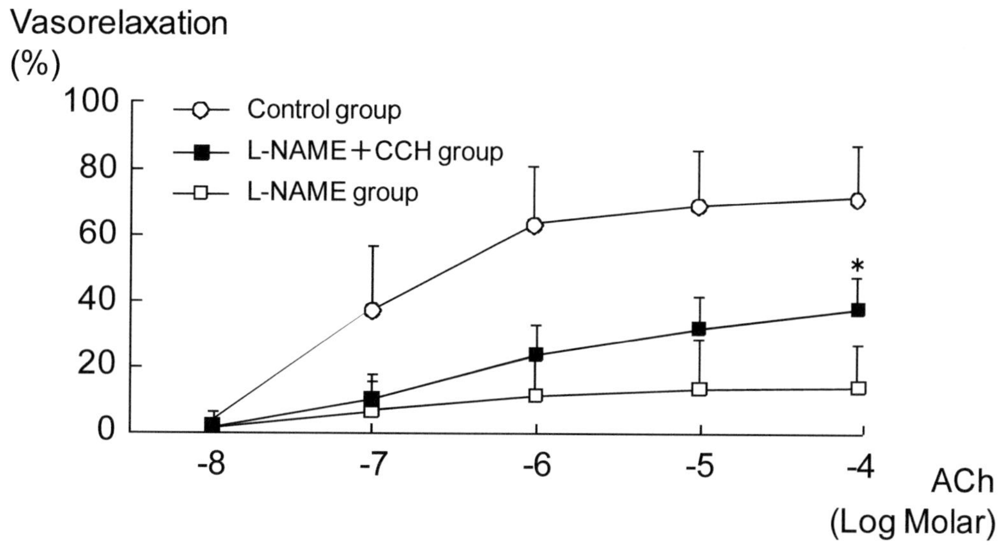


Fig. 7. Vasorelaxation of rat thoracic aortas over the 8 weeks of the test period . Treatment with acetylcholine chloride caused concentration-dependent relaxation of the thoracic aorta preparations from all groups. Especially at high acetylcholine concentrations, vasorelaxation was significantly higher in the L-NAME + CCH group than in the L-NAME group. Data are mean ± SE values (n=8-9 rats). * $P< 0.05$ versus L-NAME group.

**3.4 Discussion**

We found that CCH treatment improved vascular endothelial function. Acetylcholine activates eNOS expressed in vascular endothelial cells and induces NO production, thereby dilating blood vessels. In L-NAME-treated rats, the vasodilation response associated with NO production induced by an acetylcholine stimulus was inhibited; however, CCH treatment improved this response. As stated earlier, our previous studies have confirmed that CCH activates eNOS in vascular endothelial cells *in vitro*; this result was again supported by our study. In essence, therefore, CCH treatment strongly activated eNOS, promoted NO production, and thus triggered a vasodilatory response.

Moreover, the survival curves showed that the survival rate of L-NAME-treated rats was significantly enhanced by CCH administration. This may have been because CCH treatment alleviated the various organ failures caused by L-NAME-induced vascular disorders. We previously conducted the same experiment by using a higher concentration of L-NAME (1 g/L) and prepared tissue sections for observation. We identified substantial tissue damage associated with L-NAME treatment in the blood vessels, kidney, and heart ; this damage was alleviated by CCH treatment (Fig. 8). The substantial fibrosis observed, especially in the heart and liver, was relieved by CCH treatment. Although further investigations of this attenuation effect of CCH treatment on tissue damage are required, we consider that it results from tissue protection via the vasoprotective effects of CCH.

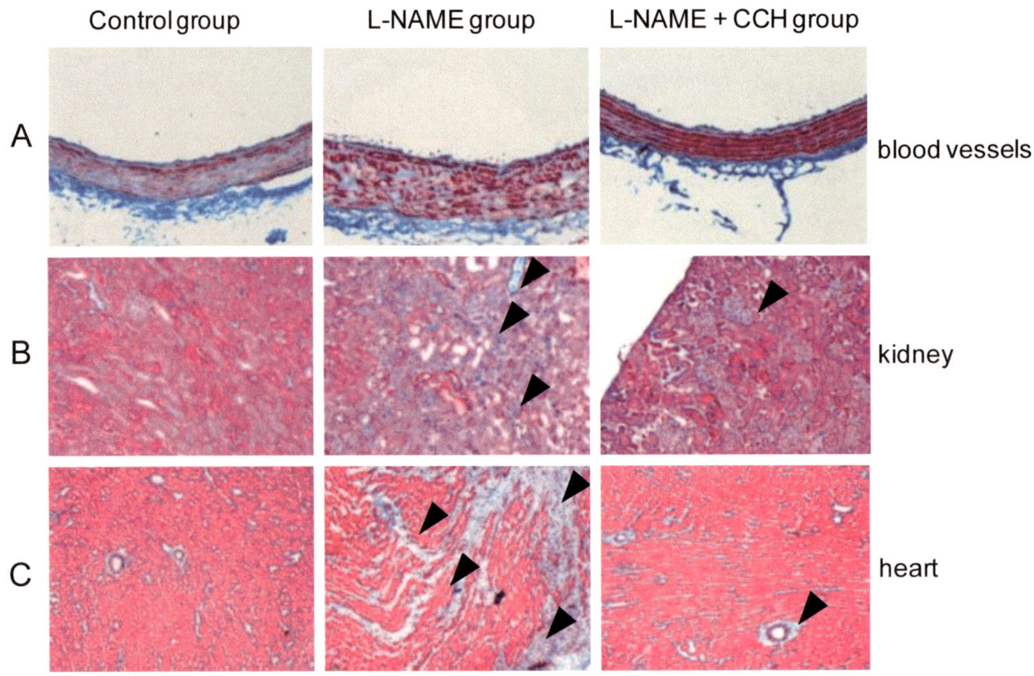


Fig. 8. Tissue sections of blood vessels (A, ×160), kidney (B, ×80) and heart (C, ×80) after treatment with L-NAME at a high concentration (1 g/L). Tissues were stained with Masson trichrome. These sections are from a similarly designed previous experiment of ours. Significant tissue damage caused by L-NAME was observed in the blood vessels, kidneys, and heart tissues, whereas CCH treatment alleviated these damages. Arrows indicate signs of fibrosis.

## 4. CCH treatment inhibits proinflammatory cytokine expression in a mouse model of arteriosclerosis

Previous studies have indicated that CCH exerts vasoprotective effects and thus organ protective effects. We therefore investigated the effects of CCH in an atherosclerosis mouse model, C57BL/6.KOR-ApoE$^{sh1}$. This mouse is spontaneously hyperlipidemic and characteristically has high total cholesterol (TC) levels and arteriosclerotic lesions. Using this mouse model, we examined the changes in blood cholesterol levels and proinflammatory cytokine expression in response to prolonged CCH treatment (Zhang, 2010).

### 4.1 Experimental animals

Eighteen male C57BL/6.KOR-ApoE$^{shl}$ mice (7 weeks old) were randomly allocated to two groups (n = 9) and fed on a normal diet or a diet supplemented with 10% CCH for 12 weeks. At the end of the 12-week experiment, the mice were sacrificed, blood was obtained from their veins, and tissues were collected for further analysis. All animal procedures were performed in accordance with the Animal Experimentation Guidelines of the Japanese Association for Laboratory Animal Science and were approved by the Animal Use and Care Committee of Nippon Meat Packers, Inc.

### 4.2 Measurement of plasma and hepatic lipids

Levels of TC, triglycerides (TG), low-density lipoprotein cholesterol (LDL-C), and high-density lipoprotein cholesterol (HDL-C) in the plasma and liver were determined. Total lipids extracted from the liver were also analyzed.

In addition, plasma levels of interleukin-6 (IL-6), soluble intercellular adhesion molecule-1 (sICAM-1), and tumor necrosis factor-α (TNF-α) were measured by ELISA.

### 4.3 Observation of tissue sections

At the end of the 12-week test period, the thoracic aorta and liver were excised from the dissected rats and were fixed in formalin, paraffin-embedded, and sliced with a microtome to prepare thin sections, which were then stained with Oil Red O or hematoxylin-eosin for histological observation.

### 4.4 Results

The mice were treated with CCH for 12 weeks and then sacrificed for analysis. Compared with those in the controls, the amounts of plasma TC and hepatic lipid and TG in the CCH group were reduced by 14.4%, 24.7%, and 42.8%, respectively (Table 1). However, CCH administration had no obvious influence on the concentrations of TG, LDL-C, and HDL-C in the plasma or of TC in the liver.

| | Plasma (mg/100ml) | | | | Liver (mg/g) | | |
|---|---|---|---|---|---|---|---|
| | TC | TG | LDL-C | HDL-C | Lipid | TC | TG |
| Control | 1208±93 | 308±72 | 678±68 | 10.2±1.5 | 75.3±6.6 | 0.31±0.11 | 4.9±2.4 |
| 10% CCH | 880±73 * | 306±64 | 550±80 | 11.3±0.9 | 56.7±4.8 * | 0.27±0.07 | 2.8±1.5 * |

Table 1. Effect of CCH treatment on plasma concentrations of TC, TG, LDL-C, and HDL-C and on hepatic total lipid, TC, and TG in C57BL/6.KOR-ApoE$^{sh1}$ mice at the end of the 12-week test period. Plasma TC, hepatic total lipid, and hepatic TG concentrations were significantly lower in the 10% CCH group than in the control group. Data are mean ± SE values (n=9 mice). * $P< 0.05$ versus L-NAME group.

We also investigated the effects of CCH treatment on plasma proinflammatory cytokine levels in C57BL/6.KOR-ApoE$^{shl}$ mice. Administration of CCH resulted in decreases in plasma levels of IL-6 (by 43.4%, $P < 0.01$), sICAM-1 (by 17.9%, $P < 0.05$), and TNF-α (by 24.1%, $P < 0.01$) (Fig.9).

To investigate whether CCH had a preventive and therapeutic effect on arteriosclerosis, atherosclerotic lesions in the aorta were observed by microscopy with Oil Red O staining (Fig.10). There were no obvious differences in the aortas of the CCH and control groups. We then tested whether CCH treatment had alleviated liver damage in the C57BL/6.KOR-ApoE$^{shl}$ mouse model. Sections of paraffin-embedded liver were stained with hematoxylin-eosin or Oil Red O. Treatment with 10% CCH for 12 weeks decreased the abundance of diffuse lipid droplets and fat vacuoles compared with that in the control group (Fig.10).

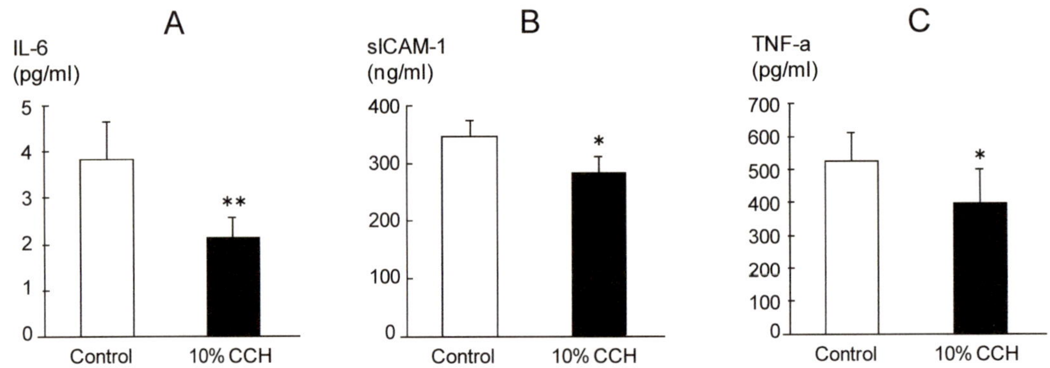


Fig. 9. Effect of CCH treatment on plasma proinflammatory cytokine levels in C57BL/6.KOR-ApoE$^{sh1}$ mice at the end of the 12-week test period. Interleukin-6 (IL-6) (A), soluble intercellular adhesion molecule-1 (sICAM-1 ) (B), tumor necrosis factor alpha (TNF-α) (C). The levels of all plasma proinflammatory cytokines were significantly lower in the 10% CCH group than in the control group. Data are mean ± SE values (n=9 mice). ＊ $P<0.05$, ＊＊ $P<0.01$ versus control group.

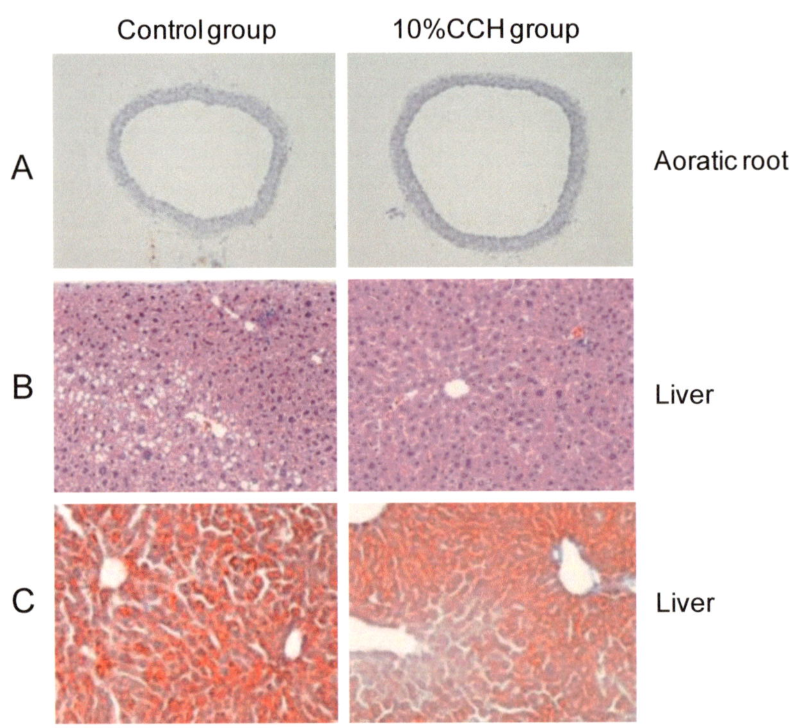


Fig. 10. Tissue sections of aortic root (A) and liver (B and C) at the end of the 12-week test period. Tissues were stained with Oil Red O (A, ×80; C, ×140) or hematoxylin-eosin (B , ×140). No obvious change was observed in the aortic root of the 10% CCH group; however, diffuse lipid droplets and fat vacuoles in the livers of the treatment group were less abundant than in those of the control group.

### 4.5 Discussion

Our results suggested that, as well as lowering plasma TC, CCH had a lipid-lowering effect through regulation of hepatic lipid biosynthesis to suppress TG levels. In humans, collagen-specific peptides are absorbed into the blood as a result of CCH treatment (Iwai, 2009). Once absorbed into the body, the CCH peptides function as regulatory factors to influence cholesterol homeostasis. This effect may have contributed to the decrease in the abundance of lipid droplets and fat vacuoles observed in the liver tissues.

Because inflammation plays an important role in the development of arteriosclerosis, inflammatory markers were also examined to investigate the anti-inflammatory function of dietary intervention. IL-6, sICAM-1, and TNF-α are the major proinflammatory cytokines secreted by adipocytes. At the same time, NO inhibits the expression of these proinflammatory cytokines in the vascular endothelium. Our previous studies indicate that orally ingested CCH induces NO production in the body. Hence, the results imply that CCH treatment downregulates several proinflammatory cytokines via NO production, thereby having beneficial effects on the fat tissues. Further detailed investigations are, however, necessary to elucidate more of the direct effects of CCH on fat cells.

Unfortunately, no direct therapeutic effect of CCH on arteriosclerotic plaques was observed in this study. Nevertheless, the data demonstrated that CCH treatment substantially reduced both the total lipid content in the liver and the production of proinflammatory cytokines such as IL-6, TNF-α, and sICAM-1 in a mouse model highly susceptible to arteriosclerosis. High levels of expression of these factors lead to the progression of arteriosclerosis. From this perspective, long-term CCH treatment may be effective as a simple dietary, rather than drug, treatment for preventing arteriosclerosis.

## 5. Conclusion: The availability of collagen peptides as a food providing anti-atherogenesis via a vasoprotective effect

It has been frequently reported that externally applied collagen peptides help to increase water retention owing to their high water retentivity. On the other hand, the functionality of orally ingested collagen is not fully understood. However, much of the evidence reported in recent years, including the results of this study, supports the specific physiological activities of collagen absorbed by the body.

In this study, we examined the impacts of collagen peptides on blood vessels from various perspectives. We demonstrated that collagen peptides exhibit vasoprotective functions via NO production and effectively protect against atherogenesis.

Functional foods will not replace pharmaceuticals. However, what humans continue to do regularly for survival is to eat. Whereas a balanced diet obviously supports healthy life, elucidation of the tertiary function of food ingredients by precisely following their mechanisms is a long-term mission for food researchers. We focused on collagen and analyzed the whole process from development of, to research into, novel chicken-derived collagen peptides. We clarified the efficacy of vasoprotection, which is a novel tertiary function of collagen peptides. We intend to continue our efforts to demonstrate the beneficial functionalities of collagen in the hope of improving the global quality of life through the consumption of this food product.

## 6. References


Katiyar SK. 2003. Skin photoprotection by green tea: antioxidant and immunomodulatory effects. Curr Drug Targets Immune Endocr Metabol Disord 3(3):234-42.

Weijer P, Barentsen R. 2002. Isoflavones from red clover (Promensil) significantly reduce menopausal hot flush symptoms compared with placebo. Maturitas 25;42(3):187-93.

Tamai T, Ikematsu H, Shionoya K, Murota I, Baba T, Hiura N, Sato R. 2004. Effect of fish sausage enriched with DHA (docosahexaenoic acid) on serum lpids (II): effect of three month-long intake on serum lipids, and safety evaluation. J Jpn Soc Clin Nutr 25(4):293-302.

Iwai K, Zhang Y, Kouguchi T, Saiga Egusa A, Shimizu M, Ohmori T, Takahata Y, Morimatsu F. 2009. Blood concentration of food-derived peptides following oral intake of chicken collagen hydrolysate and its angiotensin-converting enzyme inhibitory activity in healthy volunteers. Nippon Shokuhin Kagaku Kogaku Kaishi 56(6):326–30.

Shigemura Y, Iwai K, Morimatsu F, Iwamoto T, Mori T, Oda C, Taira T, Park E, Nakamura Y, Sato K. 2009. Effect of Prolyl-hydroxyproline (Pro-Hyp), a food-derived collagen peptide in human blood, on growth of fibroblasts from mouse skin. J Agric Food Chem 57(2):444–9.

Ohara H, Ito K, Iida H, Matsumoto H. 2009. Improvement in the moisture content of the stratum corneum following 4 weeks of collagen hydrolysate ingestion. Nippon Shokuhin Kagaku Kogaku Kaishi 56:137–45.

Arborelius M, Konttinen Y, Nordström D, Solovieva S. 1999. Gly-X-Y repeat sequences in the treatment of active rheumatoid arthritis. Rheumatol Int 18(4):129-35.

Kato T, Node K. 2004. Frontier of vascular failure. Node K. (Eds.). Concept of vasucular failure. 21-2. Tokyo. Medical review.

Taguchi Y. 2002. Development of a low allergic chicken gelatin. Packaging of foodstuff. 33(2): 35-40.

Saiga A, Iwai K, Hayakawa T, Takahata Y, Kitamura S, Nishimura T, Morimatsu F. 2008. Angiotensin I-converting enzyme inhibitory peptides obtained from chicken collagen hydrolysate. J Agric Food Chem 56:9586–91.

Gupta R, Guptha S. 2010. Strategies for initial management of hypertension. Indian J Med Res. 132(5):531-42.

Sharma JN. 2009. Hypertension and the bradykinin system. Curr Hypertens Rep 11(3):178-81.

Kouguchi T, Ohmori T, Hayakawa T, Takahata Y, Maeyama Y, Kajimoto Y, Kitakaze M, Morimatsu F. 2008. Hypotensive effects and safety of intake of lactic acid beverage containing chicken collagen hydrolysate in subjects with mild hypertension or high-normal blood pressure. Jpn Pharmacol Ther 36(6):561–75.

Zhang Y, Kouguchi T, Shimizu M, Ohmori T, Takahata Y, Morimatsu F. 2010. Chiken collagen hydrolysate protects rats from hypertension and cardiovascular damage. J Med Food 13(2):399-405.

Zhang Y, Kouguchi T, Shimizu K, Sato M, Takahata Y, Morimatsu F. 2010. Chicken collagen hydrolysate reduces proinflammatory cytokine production in C57BL/6.KOR-ApoE$^{shl}$ mice. J Nutr Sci Vitaminol 56(3):208-10.